Handbook of Parkinson's Disease

Handbook of Parkinson's Disease

Edited by

WILLIAM C. KOLLER

Department of Neurology
Movement Disorder Clinic
Parkinson Disease Center
Loyola University Stritch School of Medicine
Maywood, Illinois

MARCEL DEKKER, INC.   New York • Basel

Library of Congress Cataloging in Publication Data

Handbook of Parkinson's disease.

Includes index.
1. Parkinsonism--Handbooks, manuals, etc. I. Koller,
William C., [date] [DNLM: 1. Parkinson Disease.
WL 359 H236]
RC382.H36   1987   616.8'33   87-637
ISBN 0-8247-7678-X

MARCEL DEKKER, INC.
270 Madison Avenue, New York, New York 10016

Current printing (last digit):
10 9 8 7 6 5 4 3 2 1

PRINTED IN THE UNITED STATES OF AMERICA

Introduction

James Parkinson's description of the shaking palsy, written in 1817, is now considered a medical classic. Its acclaim derives from the author's unusually vivid and accurate description of the constellation of symptoms as well as the recognition of the evolution and progression of the disorder which now bears his name. Less well appreciated is Parkinson's motivation in undertaking the task of writing his monograph. As stated in the final section:

> Before concluding these pages, it may be proper to observe once more, that an important object proposed to be obtained by them is, the leading of the attention of those who humanely employ anatomical examination in detecting the cause and nature of diseases, particularly to this malady. By their benevolent labours its real nature may be ascertained, and appropriate modes of relief, or even of cure, pointed out.

During much of the 150 years following Parkinson's challenge to the research community few, if any, advances toward understanding the nature or providing means of effective relief from the disease occurred. However, in the past twenty years this has changed remarkably with significant and impressive progress toward reaching the goal which he had set. Indeed, there has been a virtual explosion of research interest and a continuous flow of new information about movement disorders in general, and Parkinson's disease in particular. As a result we now have a more precise delineation of Parkinson's disease as a clinical entity with established morbid anatomy and biochemical changes. The major symptoms have been correlated with a deficiency of striatal dopamine and are reversible by restoring the action of this neurotransmitter by pharmacological agents. Hence its treatment is on a sound, rational footing. Most importantly, new concepts concerning its etiogenesis and pathogenesis have come to the fore which hold the possibility of leading to methods of prevention or halting the progression of this enigmatic disorder.

This volume conceived and edited by Dr. Koller brings into sharp focus the developments of fundamental and clinical knowledge which have occurred in parkinsonism in general, and Parkinson's disease in particular, over the past two decades. Drawing on a large cadre of active investigators from a variety of disciplines of the neurosciences in the United States and abroad, an in-depth state-of-the-art volume in this field has been developed. It is in every respect a handbook, one which is as useful to the clinician responsible for the everyday care of the patient, as it is to the investigative scientist.

Melvin D. Yahr, M.D.
New York City, N.Y.
February 1987

Preface

Parkinson's disease is a common chronic neurologic illness of adult life. Its insidious onset, slow progression, and prolonged course make it likely that physicians of diverse specialities will at some time be caring for parkinsonian patients. The many difficulties associated with long-term treatment make management of Parkinson's disease exceedingly challenging even for the experienced practitioner.

Parkinson's disease is the prototypic illness in which a neurotransmitter disturbance has been identified. This discovery led to an effective therapy approach. Yet suffering and disability continue in many parkinsonian patients. Recent advances in our understanding of the pathophysiology of Parkinson's disease and the introduction of new therapies give renewed hope that Parkinson's disease may one day be controlled.

It is the purpose of this book to present up-to-date information on the many aspects of Parkinson's disease. It is hoped that this volume will serve as a reference source for those seeking answers to questions on Parkinson's disease. The recent increase in our knowledge of this disorder makes this effort timely.

Appreciation and thanks are extended to the authors and other investigators who have contributed to our knowledge of Parkinson's disease. Undoubtedly their research efforts will one day eliminate the human misery of those who suffer from Parkinson's disease.

William C. Koller

Contributors

Ellsworth C. Alvord, Jr., M.D. Professor of Pathology (Chief of Neuropathology), Department of Pathology, University of Washington School of Medicine, Seattle, Washington

Roger C. Duvoisin, M.D. Department of Neurology, University of Medicine and Dentistry of New Jersey-Robert Wood Johnson Medical School, Piscataway, New Jersey

Lysia S. Forno, M.D. Associate Professor, Department of Pathology, Veterans Administration Medical Center, Palo Alto, and Department of Pathology, Stanford University, Stanford, California

Christopher G. Goetz, M.D. Associate Professor, Department of Neurological Sciences, Rush-Presbyterian St. Luke's Medical Center, Chicago, Illinois

John H. Gordon, M.D. Department of Pharmacology, Chicago Medical School, North Chicago, Illinois

Richard E. Heikkila, Ph.D. Professor, Department of Neurology, University of Medicine and Dentistry of New Jersey-Robert Wood Johnson Medical School, Piscataway, New Jersey

Joseph Jankovic, M.D. Associate Professor, Department of Neurology, Director, Parkinson's Disease Center, Baylor College of Medicine, Houston, Texas

Susan E. Kase, B.S. Physical Therapy, Senior Physical Therapist, Parkside Home Health Services, Inc., Park Ridge, Illinois

M. Victoria Kindt, M.D.   Department of Neurology, University of Medicine and Dentistry of New Jersey-Robert Wood Johnson Medical School, Piscataway, New Jersey

Harold L. Klawans, M.D.   Professor of Neurology and Pharmacology, Departments of Neurological Science and Pharmacology, Rush Medical College, Chicago, Illinois

William C. Koller, M.D., Ph.D.   Professor of Neurology, Department of Neurology, Loyola University Stritch School of Medicine, Maywood, Illinois

Anthony E. Lang, M.D., F.R.C.P.(C)   Assistant Professor, Division of Neurology, Movement Disorders Clinic, Toronto Western Hospital, Toronto, Ontario, Canada

J. William Langston, M.D.   Director, Parkinson's Disease Research and Clinical Programs, Institute for Medical Research, San Jose, California

Andrew John Lees, M.D., M.R.C.P.   Consultant Neurologist, National Hospitals for Nervous Diseases, London, England

Bonnie E. Levin, Ph.D.   Instructor in Neurology, Director, Neuropsychology Assessment Unit, Department of Neurology, University of Miami School of Medicine, Miami, Florida

Peter A. Le Witt, M.D.   Director of Neurology, Neurology Department, Lafayette Clinic, Associate Professor of Neurology and Psychiatry, Wayne State University School of Medicine, Detroit, Michigan

J. M. Martínez-Lage, M.D.   Department of Neurology, Clínica Universitaria, University of Navarra Medical School, Pamplona, Spain

Reijo J. Marttila, M.D.   Senior Lecturer, Department of Neurology, University of Turku, Turku, Finland

Richard Mayeux, M.D.   Associate Professor of Neurology and Psychiatry, Departments of Neurology and Psychiatry, Columbia University College of Physicians and Surgeons, New York, New York

Eldad Melamed, M.D.   Sebulsky-Royce Professor of Neurology, Department of Neurology, Hadassah University Hospital, Jerusalem, Israel

Anthony G. Mlcoch, Ph.D. Speech Pathologist, Department of Speech Pathology and Audiology, Edward Hines, Jr. Veterans Administration Hospital, Hines, Illinois

Paul A. Nausieda, M.D. Director, Sleep Wake Disorders Center, St. Mary's Hospital, Milwaukee, Wisconsin

John G. Nutt, M.D. Associate Professor, Department of Neurology, Oregon Health Sciences University, Portland, Oregon

José A. Obeso, M.D. Consultant Neurologist, Department of Neurology, Clinica Universitaria, University of Navarra Medical School, Pamplona, Spain

Cheryl A. O'Riordan, M.P.H., O.T.R./L. Assistant Chief-Clinical Education Coordinator, Occupational Therapy-Rehabilitation Medicine Service, Edward Hines, Jr., Veterans Administration Hospital, Hines, Illinois

Mark J. Perlow, M.D. Professor, Department of Neurology, University of Illinois Westside Veterans Administration Hospital, Chicago, Illinois

Niall P. Quinn, M.A., M.B., M.R.C.P. Lecturer in Neurology, University Department of Neurology, Institute of Psychiatry, King's College School of Medicine and Dentistry, London, England

R. Sandyk, M.D. Department of Neurology, University of Arizona, Tucson, Arizona

George Selby, M.D., F.R.C.P., F.R.A.C.P. Head, Section of Neurology, Royal North Shore Hospital, Sydney, New South Wales, Australia

Stuart R. Snider, M.D. Clinical Scientist, Department of Neurology, University of Arizona, Tucson, Arizona

Patricia K. Sonsalla, M.D. Department of Neurology, University of Medicine and Dentistry of New Jersey-Robert Wood Johnson Medical School, Piscataway, New Jersey

Caroline M. Tanner, M.D. Assistant Professor, Department of Neurological Sciences, Rush Presbyterian St. Luke's Medical Center, Chicago, Illinois

Kenneth Laurence Tyler, M.D. Assistant Professor of Neurology, Harvard Medical School, Assistant Neurologist, Massachusetts General Hospital, Boston, Massachusetts

George R. Uhl, M.D., Ph.D.   Assistant Professor of Neurology, Department of Neurology, Harvard Medical School, Howard Hughes Medical Institute, Massachusetts General Hospital, Boston, Massachusetts

Mark M. Voigt, M.D.   Department of Neurology, Harvard Medical School, Howard Hughes Medical Institute, Massachusetts General Hospital, Boston, Massachusetts

William J. Wiener, M.D.   Professor of Neurology, Department of Neurology, Director, Movement Disorder Clinic, University of Miami School of Medicine, Miami, Florida

G. Frederick Wooten, M.D.   Mary Anderson Harrison Professor of Neurology, Department of Neurology, University of Virginia Medical School, Charlottesville, Virginia

Contents

Handbook of Parkinson's Disease

1
A History of Parkinson's Disease

KENNETH LAURENCE TYLER
Harvard Medical School, and Massachusetts General Hospital, Boston, Massachusetts

Paralysis agitans almost seems to have appeared sui generis with Parkinson's description in 1817. The nosologists of earlier centuries may have seen patients with this type of disorder and certainly recognized specific components of the disease. One can, for example, find mention of "tremor" in the Hippocratic corpus and in the works of Celsus and Galen. In his monograph on shaking palsy, Parkinson referred to earlier writings by Sylvius de la Boë, Juncker, Sauvages, and van Swieten. Sylvius de la Boë (1680) was one of the first to separate clearly a species of tremor that occurred during a voluntary act from tremor occurring at rest. In the 18th century, Sauvages (1768) and van Swieten (1749) also made similar distinctions. Parkinson credited Gaubius (1758) and Sauvages (1768) with early descriptions of the festinating gait that he saw in his patients (see Parkinson, 1817, Sanders, 1880). Rereading these early descriptions, one is struck by their essentially fragmentary nature. Physicians before Parkinson may have seen cases of "paralysis agitans" yet it was Parkinson who finally captured its essence in a fashion that is compelling and obvious to the modern reader.

The details of James Parkinson's life (1755-1824) have never been better outlined than by W.H. McMenemey in a bicentenary volume of papers on James Parkinson edited by MacDonald Critchley (1955). Parkinson was a general practitioner who regularly contributed clinical papers on various subjects to medical journals. Among the topics on which he wrote were hydrophobia, gout, the effects of lightning, and typhoid fever! A paper on "Diseased Appendix Vermiformis" (1812) dates as one of the earliest contributions on this subject (Fig. 1). Parkinson also wrote several books on medical subjects designed for popular consumption including: *Dangerous Sports* (1800), *The Villager's Friend and Physician* (1800), *Hints for the Improvement of Trusses* (1802) and *Medical*

CASE

OF

DISEASED

APPENDIX VERMIFORMIS,

By JOHN PARKINSON, Surgeon, Esq.

COMMUNICATED

By JAMES PARKINSON, Esq.

Read January 21, 1812.

A PREPARATION of diseased appendix vermiformis in my possession, was removed from a boy about 5 years of age who died under the following circumstances.

He had been observed for some time, to decline in health, but made no particular complaint, until two days before his death, when he was suddenly seized with vomiting, and great prostration of strength. The abdomen became very tumid and painful upon being pressed : his countenance pale and sunken, and his pulse hardly perceptible. Death, preceded by extreme restlessness and delirium, took place within 24 hours.

Upon examination, the whole surface of the peritoneum was found inflamed, and covered with a

FIGURE 1 Title page of article on appendicitis communicated by James Parkinson and written by his son.

Admonitions, with Observations on the Excessive Indulgence of Children (1799). He even prepared a guide for medical students (*The Hospital Pupil*, 1800). He was the author of a thoughtful monograph entitled, *Observations on the Act for Regulating Mad-Houses* (1811), produced after he was unjustly accused of falsely committing a woman to an asylum (Fig. 2).

Although Parkinson's many medical writings suggest that he had a busy career as a physician, his interests were eclectic. He was one of England's foremost early paleontologists, and his two books on the subject, *Organic Remains of a Former World* (1811) and *Outlines of Oryctology* (1822) (11) were considered

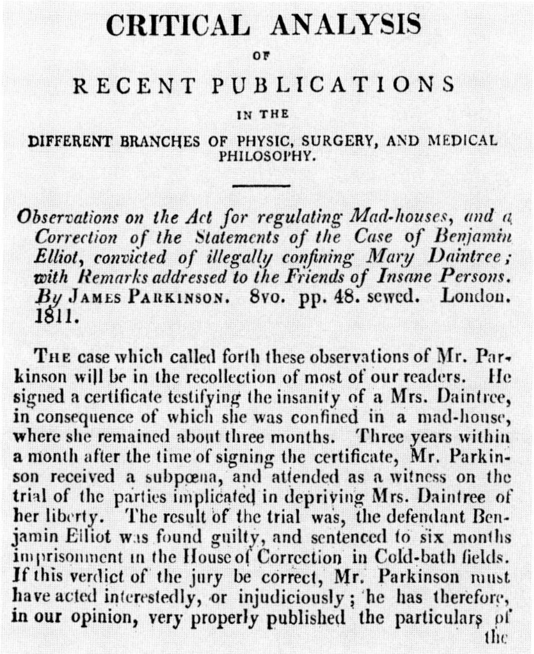

CRITICAL ANALYSIS

OF

RECENT PUBLICATIONS

IN THE

DIFFERENT BRANCHES OF PHYSIC, SURGERY, AND MEDICAL
PHILOSOPHY.

Observations on the Act for regulating Mad-houses, and a Correction of the Statements of the Case of Benjamin Elliot, convicted of illegally confining Mary Daintree; with Remarks addressed to the Friends of Insane Persons. By JAMES PARKINSON. 8vo. pp. 48. sewed. London. 1811.

THE case which called forth these observations of Mr. Parkinson will be in the recollection of most of our readers. He signed a certificate testifying the insanity of a Mrs. Daintree, in consequence of which she was confined in a mad-house, where she remained about three months. Three years within a month after the time of signing the certificate, Mr. Parkinson received a subpœna, and attended as a witness on the trial of the parties implicated in depriving Mrs. Daintree of her liberty. The result of the trial was, the defendant Benjamin Elliot was found guilty, and sentenced to six months imprisonment in the House of Correction in Cold-bath fields. If this verdict of the jury be correct, Mr. Parkinson must have acted interestedly, or injudiciously; he has therefore, in our opinion, very properly published the particulars of the

FIGURE 2 Title page of a review of Parkinson's *Observations on the Act for Regulating Mad-Houses.*

important works by his contemporaries (Fig. 3). Another contribution, *The Chemical Pocket-Book* (1799) was equally well received and went through several editions (Figs. 4,5).

Perhaps the most fascinating part of Parkinson's career was neither scientific nor medical in nature. Writing under both his own name and the pseudonym "Old Hubert," he published nearly a dozen political pamphlets in the period between 1793 and 1795. These appeared in the aftermath of the French Revolution, when England was in a state of political turmoil. "Reform societies" and "revolutionary clubs" were organized and members began to campaign for parliamentary reform. Parkinson joined several of these including the "Society for Constitutional Information" and the "London Corresponding Society." The goals of these societies seem surprisingly mild by today's standards. Members protested against the "intolerable grievance" of paying "numerous, burthensome and unnecessary" taxes. They rebelled against inequities in the system of parliamentary representation, which effectively disenfranchised millions of people. They called for an end to the specialized system of elections in which individuals voted for only a small minority of parliament, the majority of

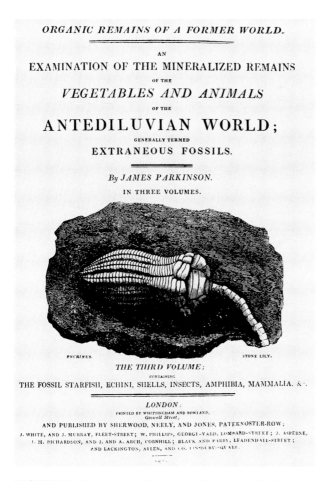

FIGURE 3   Title page of *Organic Remains of a Former World*, Parkinson's classic early work on paleontology.

members being elected by small groups of electors representing incorporated townships and other privileged groups. They noted that fewer than 500 privileged voters in the county of Cornwall elected nearly the same number of representatives to parliament as all three million people in Scotland (McMenemey, 1955).

The reaction of the established government to the reform societies was anything but tolerant. Thomas Paine's *Rights of Man* (1790, 1792) was banned, and serious consideration was given to the idea of going to war in an effort to restore the French monarchy. Edmund Burke was one of the leading supporters of the conservative policies of the established government. "Old Hubert" became one of his staunchest opponents in a battle of sarcasm and polemics. Old Hubert entitled one of his essays, "An Address to the Honorable Edmund Burke from the Swinish Multitude" (1793) and another, "Pearls Cast Before Swine by Edmund Burke—Scraped Together by Old Hubert" (1793) (Figs. 6,7).

The political situation in England reached a crisis after the execution of Louis XVI and Marie Antoinette in 1792. The House of Commons voted overwhelmingly to refuse to consider any petitions for parliamentary reform (1793); the president and several members of the London Corresponding Society were found guilty of treason against the state and sentenced to long prison terms or transported to Australia. Parkinson was subpoenaed before the Privy Council to give evidence concerning a plot to assassinate King George III, and initially declined to testify unless assured that he would not be made to incriminate himself. Attempted regicide was no light matter. In 1794 an Edinburg court had sentenced two such plotters to be hanged until dead, then disemboweled, and quartered.

Perhaps the best synopsis of Parkinson's political views comes from his pamphlet *Revolution without Bloodshed; or Reformation Preferable to Revolt* (1794) (Fig. 8). Some of the radical suggestions contained therein are worth noting:

Taxation should be in proportion to an individual's ability to pay
Excise taxes on necessities of life should be abolished
Workmen should not be imprisoned for uniting to obtain an increase in wages
Punishment should be proportional to the severity of the crime
Provisions should be made to aid the aged and disabled who could not support themselves
Tradesmen who became bankrupt should not be imprisoned

Parkinson's political writings ceased abruptly in 1795 when he was 40 years of age. He was 62 when he published the monograph, *Essay on the Shaking Palsy* (1817) for which we eponymously remember him today. Perhaps he should be more accurately remembered as an individual with tremendous breadth of interest, who was concerned not only with the broad scientific problems of his time, but also with its pressing social issues and problems.

James Parkinson became famous for his "precipitate publication of mere conjectural suggestions" which appeared in 1817 under the title, "An Essay on the Shaking Palsy" (Fig. 9). In the preface he apologized to his readers for the work's shortcomings, noting that "mere conjecture takes the place of experiment" and that "analogy is the substitute for anatomical examination." He was clearly incited to publish by the fact that he believed that the disease he called "shaking palsy" or "paralysis agitans" seemed to have "escaped particular notice." He hoped his description would excite others to "extend their

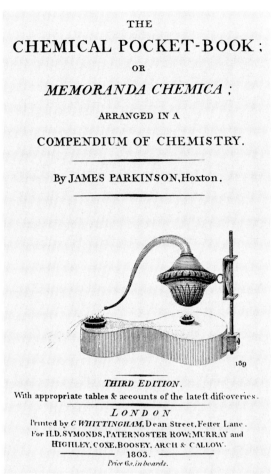

THE

CHEMICAL POCKET-BOOK;

OR

MEMORANDA CHEMICA;

ARRANGED IN A

COMPENDIUM OF CHEMISTRY.

By JAMES PARKINSON, Hoxton.

THIRD EDITION.
With appropriate tables & accounts of the lateſt diſcoveries.

L O N D O N
Printed by *C WHITTINGHAM*, Dean Street, Fetter Lane.
For H.D. SYMONDS, PATERNOSTER ROW; MURRAY and
HIGHLEY, COXE, BOOSEY, ARCH & CALLOW.
——— 1803. ———
Price 6s. in boards.

FIGURE 4 Title page of Parkinson's *Chemical Pocket-Book*, a popular synopsis of contemporary knowledge in the field of chemistry.

researches" to this disease so that they might "point out the most appropriate means of relieving a tedious and most distressing malady."

Parkinson's magnum opus of 66 pages was divided into five chapters. In the first chapter, he provided a definition of the disease and reviewed its natural history. The chapter ends with a brief precis of six "illustrative cases," which formed the basis for Parkinson's observations.

Parkinson called the disease he was describing "shaking palsy" but also provided a Latin synonym, "paralysis agitans." It is a common misconception,

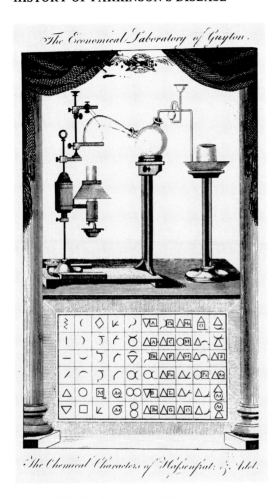

FIGURE 5   Facing page to Figure 4.

perpetuated in some neurology textbooks, that it was not Parkinson but instead Marshall Hall who initially applied the term paralysis agitans to this disease.

Parkinson's definition of shaking palsy was succinct:

Involuntary tremulous motion, with lessened muscular power, in parts not in action and even when supported; with a propensity to bend the trunk forwards, and to pass from a walking to a running pace: the senses and intellects being uninjured. (Fig. 10)

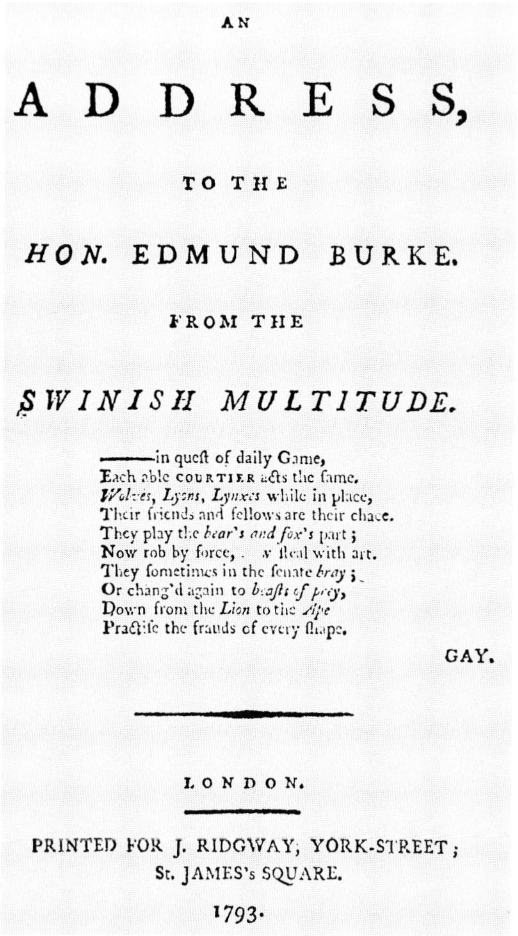

AN

A D D R E S S,

TO THE

HON. EDMUND BURKE.

FROM THE

SWINISH MULTITUDE.

———in queſt of daily Game,
Each able COURTIER acts the ſame.
Wolves, Lyons, Lynxes while in place,
Their friends and fellows are their chace.
They play the *bear's* and *fox's* part;
Now rob by force, ⋅ r ſteal with art.
They ſometimes in the ſenate *bray* ;
Or chang'd again to *beaſts of prey*,
Down from the *Lion* to the *Ape*
Practiſe the frauds of every ſhape.

GAY.

L O N D O N.

PRINTED FOR J. RIDGWAY, YORK-STREET;
St. JAMES's SQUARE.

1793.

FIGURES 6, 7 Covers from two political pamphlets written by Parkinson under the pseudonym "Old Hubert."

The definition was followed by a synopsis of the natural history of the disease. It was of insidious onset, the initial symptom usually being "a slight sense of weakness, with a proneness to trembling in some particular part; sometimes in the head, but most commonly in the hands and arms." This "first stage" typically lasted for about 2 years. During the subsequent year, the symptoms increased in the part first affected and then gradually spread, typically to involve a symmetrical part on the opposite side of the body. Within a few more months, "the patient is found to be less strict than usual in preserving an upright posture." Unsteadiness of the hand while writing or when the patient was "em-

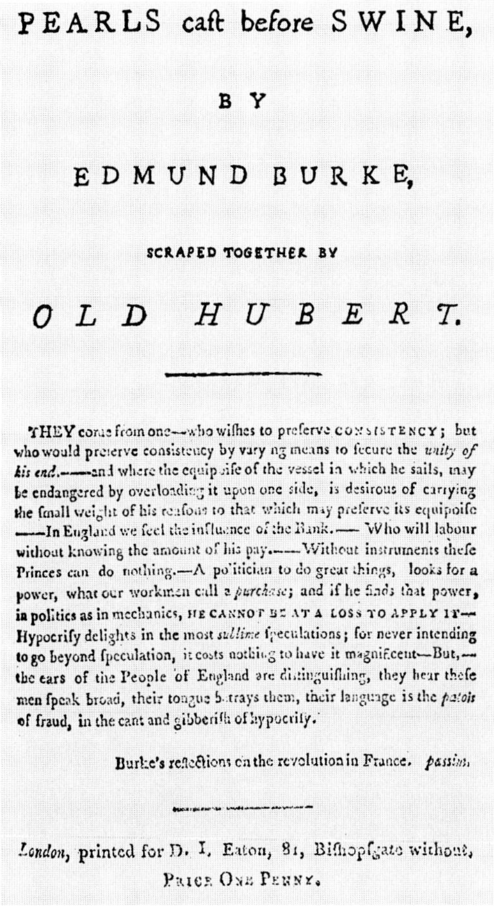

PEARLS caft before SWINE,

BY

EDMUND BURKE,

SCRAPED TOGETHER BY

OLD HUBERT.

———————

THEY come from one—who wifhes to preferve CONSISTENCY; but who would preferve consiftency by vary ng means to fecure the *unity of his end.*———and where the equip ife of the veffel in which he fails, may be endangered by overloading it upon one fide, is defirous of carrying the fmall weight of his reafons to that which may preferve its equipoife ———In England we feel the influence of the Bank.——— Who will labour without knowing the amount of his pay.———Without inftruments thefe Princes can do nothing.—A po'itician to do great things, looks for a power, what our workmen call a *purchase*; and if he finds that power, in politics as in mechanics, HE CANNOT BE AT A LOSS TO APPLY IT.— Hypocrify delights in the most *subline* fpeculations; for never intending to go beyond fpeculation, it cofts nothing to have it magnificent—But,— the ears of the People of England are diftinguifhing, they hear thefe men fpeak broad, their tongue betrays them, their language is the *patois* of fraud, in the cant and gibberifh of hypocrity.

Burke's reflections on the revolution in France. *passim.*

——————————

London, printed for D. I. Eaton, 81, Bifhopfgate without. PRICE ONE PENNY.

FIGURE 7

ploying himself in any nicer kind of manipulation" appeared next. The patient's infirmity gradually increased; the hand failed to "answer with exactness to the dictates of the will." Walking became increasingly laborious as the "legs are not raised to that height, or with that promptitude which the will directs." Falls frequently resulted. In this advanced stage, "writing can now be hardly at all accomplished" and eating was a chore—the fork "not being duly directed," the morsel of food only "with much difficulty conveyed to the mouth." The limbs seemed to be in constant agitation. The "propensity to lean forward becomes invincible," due to a "diminution of the nervous power in the extensor muscles of the head and trunk." The poor victim was "thrown on the toes and forepart

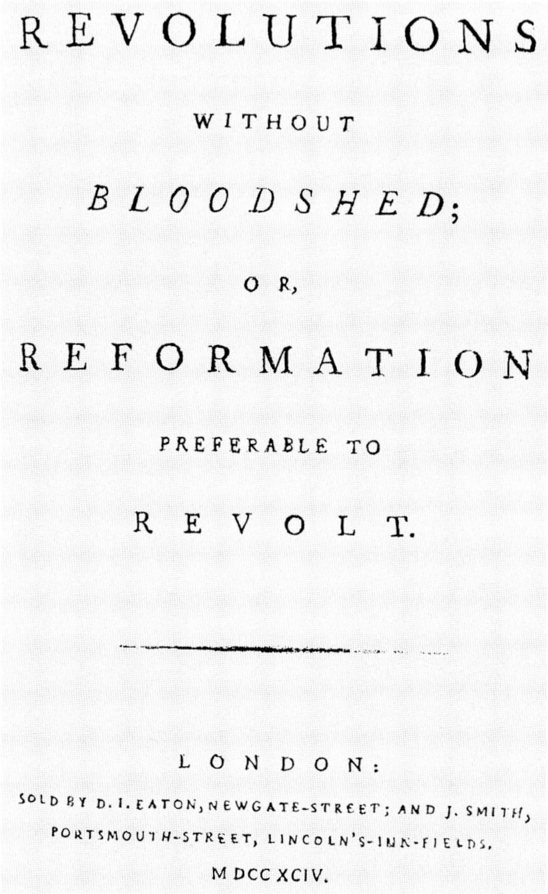

R E V O L U T I O N S

W I T H O U T

B L O O D S H E D;

O R,

R E F O R M A T I O N

PREFERABLE TO

R E V O L T.

LONDON:

SOLD BY D. I. EATON, NEWGATE-STREET; AND J. SMITH,
PORTSMOUTH-STREET, LINCOLN'S-INN-FIELDS.
M DCC XCIV.

FIGURE 8 A political pamphlet published anonymously by Parkinson in which he lists 24 beneficial results which would be produced by reforming the system of representation in Parliament.

of the feet; being, at the same time irresistibly impelled to take much quicker and shorter steps, and thereby to adopt unwillingly a running pace." As the disease's end approached, the patient's words become "scarcely intelligible." He had to be fed and "the food is with difficulty retained in the mouth until masticated; and then as difficultly swallowed." Saliva continually drained from the mouth. "The urine and faeces are passed involuntarily." Finally, at the last, "constant sleepiness, with slight delirium, and other marks of extreme exhaustion, announce the wished-for release."

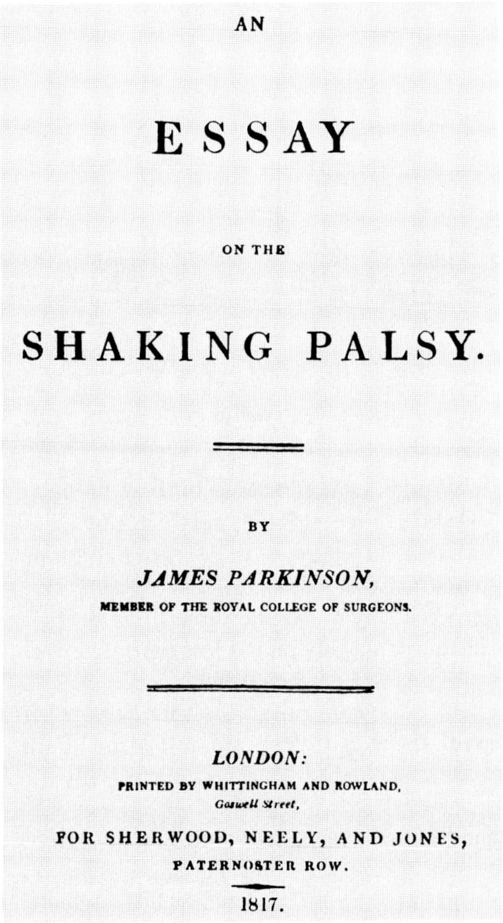

AN

E S S A Y

ON THE

SHAKING PALSY.

BY

JAMES PARKINSON,
MEMBER OF THE ROYAL COLLEGE OF SURGEONS.

LONDON:
PRINTED BY WHITTINGHAM AND ROWLAND,
Goswell Street,

FOR SHERWOOD, NEELY, AND JONES,
PATERNOSTER ROW.

1817.

FIGURE 9   Title page of Parkinson's monograph on shaking palsy (1817).

Parkinson's words provide a vivid and graphic picture of the evolution of the "shaking palsy." They appear to be the work of someone who has extensive first-hand experience with the disease. Yet, somewhat paradoxically, Parkinson apparently based his monograph entirely on six cases. The patient who initially stimulated his interest in the disease (Case I) came to his attention several years prior to the publication of his monograph. He was a man "rather more than fifty years of age" who had lived a life of "remarkable temperance and sobriety" while working as a gardener. The pattern of his illness typified that described earlier, and the case report itself contains few new or noteworthy additional

SHAKING PALSY. *(Paralysis Agitans.)*

Involuntary tremulous motion, with lessened
  muscular power, in parts not in action and
  even when supported ; with a propensity
  to bend the trunk forward, and to pass
  from a walking to a running pace : the
  senses and intellects being uninjured.

FIGURE 10   Parkinson's definition of shaking palsy as it appeared in his Essay
(1817).

details. Parkinson's "eager wish" to acquire some further knowledge of the
nature of this man's disease must have been intense, for his next two cases (Cases
II, III) were "noticed casually in the street." The first of these was a 62-year-old
man who had "suffered from the disease for 8 or 10 years. All his extremities
were considerably agitated, the speech was very much interrupted, and the body
much bowed and shaken. He walked almost entirely on the fore part of his feet,
and would have fallen every step if he had not been supported by his stick."
Parkinson was apparently not deterred from prognosticating on the basis of his
single previous case and "fully assured" the man of "the incurable nature of his
complaint" whereupon the fellow understandably "declined making any
attempts for relief."

Parkinson's second casual sighting (Case III) was a man of "about 65." He
was of interest because of the severity of his tremor, which Parkinson characterized as a vehement agitation that involved the limbs, head and "whole body."
The poor man was forced "to go on a continued run and to employ his stick
every five or six steps to force him more into an upright posture, by projecting
the point of it with great force against the pavement."

Case IV, a man about 55 years of age, came to see Parkinson for an abscess
over the ribs. Unfortunately, the chance to follow the evolution of his shaking
palsy was "lost by his removal to a distant part of the country"—perhaps the
first recorded example of "lost to follow-up" in a study of paralysis agitans.

Case V also seemed to pose insurmountable problems. The "particulars" of
the case "could not be obtained," and in fact, "the lamented subject . . . was
only seen at a distance."

The final patient (Case VI), a 72-year-old man provided a more suitable object for study. His disease was of eleven or twelve years' duration and had begun
with weakness in the left hand and arm followed soon after by trembling. Three
years later, the right arm was similarly involved, and in about 3 more years both

legs. In the tenth or eleventh year of his illness, the man awoke one night to find, "that he had nearly lost the use of his right side, and that the face was much drawn to the left side." Parkinson astutely noted that "neither the arm nor the leg of the paralytic side was in the least affected with the tremulous agitation; but as their paralysed state was removed, the shaking returned."

Parkinson's description of this patient's gait was reasonably detailed. He noted that the man was "under much apprehension of falling forwards" and he seemed to have great difficulty "raising his feet." His wife told Parkinson that she believed that her husband would consider stepping over a pin as a difficult task. It was also this patient who called Parkinson's attention to the effect of sudden changes in posture on his tremor. If he "threw himself rather violently into a chair," the "shaking completely stopped" only to return a few minutes later.

Reading the six brief case vignettes, one is struck by the fact that Parkinson's conception of paralysis agitans depended almost entirely on the information he was able to obtain by history and upon the clinical findings which were obvious by visual inspection. There is no real evidence that Parkinson actually examined any of his patients. This perhaps may account for his apparent failure to appreciate features such as the degree of muscular rigidity or the presence of "cogwheeling." It is less clear why he did not comment on the slowed movement (bradykinesia) that his patients must have experienced.

In Chapter II of his essay, Parkinson briefly expanded on what he identified as the two cardinal symptoms of paralysis agitans: the "involuntary tremulous motion" and the propensity to "pass from a walking to a running pace." In describing the tremor characteristic of shaking palsy, Parkinson specifically indicated that its distinguishing feature was the fact that it occurred "whilst the affected part is supported and unemployed" and that it ceased with the adoption of voluntary motion.

In the third chapter, Parkinson marshalled the evidence that distinguished shaking palsy "from other diseases with which it may be confounded." He was aware that some patients with palsy "consequent to compression of the brain, or dependent on partial exhaustion of the energy of that organ" developed tremor of the palsied limbs. He noted that sudden onset of weakness and the frequent presence of sensory impairment characterized these cases. In shaking palsy, there was never a "lessened sense of feeling," and even late in the disease, the dictates of the will were still "conveyed to the muscles; and the muscles act on this impulse, but their actions are perverted."

Shaking palsy could also be confounded with the

trembling consequent to indulgence in the drinking of spirituous liquors; that which proceeds from the immoderate employment of tea and coffee; that which appears to be dependent on advanced age; and all those tremblings which proceed from the various circumstances which induce a diminution of power in the nervous system.

The characteristics of the tremor enabled one to distinguish readily shaking palsy from these various ailments. In the former, "If the trembling limb was supported, and none of its muscles be called into action, the trembling will cease." In true shaking palsy, the reverse of this occurred: "The agitation continues in full force whilst the limb is at rest and unemployed; and even is sometimes diminished by calling the muscles into employment."

Parkinson's discussion of the "proximate" and "remote" causes of shaking palsy was "made under very unfavorable circumstances" because he did not have "the advantage in a single case, of that light which anatomical examination yields . . ." He used "conjecture founded on analogy, and an attentive consideration of the peculiar symptoms of the disease" as the "only guides that could be obtained for this research" and offered the resulting opinion with "hesitation." He concluded that shaking palsy was due to a diseased state of the superior part of the medulla spinalis ("that part [of the medulla] which is contained in the canal formed by the superior cervical vertebrae") and eventually extended to involve the medulla oblongata. He thought that the medulla might be affected by some prior injury as might result from trauma or inflammation. None of his patients was able to recall any injury of the type Parkinson postulated, but rather attributed the disease to a variety of factors such as "spirituous liquors" (Case II), "long lying on the damp ground" (Case III), or being engaged in work that required "considerable exertion of the involved limbs" (Case I).

As shaking palsy progressed, it tended to involve sequentially the arms followed by the legs, head, trunk and "lastly the muscles of the mouth and fauces." Parkinson believed that this extension of the disease, over so widespread an area of the body, tended to exclude peripheral sites of pathology such as the brachial nerves (which might be considered at first when the process was confined to the arms and hands). He believed that "impediment to speech, the difficulty in mastication and swallowing, the inability to retain, or freely to eject the saliva," which appeared late in the disease, indicated that the morbid process had spread from the superior portion of the medulla spinalis to involve the medulla oblongata. The "absence of any injury to the sense and to the intellect" indicated that "the morbid state does not extend to the encephalon."

The final chapter of *Essay on the Shaking Palsy* is devoted to "considerations respecting the means of cure." Parkinson hoped that "some remedial process may ere long be discovered; by which, at least, the progress of the disease may be stopped." He thought that therapy would have the greatest chance for success if initiated during the "first stage" of the disease when symptoms were typically confined to the arms.

Parkinson suggested a trial of venesection; blood was to be taken from the upper part of the neck followed by the application of vesicatories to induce a "fresh blister." The blister was made with a "caustic" and kept open by inserting an almond-shaped piece of cork. This later maneuver was designed to ensure that a "sufficient quantity" of pus would continue to discharge. Although this therapy might appear somewhat odd to the modern reader, it seemed eminently rational to Parkinson. He believed that an injury to the medulla or its surrounding membranes could produce a state of excitement or irritation in the medulla itself, which in turn triggered a local "afflux" of blood into the minute vessels within the medulla. The resulting increase in volume of the medulla, which was encased inside the unyielding bone of the spinal canal, would produce a "degree of pressure" that might "eventually interrupt the influence of the brain upon the inferior portions of the medullary column, and upon the parts on which the nerves of this portion are disposed." Local bloodletting and suppurative discharge would obviously prove valuable by reducing the degree of vascular congestion and "interstitial addition," hence decompressing the medulla. One can only wonder how many of our own equally plausible-sounding rationales for therapy will seem as bizarre to neurologists 170 years from now.

Parkinson's essay was generally well reviewed in the leading medical journals (McMenemey, 1955) and was subsequently read by many of the leading English authorities on diseases of the nervous system. John Cooke cites Parkinson's study of paralysis agitans in the second volume of his *Treatise on Nervous Disease* (1821). His description does not seem to include any new material and seems to be based entirely on Parkinson's account. In his *Lectures on the Nervous System and its Diseases* (1836), Marshall Hall also comments extensively on "paralysis agitans." Like Cooke before him, Hall adds little that is new or novel in his description. The results of autopsy in a 28-year-old man with hemiparkinsonism convinced him that many cases of paralysis agitans shared features with patients with diseases of the corpora quadrigemina of the midbrain caused by localized processes such as tuberculoma. Marshall Hall also noted similarities between the tremor of paralysis agitans and "tremor mercurialis," a species of tremor he had frequently seen in workers using mercury for silvering mirrors.

Robert Bentley Todd discussed paralysis agitans in an article on "paralysis" in 1834 and again in his *Clinical Lectures on Paralysis* (1854). He based his commentary on extensive quotations from *Essay on the Shaking Palsy* and noted that only a "few" cases of the disease had been recorded since Parkinson's account. Todd's descriptions succinctly conveyed the basic features of the disease.

The disease approaches gradually and almost imperceptibly, generally commencing with a sense of weakness and slight tremor of the hands and arms, and occasionally of the head. After a lengthened period, perhaps a year, the patient loses his balance in walking and bends forwards. The feet are power-less and tremble. The tremor becomes permanent, overpowering, and does not even cease when the parts are firmly supported. Head, hands, and feet, are in constant tremulous movement. When the patient attempts to walk, he throws himself upon the toes and front of the foot, walks hastily and inse-curely, in constant danger of falling on his face. The tremor now continues during sleep, and becomes so violent that the bedstead shakes, and the pa-tient wakes up. He is unable to read or write, and being unable to eat by him-self, requires to be fed. Mastication is difficult, the saliva flows from the mouth. There is constant constipation, the trunk is bent forwards, the chin rests on the sternum. At last, there is entire loss of speech and deglutition, in-voluntary evacuations, stupor and death. (1834)

After a time the patient finds that he cannot perform small actions with the diseased arm; he cannot button his clothes, nor pick up a pin . . . then he notices that he cannot write so well as formerly; his handwriting becomes tremulous . . . the leg goes through the same series of symptoms . . . he speaks slowly and hesitatingly, but yet his mental faculties do not seem to suffer much . . . these cases are exceedingly chronic . . . The patient begins to stoop; he finds he cannot hold himself erect; and in some instances his gait is apt to pass into that which is known as symptomatic of the disease termed "paralysis agitans." (1854)

The writings of Cooke, Todd, and Marshall Hall as well as those by Stokes, Graves (1843), and Elliotson (1839) helped disseminate information about paralysis agitans, and directed readers to Parkinson's original account. An example can be seen in Romberg's section on paralysis agitans in his *Lehrbuch der Nervenkrankheiten des Menschen* (Manual of the Nervous Diseases of Man) (1840–1846). Romberg included paralysis agitans in his chapter on "tremors" which appeared in the section of his *Lehrbuch* devoted to "Neuroses of Mo-tility." He began by quoting extensively from Todd's account and then noted, "I have often had the opportunity of observing this form of tremor." He went on to describe several cases he had evaluated. It is difficult to tell if all his patients in fact had paralysis agitans. Summarizing their tremor, Romberg states, "With every movement the tremor . . . increased considerably." Either he was wit-nessing patients with paralysis agitans and intention tremor or misdiagnosing some cases.

Romberg, like Parkinson, was at a loss to define the cause of the disease. He described one patient whose disease apparently began after he was "plundered of his clothes by Cossacks, in 1813 . . . and left lying on the damp ground for several hours." When it came to therapy, he warned that in one patient, strychnia had "increased the intensity of the disease." He was more fortunate with a second patient in whom a trial of "carbonate of iron," in association with warm baths and cold affusions applied to the head and neck, resulted in a "marked diminution of the symptoms."

Reviewing the contributions made during the first half-century following Parkinson's original description of paralysis agitans, one is impressed with how little they augment Parkinson's original report. This picture would change dramatically with the contributions of French neurologists including Trousseau, followed by Charcot and his pupils.

Trousseau devoted the fifteenth of his *Lectures on Clinical Medicine* (1859, 1868) to "senile trembling and paralysis agitans." Despite the fact that he too used the term "paralysis agitans," Trousseau noted that it seemed an inappropriate name since "there is no paralysis at the commencement of this strange form of chorea." (It might be argued that his reference to the disease as a "strange form of chorea" probably falls equally wide of the mark.) He based this opinion on his own observations, which he confirmed by using a dynamometer to measure strength in several of his patients. He admitted that "in the long run, however, real weakness supervenes, and towards the close of the disease the loss of muscular power is such that the existence of paralysis cannot be denied."

Trousseau made a number of clinical contributions that added to the understanding of important features of paralysis agitans. He noted that a type of muscular "rigidity," which he considered resembled that seen following hemorrhage or softening (infarction) of the brain, could occur in some patients. Yet the example he provided to illustrate this point seems quite atypical. It is a man with a 2-year history of disease whose fourth and fifth fingers were curled into the palm of his hand and who could barely extend his other fingers. In another case, Trousseau specifically stated "There is no rigidity of the limb, and when the patient does not exert his will, his limb is perfectly supple and I can move it in every direction."

Trousseau also offered an interesting explanation for the festinating gait seen in some afflicted patients. "His body inclines forward as he walks, and he keeps the arm on the affected side in a semiflexed attitude and closely pressed against the trunk. As his center of gravity is thus displaced, he is obliged to run after himself, as it were, so that he keeps trotting and hopping on."

He also seemed aware of bradykinesia. He found that one patient, when asked to repeatedly open and close his hand, did so quickly at first, but then more and more slowly until he was unable to do it at all. He noted that "the muscles have retained their strength, and yet their functions are nearly abolished." Trousseau also commented that intellectual deterioration could occur in paralysis agitans. "The intellect is at first unaffected, but gets weakened at last; the patient loses his memory, and his friends soon notice that his mind is not so clear as it was: precocious caducity sets in."

Trousseau found that paralysis agitans was "an inexorable complaint which terminates fatally within a shorter or longer period, in spite of all treatment." He had "not cured a single patient" with medication. Pneumonia was the ultimate cause of death in several cases under his care. These patients apparently did not come to necropsy because Trousseau later noted, "I am not aware that the anatomical lesions special to paralysis agitans have been studied in France, and it seems that those who looked out for them, did not find any." He quoted at length the details of a case of Professor Oppolzer's in Austria (1861), "The medulla oblongata and the pons varolii were found indurated, while in the lateral columns of the cord, especially in the lumbar region, the medullary substance exhibited grey opaque striae."

In 1861 and 1862, Charcot and Vulpian published a three-part article in the *Gazette Hebdomadaire* covering their initial experience with paralysis agitans at the Salpêtrière. This was followed in 1867 by a monograph by Charcot's pupil, Ordenstein, whose thesis for his doctorate in medicine was on the subject of paralysis agitans and its differentiation from disseminated (multiple) sclerosis (1867). Lecture 5 of Charcot's *Leçons Sur les Malades du Système Nerveux* (1872) provides a comprehensive summary of Charcot's teachings and is available in English translation (1877). (Quotations are from this source unless otherwise noted.)

Charcot, like Romberg before him, appeared to have learned of paralysis agitans from Todd's synopsis of Parkinson's essay (Charcot and Vulpian, 1861). Charcot also agreed with Romberg that the disease was a "neurosis" by which he meant a disease in which "no proper lesion" had been identified. He noted that "frequently the causes remain unknown," but he was impressed by the frequency with which patients gave a history of exposure to "damp cold" or had been subject to "vivid moral emotions" (émotions morales vives) such as an acute fright. Most of his patients were of advanced age ("more than 40 or 50 years") although he was aware of a case of Duchenne's "who was a youth of 16."

Charcot considered the most striking and fundamental symptom of paralysis agitans was tremor (1861, 1872). It existed "even when the individual reposes, limited at first to one member, then little by little becoming generalised" (1872). To this symptom was added "sooner or later an apparent diminution of muscular strength. The movements are slow and seem feeble, although dynamometrical experiments prove that this diminution is not real. This motor impotence appears to be due in part . . . to the rigidity which prevails in the muscles." Charcot went on to describe a "singular symptom" which "comes to complicate the situation: The patient loses the faculty of preserving equilibrium whilst walking. In some patients we notice a tendency to propulsion or to retropulsion . . . compelled to adopt a quick pace; the individual is unable, without extreme difficulty, to stop—being apparently forced to follow a flying centre of gravity." He then goes on to discuss other important symptoms including "a peculiar attitude of the body and its members, a fixed look, and immobile features."

In the immense majority of cases, the disease was insidious in its onset. The tremor was frequently "passing and transitory" and it could be suspended by walking, grasping, lifting, taking a pen, writing, "any effort at all of the will." Tremor was typically "circumscribed to the foot, the hand, or the thumb." Some patterns of tremor in the hand were "almost pathognomonic" as when "the patient closes the fingers on the thumb as though in the act of spinning wool," or "crumbling bread," or the thumb moves over the fingers as when a pencil or paper ball is rolled between them. He noted, "These are, if I do not mistake, peculiarities which belong specifically to the tremor of paralysis agitans." Charcot also called attention to the fact that in some patients "a very remarkable feeling of fatigue" or pain of a rheumatic or neuralgic type preceded the onset of tremor.

As the disease progressed, it "observed certain rules." The usual pattern of spread was from the arm to the ipsilateral leg, with this pattern repeating itself on the contralateral side. "Decussated" invasion (upper extremity to contralateral lower extremity) was the rarest pattern with "hemiplegic" and "paraplegic" types occurring infrequently. Once tremor became established, its intensity often seemed to fluctuate. It was exacerbated by emotion and attenuated by voluntary movements, and "annihilated" by natural sleep and anesthetics such as chloroform. Charcot had seen paroxysmal crises in which tremor became transiently more severe without any appreciable cause.

Tremor imparted "special characters" to the handwriting (Fig. 11), which in the earliest stage could often be perceived only after examination with a magnifying glass, a fact well-described by Charcot's pupil, Bourneville. The down-strokes of the pen appeared relatively normal, the finer up-strokes became "tremulous" with some parts of the letters being thicker and heavier than others.

Charcot insisted that tremor did not involve the face or jaws (Charcot and Vulpian, 1861–1862; Charcot, 1872): "Far from trembling, the muscles of the face are motionless, there is even a remarkable fixity of look, and the features

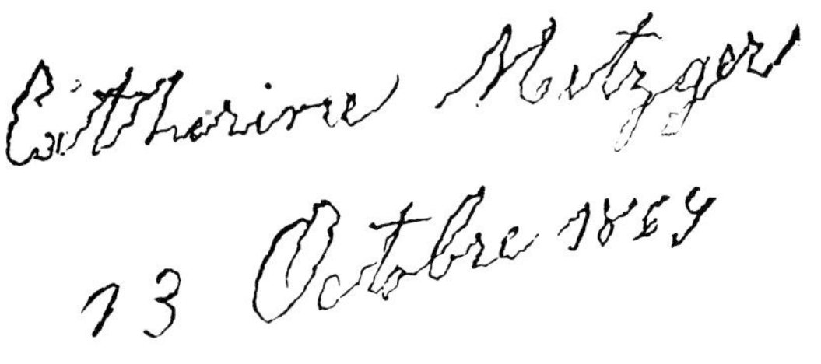

FIGURE 11 A specimen of the handwriting of a patient with paralysis agitans under the care of Professor Charcot at the Hôpital St. Louis in 1869. Note the sinuous and irregular letters. The down-strokes are nearly normal, the up-strokes are very tremulous (from Charcot, 1872).

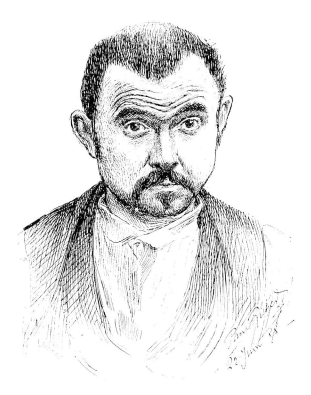

FIGURE 12   Drawing by Paul Richer, a former intern of Charcot's and later Chief of the Laboratory at La Salpêtrière and Professor of Creative Anatomy at the National School of Fine Arts. The drawing is dated June 22, 1888 and depicts the facial features of a patient with paralysis agitans (from Richer, 1888).

present a permanent expression of mournfulness, sometimes of stolidness or stupidity" (Fig. 12). The tongue could be stirred by tremor, which augmented when it was protruded. The lips appeared to be drawn or firmly pressed together and "pouting." Bourneville noted that a fine tremor could be seen at times in the lower lip.

Speech was "slow, jerky and short of phrase" and "cost a considerable effort of will." At times, if the body tremor was intense, it could affect articulation and words "jolted out as it were, like that of an inexperienced rider on horseback, when the animal is trotting."

Charcot emphasized "a characteristic which we believe was overlooked by Parkinson . . ."—the rigidity found in the muscles of the neck, body, and extremities. Patients complained of a sensation of "cramps" or "stiffness," which initially might be transient but later became fixed, although subject to some variation in intensity. The flexor muscles were always the first group to be affected by rigidity and the most intensely involved. It was this rigidity that imposed on patients their characteristic attitude (Figs. 13–17); the head gently bent forward, the body inclined forward, the elbows being held near the chest with the hands flexed on the forearm and the forearm flexed slightly on the upper arms. A characteristic "deformity" of the hand occurred (Fig. 18). The thumb and index finger extended and apposed ("as if to hold a pen") and the fingers slightly bent into the palm and deviated to the ulnar side. In advanced cases, the legs were held in semiflexion, the knees adducted, the feet extended and inverted.

Charcot believed that rigidity was also responsible for the fact that patients seem to move in one piece as if their joints were soldered together. He agreed with the German neurologist Benedikt that rigidity contributed to "rendering movement laborious" but thought it was not the only cause of this situation (see below). He had seen patients in whom rigidity was a prominent early symptom and tremor was "scarcely noticed" and of "little intensity," but believed that those were rare and exceptional.

Charcot stated that retardation and laboriousness in the execution of movements were another cardinal feature of paralysis agitans. He clearly stated that this was an independent facet of the disease "dependent neither on the existence of tremors, nor on that of muscular rigidity." Motor acts were performed with "extreme slowness" due to a "lapse of time between the thought and the act." Charcot took great pains to emphasize that in all these cases, "muscular power is retained in a remarkable degree," a fact he confirmed using a dynamometer.

When he came to describe the characteristic gait of patients with paralysis agitans, Charcot objected to Trousseau's earlier suggestion that the festinating pace was dependent on the patient's center of gravity being displaced forward by the inclination of the head and body. He cited examples of patients who ran or fell backwards, and of cases in which "propulsion" occurred before the postural changes were apparent.

Under the heading "disagreeable sensations," Charcot described patients who complained of "a nearly permanent sensation of tension and traction in most of the muscles . . . an indefinable uneasiness, which shows itself in a perpetual desire for change of posture." Other patients had an "habitual sensation of excessive heat" that "is especially felt in the epigastrium and the back." This sensation was "frequently accompanied by profuse perspiration."

During the terminal period of the disease, "the mind becomes clouded and memory is lost. General prostration sets in, the urine and faeces are passed unconsciously . . . the patients succumb to the mere progress of their disease. . ." Charcot, like Trousseau before him, noted that death was often due to pneumonia. In some patients at this terminal period, the tremor "is frequently seen to diminish and even to disappear."

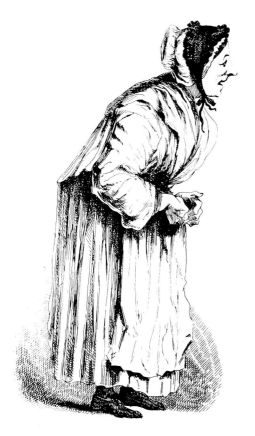

FIGURES 13, 14 Drawings by Paul Richer of the posture of a patient with paralysis agitans as it appeared in 1874 (Fig. 13) and in 1879 (Fig. 14) (from Charcot, 1872–1873).

After reviewing previously reported descriptions of pathologic investigations into paralysis agitans, Charcot summarized the results by stating that "the special lesion of paralysis agitans remains to be discovered." His own examinations would not prove exceptional; he found an "obliteration of the central canal of the spinal cord" in several cases.

When it came to therapy, Charcot stated, "Everything or almost everything had been tried against this disease." In his hands, strychnine seemed to "exasperate the trembling" rather than reduce it (Charcot and Vulpian, 1861–1862, Charcot, 1872). Ergot, belladonna, and opium "have not yielded any very profitable results." He went on to say, "Latterly I have made use of hyoscyamine, from which some patients have obtained relief; its action, however, is simply

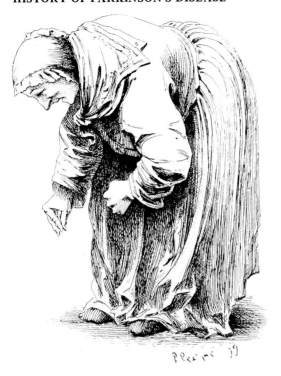

FIGURE 14

palliative." Hyoscyamine (an atropine isomer) is not mentioned by Charcot in his discussion of therapy in 1862, but does appear in Ordenstein's thesis (1867) and Charcot's *Leçons* (1872). Charcot was probably not the first to employ hyoscyamine; Handfield Jones mentions it in his book on functional nervous diseases (1864).

Charcot's successors at La Salpêtrière continued to contribute clinical insights to specific aspects of the disease that Charcot had characterized so well. Brissaud devoted two of his own *Leçons* at La Salpêtrière during 1893–1894 to the "Maladie de Parkinson" (Parkinson's disease) (1895). He was one of the first to refer to the face of patients as a "masque" (mask). In discussing rigidity, he noted that its spread bore a certain analogy to the march of jacksonian epilepsy. Brissaud commented that the immobility of these patients gave them a "mummified" appearance and made their gestures seem unduly dignified and reserved. He approvingly quoted Charcot's dictum that although the rigidity and posture of parkinsonism could occur without the presence of tremor, one never encountered persisting tremor without rigidity. His comments on tremor largely reiterated Charcot's. One particularly apt turn of phrase was the comment that tremor of

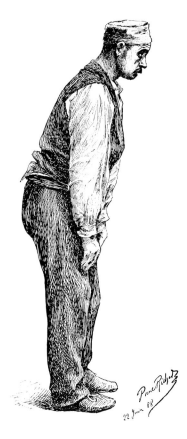

FIGURE 15   Drawing by Paul Richer of the posture of the patient whose face is shown in Figure 12. This drawing is also dated June 22, 1888 (from Richer, 1888).

the tongue between the teeth made it appear as if the patient "murmured an interminable litany" in a voice that was "weak" and without intonation.

Brissaud's comments on the ocular aspects of paralysis agitans are more detailed than Charcot's. Brissaud pointed out that although "true nystagmus" was not present, some patients had "nystagmiform" movements on lateral gaze, which he thought represented the eyes' "fashion of trembling." The eyelids were "rigid" but also animated with small fluttering movements. The pupil was "stenosed and rigid" and the eye seemed fixed in an immobile position. This immobility was not to be confused with ophthalmoplegia because patients could move their eyes, but often preferred to look at things from the corner of the eyes rather than turn the head.

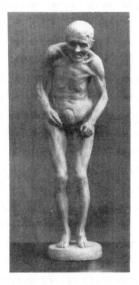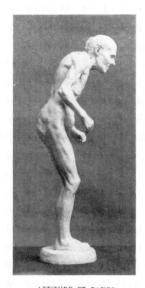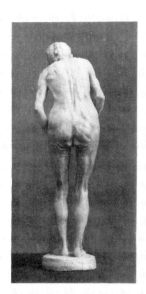

ATTITUDE ET FACIES
Dans la maladie de Parkinson.
Statuette de M. le Dʳ Paul Richer, d'après une malade de la Salpêtrière.

FIGURE 16 Statuette by Paul Richer of a patient with paralysis agitans, one of a series of sculptural representations by Richer of the principal types of neurologic disease. The subject was a 58-year-old female patient of Professor Charcot's at the Salpêtrière in 1892 (from Richer and Meige, 1895).

Brissaud thought that with the "idea" of a movement, tremor became exaggerated, but that with the movement itself, tremor ceased. He made a number of interesting observations on the synchronism of tremor in different parts of the body. The movements were "almost absolutely" in time with each other, a feature that was a "strong presumption" in favor of the central rather than peripheral nature of the disease. When movements became temporarily out of time with each other, it was usually the lower limb that lagged behind the upper. He tried to draw an analogy to the oscillation of an articulated pendulum with weights representing the different limbs swinging with two different periods and hence, at times, out of phase with each other.

Brissaud also extended Charcot's teachings when he emphasized the frequency of "psychic troubles" in patients with Parkinson's disease. Patients often "appeared in general indifferent to all that which surrounded them" and had "the same repugnance to emit their ideas as to move their limbs." Brissaud cited the work of Ball who had described different types of mental changes in these

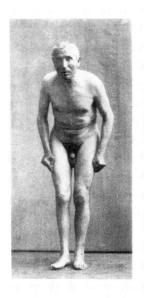
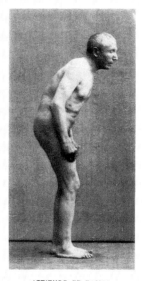
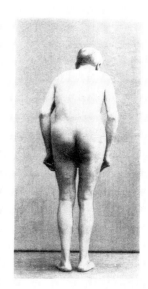

ATTITUDE ET FACIES
Dans la maladie de Parkinson.
D'après un malade de la Salpêtrière.

FIGURE 17 Photograph of a patient at La Salpêtrière with paralysis agitans, illustrating the typical posture and facial features produced by the disease. This patient was often used by Charcot in his clinical demonstrations (from Richer and Meige, 1895).

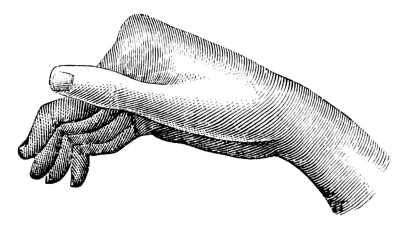

FIGURE 18 Deformity of the fingers in a patient with paralysis agitans. Charcot noted the similarity with the deformity caused by "chronic articular rheumatism." Compare with Gowers' depiction in Figure 21 (from Charcot, 1872).

patients, ranging from alterations in character and humor (such as excessive irritability) to actual "weakness of intellectual faculties" that could take any form
from obtusion to complete dementia.

Brissaud carefully reviewed the various pathologic lesions that had been reported in cases of Parkinson's disease. He was particularly impressed by a case of
hemiplegic parkinsonism described by Blocq and Marinesco (1893), in which a
sharply demarcated tuberculoma had been found in the contralateral inferior
peduncle and had "completely destroyed the locus niger [substantia nigra] ." He
commented that this structure was "very obscure" and that not much was
known either of its normal structure or of its pathologic physiology but went on
to postulate that it might be involved with voluntary and automatic movements
and muscular tone. With tremendous prescience, he hypothesized that "a lesion
of the locus niger could very well be the anatomic substrate of Parkinson's
disease."

Although many other contributions were made in the late part of the
nineteenth century, none was more important in crystallizing our modern conception of paralysis agitans than that of Sir William Gowers in England. His ideas
are summarized in his *Manual of Diseases of the Nervous System* (1886-1888).
By 1888, he had accumulated personal notes on 80 cases. He found a slight
(63%) male predominance. As to age at onset, "it usually commences after 40
years of age. Nearly half the cases begin between 50 and 60, and about one-fifth
in each of the two decades, 40-50 and 60-70 . . ." The earliest onset among his
cases was at 29 and the oldest at 69. Fifteen percent had a "hereditary influence"
but in addition to true familial cases of paralysis agitans, this figure also included
cases with "a history of insanity or epilepsy in near relatives." Gowers found
"exciting causes" in about one-third of his cases including "emotion, physical injury, and acute disease"—the latter included dysentery and typhoid fever. Under
the heading of "symptoms" came descriptions of the "anxious and fixed" face
and the characteristic body posture (Fig. 19). He noted that in two-thirds of patients tremor preceded weakness. He was clearly more impressed with weakness
than Charcot, a fact he referred to when explaining in a footnote that the name
of the disease, "paralysis agitans," was generally appropriate "since in the majority of the cases both symptoms are conspicuous."

Tremor typically began in the arms (61 of 75 cases) and more frequently on
the left (35 cases) than on the right side (26 cases). In the arm, "the tremor
usually commences in the hand, sometimes in the finger and thumb." Although
in four cases onset had been in the shoulder, symptomatic progression from the
arm to the ipsilateral leg ("hemiplegic") was "by far the most common" pattern,
and many conceivable variations existed.

Tremor resulted from "alternating contractions in opposing muscles" and was
"greatest in the hands and fingers." A metaphor Gowers used to describe the
tremor strikes the modern reader as odd: "A movement of the fingers at the

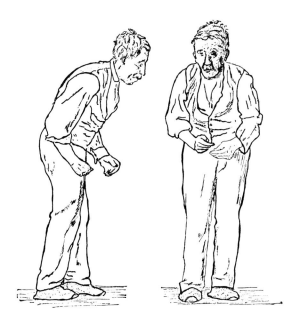

FIGURE 19 Characteristic posture of a patient with paralysis agitans as illustrated by Gowers (1886–1888). "The head is bent foward, and the expression of the face is anxious and fixed, unchanged by any play of emotion. The arms are slightly flexed at all joints, from muscular rigidity . . ."

metacarpo-phalangeal joints similar to that by which Orientals beat their small drums." We are more comfortable with: "As in the act of rolling a small object between the fingertips." In the legs, tremor was usually "greatest in the muscles moving the ankle joint, and the heel may beat the floor as the patient is sitting, it is slight in the toes, but may be distinct in the thigh, sometimes in the adductors, sometimes in the flexors of the knee." He had never seen tremor in the muscles of the abdomen or the soft palate, but had occasionally seen it in the trunk, back muscles, jaw, tongue, and "very rarely" the muscles of the face. In most cases, the "head is free from tremor except such as may be communicated to it from distant oscillation." Unlike Charcot, Gowers was willing to admit exceptions to this rule; true tremor of the head could be caused by contractions of trapezius, sternomastoids, or splenius.

The amplitude of tremor "increases with the progress of the disease." At its minimum, it was "so slight as to need close observation to detect it," but it could be so great as to "amount to 2 inches at the extremity of the fingers." To determine its frequency, Gowers made a large number of "myographic tracings" (Fig. 20). He found a variation in frequency between 4.8 and 7 oscillations/sec

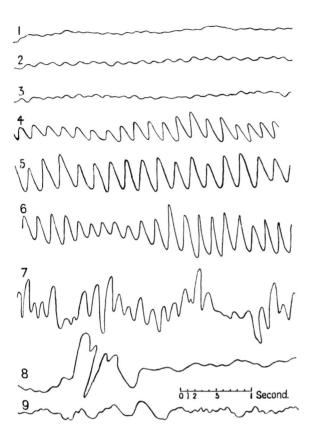

FIGURE 20 Myographic tracings of various forms of tremor. 1. posthemi-
plegic; 2–6. paralysis agitans; 7. multiple sclerosis; 8. general paresis; 9. hysteria
(from Gowers, 1886–1888).

and discovered that "the fine tremor of the early stage is often distinctly quicker
than the coarser tremor of the later period." The frequency of tremor was "nearly the same rate" in different limbs of the same patient (e.g., 6 Hz in the arm,
6.8 Hz in the leg). He contrasted the tremor in paralysis agitans to that of insular
sclerosis, general paralysis of the insane, and hysteria, stressing the importance of
tremor at rest in the former. Voluntary movement "may stop the tremor for a
few seconds, sometimes for many, but it recommences and accompanies the
movement." In rare cases, "the tremor may be distinct and even considerable on

voluntary movement, and may almost or quite cease as soon as the limbs are at rest." It could also be "fine" during rest and "coarser" during movement. Because of the tremor, "The patient's handwriting reveals his disease . . . every line is a zigzag." Like Charcot and Bourneville, he used a magnifying glass to recognize slight cases of irregularity in writing.

Gowers, like Parkinson, had seen tremor that persisted during sleep, but thought this was an exception to the general rule that "sleep usually brings stillness to the shaking limbs." He also found that paroxysmal exacerbations of tremor could occur in rare cases, especially under the influence of emotional excitement.

Muscular weakness and rigidity were "as characteristic of the disease as is the tremor." "Voluntary movement is not only feeble; it is also slow." Slowness could result either from "a delay in the commencement of movement" or in its execution. This slowness was due "in part" to rigidity. Rigidity also imposed characteristic postures on the limbs because of its preponderance in flexor muscles (Fig. 21).

Gowers's description of the gait of parkinsonian patients encapsulated all its notable features: The patient rises up slowly from the chair with head and

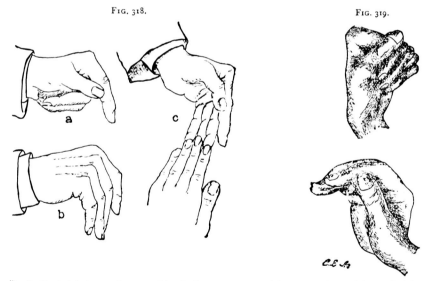

FIG. 318.   FIG. 319.

Fig. 318.—Paralysis agitans. Posture of hands from contracture of the interossei : *a*, left hand ; *b*, right hand. In the left hand the contracture is greater than in the other, and has led to some permanent shortening of the interossei, so that the fingers cannot be extended even passively. The maximum passive extension is shown at *c*.

Fig. 319.—Contraction of fingers in paralysis agitans. Maximum voluntary extension.

FIGURE 21   Hand postures in paralysis agitans (from Gowers, 1886–1888).

shoulders bent forward. His steps are short, and the first may be taken slowly and with difficulty, but they become quicker and quicker, until the patient seems about to run ("festination") and often, from the inclination of the body, to be on the point of falling forward ("propulsion").

In describing the speech of his patients, Gowers found it to be "monotonous" with "a delay in commencing a sentence" often followed by rapidly uttered words and "confluence of syllables." Gowers recalled Charcot when he noted the frequency of subjective sensory and vasomotor sensations in his patients. These could take the form of "aching pains in the limbs," a "great sense of fatigue," or an "abnormal sensation of temperature." Nearly half of his patients complained of a "sense of heat," which could be "referred to the interior of the body or localized in the most affected limb." An abnormal sensation of cold was "only half as common." The sense of heat was frequently accompanied by "increased perspiration" and sometimes was found in association with papillary miosis ("another indication of disturbed function of the sympathetic system"). Gowers also grouped with these symptoms feelings of "extreme restlessness" associated with a desire to change one's posture every few minutes.

Mental symptoms could include irritability and depression. In the later stages of the disease, there could be "mental weakness," "loss of memory," and sometimes "a tendency to delusions."

When it came to treatment, Gowers advised that "mental strain" and "physical exhaustion" were to be avoided. "Life should be quiet and regular, freed, as far as may be, from care and work." He had found that morphia, hyoscyamine, conium (hemlock), and "Indian hemp" (*Cannabis sativa* var. *indica*) "quiet the tremor for a time." Arsenic "occasionally seems to do some real good." He concluded by stating, "My own experience is to the effect that arsenic and Indian hemp, the latter sometimes combined with opium, are of most use. I have several times seen a very distinct improvement for a considerable time under their use."

In this review, we have traced the history of paralysis agitans through the nineteenth century. In an attempt to enable the reader to see paralysis agitans through the eyes of physicians of this era, we have quoted them verbatim whenever possible. Later contributions would come from clinicians such as S.A.K. Wilson, Derek Denny-Brown, F.M.R. Walshe, and others. Modern insights into the basis of many of the motor abnormalities found in parkinsonism have been admirably summarized by Marsden in his Wartenberg lecture (1982). These later contributions built upon and extended the solid pedestal of knowledge begun during the nineteenth century.

ACKNOWLEDGMENTS

Dr. Kenneth Tyler is supported by a physician–scientist award from the National Institute of Allergy and Infectious Diseases. Additional support for this work came from a grant provided by the William P. Anderson Foundation.

REFERENCES

Blocq P, Marinesco G. (1894). Sur un cas de tremblement parkinsonien hémi-plégique symptomatique d'une tumeur du péduncule cérébrale. *Rev. Neurologique* 2: 265.

Brissaud E. (1895). Vingt-Deuxième Leçon: Pathogenie et Symptoms de la maladie de Parkinson pp. 469–487; Vingt-Troisième Leçon: Nature et Pathogenie de la maladie de Parkinson pp. 488–501. In Merge H (Ed.), *Leçons sur les Maladies Nerveuses (Salpêtrière 1893–1894)*, Paris, G. Masson.

Charcot JM, Vulpian A. (1861–1862). De la paralysie agitante. *Gaz Hebdom Med Chir* 8: 765, 816; 9: 54.

Charcot JM. (1872). Cinquieme Leçon: De la paralysie agitante. In Bourneville (Ed.), *Leçons sur les maladies du système nerveux faites a la Salpêtriere*, Paris, A. Delahaye.

Charcot JM. (1877). On paralysis agitans (Lecture V). In *Lectures on the Diseases of the Nervous System*. G. Sigerson (trans). London, New Sydenham Society, pp. 129–156.

Cooke R. (1821). *History of the Method of Cure of the Various Species of Palsy* p. 207 (Vol. II, part I), *A Treatise of Nervous Diseases*. London, Longmann, Hurst, Rees, Orme and Brown.

Critchley M. (Ed.) (1955). *James Parkinson (1755–1824)*. London, MacMillan.

Denny-Brown D. (1962). *The Basal Ganglia and Their Relation to Disorders of Movement*. London, Oxford.

Gowers WR. (1886–1888). *A Manual of Diseases of the Nervous System*. London, J. & A. Churchill.

Gowers WR. (1899). Paralysis agitans. In Allbutt and Rolleston (Eds.): *A System of Medicine* (Vol. VIII). London, MacMillan.

Graves RJ. (1843). *A System of Clinical Medicine*, p. 714. Dublin, Fannin & Co.

Hall M. (1841). *On the Diseases and Derangements of the Nervous System*. London, Bailliere.

Handfield Jones C. (1864). *Studies on Functional Nervous Disorders*, p. 266–267, London, Churchill and Sons.

Marsden CD. (1982). The mysterious motor function of the basal ganglia. (The Robert Wartenberg Lecture). *Neurology* 32: 514.

McMenemey WH. (1955). James Parkinson (1755–1824). A biographical essay. In Critchley M (Ed.) *James Parkinson (1755–1824)*. London, MacMillan.

Ordenstein L. (1867). *Sur la Paralysie Agitante et la Sclérose en Plaque Généralisée*. Paris, E. Martinet.

Parkinson J. (1787). Some account of the effects of lightning. *Mem Med Soc* 2: 493.

Parkinson J. (1799). *The Chemical Pocket-book; or Memoranda Chemica; Arranged in a Compendium of Chemistry*. London, H.D. Symonds.

Parkinson J. (1799). *Medical Admonitions to Families Respecting the Preservation of Health and the Treatment of the Sick*. London, H.D. Symonds.

Parkinson J. (1800). *Dangerous Sports*. London.

Parkinson J. (1800). *The Hospital Pupil, or an Essay Intended to Facilitate the Study of Medicine and Surgery, in 4 Letters*. London, H.D. Symonds.

Parkinson J. (1800). *The Villager's Friend and Physician*. London.

Parkinson J. (1802). *Hints for the Improvement of Trusses*. London.

Parkinson J. (1811). *Observations on the Act Regulating Mad-Houses*. London, Whittingham and Rowland.

Parkinson J. (1812). Case of diseased appendix vermiformis. *Med Chir Trans* 3: 57.

Parkinson J. (1814). Cases of hydrophobia. *London Med Repository* 1: 289.

Parkinson J. (1817). *An Essay on the Shaking Palsy*. London, Sherwood, Neely, and Jones.

Parkinson J. (1822). *Outlines of Oryctology*. London, Sherwood, Neely, and Jones.

Parkinson J, Parkinson JWK. (1824). On the treatment of infections of typhoid fever. *Med Repository* (new series) 1: 197.

Parkinson J. (1833). *Organic Remains of a Former World. An Examination of the Mineralized Remains of the Vegetables and Animals of the Antediluvian World; Generally Termed Extraneous Fossils*. (3 vols.). London, Sherwood, Neely, and Jones.

Parkinson J. (Anon.). (1794). *Revolutions Without Bloodshed, or, Reformation Preferable to Revolt*. London, D.I. Eaton.

Parkinson J. ("Old Hubert"). (1793). *An Address, to the Hon. Edmund Burke From the Swinish Multitude*. London, J. Ridgway.

Parkinson J. ("Old Hubert"). (1793). *Pearls Cast Before Swine by Edmund Burke, Scraped Together by Old Hubert*. London, D.I. Eaton.

Richer P. (1888). Habitude extérieure et facies dans la paralysie agitante. *Nouv Icon Salpêtrière* 1: 213–216.

Richer P, Meige H. (1895). Étude morphologique sur la maladie de parkinson. *Nouv Icon Salpëtrière* 8: 361–371.

Romberg M. (1840–1846). *Lehrbuch der Nervenkrankheiten des Menschen*. Berlin, A. Duncker.

Romberg M. (1853). *A Manual of the Nervous Diseases of Man*. Vol. II pp. 233–235. E.H. Sieveking (trans.). London, New Sydenham Society.

Sanders WR. (1880). Paralysis agitans. In Reynolds JR (Ed.), *A System of Medicine*. Philadelphia, Henry Lea's Son & Co.

Todd RB. (1834). Paralysis. In Forbes J, Tweedie A, Conolly J (Eds.), *The Cyclopedia of Practical Medicine*, Vol. III. London.

Todd RB. (1855). *Certain Diseases of the Brain, and Other Affections of the Nervous System*. Philadelphia, Lindsay & Blakiston.

Trousseau A. (1861). Tremblement senile et paralysie agitante. In: *Clinique Médicale de l'Hôtel-Dieu de Paris*. Paris, Bailliere.

Trousseau A. (1868). Lecture XV: Senile trembling and paralysis agitans. In *Lectures on Clinical Medicine Delivered at the Hôtel-Dieu, Paris*. P. V. Bazire (trans.). London, New Sydenham Society.

Vulpian A. (1879). Paralysie agitante. In: Raymond F (Ed.), *Clinique Médicale de l'Hôpital de la Charité*. Paris, Octave Doin.

Walshe FMR. (1955). A clinical analysis of the paralysis agitans syndrome. In: Critchley M (Ed.), *James Parkinson (1755-1824)*. London, MacMillan.

Wilson SAK. (1940). *Neurology*. London, Arnold.

2
Epidemiology

REIJO J. MARTTILA
University of Turku, Turku, Finland

Epidemiology is the science concerned with defining the frequency of disease within populations, the characteristics of the persons affected, and the natural history of the disease. The segment of epidemiology investigating these aspects is known as descriptive epidemiology. Another branch of the science, analytic epidemiology, principally aims at detecting clues to the cause of disease, and does so mainly by studying differences in the exposure to various factors or conditions between those with the particular disease and those without. We will discuss both of these in this chapter.

In defining the frequency of disease, two indices are commonly used, prevalence and incidence. The prevalence is usually expressed as the prevalence rate, which is in fact a ratio, and describes the cases with a given disease in the population studied per 100,000 persons at risk. A point prevalence ratio is most often used, which refers to the prevalence ratio at a certain date. The incidence describes the occurrence of new cases of a given disease during a specified period of time, usually 1 year, and per 100,000 population at risk: the annual incidence rate. The frequency of death is similarly measured as a mortality rate, which indicates the number of annual deaths from a given disease per 100,000 population. Prevalence, incidence, and mortality calculated for the total population are known as crude rates, but these indices can be calculated for certain subgroups of the population, for example, for men and women and for different age groups, the results being the sex-specific and age-specific morbidity and mortality rates. Since different populations are not necessarily comparable in terms of ratios of age and sex, the age- and sex-specific rates can be used for comparison, or the crude rates can be adjusted to a certain reference population to enable a comparison with other rates similarly treated.

While substantial etiologic clues may be obtained from the occurrence pattern of a disease and characteristics of the affected population, analytic epidemiology specifically aims at discovering the cause of the disease, or at least at providing fresh lines for further research into the cause. To this end, analytic epidemiology searches for risk factors and associations with disease. In practice, this can be accomplished by following up persons exposed or unexposed to a given factor suspected to be connected either with a low or high risk for the disease under study, and identifying new cases with the disease in both groups. This prospective or cohort study is seldom applicable to chronic diseases, especially those with a relatively low incidence and a long risk period for onset, such as Parkinson's disease. Instead, the retrospective approach may be utilized. In this study design, the past exposures and events in pairs of cases with the disease and suitably matched controls without the disease are compared; hence the name case–control study. For further details of the methods and uses of epidemiology, and of particular problems encountered in neuroepidemiology, recent reviews are available (1–3).

DESCRIPTIVE EPIDEMIOLOGY

In investigations of the frequency of the disease within a population, two issues are critical: completeness of case identification and accuracy in the diagnosis. Most figures about the occurrence of Parkinson's disease have been obtained utilizing the community survey, a method relying on the ascertainment of all patients in a defined area who have come to medical attention. A prerequisite for this type of study is a developed medical care and registration system, despite which, however, a certain number of patients inevitably remain unidentified. Since there is usually a 1- or 2-year delay from the first symptoms to diagnosis in Parkinson's disease (4), the majority of patients remaining outside the community survey are those with early, still undiagnosed disease. Thus the result of a community survey always represents a minimum estimate of disease frequency. A population-based search is the preferable approach, but practical reasons restrict its use to small populations or samples of populations. There are two recent studies in which this approach has been applied to investigating the epidemiology of Parkinson's disease (5,6). The patients identified in community surveys have usually been diagnosed and treated at different medical centers or by private practitioners who do not necessarily use similar diagnostic criteria. Confusion resulting from this can be avoided by subsequent neurologic examination of the patients found in the preliminary search. Studies in which this has been done have indicated that 11–42% of the patients carry an incorrect diagnosis of Parkinson's disease (7–12); most of these have had essential tremor. In addition, classification of the disorders sharing the clinical signs of deficient nigrostriatal dopamine function (i.e., hypokinesia, rigidity, and tremor), and known as parkinsonism, has been refined during recent years. Many types of secondary parkinsonism or parkinsonism associated with neurologic system degenerations have been recognized as distinct from primary parkinsonism or idiopathic Parkinson's disease (13; Koller, Chap. 3). Since differential diagnosis of these disorders requires experienced clinical evaluation, the possibility of diagnostic inaccuracy in patients pooled from various sources increases further.

Due to methodologic limitations and varying diagnostic methods it is readily understandable that the morbidity figures for Parkinson's disease obtained in different epidemiologic surveys are not strictly comparable. Despite their limitations, these studies have nevertheless substantially advanced our knowledge of the epidemiologic profile of Parkinson's disease, and have identified some interesting trends that may have relevance to the search for the cause of the disease.

Prevalence

Epidemiologic surveys of Parkinson's disease (Table 1) conducted in different parts of the world suggest that the disease probably occurs throughout the world. Up to now, no population has been identified as totally protected against this disease. Most of the epidemiologic studies have investigated Caucasian populations, of Northern European or Anglo-Saxon descent, and only a limited number of studies are available of the occurrence of Parkinson's disease in other races.

In Caucasians the crude prevalence ratios vary from 84 to 187 per 100,000 population. The variation between the lowest and highest figure is thus more than twofold. In some studies, postencephalitic parkinsonism is included in the prevalence figures; the variation among different studies is not, however, reduced if postencephalitic cases are excluded. Because of the variability in the case ascertainment of the surveys, no clear geographic pattern emerges. Furthermore, as is evident from the prevalence figures, no clusters of Parkinson's disease have been detected, nor has it been possible to identify any smaller foci with a high frequency of Parkinson's disease.

Two studies, one from Baltimore (17) and one from Johannesburg, South Africa (23), have indicated a considerably lower prevalence of Parkinson's disease among the black population than among the whites resident in the same geographical area, implying a reduced risk for Parkinson's disease among blacks. In keeping with this assumption, a relatively low prevalence has been found in the Sardinian population, which is ethnically a mixture of whites, blacks, and Arabs (11). Both the U.S. and South African studies utilized community survey techniques, and thus medicosocial factors may affect the results; a population-based study of a biracial community in Mississippi failed to confirm the difference between the whites and blacks. The crude prevalence ratio was somewhat higher in the whites (18), but the prevalence ratios of the blacks and whites were identical in the population aged over 40 years (5). In Japanese and Chinese

TABLE 1 Epidemiology of Parkinson's Disease

	Prevalence (per 100,000)		Annual incidence (per 100,000)
Whites			
Rochester 1955 (14)	187	(167)[a]	23.8
Rochester 1965 (15)	157	(146)	19.3
Rochester 1967–79 (16)			18.2
Baltimore 1967–69 (17)	128	male	
	121	female	
Mississippi 1978 (18)	159		
New Zealand, Wellington 1962 (7)	106	(97)	
Australia, Victoria 1962 (19)	85	(78)	7.0
England, Carlisle 1961 (20)	112		12.2
Scotland, Aberdeen 1984 (21)	164		
Iceland 1963 (8)	169	(163)	16.0
Finland, Turku 1971 (9)	120	(114)	14.8
Denmark, Aarhus 1972 (10)	84	(79)	8.7
Sardinia 1972 (11)[b]	66	(63)	4.9
Bulgaria, Sofia 1981 (22)	166		16.3
South Africa, Johannesburg 1970 (23)	159		
Blacks			
Baltimore 1967–69 (17)	31	male	
	4	female	
Mississippi 1978 (18)	103		
South Africa, Johannesburg 1970 (23)	4		
Asians			
Japan, Kyoto 1978 (24)	46		
Japan, Kagoshima 1980 (24)	37		
Japan, Yonago 1980 (12)	81		10.2
China 1983 (6)	44		

[a]Postencephalitic cases excluded.
[b]Ethnically a mixture of whites, blacks, and Arabs.

populations, Parkinson's disease appears to occur with a lower prevalence than among Caucasians, also suggesting that racial differences in the susceptibility to Parkinson's disease may occur. However, the contribution of environmental effects cannot be excluded, since there are no studies on the prevalence of Parkinson's disease in Asian and Caucasian races sharing the same environment.

Parkinson's disease ranks among the most common chronic neurologic diseases. It is 13th in relative frequency, preceded by such major entities as headache, epilepsy, brain injury, cerebrovascular disorders, neurologic complications of alcoholism, lumbosacral pain syndromes, dementia, and sleep disorders (25).

In the U.S. population of 238 million people, calculated according to an arbitrary average prevalence ratio of 150 per 100,000, there are at least 360,000 persons affected by Parkinson's disease.

Incidence

Incidence would be a more suitable means to evaluate the risk of Parkinson's disease in different populations and races, but it has been studied less often than the prevalence. All but one of the reported annual incidence rates are for Caucasian populations; the one other study describes the incidence in a Japanese population (Table 1). Annual incidence rates vary from 5 to 24 per 100,000 population, the proportional variation among the studies being thus greater than in the prevalence rates. This, however, cannot be attributed to an unequal occurrence of Parkinson's disease, since methodologic variability, and especially the variability in the length of the period when incidence data have been gathered, seriously affect the results. If an average annual incidence of 15 per 100,000 is used, there will be some 36,000 new cases of Parkinson's disease in the United States annually. As the prevalence of Parkinson's disease is relatively stable, this also means that a comparable number of patients with Parkinson's disease die annually, from Parkinson's disease or from other causes. Accordingly, it can be seen that the duration of a disease with stable prevalence and incidence can be calculated by dividing the prevalence by the annual incidence. In Parkinson's disease such calculation produces figures from 8 to 10 years (8-10,14,15,19,20).

Age and Sex-Related Morbidity

Parkinson's disease is a disease of late middle age and beyond. The mean age at onset in the different epidemiologic series is 58-62 years (7-9,14,19). Onset before the age of 30 years is rare, and most patients develop Parkinson's disease between 50 and 79 years of age (Fig. 1). A more accurate picture of the risk of Parkinson's disease can be obtained in the age-specific incidence rates (Fig. 2). The incidence is very low before the age of 30-40 years, after which the incidence increases sharply with advancing age up to the age of 70-79 years, when the risk of being affected by Parkinson's disease is greatest: 1 or 2 persons annually out of every 1,000 persons of such age will develop Parkinson's disease. At very high ages, the incidence of Parkinson's disease again declines, a phenomenon that may give important clues about the pathogenesis of the disease, and will be discussed in detail later.

The mean age of the patients with Parkinson's disease living in the community (i.e., the prevalent cases at a certain time) is 67-68 years (7-9,12,14), 75-80% of the patients being 60-79 years old (Fig. 3). Age-specific prevalence (Fig. 4) ratios increase after the age of 50 years. The proportionally highest occurrence of Parkinson's disease concentrates in the same age group (70-79

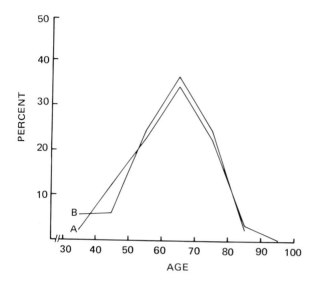

FIGURE 1   Distribution of patients with Parkinson's disease by age at onset.
Data from (A) Gudmundsson (8), (B) Marttila and Rinne (9).

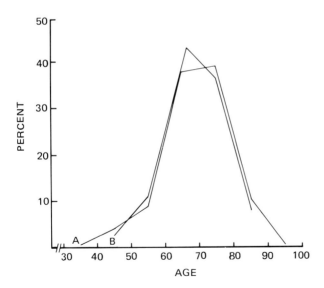

FIGURE 2   Distribution of patients with Parkinson's disease by age. Data from
(A) Gudmundsson (8), (B) Marttila and Rinne (9).

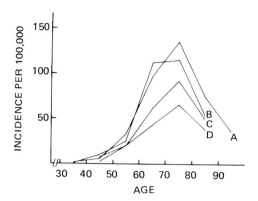

FIGURE 3   Age-specific incidence of Parkinson's disease. (A) Iceland (8); (B) Rochester (1); (C) Finland, Turku (9); (D) England, Carlisle (20).

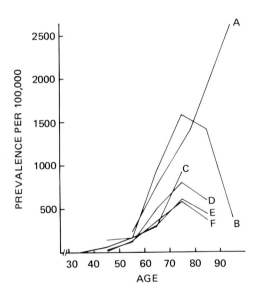

FIGURE 4   Age-specific prevalence of Parkinson's disease. (A) Rochester (14); (B) Iceland (8); (C) Australia, Victoria (19); (D) Finland, Turku (9); (E) England, Carlisle (20); (F) Denmark, Aarhus (10).

years old); in this age group up to 1.5% of the individuals have Parkinson's disease. Consistent with the incidence figures, prevalence ratios also appear to decrease in the very old, though some studies indicate increasing prevalence up to the age of over 90 years.

Clinical series have suggested that the sexes are affected differently by Parkinson's disease; a male predominance has most often been observed. However, several sources of bias may distort sex distribution in such series. More reliable data can be obtained in epidemiologic studies, and even then the crude prevalence or incidence rates are not free from bias, since female and male age structures are seldom identical. Therefore age- and sex-specific prevalence, or preferably incidence, is the most reliable indicator in estimating the risk of Parkinson's disease in the sexes. According to such estimates, there appears to be no difference between the sexes in the risk of being affected by Parkinson's disease (9,16).

Time Trends

Parkinson's disease is known to have occurred before James Parkinson's classic description in 1817, and has since been recognized as a major neurologic disease entity. Prevalence studies cover only the last three decades, but during that period of time no major temporal fluctuations have been seen. Similarly, incidence statistics from Rochester, Minnesota, from 1935 to 1979 (15,16), have not indicated any substantial changes, suggesting that Parkinson's disease has occurred at a relatively steady rate during the past five decades.

In the early 1920s an epidemic of encephalitis lethargica, first reported in Vienna in 1917, spread worldwide. This encephalitis was most probably caused by a virus, although the agent has never been isolated. As a sequel to this illness, in some cases years after the acute encephalitis, 50-70% of the victims developed a clinical syndrome characterized by the parkinsonian signs of rigidity, hypokinesia, and tremor, but also by abnormalities in ocular movements, pupillary abnormalities, cranial nerve palsies, and behavioral disturbances (23). The age at onset was remarkably low in comparison with idiopathic Parkinson's disease: it was on average, 25-30 years. After the epidemic, during the 1930s this postencephalitis parkinsonism was twice as prevalent as idiopathic Parkinson's disease, but has since then steadily declined in frequency (27). At present, only rare survivors with this condition may be encountered.

It has been suggested that even idiopathic Parkinson's disease might be caused by a subclinical infection with encephalitis lethargica during the 1920s. As the cohort subjected to the epidemic dies, Parkinson's disease would disappear as a major entity, which is predicted to happen during the 1980s (28). This suggestion, known as the cohort theory, was based on the finding that the mean age at onset of patients with parkinsonism rose almost linearly with the calendar time during 1920 to 1955. Others have, however, shown that this increase could also have resulted from the combined effects of two diseases, postencephalitic parkinsonism slowly decreasing in frequency and with onset at young ages, and idiopathic Parkinson's disease remaining essentially unchanged in frequency and age structure (15,26,29). Since 1961, when the cohort theory was proposed, evidence against it has accumulated: there is no indication of a decrease in the prevalence or incidence of Parkinson's disease, but postencephalitic parkinsonism has almost totally disappeared.

Natural History and Mortality

The mortality rates from Parkinson's disease in different countries vary from 0.5 to 3.8 per 100,000 population (30). The use of these data for comparative purposes is not reliable, since Parkinson's disease is underreported in death certificates, and there are marked differences in the coding and reporting of diseases in death certificates between countries. Before the introduction of levodopa therapy, the duration of Parkinson's disease averaged 9-10 years, though with a considerable overall range from 1 to 33 years (31,32). As noted before, indirect estimates from the epidemiologic indices also produce similar estimates, from 8 to 10 years. An excess mortality accompanies the natural course of Parkinson's disease. In a group of parkinsonian patients followed for 15 years, the relative survival as compared with the general population was only 67% (15). Hoehn and Yahr (32) found that the mortality of Parkinson's disease patients was 2.9 times that expected in the general population of comparable race, sex, and age. Because levodopa treatment substantially improves the symptoms of Parkinson's disease, and thus the quality of life, several studies have tried to elucidate whether levodopa treatment concurrently also increases life expectancy. Several studies have suggested that levodopa therapy significantly reduces the excess mortality (33-38), but this has proved difficult to assess since many factors confound the comparison of the mortality of levodopa-treated patients with the mortality pattern before the levodopa era. At the same time, however, the mean age at death of Parkinson's disease patients has increased from 67-69 years (31,32) in the prelevodopa era to 72-73 years in the levodopa-treated patients. A similar increase has been observed in the mean duration of the disease, from 9-10 years up to 13-14 years (35-39), that is, an increase of 3-4 years in the patients' life expectancy. Due to this enhanced life expectancy, the overall number of living patients with Parkinson's disease may increase in the near future, with a shift toward older ages (40).

ANALYTIC EPIDEMIOLOGY

The lifetime risk of developing Parkinson's disease can be estimated in a population if both age-specific incidence rates and life tables for that population are available. Such calculations show that in a cohort of 100,000 Caucasian individuals, there will be some 2,400 cases of Parkinson's disease during their lifetime: the risk is 2.4% (8,14). Up to now, the search for risk factors and associations has not provided any means to identify groups with a high risk of subsequent development of Parkinson's disease. Several important observations, however, have been made in the field of analytic epidemiology, particularly those concerned with the issue of exogenous or endogenous origin of Parkinson's disease, and the discovery of some associations suggesting a long subclinical period.

Genetics

A major challenge for analytic epidemiology is whether Parkinson's disease is inherited or caused by environmental effects, an issue that has been a subject of heavy debate for years and is fully discussed elsewhere in this volume. In various studies, including epidemiologic series, the proportion of patients with Parkinson's disease in their relatives varies from 2 to 62% (41). This variability derives from at least two sources. In some studies reporting a high familial incidence, diagnostic inaccuracy is apparently involved: probands and secondary cases with dominantly inherited essential tremor have been incorrectly diagnosed as having Parkinson's disease. The secondary cases have usually not been examined, but the diagnosis has been based on information received from the patients or members of their families, adding further diagnostic uncertainty. For these reasons, it has not been possible to reach any meaningful conclusion as to whether or not heredity is involved. A recent twin study (42), however, has clarified the situation. Among 43 monozygotic pairs in which an index case had definite Parkinson's disease, only one pair was concordant for Parkinson's disease. Since studying monozygotic twins is a powerful approach to the evaluation of the role of heredity in the origin of diseases, the lack of concordance observed in this very careful study clearly indicates that major factors in the cause of Parkinson's disease are nonhereditary, the disease probably being caused by some environmental factor or factors.

Risk Factors and Associations

Parkinson's disease does not associate with sex, residence, occupation, or social status (11,43). Several case–control studies have evaluated the association of Parkinson's disease with other diseases. In a large series of autopsies, no difference was found in the occurrence of arteriosclerosis, malignant tumors, or other diseases recognized in autopsy among Parkinson's disease patients and three groups of controls with craniocerebral injury, myocardial infarction, or pulmonary tuberculosis (44). In clinical comparisons, the only feature repeatedly observed is a negative association with arterial hypertension; hypertension occurs less frequently in patients with Parkinson's disease (43,45,46). This is possibly due to the autonomic dysfunction of Parkinson's disease, which tends to lower the blood pressure and thus prevent the development of hypertension. Other inconsistent associations have also been reported. Patients with early onset Parkinson's disease have exhibited thyroid disease and diabetes more often than expected (47), but this association has not been confirmed in larger series. Similarly, varicose veins of the lower extremities may occur less frequently in parkinsonian patients (46), though the significance of this finding is unknown. The relation of essential tremor to Parkinson's disease is controversial. Some clinical series suggest an increased risk of Parkinson's disease in families with essential tremor (47,48), but epidemiologic surveys of Parkinson's disease or essential tremor have not detected anything more than a chance association of these two disorders (43,49).

There appears to be no difference in the exposure of Parkinson's disease patients to various environmental effects, such as drugs, vaccinations, radiation, or animal contacts (42,45,50), but the patients may have experienced more head injuries than expected (42,51). There is no evidence that patients with Parkinson's disease have consumed any peculiar type of diet, although two studies did find that many of the patients disliked green vegetables (44,47). The alcohol consumption of the patients is no different from the general population of the same age (52). Several studies have postulated that among parkinsonian patients there are fewer smokers than in the general population (42,51,53-55) and, in particular, the number of patients who have ever smoked is significantly smaller than in the controls of comparable age and sex. Smoking, however, does not protect against Parkinson's disease, since the degree of nicotine exposure of smokers who do subsequently develop Parkinson's disease is no different from that of controls (56). Furthermore, the incidence of Parkinson's disease is similar in both sexes, though there are fewer smokers among women than men. Since many Parkinson's disease patients have been lifelong abstainers from smoking, and it is known that smoking is usually started during adolescence or early adulthood, some factor or factors operating during that time may be responsible for the abstention. Evidence from clinical observations (57) and some case–control studies (58) suggests that there may be distinct behavioral characteristics shared by many parkinsonian patients, which may antedate the clinical onset even by decades. A typical personality has been described as rigid, introverted, emotionally and attitudinally inflexible, and susceptible to depressive illness. It has been accordingly suggested that these personality features may have determined the negative attitude to smoking, or that the abstaining from smoking and behavioral characteristics may be results of the same process, possibly from the subclinical Parkinson's disease.

Etiologic Clues

In addition to Parkinson's disease probably being an acquired disease caused by some environmental effects, it may be of advantage specifically to note several other clues evident from the epidemiologic features of the disease. Parkinson's disease, and hence also its cause, appears to occur worldwide, however, with some predilection for the Caucasians. Although presently available data do not suggest any major geographic differences, such differences are not entirely excluded; it is not known whether Caucasians living in Asia, where the original population has a low prevalence, exhibit a similar risk of being affected by Parkinson's disease as Caucasian populations on other continents. Similarly, it is unknown whether inborn racial characteristics or cultural factors explain the apparent differences in susceptibility to Parkinson's disease between the races.

It is obvious from the epidemiology that the cause of Parkinson's disease has operated at a relatively fixed rate at least for several decades. Indirect evidence from mortality statistics and clinical descriptions suggests a rather similar occurrence during the nineteenth century. With these characteristics, the cause of Parkinson's disease is unlikely to be a product of modern technology.

Negative association with smoking, and the occurrence of certain behavioral characteristics, suggest that the clinical onset of Parkinson's disease is preceded by a subclinical period. This is supported by findings that incidental Lewy body nerve cell degeneration is seen in 4-7% of persons aged over 60 years and without clinical symptoms of Parkinson's disease at death (59,60). This also implies that the number of persons exposed to the cause of Parkinson's disease is probably greater than the 2.5% who develop clinical Parkinson's disease during life. A minimum proportion of the exposed may be 5-10% of the population. Neurochemical studies are also consistent with a long subclinical period, since some 70-80% of the striatal dopamine has already been lost when the motor symptoms appear (61). The length of the subclinical period is not known, but it has been estimated that the cause of Parkinson's disease may exert its action at least 20-30 years prior to clinical onset, or perhaps even earlier than that.

Epidemiology is unable to furnish any solid clues as to the nature of the cause. Infections, viral or due to other infective agents, have often tentatively been connected with the unknown cause of Parkinson's disease, mostly because of the common occurrence of parkinsonism as a sequel to encephalitis lethargica. Similarly, the recent discovery of MPTP-induced parkinsonism has renewed the interest in toxic substances as a cause of Parkinson's disease (62). Both infections and toxic substances are compatible with the epidemiologic features, as are also some of the other proposed causes, including the lack or inadequate supply of trophic factors to substantia nigra neurons during intrauterine development (63), or somatic mutation occurring early in the embryogenesis (64). All of these possibilities certainly deserve further research. Premature or accelerated aging has often been quoted as an important pathogenetic mechanism in the origin of Parkinson's disease. If such development does occur in Parkinson's disease, the incidence of the disease might be expected to show a steady increase with advancing age, yet the observed incidence pattern indicates a clear reduction after the eighth decade. This incidence pattern does not support the pathogenetic influence of aging as such; on the contrary, it is more consistent with an exogenous cause of Parkinson's disease.

REFERENCES

1. Kurtzke JF, Kurland LT. (1981). The epidemiology of neurologic disease. In: Baker AB, Baker LH (Eds.), *Clinical Neurology*, Vol. 3. New York, Harper and Row.
2. Schoenberg BS. (1977). Neuroepidemiology. Incidents, incidence, and co-incidence. *Arch Neurol* 34: 261-265.
3. Kurtzke JF. (1984). Neuroepidemiology. *Ann Neurol* 16: 265-277.
4. Marttila RJ. (1983). Diagnosis and epidemiology of Parkinson's disease. *Acta Neurol Scand* 68 (suppl. 95): 9-17.
5. Schoenberg BS, Anderson DW, Haerer AF. (1985). Prevalence of Parkinson's disease in the biracial population of Copiah County, Mississippi. *Neurology* 35: 841-845.
6. Li S, Schoenberg BS, Wang C, Cheng X, Rui D, Bolis CL, Schoenberg DG. (1985). A prevalence survey of Parkinson's disease and other movement disorders in the People's Republic of China. *Arch Neurol* 42: 655-657.
7. Pollock M, Hornabrook RW. (1966). The prevalence, natural history and dementia of Parkinson's disease. *Brain* 89: 429-448.
8. Gudmundsson KRA. (1967). A clinical survey of Parkinsonism in Iceland. *Acta Neurol Scand* 43 (suppl. 33): 9-61.
9. Marttila RJ, Rinne UK. (1976). Epidemiology of Parkinson's disease in Finland. *Acta Neurol Scand* 53: 81-102.
10. Dupont E. (1977). Epidemiology of parkinsonism: The Parkinson investigation, Aarhus, Denmark. In: Worm Petersen J, Bottcher J (Eds.), *Symposium on Parkinsonism*, Denmark, Merck, Sharp & Dohme, p. 65-75.
11. Rosati G, Granieri E, Pinna L, Aiello L, Tola R, DeBastini P, Pirisi A, Devoto MC. (1980). The risk of Parkinson disease in Mediterranean people. *Neurology* 30: 250-255.
12. Harada H, Nishikawa S, Takahashi K. (1983). Epidemiology of Parkinson's disease in a Japanese city. *Arch Neurol* 40: 151-154.
13. Fahn S. (1977). Secondary parkinsonism. In: Goldensohn ES, Appel SH (Eds.), *Scientific Approaches to Clinical Neurology*. Philadelphia, Lea & Febiger. 1189.
14. Kurland LT. (1958). Epidemiology: incidence, geographic distribution and genetic considerations. In: Field WJ (Ed.), *Pathogenesis and Treatment of Parkinsonism*. Springfield, Charles C Thomas.
15. Nobrega FT, Glattre E, Kurland LT, Okazaki H. (1969). Comments on the epidemiology of parkinsonism including prevalence and incidence statistics for Rochester, Minnesota, 1935-1966. In: Barbeau A, Brunette JR (Eds.), *Progress in Neurogenetics*. Amsterdam, Excerpta Medica.
16. Rajput AH, Offord KP, Bcard CM, Kurland LT. (1984). Epidemiology of parkinsonism: incidence, classification, and mortality. *Ann Neurol* 16: 278-282.

17. Kessler II. (1972). Epidemiologic studies of Parkinson's disease. III. A community based survey. *Am. J. Epidemiol.* 96: 242–254.

18. Schoenberg BS, Anderson DW, Haerer AF. (1982). Differences by race in the prevalence of Parkinson's disease. In VIIth International Symposium on Parkinson's Disease, Abstracts, Frankfurt.

19. Jenkins AC. (1966). Epidemiology of parkinsonism in Victoria. *Med. J. Aust.* 2: 496–502.

20. Brewis M, Poskanzer DC, Rolland C, Miller H. (1966). Neurological disease in an English city. *Acta Neurol. Scand.* 42 (suppl. 24): 1–89.

21. Mutch W. (1985). Parkinson's disease in Aberdeen; 1983–1984. In Social, Epidemiological and Therapeutic Aspects of Parkinson's Disease, Abstracts, London, 1985.

22. Chalmanov V. (1985). Personal communication.

23. Reef HE. (1977). Prevalence of Parkinson's disease in a multiracial community. In: den Hartog Jager WA, Bruyn GW, Heijstee APJ (Eds.), *11th World Congress of Neurology*. Amsterdam, Excerpta Medica.

24. Kondo K. (1981). Epidemiology of Parkinson's disease. Clues for etiology. In *12th World Congress of Neurology*. Amsterdam, Excerpta Medica.

25. Kurtzke JF. (1982). The current neurologic burden of illness and injury in the United States. *Neurology* 32: 1207–1214.

26. Duvoisin RC, Yahr MD. (1965). Encephalitis and parkinsonism. *Arch. Neurol.* 12: 227–237.

27. Dimsdale H. (1946). Changes in the parkinsonian syndrome in the twentieth century. *Q. J. Med.* 14: 155–170.

28. Poskanzer DC, Schwab, RS. (1961). Studies in the epidemiology of Parkinson's disease predicting its disappearance as a major clinical entity by 1980. *Trans. Am. Neurol. Assoc.* 86: 234–235.

29. Hoehn MM. (1976). Age distribution of patients with parkinsonism. *J. Am. Geriatr. Soc.* 24: 79–85.

30. Goldberg ID, Kurland LT. (1962). Mortality in 33 countries from disease of the nervous system. *World Neurol.* 3: 444–465.

31. Pritchard PB, Netsky MG. (1973). Prevalence of neoplasms and causes of death in paralysis agitans. *Neurology* 23: 215–222.

32. Hoehn MM, Yahr MD. (1967). Parkinsonism: onset, progression, and mortality. *Neurology* 17: 427–442.

33. Diamond SG, Markham ChH. (1976). Present mortality in Parkinson's disease: the ratio of observed to expected deaths with a method to calculate expected deaths. *J. Neural Transm.* 36: 259–269.

34. Zumstein H, Siegfried J. (1976). Mortality among Parkinson patients treated with L-dopa combined with a decarboxylase inhibitor. *Eur. Neurol.* 14: 321–327.

35. Sweet RD, McDowell FH. (1975). Five years' treatment of Parkinson's disease with levodopa. *Ann. Intern. Med.* 83: 456–463.

36. Yahr MD. (1976). Evaluation of long-term therapy in Parkinson's disease. Mortality and therapeutic efficacy. In: Birkmayer W, Hornykiewicz O. (Eds.), *Advances in Parkinsonism*. Basle, Editiones Roche.

37. Marttila RJ, Rinne UK, Siirtola T, Sonninen V. (1977). Mortality of patients with Parkinson's disease treated with levodopa. *J. Neurol.* 216: 147–153.

38. Shaw KM, Lees AJ, Stern GM. (1980). The impact of treatment with levodopa on Parkinson's disease. *Q. J. Med.* 49: 283–293.

39. Maier Hoehn MM. (1985). Result of chronic levodopa therapy and its modification by bromocriptine in Parkinson's disease. *Acta Neurol. Scand.* 71: 97–106.

40. Marttila RJ, Rinne UK. (1979). Changing epidemiology of Parkinson's disease: Predicted effects of levodopa treatment. *Acta Neurol. Scand.* 59: 80–87.

41. Marttila RJ, Rinne UK. (1981). Epidemiology of Parkinson's disease—an overview. *J. Neural Transm.* 51: 135–148.

42. Ward CD, Duvoisin RC, Ince SE, Nutt JD, Eldridge R, Calne DB. (1983). Parkinson's disease in 65 pairs of twins and in a set of quadruplets. *Neurology* 33: 815–824.

43. Marttila RJ, Rinne UK. (1976). Arteriosclerosis, heredity, and some previous infections in the etiology of Parkinson's disease. A case–control study. *Clin. Neurol. Neurosurg.* 76: 46–56.

44. Kondo K. (1984). Motor neuron disease and Parkinson's disease are not associated with other disorders at autopsy. *Neuroepidemiology* 3: 182–194.

45. Kondo K. (1984). Epidemiological clues for the etiology of Parkinson's disease. *Adv. Neurol.* 40: 345–351.

46. Rajput AH. (1983). Epidemiology of Parkinson's disease. *Can. J. Neurol. Sci.* 11: 156–159.

47. Barbeau A, Pourcher E. (1983). Genetics of early onset Parkinson disease. In: Yahr MD (Ed.), *Current Concepts of Parkinson Disease and Related Disorders.* Amsterdam, Excerpta Medica.

48. Geraghty JJ, Jankovic J, Zetusky WJ. (1985). Association between essential tremor and Parkinson's disease. *Ann. Neurol.* 17: 329–333.

49. Rautakorpi I, Marttila RJ, Takala J, Rinne UK. (1982). Occurrence and causes of tremors. A population-based investigation. *Neuroepidemiology* 1: 209–215.

50. Kessler II. (1972). Epidemiologic studies of Parkinson's disease. II. Hospital based survey. *Am. J. Epidemiol.* 95: 308–318.

51. Godwin-Austen RB, Lee PN, Marmot MG, Stern GM. (1982). Smoking and Parkinson's disease. *J. Neurol. Neurosurg. Psychiatry* 45: 577–581.

52. Lang AE, Marsden CD, Obeso JA, Parkes JD. (1982). Alcohol and Parkinson disease. *Ann. Neurol.* 12: 254–256.

53. Kessler II, Diamond EL. (1971). Epidemiologic studies of Parkinson's disease. I. Smoking and Parkinson's disease: a survey and explanatory hypothesis. *Am. J. Epidemiol.* 94: 16–25.

54. Baumann RJ, Jameson HD, McKean HE, Haack DG, Weisberg LM. (1980). Cigarette smoking and Parkinson's disease: 1. A comparison of cases with matched neighbors. *Neurology* 30: 839–843.

55. Marttila RJ, Rinne UK. (1980). Smoking and Parkinson's disease. *Acta Neurol. Scand.* 62: 322–325.
56. Haack DG, Baumann RJ, McKean HE, Jameson HD, Turbek JA. (1981). Nicotine exposure and Parkinson disease. *Am. J. Epidemiol.* 114: 191–200.
57. Todes CJ, Lees AJ. (1985). The pre-morbid personality of patients with Parkinson's disease. *J. Neurol. Neurosurg. Psychiatry* 48: 97–100.
58. Ward CD, Duvoisin RC, Ince SE, Nutt JD, Eldridge R, Calne DB. (1984). Parkinson's disease in twins. *Adv. Neurol.* 40: 341–344.
59. Lipkin LE. (1959). Cytoplasmic inclusions in ganglion cells associated with parkinsonian states: a neurocellular change studied in 53 cases and 206 controls. *Am. J. Pathol.* 35: 1117–1133.
60. Forno LS. (1969). Concentric hyalin intraneuronal inclusions of Lewy type in the brain of elderly persons (50 incidental cases): the relationship to parkinsonism. *J. Am. Geriatr. Soc.* 17: 557–575.
61. Bernheimer H, Birkmayer W, Hornykiewicz O, Jellinger K, Seitelberger F. (1973). Brain dopamine and syndrome of Parkinson and Huntington. Clinical, morphological and neurochemical correlations. *J. Neurol. Sci.* 20: 415–455.
62. Langston JW, Ballard P, Tetrud JW, Irwin I. (1983). Chronic parkinsonism in humans due to a product of meperidine-analog synthesis. *Science* 219: 979–980.
63. Eldridge R, Ince SE. (1984). The low concordance rate for Parkinson's disease in twins: a possible explanation. *Neurology* 34: 1354–1356.
64. Robbins JH, Otsuka F, Tarone RE, Polinsky RJ, Brumback RA, Nee LE. (1985). Parkinson's disease and Alzheimer's disease: hypersensitivity to X rays in cultured cell lines. *J. Neurol. Neurosurg. Psychiatry* 48: 916–923.

3
Classification of Parkinsonism

WILLIAM C. KOLLER
Loyola University Stritch School of Medicine, Maywood, Illinois

Parkinsonism is a symptom complex consisting of resting tremor, bradykinesia, rigidity, and impaired postural reflexes. The diagnosis is based on the observations of these clinical findings. Parkinsonism may be caused by a variety of different insults to the central nervous system. Parkinson's disease or idiopathic parkinsonism is the most common cause. In this chapter the diverse conditions contributing to the differential diagnosis of parkinsonism will be reviewed.

PARKINSON'S DISEASE (IDIOPATHIC PARKINSONISM)

The variable clinical expression of Parkinson's disease suggests that certain subgroups of the disorder may exist (1). The inherent heterogeneity of the condition allows for several arbitrary classifications (Table 1). Age of onset of Parkinson's disease can be quite variable. The majority of cases have their onset between age 50 and 70 years (see Chap. 2). A childhood or juvenile form of the disease has been reported (2-6). The majority of these cases had a positive family history as well as other neurologic symptoms. The accuracy of diagnosis of these cases has been questioned and it is possible that some of the cases reported to have juvenile Parkinson's disease could have been other movement disorders such as Wilson's disease, the rigid form of Huntington's disease, Hallervorden-Spatz disease, or one of the olivopontocerebellar degenerations. However, Clough and colleagues (6) reported a case of a 15-year-old girl who had parkinsonian symptoms without other neurologic signs and no family history of neurologic disease. This patient had a good response to levodopa therapy. It can be concluded that juvenile Parkinson's disease is probably a distinct entity but it is exceedingly rare. Parkinson's disease is also uncommon before age 40

TABLE 1   Possible Classification Schema
for Parkinson's Disease

Age at onset
  juvenile
  less than 40 years
  between 40 and 75 years
  greater than 75 years
Clinical symptom
  tremor predominant
  akinetic–rigidity predominant
  postural instability–gait abnormality
Mental status
  dementia present
  dementia absent
Clinical course
  benign
  progressive
  malignant

---

years and after age 75 years. Mjones (7) found that patients with onset before age 40 had a rapid progression while a later-onset group had a more benign course. Birkmayer and co-workers (8), however, reported opposite results for these two groups. Further studies are needed before conclusions regarding subtyping by age at onset can be drawn.

Several distinct clinical patterns can occur in Parkinson's disease (1). Zetusky and co-workers (1) suggested that two Parkinson's disease subgroups exist: one with postural instability and gait difficulty and a second group with tremor as the dominant feature. Other differentiating features for the tremor subgroup were a family history for tremor, an earlier age of onset, and preservation of mental status. Patients with tremor were thought to have less functional impairment and a more benign course. The presence or absence of dementia provides another possible classification. Lieberman and co-workers (9) stated that one-third of patients with Parkinson's disease display evidence of dementia. However, while it appears clear that dementia occurs with Parkinson's disease, controversy exists concerning the percentage of patients who are afflicted. More recent studies indicated that 7-15% is a more accurate estimate (10). The clinical course of Parkinson's disease is usually slowly progressive. However, a more benign course occurring in 15% of patients (11) and a "malignant" form of the disease with marked deterioration after 1 years of therapy have also been noted (12). It is possible that different neuroanatomical and neurochemical substrates may be responsible for the varying clinical manifestations.

INFECTIONS

Parkinsonism can result from infectious and postinfectious causes (Table 2). Encephalitis lethargica was an epidemic form of encephalitis in which parkinsonism was a common complication (13,14). Postencephalitic parkinsonism is mainly of historical interest at this time, since the encephalitis no longer occurs and new cases of this form of parkinsonism are not seen. Encephalitis lethargica occurred in pandemics in Europe from 1915 to 1918 and in the United States from 1918 to 1919 (15). No major outbreaks occurred after 1926 and by 1935 the disease had virtually disappeared. Several sporadic cases were, however, reported as late as the 1950s (16). The incidence of epidemic encephalitis in the United States peaked in 1923 with almost 2,000 deaths reported. The disease occurred at all ages but young adults appeared particularly susceptible. Overall mortality rates approached 40%. Only 15% of patients made a complete recovery.

The symptoms of encephalitis lethargica tended to vary (11,17). Acute manifestations frequently included fever, lethargy, somnolence, ocular nerve palsies, parkinsonism, chorea, myoclonus, restlessness, delirium, hypomania, and hallucinations. Less commonly, signs of meningitis, monoplegia, hemiplegia, aphasia, cranial nerve palsies, ataxia, and motor neuron dysfunction were present. The cerebrospinal fluid usually showed a lymphocytosis, a slight elevation of protein, and a normal sugar content. The diagnosis was based on the clinical signs and the presence of a known epidemic. Parkinsonism developed as a long-term sequelae, months to years after the encephalitis, even when the acute stages did not manifest extrapyramidal symptoms (17). It is estimated that more than 60% of patients with encephalitis lethargica developed parkinsonian features. The latency period was less than 5 years in 50% of cases and less than 10 years in 80%. The average age of onset of postencephalitic parkinsonism was about 27 years. The rate of progression was either very slow or static. Dyskinetic movements such as chorea or dystonia could also be present in addition to parkinsonism. Other features common to the postencephalitic state were lateral curvature of the spine and oculogyric crisis, a fixation of the eyes in one position usually upward. Oculogyric crisis is not seen in Parkinson's disease. Postencephalitic parkinsonism is less severe and less completely developed than the idiopathic form and can be diagnosed based on a history of encephalitis lethargica and its characteristic neurologic sequelae or by oculogyric crises without a

TABLE 2 Infectious and Postinfectious
Causes of Parkinsonism

Encephalitis lethargica
Encephalitides
Syphilis

history of encephalitis (estimated to occur in 10% of cases) (11). The pathologic features of postencephalitic parkinsonism differ from those of the acute encephalitis, in which there are areas of hyperemia in the meninges and the gray matter. The tegmentum of the midbrain is usually most severely affected with lesser involvement of the pons and the striatum (18). In the chronic state the inflammation is replaced with degeneration of neurons and gliosis throughout the central nervous system but particularly in the midbrain (19). In patients who have survived many years with postencephalitic parkinsonism the substantia nigra and globus pallidus are the most severely affected structures. Lewy bodies (neuronal inclusions common to Parkinson's disease) occasionally are present. Neurochemical changes consist of marked reduction of monoamines, particularly dopamine, in the basal ganglia. The cause of postencephalitic parkinsonism remains unknown. Treatment of parkinsonian features is achieved with levodopa or other antiparkinsonian drugs (20). Lower dosages of levodopa are needed than in the treatment of Parkinson's disease (21).

The development of parkinsonism with other encephalitides is rare. Parkinsonism has been reported after Japanese B and Western equine encephalitis and is transient, static, or improves with time (22,23). When parkinsonism does occur with these viral encephalitides, it develops during the convalescent phase and not after a latent period. Cases of parkinsonism secondary to neurosyphilis were reported when that infection was prevalent. However, the coincidental occurrence of two common diseases could account for many of these observations. However, cases of leutic mesencephalitis with parkinsonism have been described (24) as well as a patient in whom parkinsonism improved after penicillin therapy for documented neurosyphilis (25).

TOXINS

Various toxins are able to cause parkinsonism (Table 3). Manganese (Mn) intoxication is a serious occupational hazard and probably is responsible for more cases of parkinsonism than any other toxin (26). Miners, workers who grind Mn oxide, and those who process the metal are at risk. Chronic exposure to a high

TABLE 3 Toxic Causes of Parkinsonism

Manganese
Carbon monoxide
Carbon disulfide
Cyanide
Methanol
MPTP

concentration of Mn dust is needed. However, only a minority of those exposed develop symptoms. The reasons underlying individual susceptibility are unknown.

Symptoms of manganism begin insidiously after 1-2 years of exposure. Somnolence, apathy, bradykinesia, emotional lability, aggressiveness, and hallucinations (manganese madness) are frequent initial manifestations (27). A progressive parkinsonian syndrome eventually replaces these symptoms (28). Difficulty with gait, postural instability, and disturbed speech are prominent abnormalities. An action rather than a resting tremor is usually present. Other neurologic signs that may occur include dementia, depression, cerebellar dysfunction, and impotency. Muscle weakness and sensory abnormalities are usually not present. Early withdrawal from exposure may result in total recovery. However, neurologic symptoms may progress even after removal. Symptoms eventually stabilize and may partially improve over several years (29). No specific tests for the diagnosis of Mn intoxication has been documented. Pathologic studies revealed neuronal loss in the striatum, cerebral cortex, and cerebellum. The globus pallidus is the most severely affected structure. The substantia nigra is normal. Striatal dopamine was found to be reduced in one patient with Mn intoxication (30). Monkeys injected with Mn oxide developed rigidity, posturing, and tremors (31). Striatal dopamine and serotonin levels were reduced. Treatment of Mn intoxication consists of removing the worker from exposure. Chelation therapy (EDTA) and levodopa treatment have been reported to be of some benefit in manganese-induced parkinsonism (32).

Carbon monoxide (CO) is a colorless, odorless, nonirritating gas that produces damage to the central nervous system by anoxemic anoxia (33). CO combines with hemoglobin to form carboxyhemoglobin, which is unable to carry oxygen. The affinity of hemoglobin for CO is 240 times greater than for oxygen. The resultant hypoxia causes tissue damage. Toxicity results from accidental exposure and from suicide attempts involving automobile exhaust. CO poisoning can occur acutely or chronically due to repeated exposures, such as in workers in closed automobile garages. The most common manifestations of chronic CO intoxication are anorexia, apathy, weight loss, headache, dizziness, myoclonus, behavioral changes, and language difficulties (34). Acute CO poisoning occurs with inhalation of high concentrations and often results in coma. The severity of poisoning correlates with the degree of CO saturation in blood. Most cases of CO intoxication are either rapidly fatal or cause no residual effect. In one survey it was found that 20% of patients with acute poisoning died. The incidence of neurologic sequelae is low (2-10%) (35). Diffuse nervous system dysfunction with some parkinsonian features occurs (36). Dementia, confusion, aphasia, apraxia, hemiplegia, akinetic mutism, and neuropathy may be present. The parkinsonian syndrome can remain static or improve (37). A case of parkinsonism without any other neuropsychiatric manifestations has been reported following acute CO intoxication (38). Pathologic and CT scan studies reveal bilateral necrosis of the globus pallidus as the most prominent and consistent abnormality (38,39). Neurochemical studies have not been performed. Reports of treatment are limited but suggest that levodopa or anticholinergic drugs may lessen CO-induced parkinsonism (37,38).

Carbon disulfide is a colorless and highly volatile liquid used in industry. Sulfhydryl groups on proteins react with carbon disulfide. Cytochrome oxidase and cerebral respiration are inhibited by the compound. Psychosis and behavioral disturbances occur with severe acute intoxication (40). Permanent dementia may result with prolonged exposure. Parkinsonism and neuropathies, both cranial and peripheral, are also observed with chronic exposure (41). Pathologic evaluation revealed diffuse neuronal loss particularly in the cerebral cortex. Rhesus monkeys given carbon disulfide for many months develop some signs of parkinsonism (42). Pathologic study showed necrosis of the globus pallidus and the substantia nigra.

Cyanide is a potent, fast-acting toxin. It inactivates cytochrome oxidase and other oxidative enzymes, resulting in cessation of cellular respiration and anoxia. The brain is particularly susceptible, resulting in failure of the medullary respiratory center. The mortality rate is approximately 95% and death usually occurs in less than 30 min. A parkinsonian syndrome has been reported in several survivors (43). Major destructive changes occur in the globus pallidus and putamen. The substantia nigra is spared.

The case of a 13-year-old girl with parkinsonian features resulting from methanol poisoning has been reported (44). She developed bilateral optic neuropathy and after one month became rigid, akinetic, and tremulous. Mental changes were also present. The parkinsonism was said to improve with levodopa therapy.

In 1982 several young adults (aged 22–44 years) in northern California presented with a profound parkinsonian syndrome after the intravenous use of what was purported to be a synthetic heroin (45). These individuals had been taking a "designer drug" produced by an illicit laboratory. The toxin, a byproduct of the synthesis, responsible for the parkinsonism was identified as 1-methyl-4-phenyl-1,2,3,6 tetrahydropyridine (MPTP) (45). The clinical characteristics of seven of these individuals have been described in detail (46). Initially euphoria, mental disturbances, and jerking of the limbs occurred with the injections. After a few days the individuals experienced slowness, stiffness, difficulty with speaking and swallowing, and tremor. Symptoms were progressive over several days to 3 weeks, after which time they stabilized. These patients displayed all the major motor features of Parkinson's disease although clinical manifestations varied among individuals. Bradykinesis, rigidity, or tremor could be the predominant symptom. A kyphotic posture was prominent in all patients. Improvement with sleep (sleep benefit) and worsening of symptoms with fatigue and stress occurred. These alterations are also common in Parkinson's disease. Profuse sweating, axial rigidity, eyelid apraxia, and dystonic posturing were occasionally observed. Freezing episodes and kinesia paradoxia (the sudden transition from immobility to normal motion provoked by sudden external stimuli) were present early in the course of the illness. All patients had severe disease (Hoehn and Yahr, stage 4 and 5).

These patients suddenly developed parkinsonism similar to Parkinson's disease of many years' duration. There was no evidence of cognitive impairment or dysfunction of other neuroanatomic systems. The neurologic examination was normal except for the parkinsonism. Psychologic testing did, however, reveal cognitive changes similar to those seen in Parkinson's disease (47). Thus, MPTP, unlike other toxins, produces a pure parkinsonian syndrome. Examination of the cerebrospinal fluid from some of these patients revealed reduction of homovanillic acid (HVA), the major metabolite of dopamine but normal levels of 5-hydroxyindoleacetic acid, the metabolite of serotonin, and 3-methoxy-4-hydroxyphenyl ethylene glycol (MHPG), the major metabolite of norepinephrine (48). In Parkinson's disease levels of both HVA and MHPG are reduced, indicating damage to both dopaminergic and noradrenergic systems. It was suggested that MPTP produced a selective lesion of the nigrostriatal dopaminergic pathway (45). Anticholinergic and amantadine therapy caused minimal benefit in these patients. Carbidopa/levodopa and dopamine agonist therapy resulted in dramatic improvement in all patients (46). It was interesting that patients with MPTP-induced parkinsonism exhibited hallucinations, dyskinesia, and motor fluctuations such as on–off phenomena almost immediately after starting levodopa therapy. These complications are usually seen in Parkinson's disease only after many years of therapy.

Several cases of presumed MPTP-induced parkinsonism have also been reported. A young graduate student was abusing substances which he had synthesized (49). He died from drug overdose and an autopsy revealed selective loss of nerve cells in the zona compacta of the substantia nigra. In another case parkinsonism developed in a chemist, aged 37 years, who had worked with MPTP (50). A population of drug abusers has been identified in northern California who had minimal exposure to MPTP and were clinically asymptomatic. However, positron emission tomography shows significant loss of dopamine activity in the basal ganglia (51). Long-term follow-up will determine if parkinsonism will develop in this group.

The hypothesis that MPTP selectively destroys nigrostriatal dopaminergic neurons was confirmed in nonhuman primates and MPTP-induced parkinsonism thus provides an animal model of Parkinson's disease (see Chap. 13). However, the relationship of MPTP-induced parkinsonism to Parkinson's disease is unclear. Whether MPTP will provide clues to the pathophysiology and cause of Parkinson's disease remains to be determined (see Chap. 15).

PHARMACOLOGIC CAUSES

Various drugs are able to induce a parkinsonian syndrome (Table 4). It is well recognized that neuroleptics (antipsychotic drugs) produce parkinsonism as a side effect. Steck in 1954, several years after the introduction of these compounds, described parkinsonism in patients treated with chlorpromazine and reserpine (52). Parkinsonism can result from the use of any of the various classes of neuroleptics (Table 5). While these drugs are used primarily as antipsychotic agents it is important to recognize nonpsychiatric uses, such as control of nausea and vomiting. Metoclopromide, an atypical neuroleptic belonging to the benzamide class, is employed in the treatment of gastric stasis. The reported incidence of neuroleptic-induced parkinsonism varies from 5 to 60%, with clinically significant parkinsonism estimated to occur in 10–15% (53,54). However, it has been suggested that the prevalence of drug-induced parkinsonism is grossly underestimated (55).

Drug-induced parkinsonism is said to occur more commonly with the potent piperazine phenothiazines or with the butyrophenones. Thioridazine is thought to have fewer extrapyramidal side effects. However, controlled studies to substantiate these speculations have not been performed. High doses of neuroleptics were thought to be associated with a greater incidence of parkinsonism; however, attempts to correlate total drug dosage with the incidence of parkinsonism have failed to show a clear relationship (56). Dramatic examples of severe parkinsonism appearing within several days of treatment with small dosages are a common clinical experience.

The mechanisms determining individual susceptibility are unclear. Epidemiologic studies suggest that increasing age and female gender may increase risk (53). The possibility that increased susceptibility to drug-induced parkinsonism might be related to subclinical Parkinson's disease has also been considered (57). However, this hypothesis is unlikely to explain totally the varied response. It has been observed, however, that subclinical Parkinson's disease may become

TABLE 4 Pharmacologic Causes of Parkinsonism

Neuroleptics
  phenothiazines
  butyrophenones
  thioxanthines
  benzamides
Reserpine, tetrabenazine
Miscellaneous agents
  Alpha-methyldopa
  lithium

TABLE 5 Neuroleptic Agents

Trade name	Generic name
Phenothiazines	
Compazine	Prochlorperazine
Etrafon (Triavil)	Perphenazine and amitriptyline
Largon	Propromazine
Levoprome	Methotrimeprazine
Mellaril	Thioridazine
Phenergan	Promethazine
Proketazine	Carphenazine
Prolixin	Fluphenazine
Quide	Piperacetazine
Repoise	Butaperazine
Serentil	Mesoridazine
Sparine	Promaxine
Stelazine	Trifluoperazine
Thorazine	Chlorpromazine
Tindal	Acetophenazine
Torecan	Thiethylperazine
Trilafon	Perphenazine
Vesprin	Triflupromazine
Butyrophenones	
Haldol	Haloperidol
Innovar	Droperidol
Thioxanthenes	
Navane	Thiothixene
Taractan	Chlorprothixene
Benzamides	
Reglan	Metoclopromide

overt during neuroleptic therapy and apparently subside when the drug is discontinued, only to reappear years later (58). Plasma neuroleptic levels do not correlate with the severity of parkinsonism (59).

The signs of parkinsonism usually begin within a few days of neuroleptic treatment with a gradual increase in incidence so that 50–70% of cases appear by 1 month and 90% of cases within 3 months (54). It is often stated that tolerance develops to neuroleptic-induced parkinsonism. However, prospective studies of this phenomenon are lacking. The observation that withdrawal of coadministered anticholinergic drugs after several months of administration leads to the appearance of a relatively small incidence of parkinsonism is the only clinical basis for this assumption. After discontinuation of neuroleptics, the majority of patients are free of parkinsonian signs within a few weeks. However, the effects may last longer, in some cases up to several years (60). There are no convincing data to support a permanent form of drug-induced parkinsonism. Metoclopramide-induced parkinsonism has been reported to take several months after discontinuation to resolve completely (61). The long-lasting effect of neuroleptic-induced parkinsonism is important to appreciate so that one can avoid diagnostic error.

It was initially thought that neuroleptic-induced parkinsonism resembled postencephalitic parkinsonism rather than Parkinson's disease (52). However, subsequent opinions suggest that the syndrome is clinically indistinguishable from Parkinson's disease (54). Akinesia, rigidity, postural abnormalities, and tremor may occur. Bradykinesia is the earliest, most common, and frequently the only manifestation, probably accounting for the expressionless face, loss of associated movements, slow initiation of motor activity, and disturbed speech. Rigidity of the extremities, neck or trunk, usually without a "cogwheel" phenomenon, may occur after the onset of bradykinesia. The characteristic parkinsonian "pill-rolling" tremor may be present later but occurs infrequently. Recent observations suggest that a postural rather than a resting tremor is more common (61,62). While drug-induced parkinsonism may resemble Parkinson's disease, detailed observation may reveal several distinguishing characteristics (61). Neuroleptic symptoms develop subacutely or acutely, are usually bilateral, and are often accompanied by orolingual movements (tardive dyskinesia). Nonetheless, differentiating drug-induced parkinsonism from Parkinson's disease may be difficult. The drug-induced form will improve with time whereas Parkinson's disease will progressively worsen.

The mechanism of neuroleptic-induced parkinsonism appears to be related to a functional deficiency of the striatal dopaminergic system (54). The phenothiazines, thioxantheses, butrophenones, and benzamides have the pharmacologic property of blocking postsynaptic dopamine receptors (dopamine antagonists). Reserpine depletes brain dopamine and other amines by interfering with presynaptic vesicular storage mechanisms, thereby permitting increased degradation by monoamine oxidase. Tetrabenazine, a synthetic analog of reserpine, also depletes amines but may also block postsynaptic dopamine receptors (63). Tetrabenazine is not currently marketed in the United States.

Treatment of neuroleptic-induced parkinsonism is usually successful with standard antiparkinsonian drugs. Anticholinergic compounds have been most frequently used. It has been suggested that anticholinergic drugs decrease the symptoms of neuroleptic-induced parkinsonism more than in Parkinson's disease and that this responsiveness can be used as a characteristic distinguishing between the two forms of parkinsonism (64). Amantadine and levodopa therapy can ameliorate the parkinsonism but dopaminergic agonists may worsen psychiatric conditions (65).

Other drugs only rarely induce parkinsonism. Two cases of Parkinson's disease exacerbated by alpha-methyldopa (Aldomet) have been observed as well as several cases of parkinsonism reported to be induced by the drug (66,67). Alpha-methyldopa is a common antihypertensive drug and has even been employed in the treatment of Parkinson's disease (68). Therefore the significance of the few reported cases of alpha-methyldopa-induced parkinsonism is unclear. Lithium has been reported to cause parkinsonism but this is not well documented. Cogwheel rigidity has been found on examination in a small percentage of patients taking lithium (69). Two patients were reported to develop parkinsonian symptoms after lithium therapy but both had had prior exposure to neuroleptics (70). Lithium commonly produces a postural tremor but whether it can induce parkinsonism is not firmly established.

MULTIPLE-SYSTEM ATROPHIES

Diseases with significant parkinsonism in association with other neurologic signs indicating degeneration of defined neuroanatomic systems have been referred to as multiple-system atrophies or the parkinsonism-plus syndromes (Table 6). Initially these disorders may be difficult to differentiate from Parkinson's disease. However, the fully developed syndromes have distinct clinical profiles (Table 7). Striatonigral degeneration is a disorder clinically similar to Parkinson's disease (71). Initially all patients with this disorder are diagnosed as having Parkinson's disease. Tremor, however, is uncommon. Dementia is not a predominant feature. No other abnormalities exist besides the parkinsonism. The main clinical feature is a lack of responsiveness to levodopa, although some mild benefit may occur early in the disease (72). Thus patients who present with typical parkinsonian features but have no therapeutic response despite high dosages of levodopa are usually labeled as having striatonigral degeneration. The diagnosis can currently be confirmed only by postmortem examination. The characteristic pathologic findings are striking neuronal loss in the putamen and caudate nucleus. Lewy bodies are not usually found.

Progressive supranuclear palsy (PSP) was definitely identified by the classic report of Steele et al. in 1964 (73). This relatively uncommon disorder usually

TABLE 6 Multiple System Atrophies with Parkinsonian Features

Striatonigral degeneration
Shy-Drager syndrome
Progressive supranuclear palsy
Olivopontocerebellar degeneration

TABLE 7 Multiple System Atrophies with Parkinsonian Features

	Parkinson's disease	Striatonigral degeneration	Shy-Drager syndrome	Progressive supranuclear palsy	Olivopontine cerebellar degeneration
Tremor	+++	+	++	+	+++
Rigidity	+++	+++	+++	+++	+++
Bradykinesia	+++	+++	+++	+++	+++
Postural instability	+++	+++	+++	+++	+++
Pyramidal signs	0	0	0	+	+++
Cerebellar signs	0	0	++	+	+++
Autonomic dysfunction	++	++	+++	+	+
Dementia	++	+	+	+++	+++
Axial and nuchal dystonia	0	0	0	+++	0
Supranuclear gaze palsy	0	0	0	+++	0
Response to levodopa	good	absent	poor	poor	poor

0, Does not occur; +, rare; ++, common; +++, frequent

starts in the sixth or seventh decade (average age at onset, 58 years) with death occurring 2-12 years later (74). Men are affected more commonly than women. The presenting signs and symptoms of PSP differ from those of Parkinson's disease. Falling, postural instability, memory problems, speech difficulty, and axial rigidity are the predominant initial symptoms. Resting tremor is uncommon (75). The hallmark of PSP is a paralysis of vertical gaze, particularly downward, which can be overcome by the oculocephalic maneuver, which suggests a supranuclear origin for the gaze palsy. Limitation of upward conjugate gaze progressively occurs normally as a result of aging. Cerebellar, corticospinal, and personality changes may also occur. Dementia is common in PSP, particularly late in the illness. Initially, PSP is usually diagnosed as Parkinson's disease. Early diagnosis is difficult because the characteristic features, such as the vertical gaze palsy, may not occur until the disease is advanced. Pathologically, neuronal loss, gliosis, granulovacular changes, and atypical neurofibrillary changes occur in the pontomesencephalic tegmentum, tectum, vestibular nuclei, striatum, and dentate nucleus (74). The response of the parkinsonian features in PSP to antiparkinsonian medications is poor and inconsistent (75). Anticholinergics, levodopa, and dopamine agonists may provide some benefit but often the responsiveness is short-lived. No treatment exists for the gaze palsy or other symptoms of progressive supranuclear palsy.

The olivopontocerebellar atrophies (OPCA) are a heterogeneous group of disorders that share some common clinical and pathologic features (76). These multiple-system degenerative diseases link cerebellar dysfunction with parkinsonism. Various classifications of the OPCAs have been proposed based on clinical and pathologic features (77). Dominant and recessive hereditary forms as well as sporadic cases have been reported. Recent studies indicate that some types of OPCA are associated with a deficit in the enzyme glutamate dehydrogenase (76). The initial and unifying clinical manifestation is progressive cerebellar ataxia with kinetic tremor. Extrapyramidal signs (parkinsonism, dystonia) become manifest during the evolution of the illness but on occasion will predominate in the early stages, resulting in the misdiagnosis of Parkinson's disease. Corticospinal and autonomic dysfunction may also be present. Pathologic abnormalities consist of neuronal loss in the cerebellar cortex, cerebellar peduncles, inferior olives, pons, striatum, and the substantia nigra (78). Parkinsonian features may be decreased by levodopa but the response is not usually dramatic and is often transient (79). No treatment exists for the cerebellar symptoms.

The association of autonomic nervous system failure with neurologic dysfunction is the multiple-system atrophy known as the Shy-Drager syndrome (80). Abnormalities of autonomic function include orthostatic hypotension, urinary incontinence, anhydrosis, pupillary changes, and impotency. Less severe signs of autonomic dysfunction occur in Parkinson's disease (see Chap. 7). Autonomic failure without neurologic signs can occur in a variety of disease states and may be idiopathic (81). The neurologic findings in Shy-Drager syndrome are parkinsonism and/or cerebellar dysfunction. Less often, signs of corticospinal or motor neuron involvement may be present. Pathologic examination in Shy-Drager syndrome reveals cell loss in the intermediolateral cell column of the spinal cord. Neuronal loss and gliosis also occur in the striatum, cerebellar cortex, and pontine nuclei (80). The substantia nigra may show depigmentation and neuronal loss. Lewy bodies are occasionally present. The parkinsonian features of Shy-Drager syndrome have a variable response to dopaminergic drugs (82).

OTHER DEGENERATIVE DISEASES

Various degenerative diseases of the nervous system may display parkinsonian features (Table 8). In 1917 Hunt described one case of juvenile parkinsonism with progressive rigidity characterized histologically by degeneration of the globus pallidus without involvement of the substantia nigra (83). He referred to the condition as primary pallidal atrophy. Subsequently several similar clinicopathologic observations have been reported (84). Both familial and sporadic cases of this rare entity have been observed. Besides parkinsonism, dyskinesias (chorea, dystonia) may also be present.

Idiopathic dystonia–parkinsonism with marked diurnal fluctuations is another rare entity characterized by dystonic and parkinsonian features (85). The disorder has an adult onset and a benign chronic course. Levels of homovanillic acid in the cerebrospinal fluid are normal. Striking improvement of both the dystonia and parkinsonism occur with small doses of levodopa, trihexiphenidyl, amantadine, or bromocriptine. Prominent dystonic symptoms unresponsive to therapy may exist in a subgroup of patients with Parkinson's disease (86). Marked diurnal fluctuation of symptoms has been reported by Yamanura and colleagues (87) in cases labeled as having juvenile parkinsonism and by Segawa and associates (88) in hereditary progressive dystonia with a childhood onset.

TABLE 8   Other Degenerative Disease of the Nervous System with Parkinsonian Features

Primary pallidal atrophy
Idiopathic dystonia–parkinsonism
Corticodentatonigral degeneration
Hemiatrophy–hemiparkinsonism
Parkinsonism–ALS–dementia complex of Guam
"Atherosclerotic" or "senile" parkinsonism
Alzheimer's and Pick's diseases
Creutzfeld-Jacob disease

Rebeiz and colleagues (89) reported in 1968 three Irish patients, aged 59–65 years, who presented with a similar clinical syndrome of parkinsonism (tremor, rigidity), impaired convergence and upward gaze, reflex blepharospasm, dysarthria, and corticospinal signs. The initial manifestation was slowness and clumsiness in one limb. Death occurred in 6–8 years. Pathologic examination showed frontoparietal atrophy with neuronal loss, gliosis, and the presence of curious swollen, nonstaining cell bodies (achromasia). Changes were also found in the pigmented portion of the substantia nigra and the dentatorubrothalamic tracts. A fourth case confirmed pathologically with the additional clinical features of dementia has been described (90).

Klawans (91) described in 1981 a new syndrome called hemiparkinsonism as a late complication of hemiatrophy. He described four men with evidence of hemiatrophy resulting from hemispheral injury in early life who developed unilateral parkinsonism on the side of the hemiatrophy. The parkinsonism began in the fourth decade of life and slowly progressed over a period from 5 to 35 years. The patients had small, narrow extremities on one side, hyperreflexia, and hemiparkinsonism consisting of tremor, rigidity, and akinesia without masked facies or abnormal postural reflexes. The clinical response to levodopa was minimal.

Endemic occurrence with familial aggregates of parkinsonism-dementia and amyotrophic lateral sclerosis (ALS) in the Chamarro population on the island of Guam has been well documented (92). The prevalence rate for parkinsonism approximates 100 per 100,000. The disease develops insidiously with a mean age of onset of 54 years and an average duration of less than 4 years. Men are afflicted more commonly than women. Clinical findings are a combination of parkinsonism and presenile dementia. Approximately 40% of patients also develop signs of ALS. Pathologically, there is neuronal loss in the cerebral cortex, substantia nigra, and globus pallidus. The substantia nigra and locus ceruleus are depigmented. Microscopically, there are neurofibrillary changes and intracycloplasmic granulovascular bodies. Lewy bodies and senile plaques are uncommon. Loss of anterior horn cells occur in patients with ALS. Levels of cerebrospinal fluid homovanillic acid and 5-hydroxyindoleacidic acid are reduced (93).

Disturbances of calcium metabolism occur in patients with ALS and less often in parkinsonism-dementia. It has been suggested that these abnormalities may be a causative factor in the diseases (94). Features of the parkinsonism but not the dementia improve with levodopa therapy (95). Familial occurrence of ALS-parkinsonism-dementia has also been observed in a German pedigree (96). A familial disorder occurring outside of Guam with parkinsonism, pyramidal signs, mental deterioration, and abnormal eye movements has been reported (97).

Parkinsonism in the past was frequently classified into three major types: Parkinson's disease, postencephalitic, and arteriosclerotic. Whether a vascular form of parkinsonism exists is questionable. Critchley (98) introduced the concept in 1929 reporting that a flexed attitude, slowness of movement, and a festinating gait developed in the course of "cerebral arteriosclerosis." The onset was usually insidious with occurrence late in life. Tremor was said not to occur but emotional lability, dementia, pyramidal, cerebellar, and pseudobulbar signs were often present indicating extensive cerebrovascular disease. It was noted that these patients do not respond to levodopa therapy (99). The pathologic basis was thought to be multiple softening of the cerebral hemispheres due to hypertensive disease. However, pathologic confirmation of this entity is lacking. Many cases labeled as arteriosclerotic parkinsonism would now be classified as other known diseases. It has also been observed that the incidence of clinical arteriosclerosis in parkinsonism is no different than in age-matched controls (100). The term "arteriosclerotic" parkinsonism is probably best avoided.

Elderly patients, even in the absence of illness, may have mild parkinsonian features such as stooped posture, uncertainty and stiffness in turning, gait problems, and generalized slowness (101). Sometimes the clinical picture in the very elderly may be difficult to distinguish from the akinetic–rigid form of Parkinson's disease. A therapeutic trial of levodopa may, at times, be necessary (102). "Senile parkinsonism" does not respond clinically to levodopa or other antiparkinson drugs. Measurements of reaction times, slowed in the elderly, are unchanged by levodopa therapy (103).

Patients with Alzheimer's and Pick's diseases, primary dementing disorders, usually have normal motor function early in the illness (104). Extrapyramidal signs are seen, however, as the disease progresses. Hypokinesia, rigidity, and an expressionless face are the most commonly observed symptoms (105). Tremor is rarely encountered. It has been suggested that striatal dopaminergic hypofunction exists in advanced Alzheimer's disease (105). Creutzfeld-Jacob disease is another dementing illness; it has a subacute onset and a rapid course. Many neurologic systems such as the corticospinal, basal ganglia, and anterior horn cell may be involved (106). Parkinsonism is present in some patients but is not the dominant feature. Patients are in a coma and usually have myoclonus with end-stage disease. The disorder has been shown to be due to a transmissible agent, presumably a virus. Pathologic changes show a spongiform encephalopathy.

CENTRAL NERVOUS SYSTEM DISORDERS

Some primary diseases of the central nervous system may present with parkinsonism as a rare symptom (Table 9). Normal pressure hydrocephalus (NPH) is a syndrome consisting of progressive dementia, gait difficulty, and urinary incontinence (107). Computed tomographic (CT) scans show enlarged ventricles without cortical atrophy. Cerebrospinal fluid shunting procedures will relieve the symptoms in some of the patients. Unfortunately no tests are available to

TABLE 9 Central Nervous System
Disorders That May Cause Parkinsonism

Normal pressure hydrocephalus
Stroke
Tumor
Trauma
Subdural hematoma
Syringomesencephalia

confirm the diagnosis or to predict which patients will respond favorably to shunting. The gait abnormality at times bears some resemblance to the gait of Parkinson's disease (108). Urinary incontinence and dementia can also occur in Parkinson's disease. Rigidity and hypokinesia may be present in NPH. Thus the clinical features of the two disorders may overlap and occasionally cause a diagnostic problem. However, the CT scan in Parkinson's disease is normal or shows cerebral atrophy.

Cerebral infarction is an exceedingly uncommon cause of parkinsonism. There are only a few well-documented cases. Tolosa and Santamaria (109) reported three patients who developed a subacute parkinsonian syndrome with CT evidence of multiple basal ganglia infarcts. The symptoms spontaneously improved over many months. Dementia and other major neurologic signs were absent. There was no history of previous strokes. Antiparkinson drugs were of minimal benefit. It is well known, however, that basal ganglia infarction commonly occurs without signs of parkinsonism (110).

Brissaud (111) in 1895 described a case of parkinsonism due to a tuberculoma in the midbrain and was the first to suggest that the substantia nigra was involved in the pathogenesis of parkinsonism. Subsequently there have been numerous reports of parkinsonism secondary to brain tumors (112–114). Both meningiomas and gliomas have been reported in both supratentorial and infratentorial compartments. Only a small percentage of tumors involving the striatum will produce parkinsonism. Clinically, patients usually have contralateral tremor and rigidity associated with signs of increased intracranial pressure. Parkinsonism is not the main clinical feature; pyramidal and sensory changes also exist. Parkinson's disease most often presents with unilateral symptoms that are not associated with other neurologic findings. Removal of the meningioma may result in the relief of all symptoms (112). The mechanism of tumors producing parkinsonism has been postulated as due to infiltration or compression of the basal ganglia or due to involvement of the premotor frontal fibers projecting to the basal ganglia.

Trauma is a controversial cause of a pure parkinsonian syndrome. Many reports exist of parkinsonism developing after trauma. Some of the previous cases involved peripheral limb injuries "producing an ascending neuritis," that can readily be discounted. Grimberg (115) in 1934 reviewed the reported cases and found that a cause and effect relationship could not be documented. He suggested that for a positive association, trauma had to be severe enough to produce definite brain damage and a short interval had to occur between the head trauma and the onset of parkinsonism. It is also possible that trauma may unmask latent subclinical Parkinson's disease or aggravate a preexisting condition. It is clear that parkinsonism in association with marked cognitive and other neurologic impairment can result as an aftermath of severe head injury or anoxic encephalopathy due to diffuse damage to the nervous system. Lindenberg (116) reported several cases of traumatic parkinsonism with the pathologic finding of hemorrhagic lesions in the region of the substantia nigra. Development of parkinsonian features following blunt head trauma in a 37-year-old man has been described with the CT correlation of a low-density area in the substantia nigra (117). Levodopa improved the parkinsonism but not other symptoms in this patient. Parkinsonism occurs in the chronic traumatic encephalopathy of boxers known as pugilistic dementia or punch-drunkenness (118). Clinically there are personality changes, memory impairment, dysarthria, tremor, and ataxia. Parkinsonian features are a part of widespread neurologic dysfunction. The former heavyweight champion Muhammed Ali is said to have parkinsonism related to this disorder. It can be concluded that trauma can, on rare occasions, cause sufficient damage to the nigrostriatal dopamine system to induce parkinsonian signs.

Two cases of parkinsonism thought to be secondary to electrical injuries have been reported (119). These types of accidents are not uncommon yet there are no other reports. Parkinson's disease could have been present in a subclinical form prior to the accident. Electrical injury as a cause of parkinsonism is therefore not established.

Cases of parkinsonism associated with subdural hematoma (120) and mesencephalia (121) have been described. In the latter case a patient with unilateral rigidity and tremor was found at autopsy to have a syrinx in the contralateral substantia nigra.

METABOLIC CAUSES

Metabolic conditions only rarely cause parkinsonism (Table 10). Disorders of calcium metabolism may result in basal ganglia calcification and sometimes parkinsonian symptoms. Pseudohypoparathyroidism, idiopathic hypoparathyroidism, postoperative hypoparathyroidism, and pseudopseudohypoparathyroidism are specific entities that may be responsible (122,123). A review in 1968 of the clinical manifestations of basal ganglia calcifications seen on skull films found that dyskinesias, parkinsonism, mental changes, cerebellar dysfunc-

TABLE 10 Metabolic Causes of Parkinsonism

Hypoparathyroidism and basal ganglia calcification
Chronic hepatocerebral degeneration

tion, seizures, and corticospinal signs were possible symptoms (123). A reversible parkinsonian syndrome is an occasional complication of postoperative hypoparathyroidism (124). Basal ganglia calcifications particularly in the globus pallidus are frequently seen on CT scan and are of no clinical significance (125). A single case of basal ganglia calcification and levodopa-resistant parkinsonism has been reported (126). Calcification of the basal ganglia results from deposition of calcium on a matrix of pericapillary acid mucopolysaccharide. The globus pallidus, striatum, and dentate nucleus are frequently involved sites.

A chronic progressive neurologic syndrome that may include resting tremor, rigidity, unsteadiness, akinesia, and monotonous speech develops in some patients with repeated episodes of hepatic coma (127). Dementia, intention tremor, ataxia, dyskinesia, weakness, and upper motor neuron signs may also be present. Parkinsonism therefore occurs as a part of a more diffuse syndrome. Pathologically, there is necrosis of the cerebral cortex and the basal ganglia.

HEREDITARY DISEASES

Various hereditary conditions are associated with parkinsonism (Table 11). Wilson's disease (hepatolenticular degeneration) is a rare disorder inherited as an autosomal recessive that, which results in degeneration of the basal ganglia and cirrhosis of the liver due to an inborn error of copper metabolism (128). Onset is usually in adolescence (mean age of onset about 15 years). The symptoms start insidiously and slowly progress. The course is often fluctuating. Behavioral changes, drooling, choreoathetosis, incoordination, rigidity, akinesia, loss of postural reflexes, and dystonia are possible symptoms (129). Tremor is

TABLE 11 Hereditary Disease of the Nervous System Associated with Parkinsonism

Wilson's disease
Huntington's disease
Hallervorden-Spatz disease
Disorders with diffuse pathology
  Spinocerebellarnigral degeneration
  Parkinsonism with ataxia and neuropathy
  Parkinsonism with alveolar hypoventilation

common but is postural or kinetic rather than resting. Dementia and seizures may also occur. Occasionally parkinsonism may be the initial manifestation. Many patients present first with liver disease. A hallmark of the condition is Kayser-Fleischer rings: deposits of greenish pigment at the limbus of the cornea. The pathogenesis of Wilson's disease is thought to be a deficiency of ceruloplasmin, which results in deposition of copper in tissues. Pathologically there is neuronal loss and astrocytosis in the striatum. The liver may show changes characteristic of postnecrotic cirrhosis. Laboratory confirmation of the disease includes decreased serum ceruloplasmin and copper levels and increased 24-hr urinary excretion of copper. Chelation with penicillamine provides effective therapy (130).

Huntington's disease is an autosomal dominantly inherited disease of the nervous system characterized by mental disturbances and hyperkinesias (131). Psychological alterations may include behavioral changes, dementia, and schizophrenia. Chorea is the dominant movement disorder. Dystonia may also be present. Dysarthria, dysphagia, and a gait abnormality become evident as the disease progresses. The average age at onset is 40 years. Huntington's disease is predominantly a hyperkinetic disorder, however, close examination may reveal mild parkinsonian signs such as rigidity and akinesia. The gait disturbance in Huntington's disease is unique to that disorder and includes some parkinsonian features (132). The disease is progressive with death occurring after approximately 10 years. There is no effective treatment. Chorea can, however, be reduced with neuroleptic drugs (132).

A variant of Huntington's disease having its onset in childhood or young adults is the rigid-akinetic form (133). Onset before age 20 years occurs in 5-10% of all cases of Huntington's disease and approximately half of these cases develop the rigid-akinetic variant either initially or after a brief period of dyskinesias. An unexplained observation is that about 80% of juvenile cases receive the abnormal gene from the father. Juvenile Huntington's disease is characterized by mental disturbances similar to the adult form. There is also a high incidence of seizures. Prominent parkinsonian signs are rigidity and hypokinesia. An action rather than a resting tremor is usually observed. Neuropathologic findings are severe neuronal loss in the striatum and cerebral cortex. The large striatal neurons appear to be spared (134). Striatal dopamine content is normal or elevated. Levodopa therapy may relieve the rigidity and akinesia (135).

Since the original family description by Hallervorden and Spatz (136) in 1922, several other families with this very rare disorder have been reported (137). Most commonly the onset is between the ages of 5 and 15 years. However, both infantile and adult cases have been documented (137,138). The course is slowly progressive with death occurring in about 10 years. The syndrome is characterized clinically by mental retardation, optic atrophy, rigidity, dystonia, choreoathosis, akinesia, or resting tremor. Infrequently, parkinsonism is the presenting manifestation. The pathologic changes in Hallervorden-Spatz disease are unique, consisting of neuronal loss and gliosis in the globus pallidus and the zona reticulata of the substantia nigra with discolorations in those structures due to deposits of an iron pigment. Axonal swelling (spheroids) are also seen. The cause of the disorder is unknown. Parkinsonian features may respond to levodopa therapy (138).

Several familial disorders have been described in which parkinsonism was part of a syndrome of widespread neurologic dysfunction. These diseases are exceedingly rare; only several kindreds have been reported. An entity referred to as spinocerebellarnigral degeneration has been documented in one family with inheritance by a dominant pattern (139). Onset occurred between age 20 and 30 years. The disorder began with gait difficulty and tremor of the hands. The fully developed clinical syndrome consists of parkinsonism, amyotrophy, corticospinal tract signs, and cerebellar ataxia. Pathologic examination in one patient revealed demyelination of the spinocerebellar tract, posterior column and cerebellar white matter, and neuronal loss in the substantia nigra and anterior horn cells. There were no changes in the cerebellar cortex and nuclei. A 54-year-old woman without a family history of neurologic disease suffering from weakness, wasting, and fasciculations associated with parkinsonism has also been reported. Autopsy showed neuronal loss in anterior horn cells, pallidum, and substantia nigra (140). A Portuguese family with a dominantly inherited syndrome of ataxia, hyperreflexia, motor weakness, rigidity, bulbar signs, and ophthalmoplegia has been studied (141). Pathologic findings in one patient were degeneration of the anterior horn cells, spinocerebellar tracts, pons, dentate nucleus, substantia nigra, and oculomotor nuclei. The parkinsonian features responded to levodopa treatment. A family with a late adult-onset syndrome consisting of cerebellar ataxia, rigidity, bradykinesia, dysarthria, fasciculations, atrophy, and spasticity occurring in various combinations in affected individuals has been observed (142). The condition was transmitted as an autosomal dominant trait. Pathologic studies revealed degeneration of the spinocerebellar tract, dentate nuclei and Purkinje cells of the cerebellum, and the dorsal root ganglion. Levodopa alleviated the parkinsonism in some patients. A familial syndrome occurring in three generations with mental depression, mild parkinsonism, and alveolar hypoventilation has been reported (143). Brain taurine levels were found to be reduced and it was suggested that this deficiency was the cause of the symptoms. A pair of identical twins with a similar syndrome has also been reported (144). Failure of respiratory control resulted in sudden death in both patients. Pathologically, there was degeneration of the striatum and substantia nigra and focal gliosis in the medulla. The mild degree of clinical parkinsonism did not correlate with the severe degenerative changes observed. Brain taurine levels were normal. There was no clinical improvement with levodopa.

ESSENTIAL TREMOR

Sometimes disorders that are not Parkinson's disease are labeled as Parkinson's disease. The most common condition misdiagnosed as Parkinson's disease is essential tremor. Hoehn and Yahr (11) found that 4.6% (39 of 856) of their population were so misdiagnosed. There are, however, many distinguishing characteristics that allow proper diagnosis (Table 12). Essential tremor is a very common disorder characterized by the sole symptom of tremor (145). Tremor is classified as resting, postural (during sustained posture), or kinetic (during motion). The parkinsonian tremor is mainly of the resting type, whereas essential tremor is postural and kinetic. Tremor is usually the flexion–extension type as opposed to the supination–pronation seen in parkinsonism. Essential tremor has a faster frequency (5-9 Hz) than the parkinsonian tremor (3-6 Hz). The onset of essential tremor can be in childhood, midadult, or late-adult ("senile tremor") life (146). There will be a positive family history in approximately 50% of cases. The disorder progresses very slowly and may remain static for long periods of time. It is not uncommon for patients to seek medical attention for the first time with a history of tremor as long as 30 years. A key historical feature of essential tremor is the recognition that ingestion of alcohol, even in small amounts, will cause marked tremor reduction for a short period (147). Alcohol does not alter parkinsonian symptoms. Essential tremor affects the hands, usually asymmetrically, and the head (yes-yes or no-no tremor). Patients complain of difficulty with handwriting, drinking liquids, and eating. Head

TABLE 12 Comparison of Parkinson's Disease and Essential Tremor

	Parkinson's disease	Essential tremor
Characteristic		
Family history	Usually negative	Positive in 50%
Alcohol	No effect	Marked tremor reduction
Medical attention sought	Early in course	Often late in course
Age at onset	Midadult	Childhood, adult, or elderly
Tremor type	Resting	Postural, kinetic
Body part affected	Hands, legs	Hands, head, voice
Disease course	Progressive	Slowly progressive, static for long periods
Bradykinesia, rigidity, postural instability	May be present	Never present
Treatment		
Levodopa	Effective	No effect
Propranolol	May decrease tremor	Effective
Primidone	No effect	Effective

tremor results in embarrassment. A voice tremor may also be present, resulting in a quavering intonation of speech. This pattern is much different from the dysfluency of Parkinson's disease, which consists of a low volume, monotonous speech, or stuttering. It is important to note that parkinsonian signs are absent in essential tremor. The need for accurate diagnosis of essential tremor is underscored by the fact that specific treatment, propranolol and/or primidone, exists (148). Levodopa and other antiparkinsonian drugs are without effect. On rare occasions, essential tremor and Parkinson's disease will coexist in the same patient.

REFERENCES

1. Zetuskay WJ, Jankovic J, Pizozzola FJ. (1985). The heterogeneity of Parkinson's disease. Clinical and prognostic implications. *Neurology* 35: 522–526.
2. Martin WE, Resch JA, Baker AB. (1971). Juvenile parkinsonism. *Arch Neurol* 25: 494–500.
3. Kilroy AW, Paulson WA, Fenichel GM. (1972). Juvenile parkinsonism treated with levodopa. *Arch Neurol* 27: 350.
4. Cartier G. (1979). Familial juvenile parkinsonism. *Acta Paediatr Belg* 32: 123–127.
5. Naidu S, Wolfson LI, Sharpless NS. (1978). Juvenile parkinsonism. A patient with possible primary striatal dysfunction. *Ann Neurol* 3: 453–455.
6. Clough CG, Mendoza M, Yahr MD. (1981). A case of sporadic juvenile Parkinson's disease. *Arch Neurol* 38: 730–731.
7. Mjones H. (1949). Paralysis agitans. A clinical and genetic study. *Acta Psychiatry Neurol Scand* (Suppl) 54: 1–195.
8. Birkmayer W, Reiderer P, Yondum JBA. (1979). Distinction between benign and malignant type of Parkinson's disease. *Clin Neurol Neurosurg* 81: 158–164.
9. Lieberman A, Dziarolowski M, Kupersmith M. (1979). Dementia in Parkinson's disease. *Ann Neurol* 6: 355–359.
10. Taylor A, Saint-Cyr JA, Lang AE. (1985). Dementia prevalence in Parkinson's disease. *Lancet* 2: 1037.
11. Hoehn MM, Yahr MD. (1967). Parkinsonism, onset, progression, and mortality. *Neurology* 17: 427–442.
12. Rinne UK, Sonniwen V, Siirtola T, Marttila R. (1980). Long-term responses of Parkinson's disease to levodopa therapy. *J Neurol Trans* (Suppl) 16: 149–156.
13. Von Economo C. (1931). *Encephalitis Lethargica: Its Sequelae and Treatment* (translated by K. O. Newman). London, Oxford University.
14. Duvoisin RC, Yahr MD. (1965). Encephalitis and parkinsonism. *Arch Neurol* 12: 227–239.
15. Eadie MJ, Sutherland JM, Doherty RL. (1965). Encephalitis: etiology of parkinsonism in Australia. *Arch Neurol* 12: 240–245.

16. Espir MLE, Spalding JMK. (1956). Three recent cases of encephalitis lethargica. *Br Med J* 1: 1141–1144.

17. Duvoisin RC, Yahr MD, Schweitzer MA, Merritt HH. (1963). Parkinsonism before and since the epidemic of encephalitis lethargica. *Arch Neurol* 9: 232–236.

18. Buzzard EF, Greenfield JG. (1919). Lethargica encephalitis: Its sequelae and morbid anatomy. *Brain* 42: 305–338.

19. Hohman LB. (1925). The histopathology of postencephalitic Parkinson's syndrome. *Bull Johns Hopkins Hosp* 36: 403–410.

20. Duvoisin RC, Labo-Amtanes J, Yahr MD. (1972). The response of patients with postencephalitic parkinsonism to levodopa. *J Neurol Neurosurg Psychiatry* 35: 487–495.

21. Calne DB. (1969). L-dopa in postencephalitic parkinsonism. *Lancet* 1: 744–746.

22. Finley FH. (1958). Postencephalitic manifestations of viral encephalitides. In: Fields W, Blaltner RJ (Eds.), *Viral Encephalitides*. Springfield, Charles C Thomas.

23. Mulder DW, Parro HM, Thalor M. (1951). Sequelae of Western equine encephalitis. *Neurology* 1: 318–327.

24. Wilson SAK, Cobb S. (1924). Mesencephalitic syphilitica. *J Neurol Psychopathol* 5: 44–51.

25. Neill KG. (1953). An unusual case of syphilitic parkinsonism. *Br Med J* 2: 320–322.

26. Cotzias GC. (1958). Manganese in health and disease. *Physiol Rev* 38: 503–529.

27. Mena I, Marin O, Fuenzalida S, Cotzias GC. (1967). Chronic manganese poisoning. Clinical picture and manganese turnover. *Neurology* 17: 128–136.

28. Cook DG, Fahn S, Brart KA. (1974). Chronic manganese intoxication. *Arch Neurol* 30: 59–64.

29. Rosenstock HA, Simons DG, Meyer JS. (1971). Chronic manganism. Neurologic and laboratory studies during treatment with levodopa. *JAMA* 217: 1354–1358.

30. Hornykiewicz O. (1970). Report to the Association for Research in Neurons and Mental Disease, New York.

31. Neff NH, Barett RE, Costa E. (1969). Selective depletion of caudate nucleus dopamine and serotonin during chronic manganese dioxide administration to squirrel monkeys. *Experientia* 25: 1140–1141.

32. Mena I. (1970). Modification of chronic manganese intoxication. Treatment with L-dopa or 5-OH tryptophan. *N Engl J Med* 282: 5–10.

33. Schwab RS, England AC. (1968). Parkinsonism syndrome due to various specific causes. In: Vinken PJ, Bruyn GW (Eds.), *Handbook of Clinical Neurology*. Amsterdam, North-Holland Publishing Co, p. 227.

34. Gilbert GJ, Glaser GH. (1959). Neurologic manifestations of chronic carbon monoxide poisoning. *N Engl J Med* 261: 1217–1220.

35. Richardon JC, Chambers RA, Heywood PM. (1959). Encephalopathies of anoxia and hypoglycemia. *Arch Neurol* 1: 178–190.
36. Garland H, Pearce J. (1967). Neurologic complications of carbon monoxide poisoning. *Q J Med* 56: 445–455.
37. Ringel SP, Klawans HL. (1972). Carbon monoxide induced parkinsonism. *J Neurol Sci* 16: 245–251.
38. Klawans HL, Stein RW, Tanner CM, Goetz CG. (1982). A pure parkinsonian syndrome following acute carbon monoxide intoxication. *Arch Neurol* 39: 302–304.
39. Kubik S. (1949). Pathological findings in five cases of carbon monoxide poisoning. *J Neuropathol Exp Neurol* 8: 112–113.
40. Braceland FJ. (1942). Mental symptoms following carbon disulphide absorption and intoxication. *Ann Intern Med* 16: 246–261.
41. Lewy FH. (1941). Neurological, medical, and biochemical signs and symptoms indicating chronic industrial carbon disulphide absorption. *Ann Intern Med* 15: 869–883.
42. Richter R. (1945). Degeneration of the basal ganglia in monkeys from chronic carbon-disulfide poisoning. *J Neuropathol Exp Neurol* 4: 324–353.
43. Qitti RJ, Rajput AH, Ashenhurst EM, Rozdilsky B. (1985). Cyanide-induced parkinsonism. A clinicopathologic report. *Neurology* 35: 921–925.
44. Guggenheim MA, Couch JR, Weinberg W. (1971). Motor dysfunction as a permanent complication of methanol ingestion. *Arch Neurol* 24: 550–554.
45. Langston JW, Ballard P, Tetrud JW. (1983). Chronic parkinsonism in humans due to a product of meperidine-analog synthesis. *Science* 219: 979–980.
46. Ballard PA, Tetrud JW, Langston JW. (1985). Permanent human parkinsonism due to 1-methyl-4-phenyl-1,2,3,6-tetrahydropyridine (MPTP). *Neurology* 35: 949–956.
47. Stern Y, Langston JW. (1985). Intellectual changes in patient with MPTP-induced parkinsonism. *Neurology* 36: 1506–1509.
48. Burns RS, LeWitt P, Ebert MH, Pakkenberg H, Kopin IJ. (1985). The clinical syndrome of striatal dopamine deficiency. Parkinsonism induced by MPTP. *N Engl J Med* 312: 1418–1421.
49. Davis GC, Williams AC, Markey SP. (1979). Chronic parkinsonism secondary to intravenous injection of meperidine analogues. *Psychiatry Res* 1: 249–254.
50. Langston JW, Ballard PA. (1983). Parkinson's disease in a chemist working with 1-methyl-4-phenyl-1,2,3,6-tetrahydropyridine. *N Engl J Med* 309: 310.
51. Calne DB, Langston JW, Martin WRW, Stoessl AJ, Ruth FJ, Adams MJ, Pate BD, Schulzer M. (1985). Positron emission tomography after MPTP: observations relating to the cause of Parkinson's disease. *Nature* 317: 246–249.
52. Steck H. (1954). Le syndrome extra-pyramidal et diencephalique au cours des traitements au forgactil au Serpasil. *Ann Med Psychol* 1/2: 737–743.

53. Ayd FJ Jr. (1961). A survey of drug-induced extrapyramidal reactions. *JAMA* 175: 1054–1060.

54. Marsden CD, Tarsy D, Baldessarini RJ. (1975). Spontaneous and drug-induced movement disorders. In: Benson DF, Blumer D (Eds.), *Psychiatric Aspects of Neurologic Disease*. New York, Grune and Stratton.

55. McClelland HA. (1976). Discussion on assessment of drug-induced extrapyramidal reactions. *Br J Clin Pharmacol* 3: 401–403.

56. Hall RA, Jackson RB, Swan JM. (1956). Neurotoxic reactions resulting from chlorpromazine administration. *JAMA* 161: 214–218.

57. Gelay J, Deniker P. (1968). Drug-induced extrapyramidal syndromes. In: Vinken PJ, Bruyn GW (Eds.), *Handbook of Clinical Neurology*, Vol 6, *Diseases of the Basal Ganglia*. Amsterdam, North-Holland.

58. Duvoisin RC. (1977). Problems in the treatment of parkinsonism. *Adv Exp Med Biol* 90: 131–155.

59. Crowley TJ, Hoehn MM, Rutledge CD, Stallings MA, Heaton RK, Sandell S, Stilson D. (1978). Dopamine excretion and vulnerability to drug-induced parkinsonism. *Arch Gen Psychiatry* 35: 97–104.

60. Klawans HL, Bergen D, Bruyn GW. (1973). Prolonged drug-induced parkinsonism. *Cont Neurol* 35: 368–377.

61. Indo T, Ando K. (1982). Metoclopromide induced parkinsonism. *Arch Neurol* 39: 494–496.

62. Herskey LA, Gift T, Rivera-Calminlin L. (1982). Not Parkinson disease. *Lancet* 2: 49.

63. Reches A, Burke RE, Kahn C, Fahn S. (1983). Tetrabenazine, an amine depleting agent, also blocks dopamine receptors in rat brain. *J Pharmacol Exp Ther* 225: 515–521.

64. Hornykiewicz O. (1975). Parkinsonism induced by dopaminergic agonists. In: Calne DB, Barbeau A (Eds.), *Advances in Neurology*. Vol 7. New York, Raven Press.

65. Hausner RS. (1980). Amantadine-associated recurrence of psychosis. *Am J Psychiatry* 137: 240–242.

66. Rosenblum AM, Montgomery EB. (1980). Exacerbation of parkinsonism by methyldopa. *JAMA* 244: 2727–2728.

67. Gillman MA, Sandyk R. (1984). Parkinsonism induced by methyldopa. *S Afr Med J* 65: 194.

68. Fermaglich J, Chase TN. (1973). Methyldopa or methyldopahydrazine as levodopa synergists. *Lancet* 1: 1261–1262.

69. Kane J, Rifkin A, Quitkin F, Klein D. (1978). Extrapyramidal side effects with lithium treatment. *Am J Psychiatry* 135: 851–853.

70. Tyrer P, Alexander MS, Regan A, Lee I. (1980). An extrapyramidal syndrome after lithium therapy. *Br J Psychiatry* 136: 191–194.

71. Adams RD, VanBogaert C, VanderEecken H. (1964). Striato-nigral degeneration. *J Neuropathol Exp Neurol* 23: 584–608.

72. Fahn S, Greenberg J. (1972). Striato-nigral degeneration. *Trans Am Neurol Assoc* 97: 275–277.

73. Steele JC, Richardson JC, Olszewski J. (1964). Progressive supranuclear

palsy: a heterogenous degeneration involving the brain stem, basal ganglia and cerebellum with vertical gaze and pseudobulbar palsy, nuchal dystonia, and dementia. *Arch Neurol* 10: 333–359.

74. Steele JC. (1972). Progressive supranuclear palsy. *Brain* 95: 693–704.

75. Jackson JA, Jankovic J, Ford J. (1983). Progressive supranuclear palsy: Clinical features and response to treatment in 16 patients. *Ann Neurol* 13: 273–278.

76. Plaitakis A. (1982). The olivopontocerebellar atrophies. In: Joynt RJ (Ed.), *Seminars in Neurology*. Vol 2. New York, Thieme-Stratton.

77. Koningsmark BW, Weiner JP. (1970). The olivopontocerebellar atrophies. A review. *Medicine* 49: 227–241.

78. Greenfield JG. (1971). *The Spinocerebellar Degenerations*. Oxford, Blackwell Scientific Publications.

79. Klawans HL, Zeithin B. (1971). L-dopa in parkinsonism associated with cerebellar dysfunction probable olivopontocerebellar degeneration. *J Neurol Neurosurg Psychiatry* 34: 14–19.

80. Shy GM, Drager GA. (1960). A neurological syndrome associated with orthostatic hypotension. *Arch Neurol* 2: 511–527.

81. Bannister R, Oppenheimer DR. (1972). Degenerative diseases of the nervous system associated with autonomic failure. *Brain* 95: 457–474.

82. Aminoff MJ, Wilcox CS, Workes MM, Kremer M. (1973). Levodopa therapy for parkinsonism in the Shy-Drager syndrome. *J Neurol Neurosurg Psychiatry* 36: 350–353.

83. Hunt JR. (1917). Progressive atrophy of the globus pallidus (primary atrophy of the pallidal system): a system disease of the motor cells of the corpus striatum. *Brain* 40: 58–148.

84. Jellinger K. (1968). Progressive pallidum atrophie. *J Neurol Sci* 6: 19–44.

85. Sunohara N, Mano Y, Ando K, Satoyoshi B. (1985). Idiopathic dystonia–parkinsonism with marked diurnal fluctuations of symptoms. *Ann Neurol* 17: 39–45.

86. Klawans HL. (1985). Parkinson's disease and dystonia. Eighth International Parkinson's Disease Symposium, New York City.

87. Yamamura Y, Sobue I, Ando K. (1973). Paralysis agitans of early onset with marked diurnal fluctuations of symptoms. *Neurology* 23: 239–244.

88. Segawa M, Hosaka A, Miyagawi T. (1976). Hereditary progressive dystonia with marked diurnal fluctuation. *Neurology* 14: 215–233.

89. Rebeiz JJ, Kolodny EH, Richardson EP. (1968). Corticodentatonigral degeneration with neuronal achromasia. *Arch Neurol* 18: 20–33.

90. Case reports of the Massachusetts General Hospital. *N Engl J Med* 1984; 313: 732–748.

91. Klawans HL. (1981). Hemiparkinsonism as a late complication of hemiatrophy. A new syndrome. *Neurology* 31: 625–628.

92. Hirano A, Kurland LT, Krooth BS, Lesseil S. (1961). Parkinsonism-dementia complex, and endemic disease of the island of Guam. *Brain* 84: 642–661.

93. Brody JA, Chase TN, Gordo EK. (1970). Depressed monoamine metabolite levels in cerebrospinal fluid of paients with parkinsonism-dementia complex of Guam. *N Engl J Med* 282: 947–952.

94. Yanagihara R, Garreto RM, Gajdusek DC. (1984). Calcium and vitamin D metabolism in Guamanian Chamarros with amyotrophic lateral sclerosisparkinsonism–dementia. *Ann Neurol* 15: 42–48.

95. Schnur JA, Chase TN, Brody JA. (1971). Parkinsonism–dementia of Guam. Treated with levodopa. *Neurology* 21: 1236–1242.

96. Schmitt H, Enser E, Hemmes L. (1984). Familial occurrence of amyotrophic lateral sclerosis–parkinsonism–dementia. *Ann Neurol* 16: 642–648.

97. Mata M, Doruini T, Zis K, Wilson R, Young A. (1981). A new form of parkinsonism–dementia syndrome; clinical and pathologic findings. *Neurology* 31: 50.

98. Critchley M. (1929). Arteriosclerotic parkinsonism. *Brain* 52: 23–83.

99. Parkes JD, Marsden CD, Rees JE, Carjon M. (1974). Parkinson's disease, cerebral arteriosclerosis, and senile dementia. *Q J Med* 43: 49–61.

100. Eadie MJ, Sutherland JM. (1964). Arteriosclerosis in parkinsonism. *J Neurol Neurosurg Psychiatry* 27: 237–240.

101. Jenkyn CR, Reeves AG. (1981). Neurologic signs in uncomplicated aging (senescence). *Semin Neurol* 7: 21–30.

102. Koller WC. (1984). The diagnosis of Parkinson's disease. *Arch Intern Med* 144: 2146–2147.

103. Neuman RP, LeWitt PA, Jaffe M, Calne DB, Larsen TA. (1972). Motor function in the normal aging population. Treatment with levodopa. *Neurology* 35: 571–573.

104. Koller WC, Glatt S, Wilson R, Fox J. (1984). Motor signs are infrequent in dementia–Alzheimer type. *Ann Neurol* 16: 514–516.

105. Moka RK, Marttila RJ, Rinne UR. (1984). Extrapyramidal signs in Alzheimer's disease. *Neurology* 34: 1114–1116.

106. Roos R, Gibbs CJ, Gajdusek CJ. (1973). The clinical characteristics of transmissible Creutzfeld-Jacob disease. *Brain* 96: 1–20.

107. Hakim S, Adams RD. (1963). The special clinical problem of symptomatic hydrocephalus with normal cerebrospinal fluid pressure. *J Neurol Sci* 2: 307–327.

108. Messert B, Wanamaker BB. (1974). Reappraisal of the adult occult hydrocephalus syndrome. *Neurology* 24: 224–231.

109. Tolosa ES, Santamaria J. (1984). Parkinsonism and basal ganglia infarcts. *Neurology* 34: 1516–1518.

110. Fisher CM. (1965). Lacunes: small deep cerebral infarcts. *Neurology* 151: 774–784.

111. Brissaud E. (1890). *Leçons sur les Maladies Nerveuses*. Paris, Masson et Cie.

112. Oliver L. (1959). Parkinsonism due to midbrain compression. *Lancet* 2: 817–819.

113. Sciarra D, Sprofkin BE. (1953). Symptoms and signs referable to the basal ganglia in brain tumor. *Arch Neurol Psychiatry* 69: 450–461.

114. Polyzoidis KS, McQueen JP, Rajput AM, MacFadyer DJ. (1985). Parkinsonism as a manifestation of brain tumor. *Surg Neurol* 23: 59–63.

115. Grimberg L. (1934). Paralysis agitans and trauma. *J Nerv Ment Dis* 79: 14–42.

116. Lindenberg R. (1964). Die schadigunjs-mechanismen der substantia nigra Gei Hirntraumen und das problem des post traumatischen Parkinsonismus. *Dtsch Z Nerbenheilkd* 185: 637–663.

117. Nayenouri T. (1985). Posttraumatic parkinsonism. *Surg Neurol* 24: 263–264.

118. Critchley M. (1957). Medical aspects of boxing. *Br Med J* 1: 357–362.

119. Weinberg MH. (1939). Two cases of parkinsonian syndrome resulting from electrical injury. *J Neurol Ment Dis* 90: 738–746.

120. Sandyk R, Kahn I. (1983). Parkinsonism due to subdural hematoma. *J Neurosurg* 58: 298–299.

121. Hardy RC, Stevenson LD. (1957). Syringomesencephalia. Report of a case with signs of Parkinson's disease having a syrinx of the substantia nigra. *J Neuropathol Exp Neurol* 16: 365–370.

122. Moskowitz MA, Winickoff RN, Heinz ER. (1971). Familial calcification of the basal ganglions. A metabolic and genetic study. *N Engl J Med* 280: 72–77.

123. Muenter MD, Whisnant JP. (1968). Basal ganglia calcifications, hypoparathyroidism, and extrapyramidal motor manifestations. *Neurology* 18: 1075–1083.

124. Berger JR, Ross DB. (1981). Reversible parkinsonian syndrome complicating postoperative hypoparathyroidism. *Neurology* 31: 881–882.

125. Koller WC, Cochran J, Klawans HL. (1979). Basal ganglia calcifications: computed tomography and clinical correlations. *Neurology* 29: 328–333.

126. Klawans HL, Lupton M, Simon L. (1976). Basal ganglia calcification as a cause of levodopa resistant parkinsonism. *Neurology* 26: 221–225.

127. Victor M, Adams RD, Cole M. (1965). The acquired (non-Wilsonian) type of chronic hepatocerebral degeneration. *Medicine* 44: 345–396.

128. Wilson SAK. (1971). Progressive lenticular degeneration. A familial necrosis disease associated with cirrhosis of the liver. *Brain* 34: 295–509.

129. Walshe JW. (1976). Wilson's disease. In: Vinken PJ, Bruyn GW (Eds.) *Handbook of Clinical Neurology*. Amsterdam, North-Holland Publishing Co.

130. Goldstein NP, Gross JB. (1976). Treatment of Wilson's disease. *Clin Neuropharm* 2: 99–112.

131. Shoulson I, Chase TN. (1975). Huntington's disease. *Ann Rev Med* 26: 419–426.

132. Koller WC, Trimble J. (1985). The gait abnormality of Huntington's disease. *Neurology* 35: 1450–1455.

133. Bird MT, Paulson GW. (1971). The rigid form of Huntington's chorea. *Neurology* 21: 271–276.

134. Bayiani O, Tabalin M, Cammaitin S. (1984). Huntington disease: Survival of large striatal neurons in the rigid variant. *Ann Neurol* 15: 154–156.

135. Barbeau A. (1969). L-dopa and juvenile Huntington's disease. *Lancet* 2: 1066.

136. Hallervorden J, Spatz H. (1922). Eigenartige Erkiankung in extrapyramidalen system mit besonderer Beteiligung des globus pallidus and der substantia nigra. *Z Ges Neurol Psychiatry* 79: 259–268.

137. Jellinger K, Naumayer E. (1971). Unusual late-onset type of Hallervorden-Spatz disease. Clinico-pathological study of a case presenting as parkinsonism. *Z Neurol* 203: 105–109.

138. Jankovic J, Kirkpatrick JB, Blomquist KA, Langlais PJ, Bird ED. (1985). Late-onset Hallervorden-Spatz disease presenting as familial parkinsonism. *Neurology* 35: 227–234.

139. Biemond A, Sinnege JLM. (1955). Tabes of Friedreich with degeneration of the substantia nigra, a special type of hereditary parkinsonism. *Confirm Neurol* 15: 129–138.

140. Serratrice GT, Toga M, Pellissier JF. (1983). Chronic spinal muscular atrophy and pallidonigral degeneration, report of a case. *Neurology* 33: 306–310.

141. Woods BT, Schaumberg HH. (1972). Nigro-spino-dentatal degeneration with nuclear ophthalmoplegia: A unique and partially treatable clinico-pathological entity. *J Neurol Sci* 17: 149–166.

142. Ziegler DK, Schimke RN, Kepes JJ, Rose DZ, Klinkerfuss G. (1972). Late-onset ataxia, rigidity, and peripheral neuropathy a familial syndrome with variable therapeutic response to levodopa. *Arch Neurol* 27: 52–66.

143. Perry TZ, Bratty PJA, Hansen S. (1975). Hereditary mental depression and parkinsonism with taurine deficiency. *Arch Neurol* 32: 108–113.

144. Purdy A, Hahn A, Barnett HJR. (1979). Familial fatal parkinsonism with alveolar hypoventilation and mental depression. *Ann Neurol* 6: 523–531.

145. Critchley M. (1949). Observations on essential tremor. *Brain* 12: 113–139.

146. Critchley E. (1972). Clinical manifestations of essential tremor. *J Neurol Neurosurg Psychiatry* 35: 365–372.

147. Koller WC, Biary N. (1984). Effect of alcohol on tremor. Comparison to propranolol. *Neurology* 34: 221–222.

148. Koller WC. (1984). Diagnosis and treatment of tremors. *Neurol Clin* 2: 499–514.

4
Genetics

ANTHONY E. LANG
Toronto Western Hospital, Toronto, Ontario, Canada

The importance of genetic factors in causing Parkinson's disease is a source of long-standing and continuing controversy. Various authors have espoused every possible site on a spectrum between the extremes of a strongly positive genetic influence and no genetic influence whatsoever. These differences in beliefs span the past century of literature on Parkinson's disease. In 1880 Charcot (1) denied the possibility of "une maladie de famille" in the same fashion that Duvoisin in 1984 concluded that "the role of genetic factors in the cause of Parkinson's disease is negligible" (2). On the other hand, many early authors have discussed the familial occurrence of the disease and a review of the literature up to 1958 suggested to Kurland (3) that "the weight of evidence now available seems to favour a genetic hypothesis for at least a large segment of the idiopathic cases." Autosomal dominant (see Table 2), autosomal recessive (4), and sex-linked (5) monogenetic modes of inheritance have all been proposed. More recently, authors such as Kondo (6) and Barbeau (7-9) and their colleagues have emphasized the contribution of inherited predisposing factors. Martin et al.'s (10) "polygenetic model with a threshold" could also be included here. This concept suggests that rather than inheriting or not inheriting the disease per se, patients are born with a genetic susceptibility to developing Parkinson's disease which is later influenced to a variable extent by other (mainly environmental) factors. The size of the "heritability" factor (the degree to which heredity contributes: 0, no contribution; 1, 100%, that is, entirely inherited) of the disease is a further source of controversy among these investigators.

DIAGNOSIS

One simple explanation for some of the extreme differences of opinion is diagnostic inaccuracy. The distinct pathologic entity of idiopathic Parkinson's disease with Lewy body formation is the most common cause for the clinical syndrome of "parkinsonism." However, as outlined in Chapter 3, this symptom complex also may be caused by a number of different pathologic disorders that interfere with the function of the nigrostriatal dopaminergic system. Several of these diseases have a clear hereditary basis (Table 1). Patients with parkinsonism beginning in childhood or adolescence have been included in several early studies that claim the importance of genetic factors in "Parkinson's disease." However, most if not all of these patients will have one of the other disorders listed in Table 1 (see footnote). In the older age group, several conditions may mimic Parkinson's disease particularly early in their course. The olivopontocerebellar atrophies (OPCA) are probably the most common inherited diseases in this category. Here, even experienced physicians may be unable to distinguish the disorder from idiopathic Parkinson's disease for many years. The inclusion of these and other cases of familial atypical parkinsonism, such as that associated with depression and alveolar hypoventilation described first by Perry et al. (12), will obviously bias reports of the genetic aspects of Parkinson's disease.

TABLE 1   Familial Non-Lewy Body Parkinsonism

Inherited disorders
    Juvenile paralysis agitans +/- diurnal variation[a]
    Olivopontocerebellar degeneration
    Joseph disease
    Parkinsonism with mental depression and alveolar hypoventilation
    Wilson's disease
    Hallervorden-Spatz disease
    Huntington's disease
    Other rare variants of various genetic disorders: spinocerebellar degeneration,
        lipidosis, familial Alzheimer's, others
Nongenetic disorders that may affect multiple family members
    Parkinson–dementia–ALS complex of Guam
    Postencephalitic parkinsonism
    Toxic (e.g., MPTP, Mn)

---

[a]This term is used variably in the literature. Some patients have very early onset parkinsonism often associated with dystonic features or diurnal variation and a strongly positive family history. Pathology is not well defined in this group. Some may have a form of pallidopyramidal degeneration. Others may demonstrate loss of nigral pigmentation without cell loss (11). Still others have an alternative diagnosis listed above. Other authors have used the term to describe any patient with parkinsonism beginning before the age of 40. The majority of those beginning in their late 20s and 30s probably have Parkinson's disease.

Probably the most common condition misdiagnosed as Parkinson's disease is essential tremor. Marttila and Rinne (13) found that 26% of all patients examined for suspected Parkinson's disease had essential tremor instead. Although it is usually easy to distinguish the two conditions clinically, in some cases the differentiation is not as certain even after 2 years of follow-up. Duvoisin and his colleagues (17) were forced to use a separate category of "indeterminate cases of parkinsonism" to describe these patients. The inclusion of patients (and families) with essential tremor has complicated several studies dealing with the genetics of Parkinson's disease, particularly since essential tremor is more common than Parkinson's disease and frequently dominantly inherited. A probable example of this misdiagnosis in the index case is the 1937 study of Allan, who found that 45 of 65 consecutive cases of apparent idiopathic Parkinson's disease had immediate relatives also affected by the "shaking palsy" (14). He concluded that in "about two-thirds of the cases studied in North Carolina shaking palsy was inherited as a dominant trait, probably conditioned by a single autosomal gene."*

Further confusion in this field has been created by other authors who have recognized the clinical distinction between the two disorders but have espoused Critchley's (15) belief that essential tremor is a "forme fruste" of Parkinson's disease. The often quoted study of Mjones (16) best exemplifies this problem. In 1949 Mjones reported the first major genetic analysis of Parkinson's disease. In a very careful and detailed study he found 162 secondary cases of parkinsonism among the relatives of 79 of his 194 probands (40.7%), and concluded that the disease is inherited in an autosomal dominant fashion with 60% penetrance. Although he carefully excluded index cases with "hereditary tremor" and isolated tremor, he did accept a large number of relatives with long-standing isolated tremor as secondary cases. Relationship to the proband served as a "diagnostic indication" without which "a number of abortive or incipient secondary cases would undoubtedly have been interpreted as, for example, essential tremor." If one eliminates the secondary cases with doubtful diagnosis, including those relatives with isolated tremor, the conclusions of this study are altered considerably (2,17).

Although now most investigators do not believe that essential tremor is a "forme fruste" of Parkinson's disease, the number of "secondary cases" with solitary tremor in Mjones' study does suggest that the two disorders might be genetically related in some fashion. The question of whether a family history of essential tremor or essential tremor itself might predispose to the development of Parkinson's disease will be considered later in this chapter.

---

*Duvoisin (2) has suggested that these families had OPCA; however, the large number of patients (two-thirds of Allan's cases) and the author's emphasis on "shaking" favor a diagnosis of essential tremor.

Finally a small number of well-recognized environmental factors may cause a parkinsonian syndrome in humans. Viruses (e.g., encephalitis lethargica), toxins (manganese, MPTP) and deficiency states (soil minerals in Parkinson's disease–amyotrophic lateral sclerosis–dementia complex of Guam (18)) all have been implicated. Occasionally multiple family members are affected. If these cases are mistaken for idiopathic Parkinson's disease, genetic studies are confounded further. Postencephalitic parkinsonism probably has been the most notable offender in this category.

The degree to which diagnostic inaccuracy in index and secondary cases could alter the interpretation of studies in parkinsonism is emphasized by Marttila and Rinne's (13) finding that more than 40% of the "Parkinson's disease" patients they reviewed had been misdiagnosed. Duvoisin (2) points out that "examination of parents reported to have parkinsonism reveals another diagnosis in at least one half." In the Parkinson's disease twin study (see below) carried out by Duvoisin and colleagues (19,20), the importance of examining index and secondary cases was further emphasized by the finding that several probands claiming or assumed to have Parkinson's disease were found to have essential tremor, multiple system atrophy, or some other disorder. Thus, the possibility of misdiagnosis both in the index case and relatives (secondary cases) must be strongly considered when one is reviewing the literature. By the nature of their methodologies it is likely that many reports have included other causes for parkinsonism and/or essential tremor. Secondary cases rarely have been examined to confirm the diagnosis and "affected" parents are usually unavailable even if this were attempted. Most studies record the numbers of secondary cases identified anamnestically from the histories of index cases with well-documented Parkinson's disease. Chart reviews without follow-up confirmatory examination of the index cases are at even further risk of diagnostic inaccuracy.

FAMILY HISTORY

Table 2 reviews several studies that provide figures for the proportion of index cases with a positive family history of parkinsonism. The size of the population at risk varies considerably from one study to another. Some authors limit themselves to immediate relatives while others include all distant kinsmen of which the patient has knowledge (often this distinction is not stipulated by the authors). In the former situation, the numbers are usually well defined while in the latter it is impossible to ascertain the total number at risk; it is likely that the proband is more aware of relatives similarly affected than of those who are not. In addition, most studies have not provided control population figures for comparison purposes. Averaging the figures in Table 2 is meaningless because of the methodologic differences among studies. It seems fair to state that a positive family history of parkinsonism will be obtained in 10-20% of patients, if one includes all relatives and somewhat less than 10% if only immediate family members are considered.

Another more useful method of determining the importance of genetic factors is to consider the prevalence of Parkinson's disease in immediate relatives (i.e., a well-defined population number) of index cases with idiopathic Parkinson's disease. Table 3 reviews six studies that provided such data. As Duvoisin (2) points out, it is inappropriate to compare these results to figures commonly quoted for the prevalence of Parkinson's disease in the general population (e.g., 2 in 1000) since the latter are determined at one moment in time (point prevalence) while the former span many years. Indeed affected relatives, especially parents, may be long since deceased at the time of inclusion. Kurland's (3) estimate that 1 in 40 (2.8%) will develop Parkinson's disease during their lifetime could be compared to prevalence figures of parkinsonism in parents of index cases, while a figure somewhat less than this should be used for the siblings of probands (more likely to be still living). Ideally, the immediate families of age- and sex-matched nonparkinsonian controls should be used for comparison. As can be seen from Table 3, the prevalence of Parkinson's disease in the immediate families of Parkinson's disease patients is approximately twice that of the control group. However, the prevalence in both parents and siblings is only slightly higher than one would have expected if the occurrence of Parkinson's disease in these secondary cases were simply due to chance alone. One possible interpretation is that misdiagnosis in index and secondary cases as outlined above could entirely account for this difference. Alternatively, although these figures are much lower than those seen in diseases with monogenetic transmission, they do suggest that genetic factors may contribute in some undefined fashion to the development of Parkinson's disease. The small increased prevalence in Parkinson's disease families indicates that if genetics play a causative role, it is considerably less than that of environmental factors.

In addition to a possible genetic predisposition, Barbeau and his colleagues (7-9) have suggested that higher prevalence figures in their Parkinsonian patients are partly due to the presence of subsets of "familial parkinsonism." Analyzing patients whose Parkinson's disease began before the age of 40, they found a positive family history of parkinsonism and/or tremor more often than in controls (7). Reviewing their larger general Parkinsonian population, they found further evidence for two major subgroups: "essential tremor related parkinsonism" and familial akinetic–rigid syndrome (8,9). The former was found to have an autosomal dominant transmission and occurred in 10% of all cases of Parkinson's disease. (Later in this chapter the possible relationship between essential tremor and Parkinson's disease will be discussed further.) The latter (accounting for 3-4% of all parkinsonians) was thought to be inherited in an autosomal recessive fashion with a high degree of consanguinity in the parents of the affected siblings. However, some of the authors' conclusions were based on an

TABLE 2 Selected Studies of Familial Aggregation in Idiopathic Parkinson's Disease

Authors	Year	Relatives included[a]	% Patients with positive family history	Mode of inheritance	Comments
Gowers (21)	1903	? All	15	Not stated	
Hart (22)	1904	? All	16	Not stated	"Neuropathic" hereditary in 25%, direct heredity in 4%
Patrick and Levy (23)	1922	? Immediate	4	—	
Allan (14)	1937	All	62	Autosomal dominant with incomplete penetrance	Diagnosis of index cases questionable (? essential tremor or OPCA)
Mjones (16)	1949	All	41	Autosomal dominant with 60% penetrance	Secondary cases with isolated tremor accepted
Kurland (3)	1958	All	16	Autosomal dominant with incomplete penetrance	Chart review
Schwab and England (24)	1958	Siblings, parents, grandparents, and offspring	4	—	
Mundinger and Riechert (25)	1963	? Immediate	1.9	—	Questionable heredity factor in another 0.5%
Pollock and Hornabrook (26)	1966	? All	14	Not stated	
Jenkins (27)	1966	? All	12.9	Not stated	
Selby (28)	1967	Direct antecedant or sibling	5	—	
Gudmundsson (29)	1967	Predominantly immediate	22	Autosomal dominant with incomplete penetrance	Likely includes other diagnoses; e.g., one family with Huntington's disease

Reference	Year	Relatives	Value	Inheritance	Comments
Strang (30)	1970	Immediate	94.5	Autosomal dominant	Includes all forms of parkinsonism as single disease. Clinical diagnostic criteria not stated but probably quite broad ("the illness has little to learn from syphilis in the art of mimicry")
Martin et al. (10)	1973	All Parents Siblings	26 13 }16.9 7.7		Controls: 14.8% 4.3% }9.5% 6.1%
Kondo et al. (6)	1973	Parents Siblings	13.3 }19.8 10.2	Polygenic	Chart review
Marttila and Rinne (31)	1976	All	6.3	Multifactorial with heritability of 80%	Controls: 4.3%
Hoehn (32)	1976	? All	19		
Roy et al. (8)	1983	All	3.4[b,c]		Controls: 10%[d]
Duvoisin (2)	1984	All	17.9[b]		23% if relatives with isolated tremor included; nearly half of secondary cases were not immediate relatives
Lang et al. (33)	1985	All Parents Siblings	9.4[b] 2.5 }3.8 1.3		Controls: 5.8%[b] 2.9% }3.8% 1.0%

[a] "All" indicates that all relatives, immediate and distant, known to the patient were included to give frequency of positive family history.

[b] Secondary cases with isolated tremor excluded (most studies fail to state this criteria).

[c] Calculated from figures given on p. 38 of Ref 8. Twenty-two cases with another family member with Parkinson's disease from a roster of 643 parkinsonian patients.

[d] Calculated assuming that kindreds had only one affected member (5 affected family members in 50 kindreds).

87

TABLE 3 Prevalence of Parkinson's Disease among Relatives of Probands with Parkinson's Disease

Authors	No. of probands	No. controls	Parents of		Sibs of	
			Proband	Control	Proband	Control
Mjönes (16)[a]	194	—	11/388[a] (2.8)	—	21/674[a] (3.1)	—
Duvoisin et al. (17)[b]	85	145[c]	—		4/146 (2.8)	3/145[c] (2.1)
Martin et al. (10)	130	115[d]	15/244 (6.2)	5/218 (2.3)	16/488 (3.3)	7/450 (1.6)
Kondo et al. (6)	263	—	35/479 (7.3)	—	27/946[e] (2.9)	—
Duvoisin (2)	207	—	15/414 (3.6)	—	11/590 (1.9)	—
Lang et al. (33)	159	104[f]	4/316 (1.3)	3/196 (1.5)	2/536 (0.4)	1/354 (0.3)
			80/1841 (4.3)	8/414 (1.9)	81/3380 (2.4)	11/969 (1.2)

Figures in parentheses are percentages.
[a] Figures taken from Duvoisin et al.'s recalculation of Mjones' data to exclude family members with monosymptomatic tremor (17).
[b] Duvoisin et al.'s study is one of the very few that examined all relatives of probands and controls.
[c] Controls include patients' spouses and their siblings.
[d] Controls were spouses of the probands.
[e] This figure is an underestimation that assumes the presence of only one affected sibling in each of the "multiplex" families (which contained "one or more affected siblings other than the proband").
[f] A hospital-based control population examined to exclude cases of Parkinson's disease.

inappropriate comparison between preselected cases of parkinsonism with other affected family members and control kindreds without the predeterminant of at least one affected relative. Analysis of the data given in these studies by other authors (reference 2, and Table 2, footnotes a and b) does not suggest a familial concentration of parkinsonism. Duvoisin has suggested that the two familial syndromes "probably represent new disorders distinct from idiopathic parkinsonism" (2).

One of the most useful methods of clarifying the genetic aspects of any disease is to compare concordance rates in monozygotic (MZ) and dizygotic twins (DZ). In a nationwide collaborative study Duvoisin and colleagues (19,20) collected data on 43 MZ and 19 DZ twin pairs in which an index case had definite Parkinson's disease. Only one MZ pair was definitely concordant for Parkinson's disease, with a second pair "possibly concordant." If questionable cases (further emphasizing the need for clinical examination in cases purported to have the disease) were included, only 4 of 48 MZ and 1 of 19 DZ pairs were concordant. These figures, which are not much different from those obtained for the occurrence of Parkinson's disease in nontwin siblings (see Table 3), provide a strong argument against the importance of genetic factors in Parkinson's disease. However, two more concordant MZ twin pairs have been reported recently (34,35) and two of the coauthors of the original twin study have since emphasized the need for a thorough study of many more twin pairs (36). Reviewing the twin data, these authors noted that the prevalence of Parkinson's disease in the families of the index twins was higher than both that of the cotwin and that expected for the general population (5.7% of parents and 5.7% of siblings were affected compared to 2.3% of monozygotic cotwins). Contrary to the original conclusion of the twin study, these authors suggest that there may indeed be a genetic predisposition to Parkinson's disease (possibly a genetically programmed low initial number of dopaminergic nigral neurons) from which the unaffected cotwin has somehow been protected in utero.

To date, it would seem that the study of Parkinson's disease in twins has not provided as definitive an answer as one would like. However, it has indicated that if genetic factors are important, they play only a minor role in causing the disorder. Based on the "NIH twin data" Kondo recently has recalculated his estimate of heritability in Parkinson's disease. As mentioned earlier, this figure, with a range from 0 to 100%, is an estimate of genetic determination; the greater the value, the greater the additive genetic component. In 1973 (3) he originally proposed a heritability factor of about 80% for Parkinson's disease (see Table 2). In 1985, when he used the twin data, the figure became 22%, which suggests that genetic factors do play a role but that environmental factors are considerably (four times) more important (37).

ESSENTIAL TREMOR

One factor that might contribute to the heritability of Parkinson's disease (if this is truly greater than zero) is a family history of essential tremor. In 1893 Gowers first commented that "nonprogressive tremor occasionally exists throughout life in some near relation" of patients with Parkinson's disease (38). He also described overlap cases with features intermediate between the two disorders. Since then a number of studies have attempted to define the connection between essential tremor and Parkinson's disease (Table 4). Unfortunately, controversy abounds here as well. Several authors report no association between the two conditions (Table 4A); some of them have compared the family histories of Parkinson's disease patients to those of controls. Examining all family members included in their study, Duvoisin and his colleagues (17) found the same frequency of essential tremor (3.4%) in siblings of Parkinson's disease patients as in patients' spouses and their siblings.

Contrary to these results other investigators have found an increased incidence of essential tremor in families of Parkinson's disease patients. As discussed above, Barbeau and colleagues claim that a dominantly inherited "essential tremor related parkinsonism" makes up 10% of all Parkinson's disease (8,9). Others report that essential tremor itself predisposes to the development of Parkinson's disease. Hornabrook and Nagurney (43) found a 35-fold increased risk of developing parkinsonism in essential tremor patients from Papua, New Guinea. More recently Geraghty and colleagues (44) from Houston reported that the prevalence of Parkinson's disease was 24 times greater than that expected in patients with long-standing essential tremor. Lang and colleagues (33) also found a positive family history of essential tremor more often in Parkinson's disease patients than in controls (17% vs. 5.6%). However, unquestionable autosomal-dominant transmission occurred in only 3.8% of the Parkinson's disease group (none of controls) and essential tremor predating the development of Parkinson's disease occurred in only 1.3%. Further studies will be required to resolve this controversy. Prevalence figures for essential tremor in different regions of the world vary markedly. Greater than 14-fold differences exist between certain locations such as Finland and Copiah County, Mississippi (10). The poorly understood population (and/or environmental) factors that account for these differences could also contribute to the discrepancies recorded for the association between essential tremor and Parkinson's disease.

Apart from essential tremor, there are other clues that hereditary factors may play a role in Parkinson's disease. Patients who develop parkinsonism induced by phenothiazine drugs have been found to have lower levels of cerebrospinal fluid homovanillic acid (HVA, the major metabolite of dopamine) during treatment than those who do not (46). Hereditary factors are suggested by Myrianthopoulos and colleagues' (47) finding of a higher incidence of parkinsonism in the relatives

TABLE 4 Studies of Possible Association Between Essential Tremor (ET) and Parkinson's Disease (PD)

Authors	Study	Comments
No Association		
Larsson and Sjogren, 1960 (39)	ET patients and families	17/80 patients had other extrapyramidal signs
Jenkins, 1966 (27)	FH$_x$ of PD patients	Figures not given, no controls
Duvoisin et al., 1969 (17)	Siblings of PD patients and their spouses	Equal number of ET cases found in each group
Marttila and Rinne, 1976 (31)	FH$_x$ of PD patients and controls	5.8% PD patients and 8.1% controls had "relatives" with probable ET
Rajput et al., 1984 (40)	Retrospective study ET patients	2% had later development of PD. Chart review: patients not examined. Duration of follow-up from symptom onset unknown. Once ET diagnosed, especially with positive FH$_x$, physicians might have been less prone to make additional diagnosis of PD especially if features of parkinsonism were mild.
Marttila et al., 1984 (41)	FH$_x$ of ET patients and controls	1.2% ET patients and 0.9% controls had an immediate relative with PD. Family included parents, siblings *and* children with no breakdown in numbers.
Findley and Cleeves (42)	FH$_x$ of ET patients	Uncontrolled observations. No figures given.

TABLE 4 (Continued)

Authors	Study	Comments
Positive Association		
Hornabrook and Nagurney, 1976 (43)	ET patients	ET patients in Papua, New Guinea had 35 times the risk of developing PD than individuals without ET
Barbeau and Pourcher, 1982 (7)	FH_x in young onset (<40 years) PD patients and controls	Tremor significantly more frequent in first and second degree relatives of PD patients. Defined a subgroup of tremor-dominant PD with high incidence of familial tremor.
Roy et al., 1983 (8)	Kindreds with "familial parkinsonism," ET, and controls	10% of all parkinsonians had "essential tremor related parkinsonism" with dominant inheritance. However, incidence of PD in families of ET patients and controls did not differ.
Geraghty et al., 1985 (44)	Long-term follow-up of ET patients	25 of 130 developed parkinsonism 13 years after onset of ET. Prevalence of PD in ET patients 24 times greater than expected.
Lang et al., 1985 (33)	FH_x of ET in PD, idiopathic dystonia, and controls	Frequency of a positive FH_x of tremor and prevalence of tremor in immediate family members of PD patients significantly higher than controls (17% vs. 5.6% and 3.7% vs. 1.1%, respectively).

FH_x, family history

of individuals apparently predisposed to drug-induced parkinsonism. The presence of inherited protective factors might be suggested by the common observation that Parkinson's disease is less prevalent in pigmented races, particularly blacks (48-52). However, in a careful study of a biracial community in Mississippi, Schoenberg and colleagues (53) did not confirm the previously reported dramatic differences between blacks and whites. Nevertheless, study of family history and environmental exposure comparing age- and sex-matched black and white patients might provide helpful clues about the causes of Parkinson's disease.

A possible genetic susceptibility to Parkinson's disease has been studied further through the evaluation of the histocompatibility complex (HLA system). Once again, variable results have been obtained. Some reports describe increased association with HLA antigens A_2 (54), A_3 (55), A_{28} (54), Aw24 (56), B_7 (57), B_{17} (58), B_{18} (58), and Bw21 (55). One study found the presence of Cw3 antigen in patients with a slowly progressive course more often than in patients with a rapid progression (57). A decreased incidence of certain HLA antigens has also been reported, including A_{11} (57), Bw35 (57,58), and C_{W4} (57). However, correcting for the number of antigens tested, others have not found an association between HLA antigens and Parkinson's disease (55,57,59). Barbeau and Roy (9), pooling the results of a large number of patients and correcting for the number of antigens tested, found that only the A_9 antigen was significantly decreased in Parkinson's disease patients. Studying haplotype disequilibrium, they found a significant reduction in HLA haplotype $A_2 B_5$. They propose that this haplotype, present in 11-12% of whites, confers some type of evolutionary positive gain or biologic advantage. Only 5% of tested parkinsonian patients had this haplotype; the authors suggest that this could correspond to the loss of a "protective factor" for Parkinson's disease. They also found the presence of "augmentation factors" such as occurrence of goiter and hyperthyroidism in families of parkinsonians. Recently, these same authors (60) have reported a difference in hydroxylation status (using debrisoquin) between controls and parkinsonian patients, the patient group with much fewer "extensive" and many more "intermediate" metabolizers than the controls. They propose that this inherited hydroxylation status predisposes to the development of parkinsonism in those exposed to causative environmental factors.

CONCLUSIONS

Despite extensive studies of the hereditary aspects of Parkinson's disease, no definitive answers are available. Misdiagnosis hampers the interpretation of much of the earlier literature. This is still a potential source of error in modern studies that do not provide for examination of secondary cases or a prolonged period of follow-up. Parkinson's disease may occur slightly more often in immediate relatives of patients than in controls but the increased frequency in these individuals is not great. Study of Parkinson's disease in twins provides the strongest argument against genetic etiologic factors; however, a larger number of twins needs to be studied and review of the available twin data does suggest a higher incidence of Parkinson's disease in other family members. The relationship between Parkinson's disease and essential tremor remains controversial. The possibility that essential tremor in the family or patient may predispose to the later development of Parkinson's disease requires further study. Other potential hereditary "augmenting" and "protective" factors also need confirmation and further elucidation.

Although the overall magnitude of heritability in Parkinson's disease is small, it is also quite possible that the degree of genetic contribution varies considerably from case to case. Eventually we may find that idiopathic Parkinson's disease is precipitated by a number of different environmental agents. Some of these may require the additional presence of certain genetic predisposing factors to produce their pathologic effects.

REFERENCES

1. Charcot JM. (1880). De la paralysie agitante. Leçons sur les maladies du système nerveux, recueillies et publiées par Bourneville. 1: 155–188, Paris.
2. Duvoisin RC. (1984). Is Parkinson's disease acquired or inherited? *Can J Neurol Sci* 11: 151–155.
3. Kurland LT. (1958). Epidemiology: incidence, geographic distribution and genetic considerations. In: Fields WS (Ed.), *Pathogenesis and Treatment of Parkinsonism*. Springfield, Charles C Thomas.
4. Dastur DK. (1956). A family with three cases of parkinson's syndrome. *Ind J Med Sci* 10: 281–285.
5. Johnston AW, McKusick VA. (1963). Sex-linked recessive inheritance of spastic paraplegia and of parkinsonism. *Proceedings of the Second International Conference of Human Genetics* (Rome, September 6–12, 1961). Vol 3. Rome, Instituto G. Mendel.
6. Kondo K, Kurland LT, Schull WJ. (1973). Parkinson's disease. Genetic analysis and evidence of a multifactorial etiology. *Mayo Clin Proc* 48: 465–475.
7. Barbeau A, Pourcher E. (1982). New data on the genetics of Parkinson's disease. *Can J Neurol Sci* 9: 53–60.
8. Roy M, Boyer L, Barbeau A. (1983). A prospective study of 50 cases of familial Parkinson's disease. *Can J Neurol Sci* 10: 37–42.
9. Barbeau A, Roy M. (1984). Familial subsets in idiopathic Parkinson's disease. *Can J Neurol Sci* 11: 144–150.
10. Martin WE, Young WI, Anderson VE. (1973). Parkinson's disease. A genetic study. *Brain* 96: 495–506.

11. Yokochi M, Narabayashi H, Iizuka R, Nagatsu T. (1984). Juvenile parkinsonism—some clinical, pharmacological and neuropathological aspects. *Adv Neurol* 40: 407–413.

12. Perry TL, Bratty PJA, Hansen S, Kennedy J, Urquhart N, Dolman CL. (1975). Hereditary mental depression and parkinsonism with taurine deficiency. *Arch Neurol* 32: 108–113.

13. Marttila RJ, Rinne UK. (1976). Epidemiology of Parkinson's disease in Finland. *Acta Neurol Scand* 53: 81–102.

14. Allan W. (1937). Inheritance of the shaking palsy. *Arch Intern Med* 60: 424–436.

15. Critchley M. (1949). Observations on essential (heredofamilial) tremor. *Brain* 72: 113–139.

16. Mjönes H. (1949). Paralysis agitans. A clinical and genetic study. *Acta Psychiatr Neurol Scand* 25 (suppl 54): 1–195.

17. Duvoisin RC, Gearing FR, Schweitzer MD, Yahr MD. (1969). A family study of parkinsonism. In: Barbeau A, Brunett JR (Eds.), *Progress in Neurogenetics.* Amsterdam, Excerpta Medica.

18. Garruto RM, Yanagihara R, Gajdusek DC. (1985). Disappearance of high incidence amyotrophic lateral sclerosis and parkinsonism–dementia on Guam. *Neurology* 35: 193–198.

19. Duvoisin RC, Eldridge R, Williams A, Nutt J, Calne D. (1981). Twin study of Parkinson disease. *Neurology* 31: 77–80.

20. Ward CD, Duvoisin RC, Ince SE, Nutt JD, Eldridge R, Calne DB. (1983). Parkinson's disease in 65 pairs of twins and in a set of quadruplets. *Neurology* 33: 815–824.

21. Gowers WR. (1903). *A Manual of Diseases of the Nervous System,* 2nd edition. Philadelphia, Blakiston.

22. Hart TS. (1904). Paralysis agitans: Some clinical observations based on a study of 219 cases seen at clinic of Professor M Allen Starr. *J Nerv Ment Dis* 31: 177–188.

23. Patrick HT, Levy DM. (1922). Parkinson's disease. A clinical study of one hundred-forty-six cases. *Arch Neurol Psychiatry* 7: 711–720.

24. Schwab RS, England AC. (1958). Parkinson's disease. *J Chron Dis* 8: 488–509.

25. Mundinger F, Riechert T. (1963). Die stereotaktischen Hirnoperationen zur Behandlung extrapyramidaler Bewegungsstörungen (Parkinsonismus und Hyperkinesen) und ihre Resultate. *Fortschr Neurol Psychiatr* 31: 1–120.

26. Pollock M, Hornabrook RW. (1966). The prevalence, natural history and dementia of Parkinson's disease. *Brain* 89: 429–448.

27. Jenkins AC. (1966). Epidemiology of parkinsonism in Victoria. *Med J Aust* 53: 496–502.

28. Selby G. (1968). Parkinson's disease. In: Vinken PJ, Bruyn GW, (Eds.), *Handbook of Clinical Neurology,* vol 6, *Diseases of the Basal Ganglia.* Amsterdam, North-Holland.

29. Gudmundsson KR. (1967). A clinical survey of parkinsonism in Iceland. *Acta Neurol Scand* 43 (suppl 33): 9–61.

30. Strang RR. (1970). The etiology of Parkinson's disease. *Dis Nerv Syst* 6: 381–390.

31. Marttila RJ, Rinne UK. (1976). Arteriosclerosis, heredity and some previous infections in the etiology of Parkinson's disease. A case-control study. *Clin Neurol Neurosurg* 79: 46–56.

32. Hoehn MM. (1976). Quoted in reference 2.

33. Lang AE, Kierans C, Blair RDG. (1986). Family history of tremor in Parkinson's disease compared to controls and patients with idiopathic dystonia. *Adv Neurol* (in press).

34. Jankovic J, Reches A. (1986). Parkinson's disease in monozygotic twins. Presented at the 8th International Symposium on Parkinson's Disease, New York City, New York, June 9–12th, p 13.

35. Koller WC, O'Hara R, Rubino F. (1985). Monozygotic twins with Parkinson's disease. *Ann Neurol* 18: 136.

36. Eldridge R, Ince SE. (1984). The low concordance rate for Parkinson's disease in twins: A possible explanation. *Neurology* 34: 1354–1356.

37. Kondo K. (1986). Epidemiological evaluation of the risk factors to Parkinson's disease. *Adv Neurol* (in press).

38. Gowers WR. (1893). Paralysis agitans. *A Manual of Diseases of the Nervous System* II. London.

39. Larsson T, Sjogren T. (1960). Essential tremor: A clinical and genetic population study. *Acta Psychiatr Neurol Scand* 36 (suppl 144): 1–176.

40. Rajput AH, Offord KP, Beard CM, Kurland LT. (1984). Essential tremor in Rochester, Minnesota: A 45-year study. *J Neurol Neurosurg Psychiatry* 47: 466–470.

41. Marttila RJ, Rautakorpi I, Rinne U. (1984). The relation of essential tremor to Parkinson's disease. *J Neurol Neurosurg Psychiatry* 47: 734–735.

42. Findley LJ, Cleeves L. (1985). The relation of essential tremor to Parkinson's disease. *J Neurol Neurosurg Psychiatry* 48: 192.

43. Hornabrook RW, Nagurney JT. (1976). Essential tremor in Papua, New Guinea. *Brain* 99: 654–672.

44. Geraghty JJ, Jankovic J, Zetusky WJ. (1985). Association between essential tremor and Parkinson's disease. *Ann Neurol* 17: 329–333.

45. Haerer AF, Anderson DW, Schoenberg BS. (1982). Prevalence of essential tremor—results from the Copiah County study. *Arch Neurol* 39: 750–751.

46. Chase TN, Schnur JA, Gordon EK. (1970). Cerebrospinal fluid monoamine catabolites in drug-induced extrapyramidal disorders. *Neuropharmacology* 9: 265–268.

47. Myrianthopoulos NC, Waldrop FN, Vincent BL. (1969). A repeat study of hereditary predisposition in drug-induced parkinsonism. In: Barbeau A, Brunette JR (Eds.), *Progress in Neurogenetics*. Amsterdam, Excerpta Medica.

48. Kessler II. (1972). Epidemiological studies of Parkinson's disease: II. A hospital-based study. *Am J Epidemiol* 95: 308–318.

49. Kessler II. (1972). Epidemiological studies of Parkinson's disease: III. A community-based survey. *Am J Epidemiol* 96: 242–254.
50. Lombard A, Gelfand M. (1978). Parkinson's disease in the African. *Cent Afr J Med* 24: 5–8.
51. Reef HE. (1977). Prevalence of Parkinson's disease in a multiracial community. In: Jager HWA, Bruyn GW, Heijstee APJ (Eds.), *11th World Congress of Neurology*. Amsterdam, Excerpta Medica.
52. Harada H, Nishikawa S, Takahashi K. (1983). Epidemiology of Parkinson's disease in a Japanese city. *Arch Neurol* 40: 151–154.
53. Schoenberg BS, Anderson DW, Haerer AF. (1985). Prevalence of Parkinson's disease in the biracial population of Copiah County, Mississippi. *Neurology* 35: 841–845.
54. Davidovitz S, Zamir R, Kott E. (1977). HLA antigens in Parkinson's disease. In: Den Hartog Jager WA, Bruyn GW, Heijstee APJ (Eds.), *11th World Congress of Neurology*. Amsterdam, Excerpta Medica.
55. Leheny WA, Davidson DLW, De Vane P, House AO, Lenman JAR. (1983). HLA antigens in Parkinson's disease. *Tissue Antigens* 21: 260–261.
56. Reed E, Lewison A, Mayeaux R, Suciu-Foca N. (1983). HLA antigens in Parkinson's disease. *Tissue Antigens* 21: 161–163.
57. Marttila RJ, Rinne UK, Thlikainen A. (1981). Histocompatibility types in Parkinson's disease. *J Neurol Sci* 51: 217–221.
58. Emile J, Truelle JL, Pouplard A, Hurez D. (1977). Association maladie de parkinson-antigenes HLA-B_{17} et B_{18}. *Nouv Presse Med* 6: 4144.
59. Takagi S, Shinohara Y, Tsuji K. (1982). Histocompatibility antigens in Parkinson's disease. *Acta Neurol Scand* 66: 590–593.
60. Barbeau A, Roy M. (1986). Genetic susceptibility, environmental factors and Parkinson's disease. *Adv Neurol* (in press).

5

Pathophysiology and Clinical Assessment of Motor Symptoms in Parkinson's Disease

JOSEPH JANKOVIC
Baylor College of Medicine, Houston, Texas

In his 1817 "Essay on the Shaking Palsy," James Parkinson recorded many of the features of the condition that now bears his name (Parkinson, 1817). Parkinson emphasized the tremor at rest, flexed posture, festinant gait (Fig. 1), dysarthria, dysphagia, and constipation. He failed to recognize other important motor signs such as rigidity, bradykinesia, and hypomimia. Charcot and others later pointed out that the term "paralysis agitans" used by Parkinson was inappropriate, because in Parkinson's disease the strength was usually well preserved and many patients with Parkinson's disease did not shake.

Although usually regarded as a motor system disorder, Parkinson's disease is now considered to be a much more complex syndrome involving the motor as well as the nonmotor systems. For example, oily skin, seborrhea, pedal edema, fatigability, and weight loss are recognized as nonspecific but nevertheless typical parkinsonian features (Van Der Linden et al., 1985). The autonomic involvement is responsible for orthostatic hypotension, paroxysmal flushing, diaphoresis, problems with thermal regulation, constipation, and bladder, sphincter, and sexual disturbances (Aminoff and Wilcox, 1971; Appenzeller and Goss, 1971). The involvement of the thalamus and the spinal dopaminergic pathway may explain some of the sensory complaints, such as pains, aches, and burning–tingling paresthesias (Koller, 1984). The special sensory organs may be also involved in Parkinson's disease and cause visual, olfactory, and vestibular dysfunction (Ward et al., 1983; Reichert et al., 1982; White et al., 1983; Bodis-Wollner and Onofrj, 1986).

Recent studies have focused on the protean neurobehavioral abnormalities in Parkinson's disease, such as apathy, fearfulness, anxiety, emotional lability,

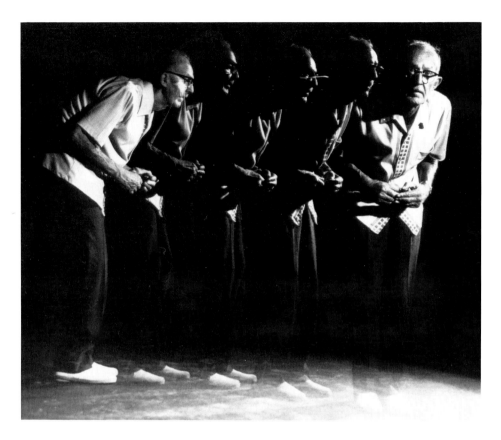

FIGURE 1 A 74-year-old man with 9 years of bilateral parkinsonism demonstrated by hypomimia, hand tremor and posturing, stooped posture, and a shuffling gait.

social withdrawal, increasing dependency, depression, dementia, bradyphrenia, a type of anomia termed the "tip-of-the-tongue phenomenon," visual–spatial impairment, sleep disturbance, psychosis, and other psychiatric problems (Mayeux, 1984).

The rich and variable expression of Parkinson's disease often causes diagnostic confusion and a delay in treatment (Koller, 1984a). In the early stages, Parkinsonian symptoms are often mistaken for arthritis or bursitis, normal aging, Alzheimer's disease, or stroke-related hemiparesis (Fig. 2). Parkinson's disease often begins on one side of the body, but usually becomes bilateral within a few months or years. However, parkinsonism may remain unilateral, particularly when it is a late sequela of posttraumatic hemiatrophy, or when it is due to a structural lesion in the basal ganglia (Klawans, 1981). In a survey of 181 treated Parkinson's disease patients, Bulpitt et al. (1985) found at least 45 different symptoms attributable to Parkinson's disease. However, only nine of these symptoms were reported by the patients with more than fivefold excess compared with those of a control population of patients randomly selected from a general practice. These common symptoms included being frozen or rooted to a spot, grimacing, jerking of arms and legs, shaking hands, clumsy hands, salivation, poor concentration, severe apprehension, and hallucinations. However, even these frequent symptoms are relatively nonspecific and do not clearly differentiate Parkinson's disease patients from diseased controls.

While systemic, mental, sensory, and other nonmotor symptoms of Parkinson's disease are often quite disabling, Parkinson's disease patients are usually most concerned about the symptoms that relate to their disturbance of movement (Jankovic, 1984). This review will focus on these motor manifestations. The emphasis will be on the pathophysiology and clinical assessment of the cardinal signs of Parkinson's disease: bradykinesia, tremor, rigidity, and postural instability (Table 1).

The specific mechanisms underlying the various Parkinson's disease symptoms are poorly understood. An accurate assessment of the disorder's motor signs should help to differentiate them from the motor changes associated with normal aging (Sudarsky and Konthal, 1983). Normal elderly subjects may have a mild extrapyramidal impairment, including slow movement and a shuffling gait. Other signs often attributed to Parkinson's disease also have been described with increased frequency among normal elderly subjects. These include disinhibition of the nuchocephalic reflex, glabellar blink reflex, snout reflex, head-retraction reflex, and the presence of paratonia, impaired vertical gaze, and cogwheel visual pursuit (Sandyk et al., 1982; Jenkyn et al., 1985). Although these signs occur more frequently in parkinsonian patients than other aged individuals, they are not specific for Parkinson's disease. However, they may indicate aging of subcortical structures, such as the basal ganglia, associated with an age-dependent loss of dopamine receptors (Wagner, 1985). The receptor loss may explain why these age-related motor signs do not improve with levodopa treatment (Newman et al., 1985).

The postulated clinical–biochemical correlations for the cardinal signs of Parkinson's disease are summarized in Table 2. Tremor and rigidity are considered "positive" signs of Parkinson's disease because they are presumably produced by a release, or disinhibition, of intact brain regions as a result of a disturbance in another part of the brain. Thus, these "positive" signs do not specifically indicate a dysfunction of the basal ganglia, and they respond well to thalamotomy. In contrast, postural instability and bradykinesia, the two "negative" signs, more specifically reflect a basal ganglia dysfunction and are unaffected by a surgical thalamic lesion.

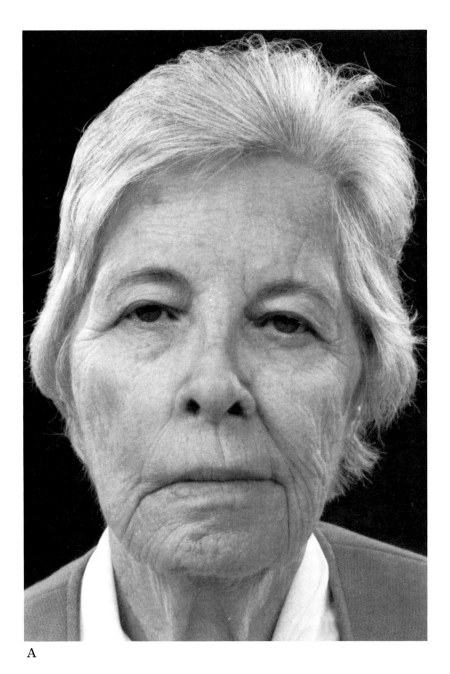

A

FIGURE 2 A. 74-year-old woman with facial asymmetry and right hemiatrophy
for 5 years associated with right hemiparkinsonism.

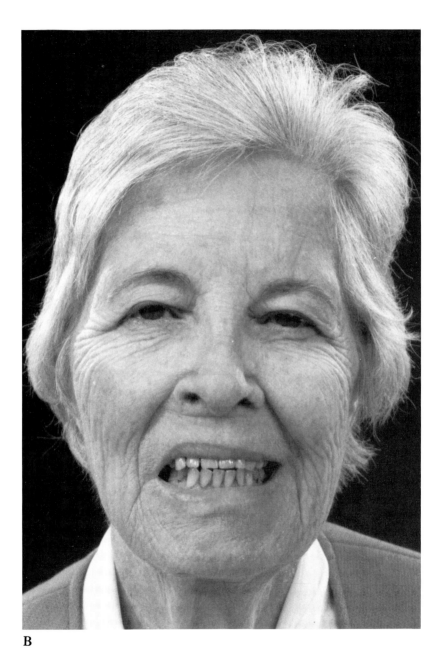

B

B. Voluntary facial contraction reveals no evidence of slight facial weakness.

TABLE 1 Motor Features of Parkinsonism

Cardinal signs
Tremor at rest
Rigidity
Bradykinesia
Loss of postural reflexes
Other motor findings
Hypomimia ("masked facies")
Speech disturbance (hypokinetic dysarthria)
Hypophonia
Dysphagia
Sialorrhea
Respiratory difficulties
Loss of associated movements
Shuffling, short-step gait, festination, freezing
Micrographia
Difficulty turning in bed
Difficulties with activities of daily living
Stooped posture, kyphosis, and scoliosis
Dystonia, myoclonus, orofacial dyskinesia
Neuroophthalmologic findings
Impaired visual contrast sensitivity
Visuospatial impairment
Impaired upward gaze
Impaired convergence
Oculogyric crises
Impaired smooth pursuit
Impaired vestibuloocular reflex
Hypometric saccades
Decreased blink rate
Spontaneous and reflex blepharospasm (glabellar or Myerson's sign)
Lid apraxia (opening or closure): involuntary levator inhibition
Motor findings related to dopaminergic therapy (see Table 5)
Levodopa-induced dyskinesias (chorea, dystonia, myoclonus, tic)

TABLE 2 Clinical-Biochemical Correlation

Symptom	Postulated localization or pathway of dominant neurotransmitter deficiency
Motor	
Tremor	Globus pallidum, DA
Rigidity	Mesocorticolimbic, DA
Bradykinesia	Nigrostriatal and meso-limbic, DA
Freezing	Locus ceruleus, NE
Postural instability	Globus pallidum, DA Vestibular nuclei, ?
Mental	
Depression	Raphe nuclei, 5-HT Locus ceruleus, NE
Bradyphrenia	Mesocortical, DA Raphe nuclei, 5-HT
Dementia, anomia	Nucleus basalis, ACH Mesocortical, DA Locus ceruleus, NE Cortical hippocampal, somatostatin
Sleep disturbance	Raphe nuclei, 5-HT
Sensory	
Pain and paresthesias	Diencephalospinal, DA
Autonomic	
Orthostasis, weight loss, constipation, impaired thermal regulation, sphincter and sexual dysfunction, seborrhea	Diencephalospinal, DA Hypothalamus, NE

DA, dopamine; NE, norepinephrine; ACH, acetylcholine; 5-HT, serotonin

BRADYKINESIA

Bradykinesia, or slowness of movement, is often used interchangeably with hypokinesia (poverty of movement) and akinesia (absence of movement). Bradykinesia is the most characteristic symptom of basal ganglia dysfunction in Parkinson's disease (Marsden, 1984a). It may be manifested by a delay in the initiation, and by slowness of execution, of a movement. Other aspects of bradykinesia include a delay in arresting movement, a decrementing amplitude and speed of repetitive movement, an intermittent immobility or "freezing," and an inability to execute simultaneous or sequential actions (Schwab et al., 1959).

An extreme degree of bradykinesia is akinesia, a state of complete immobility. This state of frozen helplessness may last seconds, minutes, or hours, and is most evident at the onset of gait ("start hesitation"), when patients arise from a chair, or when they turn or walk through narrow passages. Patients often learn a variety of tricks to overcome the freezing attacks: marching to command ("left, right, left, right"), stepping over objects (end of a walking stick, pavement stone, cracks in the floor, etc.), walking to music or metronome, shifting body weight, rocking movements, and others (Stern et al., 1980). The frequency and the severity of the freezing attacks seem to correlate with the duration of the disease, and the freezing is not amenable to levodopa or other antiparkinson therapy. Earlier reports of favorable response of "freezing" to DL-threoserine, a norepinephrine precursor, have not been confirmed by more recent clinical trials (Reches, 1985).

After recording electromyographic (EMG) patterns in the antagonistic muscles of parkinsonian patients during a brief ballistic elbow flexion, Hallett and Khoshbin (1980) concluded that the most characteristic feature of brady-kinesia was the inability to "energize" the appropriate muscles to provide a sufficient rate of force required for the initiation and the maintenance of a large, fast (ballistic) movement. Therefore, Parkinson's disease patients need a series of multiple agonist bursts to accomplish a larger movement. The impaired genera-tion and velocity of ballistic movement can be ameliorated with levodopa (Flowers, 1976; Jankovic and Frost, 1981; Baroni et al., 1984). The observed improvement of motor signs with levodopa strongly supports the notion that dopamine plays a key role in motor control. Measuring brain dopamine metab-olism of rats running on straight and circular treadmills, Freedman and Yama-moto (1985) found that dopamine metabolism in the caudate nucleus was more affected by posture and direction of movement, whereas dopamine metabolism in the nucleus accumbens was more linked to the speed and direction of move-ment. The timing of contraction, first of the agonists and then of the antagonists, appears to be normal in Parkinson's disease, and is probably more under cerebel-lar than basal ganglia control (Hallett and Khoshbin, 1980; Ito, 1984). In other words, in Parkinson's disease the simple motor program to execute a fast ballistic movement is intact, but it fails because the initial agonist burst is insufficient. Micrographia, a typical Parkinson's disease symptom, is an example of a muscle-energizing defect (Hallett and Khoshbin, 1980).

Bradykinesia, like other parkinsonian symptoms, is dependent on the emo-tional state of the patient. With a sudden surge of emotional energy, the immobile patient may catch a ball or make other fast movements. This curious phenomenon, called "kinesia paradoxica," demonstrates that the motor pro-grams are intact in Parkinson's disease, but that patients have difficulty utilizing the programs without the help of an external trigger (Marsden, 1982a; Bloxham ct al., 1984). Therefore, parkinsonian patients are able to make use of prior information to perform an automatic or a preprogrammed movement, but they cannot use this information to initiate or select a movement.

Marsden (1982a) contends that the fundamental defect in Parkinson's disease is the inability to execute learned sequential motor plans automatically. This impairment of normal sequencing of motor programs probably results from a disconnection between the basal ganglia and the supplementary motor cortex, an area that subserves planning function for movement. The supplementary motor cortex receives projections from the motor basal ganglia (via the globus pallidus and ventrolateral thalamus) and, in turn, projects the motor cortex. However, the cortical readiness potential recorded over the supplementary motor cortex of Parkinson's patients is normal, while it is markedly attenuated over the primary motor cortex (Deecke, 1977; Schultz, 1984). This suggests possible involvement of the primary motor cortex in Parkinson's disease, but no morphologic abnormalities are observed in this area. In Parkinson's disease there also seems to be an abnormal processing of the sensory input necessary for the generation and execution of movement. This was the interpretation of a study by Tatton et al. (1984) in MPTP-treated monkeys. Recording from the motor cortex, they showed markedly increased gain of the long-latency (M2) segments of the mechanoreceptor-evoked responses.

Most of the neurophysiological and neurobehavioral studies in Parkinson's disease have concluded that the basal ganglia (and possibly the supplementary motor cortex) play a critical role in planning and in sequencing voluntary movements (Stern et al., 1983). For example, when a patient arises from a chair, he or she may "forget" any one of the sequential steps involved in such a seemingly simple task: to flex forward, place hands on the arm rests, place feet under the chair and then push out of the chair into an erect posture. Similar difficulties may be encountered when sitting down, squatting, kneeling, turning in bed, and walking. Lakke (1985) suggests that since the patient can readily perform these activities under certain circumstances, such as when emotionally stressed ("akinesia paradoxica"), the intrinsic program is not disturbed, and therefore these axial motor abnormalities are a result of apraxia. Thus, the Parkinson's patient has an inability to "call up" the axial motor program on command (Lakke, 1985).

The inability to combine motor programs into complex sequences seems to be a fundamental motor deficit in Parkinson's disease. The study of a reaction time and a velocity of movement provides some insight into the mechanisms of the motor deficits at an elementary level. Evarts et al. (1981) showed that both reaction (RT) and movement (MT) times are independently impaired in Parkinson's disease. In patients with asymmetrical findings, the RT is slower on the more affected side (Yokochi et al., 1985). RT is influenced not only by the degree of motor impairment but also by the interaction between the cognitive processing and the motor response. This is particularly evident when choice RT is used and compared to simple RT (Rafal et al., 1984). Bradykinetic patients with Parkinson's disease have more specific impairment in choice RT, which involves a stimulus categorization and a response selection, and reflects disturbance at more complex levels of cognitive processing (Pirozzollo et al., 1985). While bradykinesia correlated with slow choice RT and with cognitive dysfunction, we found no such correlation in patients who had tremor as the dominant symptom. Other studies of cognitive and motor performance revealed a rough correlation between the two processes. For example, in patients with levodopa-induced motor fluctuations, the cognition (largely determined by a state of arousal and affect) seemed more impaired during the "off" periods than during the "on" periods condition (Brown et al., 1984). However, bradyphrenia (slow thinking and information processing) does not always correlate with bradykinesia, and therefore different biochemical mechanisms probably underlie these two neurobehavioral disturbances (Rafal et al., 1984).

MT, particularly when measured for proximal muscles, is less variable than RT and more consistent with the clinical assessment of bradykinesia. Both MT and RT are better indicators of bradykinesia than the speed of rapid alternating movements. Ward et al. (1983) attempted to correlate the median MT and RT with tremor, rigidity, or manual dexterity in 10 patients rated on a 0–4 modified Columbia scale. The only positive correlations were found between MT and rigidity and between RT and manual dexterity.

In another experiment, Ward and colleagues (1983) asked their patients to walk along a 7-m pressure-sensitive mat, which recorded the number of steps and the length and the duration of each step. The median step length and the length variant were computed and compared to clinical gait score. A weak, but significant, correlation was found between the objective and clinical scores. Thus, both quantitative and clinical evaluation of gait seemed to provide an index of bradykinesia. Teräiväinen et al. (1980) found that counting the number of steps and the time taken to walk over a specified distance correlated better with clinical bradykinesia than with electromechanical quantification of error in a visual-pursuit tracking task. Day et al. (1984) also found that, despite obvious bradykinesia, Parkinson's disease patients may exhibit normal tracking by using a predictive motor strategy. Using a metal walkway, foil shoe contacts, and ultraviolet and video recorder, Stern et al. (1983) analyzed the gait and mobility in 50 patients with idiopathic Parkinson's disease. They were unable to differentiate the specific abnormalities associated with the parkinsonian gait from the other gait disorders. Therefore, while clinical assessment of gait seems rather crude, the objective gait measurements do not offer any advantage over the clinical rating.

Of the various objective assessments of bradykinesia, the MT correlates best with the total clinical score, but it is not as sensitive an indicator of the overall motor deficit as is the clinical rating. Ward et al. (1983) concluded that although MT was a useful measurement, it alone did not justify the use of elaborate and expensive technology. The clinical rating scale probably more accurately reflects the patient's disability because it includes more relevant observations.

TREMOR

Tremor, while less specific than bradykinesia, is one of the most recognizable symptoms of Parkinson's disease. However, only half of all patients present with tremor as the initial manifestation of Parkinson's disease, and 15% never have tremor during the course of the illness (Martin et al., 1983). Although tremor at rest (4-6 Hz) is the typical parkinsonian tremor, most patients also have tremor during activity, and this postural tremor (5-8 Hz) may be more disabling than the resting tremor. It has been postulated that the typical tremor at rest results from nigrostriatal degeneration and consequent disinhibition of the pacemaker cells in the thalamus (Findley and Gresty, 1984). These thalamic neurons discharge rhythmically at 5-6 Hz, a frequency similar to the typical parkinsonian tremor at rest (Llinas and Johnsen, 1982; Lamarre, 1984). Some support for the thalamic pacemaker theory of the Parkinson's disease tremor also comes from the studies of Lee and Stein (1981), which show that the resting 5-Hz tremor is remarkably constant and relatively resistant to resetting by mechanical perturbations. Furthermore, during stereotactic thalamotomy, 5-Hz discharges are usually recorded in the nucleus ventralis intermedius of the thalamus in parkinsonian as well as in normal subjects, even in the absence of visible tremor. This rhythmic bursting is not abolished by deafferentation or paralysis (Marsden, 1984a).

The biochemical defect underlying either resting or postural parkinsonian tremor is unknown. Bernheimer and colleagues (1973) showed that the severity of tremor paralleled the degree of homovanillic acid (HVA) reduction in the pallidum. In contrast, bradykinesia correlated with dopamine depletion in the caudate nucleus. In an experimental monkey model of Parkinsonian tremor, a pure lesion in the ascending dopaminergic nigrostriatal pathway is not sufficient to produce the alternating rest tremor (Pechadre et al., 1976). Experimental parkinsonian tremor requires nigrostriatal disconnection combined with a lesion involving the rubrotegmentospinal and the dentatorubrothalamic pathways. A typical Parkinson's disease tremor is observed in humans and in experimental animals exposed to MPTP, a neurotoxin that presumably affects, rather selectively, the nigrostriatal dopaminergic system (Ballard et al., 1985; Calne et al., 1985; Snyder and D'Amato, 1986). However, the cerebellorubrothalamic system has not been examined in detail in this MPTP model. Furthermore, in MPTP subjects, a prominent action tremor was more typically seen than a tremor at rest.

The mechanism of the parkinsonian action tremor is unknown. The frequency (6 Hz) of the postural (action) tremor is the same as the frequency of the cogwheel phenomenon, elicited during passive movement (Lance et al.,

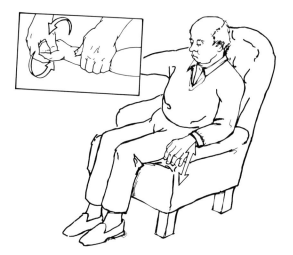

FIGURE 3 Parkinsonian cogwheel rigidity elicited by passive rotation of the wrist is enhanced by voluntary repetitive movement of the contralateral hand.

1963; Jankovic and Fahn, 1980; Findley et al., 1981) (Fig. 3). The postural tremor in Parkinson's disease resembles the essential tremor (ET), and this can lead to diagnostic confusion. The problem is further complicated by the observation that Parkinson's disease and ET can coexist. We found that 6.7% of all Parkinson's disease and 20% of all ET patients had the combination of Parkinson's disease and ET (Geraghty and Jankovic, 1985; Jankovic, 1986a). The expected prevalence is 0.41% for ET and 0.35% for Parkinson's disease (Haerer et al., 1982; Schoenberg et al., 1985). While there is some overlap in the clinical manifestations, there should be no problem in the differential diagnosis between ET and Parkinson's disease tremor (Table 3).

In the early studies, mechanical and optic devices were used to record tremor (Holmes, 1922). EMG recordings and accelerometers, assisted by computer analysis, have been utilized recently to measure the characteristics of tremor. However, most accelerometers record tremor in a single plane. By using computed triaxial accelerometry, we recorded the distortion of the normal motion characteristics in patients with Parkinson's disease and ET during voluntary arm abduction–adduction movement (Jankovic and Frost, 1981). There was a good correlation between the reduction in the distortion and the clinical improvement in response to medications. However, the quantitative recordings of tremor, although accurate, are time-consuming, costly, and influenced by the emotional state of the patient. Moreover, it is questionable whether such recordings provide a reliable index of a meaningful therapeutic response.

TABLE 3 Differential Diagnosis of Parkinson and Essential Tremor

	Parkinsonian tremor	Essential tremor
Age at onset (years)	55–75	10–80
Sex	M>F	M≤F
Family history	−	+
Site of involvement	Hands, legs, jaw, chin, tongue	Hands, head, voice, tongue
Characteristics	Supination–pronation	Flexion–extension
Influencing Factors		
Rest	↑	→
Action	→	↑
Mental concentration, walking	↑	→
Frequency (hz)	4–7	8–12
Electromyography (contraction of antagonists)	Alternating parkinsonism	Simultaneous
Associated features		Cogwheel rigidity (±) Dystonia Myoclonus Charcot-Marie-Tooth disease
Neuropathology	Nigrostriatal degeneration, Lewy bodies	No discernible pathology
Treatment	Anticholinergics, amantadine, dopa-minergic drugs, surgery (thalamotomy)	Beta blockers, benzodiazepines, pyrimidone, phenobarbital, amantadine, alcohol

RIGIDITY

Rigidity is less variable than tremor, and it probably better reflects the patient's functional disability. Rigidity may contribute to subjective stiffness and tightness, a common complaint in patients with Parkinson's disease. However, there is relatively poor correlation between the sensory complaints experienced by most patients, and the degree of rigidity (Snider et al., 1976; Koller, 1984b). In mild cases, cogwheel rigidity can be brought out by a passive rotation of the wrist or flexion-extension of the forearm, while the patient performs a repetitive voluntary movement in the contralateral arm (Matsumoto et al., 1963) (Fig. 3).

The neurophysiological mechanisms of rigidity are still poorly understood. Spinal monosynaptic reflexes are usually normal in Parkinson's disease. Recordings from muscle spindle afferents revealed an activity in rigid parkinsonian patients not seen in normal controls. This suggested an increased fusimotor drive due to hyperactivity of both alpha and gamma motor neurons. However, this fusimotor overactivity probably is an epiphenomenon, reflecting the inability of Parkinson's patients to relax fully. Passive shortening of a rigid muscle, due to Parkinson's disease or seen in tense subjects, produces an involuntary contraction, called the Westphal phenomenon. While the mechanism of this sign is unknown, it probably is the result of excessive supraspinal drive on normal spinal mechanism. This shortening reaction may be abolished by procain infiltration of the muscle. Thus, there is no convincing evidence of primary defect of fusimotor function in parkinsonian rigidity (Burke, 1984).

The measurement of torque or of resistance during passive flexion-extension movement has been used most extensively as an index of rigidity. Utilizing these techniques, it has been demonstrated that rigidity correlated with increased amplitude of the long-latency (transcerebral) responses to sudden stretch. These long-latency stretch reflexes represent a positive (release) phenomenon, mediated by motor pathways that do not traverse the basal ganglia. The earlier techniques of passively flexing and extending the limbs were later refined by Mortimer and Webster (1979), who designed a servocontrolled electronic device to move the limb at a constant angular velocity. They and others (Lee and Tatton, 1975; Berardelli et al., 1983; Rothwell et al., 1983) demonstrated a close relationship between the enhanced long-latency stretch reflexes and the degree of activated rigidity. The opposite is true in Huntington's disease, in which these long-latency stretch reflexes are diminished or absent. Using measurements of the tonic stretch reflex as an index of rigidity, Meyer and Adorjani (1983) found an *inverse* correlation between the "dynamic sensitivity" (ratio between the increase in reflex EMG at a high versus low angular velocity) and the severity of parkinsonian rigidity. On the other hand, the "static" component of the tonic stretch reflex (the maximum reflex activity at greatest stretch or at sustained stretch) *positively* correlated with the severity of rigidity. Both the dynamic and the static components of the tonic stretch reflex may be reduced by antiparkinson drugs (Meyer and Adorjani, 1983). Although Lee and Tatton (1975) showed diminution of the amplitude of the reflex after treatment, correlating it with improvement in rigidity, the measurement of long-latency responses is quite cumbersome, time-consuming, and possibly unreliable (Marsden and Schacter, 1981). Moreover, a marked overlap in the long latency response between Parkinson's and normal subjects has been noted (Teräväinen and Calne, 1980).

POSTURAL INSTABILITY

The loss of balance associated with propulsion and retropulsion is probably the least specific, but most disabling, of all parkinsonian symptoms. Purdon-Martin (1967), after studying nine brains of patients with postencephalitic parkinsonism, concluded that the globus pallidum degeneration was most responsible for the loss of righting reflexes and of postural instability in parkinsonian patients. Reichert et al. (1982) correlated postural instability in Parkinson's disease patients with reduced or absent vestibular responses.

Traub et al. (1980) studied postural reflexes in 29 Parkinson's disease patients by recording anticipatory postural responses in the legs (triceps surae) in response to perturbations of one of the arms. In normal subjects, a burst of activity can be recorded from the calf muscles at a latency of 80 msec after the perturbation. This postural adjustment occurs even before any movement can be recorded in the legs (latency, 150 msec). Therefore, this reflex adjustment is anticipatory and centrally generated. In Parkinson's disease, the anticipatory postural reflexes are absent or markedly diminished. Such abnormalities were present in 10 of the 18 patients with moderately severe Parkinson's disease and in 2 of 11 Parkinson's disease patients without obvious postural instability. Since some patients with normal anticipatory reflexes can still fall, it is likely that other mechanisms contribute to the falls of parkinsonian patients (Aita, 1982). Furthermore, patients with progressive supranuclear palsy, who are much more prone to falling than Parkinson's disease patients, have normal anticipatory postural responses (Traub, 1980; Jankovic, 1984).

Weiner et al. (1984) found moderate or severe loss of balance in response to a standing postural perturbation in 68% of 34 patients in a geriatric care facility. They suggested that a postural reflex dysfunction was largely responsible for the unexplained falls in the elderly.

The parkinsonian gait reveals some features common with the gait disturbance associated with normal-pressure hydrocephalus (Fisher, 1982; Knutsson, 1985). In a study of 50 subjects older than 70 years, Sudarsky and Ronthal (1983) established a principal cause of the gait disorder in all but 7 subjects ("essential gait disorder"). They but not others (Koller et al., 1983) suggested that this senile gait is related to normal-pressure hydrocephalus.

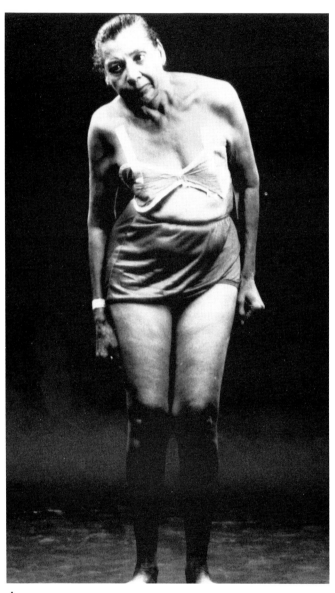

A

FIGURE 4   A 63-year-old woman with progressive scoliosis to the right side for 20 years and left hemiparkinsonism manifested by hand and leg tremor, rigidity, and bradykinesia. A. Front view. B. Back view.

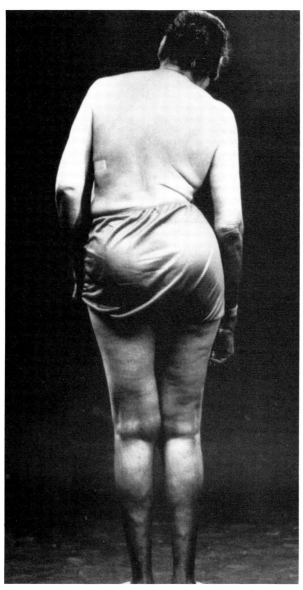

B

The gait and postural problems associated with Parkinson's disease probably result from a combination of bradykinesia, rigidity, loss of anticipatory proprioceptive reflexes, loss of protective reaction to a fall, gait and axial apraxia, ataxia, vestibular dysfunction, and orthostatic hypotension.

OTHER MOTOR MANIFESTATIONS

There are many other motor findings in Parkinson's disease (Table 1), most of which are directly related to one of the cardinal signs. For example, the loss of facial expression ("hypomimia," "masked facies") and the bulbar symptoms (dysarthria, hypophonia, dysphagia, and sialorrhea) result from orofacial-

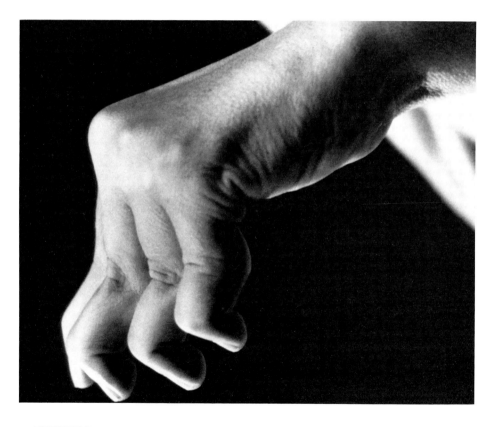

FIGURE 5   A 44-year-old woman with Parkinson's disease showing typical dystonic ("striatal") hand with flexion at the metacarpophalangeal joints, extension at the proximal interphalangeal joints, and flexion at the distal interphalangeal joints. The dystonia completely resolves with levodopa. (From Fahn and Jankovic, 1984.)

laryngeal bradykinesia and rigidity (Critchley, 1981; Hunker et al., 1982; Van Der Linden et al., 1985). Respiratory difficulties result from a variety of mechanisms, including a restrictive component due to rigid respiratory muscles and levodopa-induced respiratory dyskinesias (Jankovic, 1986b). Abnormal axial posture (Figs. 1, 4) (kyphosis, scoliosis) and distal deformities due to dystonia or "striatal" hand (Fig. 5) or foot may occur in de novo (untreated) and treated parkinsonian patients (Gortvai, 1963; Nausieda et al., 1980; Jankovic, 1982; Fahn and Jankovic, 1984; Sunohara et al., 1985). Duvoisin and Marsden (1975) studied 20 Parkinson's disease patients with scoliosis and found that 16 of the patients tilted away from the side with predominant parkinsonian symptoms. However, subsequent studies could not confirm this interesting observation (Grimes et al., 1986).

Of the various oculomotor problems characteristically seen in Parkinson's disease, the following are most common: impaired saccadic and smooth pursuit, limitation of upward gaze and convergence, oculogyric crises, spontaneous and reflex blepharospasm, apraxia of lid opening (involuntary levator inhibition), and apraxia of eyelid closure (Jankovic, 1985; Leport and Duvoisin, 1985). Although supranuclear ophthalmoplegia is often used to differentiate progressive supranuclear palsy from Parkinson's disease, this oculomotor abnormality has also been described in otherwise typical parkinsonian (Guiloff, 1980; Jankovic, 1984).

ASSESSMENT OF DISABILITY

The assessment of Parkinson's disease is difficult, because the movement disorder is expressed variably in an individual patient (intrapatient variability) at different times, and it is influenced by emotional state, response to medication, and other variables. Moreover, there is a marked interpatient variability of symptoms and signs. To study this heterogeneity and to determine possible patterns of clinical associations, we analyzed the clinical findings in 334 patients with idiopathic Parkinson's disease. Using the Spearman rank order coefficients for the different signs and symptoms, we identified at least two distinct clinical populations of parkinsonian patients (Zetusky et al., 1985). One subtype was characterized by a prominent tremor, an early age at onset, and a greater familiar tendency (Table 4). Another subtype was dominated by postural instability and gait difficulty (PIGD), and was associated with greater degree of dementia, bradykinesia, functional disability, and a less favorable long-term prognosis. Thus Parkinson's disease should not be considered a unitary disorder, but a syndrome with characteristic patterns of symptoms, course, response to therapy and different etiologies (Jankovic and Calne, 1987). The different subsets of Parkinson's disease may have different pathogenesis and even different genetic predisposition (Barbeau, 1984; Jankovic and Reches, 1986). The tremor-dominant Parkinson's disease may be related to an autosomal-dominant essential tremor (Barbeau and Roy, 1984; Geraghty et al., 1985) (Table 4).

TABLE 4 Clinical Patterns in Parkinson's Disease: Relationship of Clinical Features in 334 Patients

	Tremor	Postural instability and gait difficulty (PIGD)
Tremor	+	0
Rigidity	+	+
Bradykinesia	0	+
PIGD	0	+
Functional disability	0	+
Mental deterioration	0	+
Late age at onset	0	+
Family history	+	0
Prognosis	Better	Worse

+, Significant correlation; 0, no significant correlation

The accurate and reliable evaluation of motor dysfunction is essential for an objective assessment of the efficacy of potentially useful drugs. Various mechanical, electrophysiological, and clinical methods have been utilized to measure the motor findings in Parkinson's disease objectively. Some of the techniques are designed to measure the frequency, amplitude, force, velocity, acceleration of contraction, and other quantitative parameters of the abnormal movement. However, such measurements may have little relevance to the actual functional disability of the patient.

In assessing the motor symptoms and signs of Parkinson's disease, two approaches have been used, both of which strive to quantitate the motor findings (Marsden and Schacter, 1981). One method utilizes neurologic history and an examination with subjective rating of symptoms, signs and functional disability, and the other method utilizes timing of specific tasks or neurophysiological tests of particular motor disturbances. While the latter method is considered to be more "objective" and "scientific," it is not necessarily more accurate, reliable, or relevant than the clinical rating. However, both approaches have certain advantages and disadvantages and, when combined, they may provide a useful method of assessing the severity of the disability and the response to therapy.

Most of the subjective methods of assessment of parkinsonian disability utilize rating scales of various symptoms and disabilities. Probably the most widely used method of staging Parkinson's disease is the Hoehn-Yahr scale (Hoehn and Yahr, 1967). While this staging scale is useful in comparing populations of Parkinson's disease patients, it is relatively insensitive to changes in a paticnt's clinical state. Therefore, the Hoehn-Yahr scale is not useful in monitoring the response of individual patients to therapy. Diamond and Markham (1983) used four rating scales, the Hoehn-Yahr staging, the New York University Parkinson's Disease Disability Scale, the Northwestern University Disability Scale, and the UCLA Disability Scale, to evaluate eight patients with Parkinson's disease treated with pergolide for 1 year. The patients were rated on all four scales by the same neurologists at each of 11 visits and prior ratings were not available to the examiner. The disability scores were converted to percentage improvement relative to baseline. There was a remarkable correlation between the four scales at 1 month, but the values varied considerably after the initial period. For example, at 5 months the improvement in disability varied between 13 and 58%, and at 9 months the Hoehn-Yahr stage showed 6% worsening, whereas the other scales showed approximately 30% improvement.

There are obvious limitations to each of these scales. As previously stated, the Hoehn-Yahr scale lacks precise sensitivity. The NYU Parkinson's Disease Scale utilizes 0-4 scoring. Rigidity and tremor are most significantly represented, because the four limbs and neck are each rated 0-4, possibly achieving the maximum score of 20. Thus, a barely perceptible tremor in all four limbs could result in a score of 4, which would be the same score assigned to a patient without tremor, but with a disabling gait disorder or postural instability. Furthermore, a more impressive improvement would have to occur in the second patient by comparison with the first in order to demonstrate a significant change in the score. The Northwestern University Disability Scale rates activities of daily living, such as dressing, hygiene, speech, and walking, on a scale of 0-10, and eating and feeding on a scale of 0-5. The UCLA Scale assigns rating factors for the 17 signs observed by the physician and 8 activities by history. For example, hypomimia is given a rating factor of 1, and akinesia a rating factor of 9. Each of the 25 items is then rated on a 0-3 scale (absent to severe), and each is then multiplied by its rating factor. While each scale has some advantages and disadvantages, because of the different methods of assessing the clinical disability, the results among clinical studies that use the different scales of disability cannot be compared. Therefore, a unified standard of ranking for parkinsonian disability is needed.

The Columbia Rating Scale is most widely used in clinical studies. Using a modified Columbia Scale in 70 Parkinson's patients, Montgomery et al. (1985) found good interobserver correlation in all the items tested (bradykinesia, gait, posture, resting tremor, and postural tremor) and in the Hoehn-Yahr stage. However, the most useful indicator of clinical disability in a patient with levodopa-induced clinical fluctuations is not necessarily the degree of tremor, rigidity, bradykinesia or postural instability observed in the office, but the percentage of time "off" during the total waking time. The difference in function between the "on" time and the "off" time is most relevant to the patient

TABLE 5 Clinical Fluctuations and Hyperkinesias in Parkinson's Disease[a]

Clinical conditions	Treatment
Fluctuations	
End-of-dose deterioration ("wearing-off")	Decreased interval between levodopa doses, dopamine agonists
Drug-resistant "off" periods	Increase levodopa, give before meals
Random oscillations ("on–off" or "yo-yo")	Decrease interval between levodopa doses, dopamine agonists, drug holidays
Freezing[b] (start hesitation and akinesia paradoxica)	Levodopa, dopamine agonists, DOPS Tapping, rhythmic commands, stepping over objects, rocking, gait modification
Hyperkinesia (dyskinesia)	
Peak dose dyskinesias ("I-D-I" response)	Reduce each (and total dose of levodopa, increase frequency of levodopa
Diphasic dyskinesias ("D-I-D" response)	Reduce anticholinergic drugs Reduce each dose of levodopa, increase frequency of levodopa
Early morning dystonia	Baclofen, nighttime levodopa, dopamine agonists, anticholinergics, tricyclics
Myoclonus	Clonazepam, methysergide, reduce levodopa
Dystonic movements and postures[b]	Anticholinergics, thalamotomy
Orofacial dyskinesia[b]	Reduce levodopa and anticholinergics
Kinesia paradoxica[b]	

[a]May be influenced by emotion, awareness, sleep, fatigue, stress.
[b]Possibly unrelated to levodopa.
DOPS = L-threo-3,4-dihydroxyphenylserine; I-D-I = improvement-dyskinesia-improvement; D-I-D = dyskinesia-improvement-dyskinesia.

(Table 5) (Jankovic, 1982; Marsden et al., 1982b; Fahn, 1982). Likewise, the duration of benefit from each dose of Sinemet is a useful index of therapeutic response. Thus, any rating scale must not only assess the motor signs but also take into account the patient's ability to perform activities of daily living and to ambulate in relationship to the total waking time. In addition to the typical motor signs, the clinical scales should include an assessment of other parkinsonian symptoms, such as dementia, depression, motivation, hallucinations, sensory symptoms, freezing, falling, and dyskinesia. Such a unified parkinsonian rating scale is currently being developed and validated as part of multicenter study of protective therapy in Parkinson's disease. The current version of the Unified Parkinson Rating Scale is listed in the Appendix.

REFERENCES

Aita JF. (1982). Why patients with Parkinson's disease fall. *JAMA* 247: 515–516.

Aminoff MJ, Wilcox CS. (1971). Assessment of autonomic function in patients with a parkinsonian syndrome. *Br Med J* 4: 80–84.

Appenzeller O, Goss JE. (1971). Autonomic deficits in Parkinson's syndrome. *Arch Neurol* 24: 50–57.

Ballard PA, Tetrud JW, Langston JW. (1985). Permanent human parkinsonism due to 1-methyl-4-phenyl-1,2,3,6-tetrahydropyridine (MPTP): seven cases. *Neurology* 35: 949–956.

Barbeau A, Roy M. (1984). Familial subsets in idiopathic Parkinson's disease. *Can J Neurol Sci* 11: 144–150.

Baroni A, Benvenuti F, Fantini L, Pantaleo T, Urbani F. (1984). Human ballistic arm abduction movements: effects of L-dopa treatment in Parkinson's disease. *Neurology* 34: 868–876.

Berardelli A, Sabra AF, Hallett M. (1983). Physiologic mechanisms of rigidity in Parkinson's disease. *J Neurol Neurosurg Psychiatry* 46: 45–53.

Bernheimer H, Birkmayer W, Hornykiewicz O, Jellinger K, Seitelberger F. (1973). Brain dopamine and the syndromes of Parkinson and Huntington: clinical morphological and neurochemical correlations. *J Neurol Sci* 20: 415–455.

Bloxham CA, Mindel TA, Frith CD. (1984). Initiation and execution of predictable and unpredictable movements in Parkinson's disease. *Brain* 107: 371–384.

Bodis-Wollner I, Onofrj M. (1986). The visual system in Parkinson's disease. In: *VIII International Symposium on Parkinson's Disease*. New York, Raven Press.

Brown RG, Marsden CD, Quinn N, Wyke MA. (1984). Alterations in cognitive performance and affect-arousal state during fluctuations in motor function in Parkinson's disease. *J Neurol Neurosurg Psychiatry* 47: 454–465.

Bulpitt CJ, Shaw K, Clifton P, Stern G, Davies JB, Reid JL. (1985). The symptoms of patients treated for Parkinson's disease. *Clin Neuropharmacol* 8: 175–183.

Calne DB, Langston JW, Martin WRW, Stoessl AJ et al. (1985). Positron emission tomography after MPTP: observations relating to the cause of Parkinson's disease. *Nature* 317: 246–249.

Critchley M. (1981). Speech disorders of parkinsonism: A review. *J Neurol Neurosurg Psychiatry* 44: 757–758.

Day BL, Dick JPR, Marsden CD. (1984). Patients with Parkinson's disease can employ a predictive motor strategy. *J Neurol Neurosurg Psychiatry* 47: 299–1306.

Diamond SG, Markham CH. (1983). Evaluating the evaluations: Or how to weigh the scales of parkinsonian disability. *Neurology* 33: 1098–1099.

Duvoisin RC, Marsden CD. (1975). Note on the scoliosis of parkinsonism. *J Neurol Neurosurg Psychiatry* 38: 787–793.

Evarts EV, Teravainen M, Calne DB. (1981). Reaction time in Parkinson's disease. *Brain* 104: 167–861.

Fahn S. (1982). Fluctuations of disability in Parkinson's disease: pathophysiological aspects. In: Marsden CD, Fahn S (Eds.), *Movement Disorders*. London, Butterworth.

Fahn S, Jankovic J. (1984). Practical management of dystonia. In: Jankovic J (Ed.), *Neurologic Clinics*, Vol 2. Philadelphia, WB Saunders.

Findley LJ, Gresty MA, Halmagyi GM. (1981). Tremor, the cogwheel phenomenon and clonus in Parkinson's disease. *J Neurol Neurosurg Psychiatry* 44: 534–46.

Findley LJ, Gresty MA. (1984). Tremor and rhythmical involuntary movements in Parkinson's disease. In: Findley LJ, Capildeo R (Eds.), *Movement Disorders: Tremors*. New York, Oxford University Press.

Fisher CM. (1982). Hydrocephalus as a cause of disturbance of gait in the elderly. *Neurology* 32: 1358–1363.

Flowers KA. (1976). Visual "closed-loop" and "open-loop" characteristics of voluntary movement in patients with parkinsonism and intention tremor. *Brain* 99: 269–310.

Freed CR, Yamamoto BK. (1985). Regional brain dopamine metabolism: a marker for the speed, direction, and posture of moving animals. *Science* 229: 62–65.

Geraghty JJ, Jankovic J, Zetusky WJ. (1985). Association between essential tremor and Parkinson's disease. *Ann Neurol* 17: 329–333.

Gortvai P. (1963). Deformities of the hands and feet in parkinsonism and their reversibility by operation. *J Neurol Neurosurg Psychiatry* 26: 33–36.

Grimes JD, Halle D, Hassan MN, Trent G, Armstrong G. (1986). Incidence and clinical features of scoliosis in Parkinson's disease. In: *VIII International Symposium on Parkinson's Disease*. New York, Raven Press.

Grimm RJ. (1984). Disorderly walks. In: Jankovic J (Ed.), *Movement Disorders*, Vol 2, *Neurologic Clinics*. Philadelphia, WB Saunders.

Haerer AF, Anderson DW, Schoenberg BS. (1982). Prevalence of essential tremor: results from the Copiah County study. *Arch Neurol* 39: 750–751.

Hallett M, Khoshbin S. (1980). A physiological mechanism of bradykinesia. *Brain* 103: 301–314.

Hoehn MM, Yahr MD. (1967). Parkinsonism: onset, progression and mortality. *Neurology* 17: 427–442.

Holmes G. (1922). Clinical symptoms of cerebellar disease and their interpretation. *Lancet* 1: 1231–1237.

Hunker CJ, Abbs JH, Barlow SM. (1982). The relationship between parkinsonian rigidity and hypokinesia in the orofacial system: a quantitative analysis. *Neurology* 32: 749–755.

Ito M. (1984). *The Cerebellum and Neural Control*. New York, Raven Press.

Jankovic J. (1982). Management of motor side effects of chronic levodopa therapy. *Clin Neuropharmacol Suppl* 1: S19–S28.

Jankovic J. (1984). Parkinsonian disorders. In: Appel SH (Ed.), *Current Neurology*, Vol 5. New York, John Wiley.

Jankovic J. (1985). Clinical features, differential diagnosis and pathogenesis of blepharospasm and cranial-cervical dystonia. *Adv Ophthal Plastic Reconstruct Surg* 4: 67–82.

Jankovic J. (1986a). Association between essential tremor and Parkinson's disease: A reply. *Ann Neurol.*

Jankovic J. (1986b). Respiratory dyskinesia in Parkinson's disease. *Neurology.*

Jankovic J, Fahn S. (1980). Physiologic and pathologic tremors: diagnosis, mechanism and management. *Ann Intern Med* 93: 460–465.

Jankovic J, Calne DB. (1987). Parkinson's disease: etiology and treatment. In: Appel SH (Ed.) *Current Neurology*, Vol. 7, Chicago, Year Book Medical Publishers (in press).

Jankovic J, Reches A. (1986). Parkinson's disease in monozygotic twins. *Ann Neurol* 19: 405–408.

Jankovic J, Frost JD. (1981). Quantitative assessment of parkinsonian and essential tremor: clinical application of triaxial accelerometry. *Neurology* 31: 1235–40.

Jenkyn LR, Reeves AG, Warren T, et al. (1984). Neurologic signs in senescence. *Arch Neurol* 42: 1154–1157.

Klawans HL. (1981). Hemiparkinsonism as a late amplification of hemiatrophy: a new syndrome. *Neurology* 31: 625–628.

Koller WC. (1984a). Diagnosis of Parkinson's disease. *Arch Intern Med* 144: 2146–2147.

Koller WC. (1984b). Sensory symptoms in Parkinson's disease. *Neurology* 34: 957–959.

Koller WC, Wilson RS, Glatt SL, Huckman MS, Fox JH. (1983). Senile gait: correlation with computer tomographic scans. *Ann Neurol* 13: 343–344.

Lakke JPWF. (1985). Axial apraxia in Parkinson's disease. *J Neurol Sci* 69: 37–46.

Lakke JPWF, Burg W, Wiegman J. (1982). Abnormalities in postural reflexes and voluntarily induced automatic movements in Parkinson patients. *Clin Neurol Neurosurg* 84: 227–235.

Lance JW, Schwab RS, Peterson EA. (1963). Action tremor and the cogwheel phenomenon in Parkinson's disease. *Brain* 86: 95–110.

Lee RG, Tatton WG. (1975). Motor responses to sudden limb displacements in primates with specific CNS lesions and in human patients with motor system disorders. *Can J Neurol Sci* 2: 285–293.

Lee RG, Stein RB. (1981). Resetting of tremor by mechanical perturbations: a comparison of essential tremor and parkinsonian tremor. *Ann Neurol* 10: 523–531.

Lee RG, Murphy JT, Tatton WG. (1983). Long-latency myotactic reflexes in man: mechanisms, functional significance, and changes in patients with

Parkinson's disease or hemiplegia. In: Desmedt J (Ed.), *Motor Control Mechanisms in Health and Disease*. New York, Raven Press.

Leport FE, Duvoisin RC. (1985). Apraxia of eyelid opening: an involuntary levator inhibition. *Neurology* 35: 423–427.

Llinas R, Jahnsen H. (1982). Electrophysiology of mammalian thalamic neurons in vitro. *Nature* 297: 406–408.

Marsden CD, Schachter M. (1981). Assessment of extrapyramidal disorders. *Br J Clin Pharmacol* 11: 129–151.

Marsden CD. (1982). The mysterious motor function of the basal ganglia. *Neurology* 32: 514–539.

Marsden CD, Parkes JD, Quinn N. (1982). Fluctuations of disability in Parkinson's disease: clinical aspects. In: Marsden CD, Fahn S (Eds.), *Movement Disorders*. London, Butterworth.

Marsden CD. (1984a). The pathophysiology of movement disorders. In: Jankovic J (Ed.), *The Neurologic Clinics*, Vol 2. Philadelphia, WB Saunders.

Marsden CD. (1984b). Function of the basal ganglia as revealed by cognitive and motor disorders in Parkinson's disease. *Can J Neurol Sci* 11: 129–135.

Martin WE, Loewenson RB, Resch JA, Baker AB. (1983). Parkinson's disease. Clinical analysis of 100 patients. *Neurology* 23: 783–790.

Matsumoto K, Rossomann F, Lin TH, Cooper IS. (1963). Studies on induced exacerbation of parkinsonian rigidity. The effect of contralateral voluntary activity. *J Neurol Neurosurg Psychiatry* 26: 27–32.

Mayeux, R. (1984). Behavioral manifestations of movement disorders. Parkinson's and Huntington's disease. In: Jankovic J (Ed.), *Neurologic Clinics*, Vol 2. Philadelphia, WB Saunders.

Meyer M, Adorjani C. (1983). Quantification of the effects of muscle relaxant drugs in man by tonic stretch reflex. In: Desmedt JE (Ed.), *Motor Control Mechanisms in Health and Disease*. New York, Raven Press.

Montgomery GK, Reynolds NC, Warren RM. (1985). Qualitative assessment of Parkinson's disease: study of reliability and data reduction with an abbreviated Columbia scale. *Clin Neuropharmacol* 8: 83–921.

Mortimer JA, Webster DD. (1979). Evidence for a quantitative association between EMG stretch responses and parkinsonian rigidity. *Brain Res* 162: 169–173.

Narabayashi H. (1980). Clinical analysis of akinesia. *J Neurol Trans* Suppl 16: 129–136.

Nausieda PA, Weiner WJ, Klawans HL. (1980). Dystonic foot response of parkinsonism. *Arch Neurol* 37: 132–136.

Newman RP, LeWitt PA, Jaffe M, Calne DB, Larsen TA. (1985). Motor function in the normal aging population: treatment with levodopa. *Neurology* 35: 571–573.

Parkinson J. (1817). *An Essay on the Shaking Palsy*. London, Sherwood, Neely, and Jones.

Pechadre JC, Larochelle L, Poirier LJ. (1976). Parkinsonian akinesia, rigidity and tremor in the monkey. Histopathological and neuropharmacological study. *J Neurol Sci* 28: 147–157.

Pirozzolo FJ, Jankovic J, Mahurin RK. (1985). Differentiation of choice reaction time performance in Parkinson's disease on the basis of motor symptoms. *Neurology* 35 (Suppl 1): 222.

Purdon-Martin J. (1967). *The Basal Ganglia and Posture*. Philadelphia, Lippincott.

Rafal RD, Posner MI, Walker JA, Friedrich FJ. (1984). Cognition and the basal ganglia: separating mental and motor components of performance in Parkinson's disease. *Brain* 107: 1083–1094.

Reches A. (1985). Noradrenergic influences on dopaminergic function and the pharmacology of dihydroxyphenyl serine (DOPS): implications for Parkinson's disease. *Clin Neuropharmacol* 8: 249–259.

Reichert WH, Doolittle J, McDowell FM. (1982). Vestibular dysfunction in Parkinson's disease. *Neurology* 32: 1133–1138.

Rothwell JL, Obeso JA, Traub MM, et al. (1983). The behavior of the long-latency stretch reflex in patients with Parkinson's disease. *J Neurol Neurosurg Psychiatry* 76: 35–44.

Sandyk R, Fleming J, Brennan MJW. (1982). The head retraction reflex—its specificity in Parkinson's disease. *Clin Neurol Neurosurg* 84: 157–160.

Schoenberg BS, Anderson DW, Haerer AF. (1985). Prevalence of Parkinson's disease in the biracial population of Copiah County, Mississippi. *Neurology* 35: 841–846.

Schwab RS, England AC, Peterson AC. (1959). Akinesia in Parkinson's disease. *Neurology* 9: 65–72.

Schultz W. (1984). Recent physiological and pathophysiological aspects of parkinsonian movement disorders. *Life Sci* 34: 2213–2223.

Snider SR, Fahn S, Isgreen WP, et al. (1979). Primary sensory symptoms in parkinsonism. *Neurology* 26: 423–429.

Snyder SH, D'Amato RJ. (1986). MPTP: a neurotoxin relevant to the pathophysiology of Parkinson's disease. *Neurology* 36: 250–258.

Stern GM, Lander CM, Lees AM. (1980). Akinetic freezing and trick movements in Parkinson's disease. *J Neurol Trans* Suppl 16: 137–141.

Stern Y, Mayeux R, Rosen J, Ilson J. (1983). Perceptual motor dysfunction in Parkinson's disease: a deficit in sequential and predictive voluntary movement. *J Neurol Neurosurg Psychiatry* 46: 145–151.

Sudarsky L, Ronthal M. (1983). Gait disorders among elderly patients. A survey study of 50 patients. *Arch Neurol* 40: 740–743.

Sunohara N, Mano Y, Ando K, Satoyoshi E. (1985). Idiopathic dystonia-parkinsonism with marked diurnal fluctuation of symptoms. *Ann Neurol* 17: 39–45.

Tatton WG, Eastovan MJ, Bedingham W, Verrier MC, Bruce IC. (1984). Defective utilization of sensory input as the basis for bradykinesia, rigidity and decreased movement repertoire in Parkinson's disease: a hypothesis. *Can J Neurol Sci* 11: 136–147.

Teräväinen H, Calne DB. (1980). Quantitative assessment of parkinsonian deficits. In: Rinne UK, Klingler M, Stamm G (Eds.), *Parkinson's Disease*.

Current Progress, Problems and Management. Amsterdam, Elsevier/North-Holland Biomedical Press.

Van der Linden C, Jankovic J, Jansson B. (1985). Lateral hypothalamic dysfunction in Parkinson's disease. *Ann Neurol* 18: 137-138.

Wagner HN. (1985). Probing the chemistry of the mind. *N Engl J Med* 312: 44-46.

Ward CD, Hess WA, Calne DB. (1983). Olfactory impairment in Parkinson's disease. *Neurology* 33: 943-946.

Ward CD, Sanes JN, Dambrosia JM, Calne DB. (1983). Methods for evaluating treatment in Parkinson's disease. In: Fahn S, Calne DB, Shoulson I (Eds.), *Experimental Therapeutics of Movement Disorders.* New York, Raven Press.

Weiner WJ, Nora LM, Glantz RH. (1984). Elderly inpatients: postural reflex impairment. *Neurology* 34: 945-947.

White OB, Saint-Cyr JA, Shapre JA. (1983). Ocular motor deficits in the early stages of Parkinson's disease. *Brain* 106: 555-570; 571-589.

Yokochi F, Nakamura R, Narabayashi H. (1985). Reaction time of patients with Parkinson's disease with reference to asymmetry of neurological signs. *J Neurol Neurosurg Psychiatry* 48: 702-705.

Zetusky WJ, Jankovic J, Pirozzolo FJ. (1985). The heterogeneity of Parkinson's disease: clinical and prognostic implications. *Neurology* 35: 522-526.

6
Mental State

RICHARD MAYEUX
Columbia University College of Physicians and Surgeons, New York, New York

Changes in the mental states of patients with Parkinson's disease are so frequently encountered that they are universally accepted as part of the disease and anticipated by most clinicians. During the last 15 years, a variety of behavioral syndromes have been described in Parkinson's disease. These disorders of intellectual and emotional function span the fields of neurology, neuropsychology, and psychiatry. However, there has been no attempt to develop a nosology of these syndromes in Parkinson's disease nor have diagnostic criteria been suggested by clinicians and investigators to aid in their recognition. A substantial amount of clinical and experimental data have been generated to formulate such an approach. This is a crucial step because future studies will need uniform research criteria to describe alterations in behavior, and individuals who assume responsibility for the care of these patients should have guidelines for diagnosis.

This chapter describes commonly encountered changes in the mental state of parkinsonian patients and offers a pertinent brief review of the literature concerning each syndrome, describing its clinical features and presumed pathogenesis. It is hoped that this review will provide the reader with suggested diagnostic criteria for mental changes in Parkinson's disease.

PSYCHIATRIC DISORDERS

Affective Disorders

Depression

Dysphoric mood is commonly encountered in Parkinson's disease (1–8). Naturally, it might be assumed that depression would occur frequently in a patient with a chronic disabling disease (9,10). However, several studies indicate that depression is more likely to be seen in parkinsonian patients than in other equally disabled individuals (1,4,5). Although Mindham et al. (11) consider Parkinson's disease unique compared to other degenerative diseases because of its biochemistry, controls matched for age and disability are not found to be depressed as often as are parkinsonian patients. This fact, combined with the observation that severity of depression does not relate to the degree of disability resulting from Parkinson's disease (7,12) has led some investigators to a search for an explanation for depression in Parkinson's disease.

Usually depression is of moderate to mild intensity as noted in Table 1, and suicide is rare. Depression is occasionally, but not consistently, related to age, duration of disease, treatment, and sex of the patient (7). In several studies (7), depression was assessed by clinical inquiry or by the use of a depression rating scale, such as the Hamilton Depression Scale (13); these may not be diagnostically accurate in Parkinson's disease because certain symptoms and signs of parkinsonism occur with depression. Nevertheless, these studies suggest that about 40% of patients with Parkinson's disease will become depressed during their illness. However, as many as 25% of these patients may experience depression prior to the onset of overt motor manifestations of Parkinson's disease or within a year of their onset. In some, depression can be associated with mild intellectual dysfunction (6).

Depression in Parkinson's disease does not consistently respond to any of the usual forms of therapy including dopamine agonists, tricyclic antidepressants, or electroconvulsive therapy (14-20). In view of some recent biochemical observations relating to this syndrome in Parkinson's disease, trials of serotonergic agonists may be warranted.

Mayeux and associates (21) found two depression syndromes in a group of parkinsonian patients: major depression: a chronic dysphoric mood associated

TABLE 1 Characteristics of Depression in Parkinson's Disease

Prevalence: 25–40%

Precedes or develops within 1 year of onset of motor manifestations in 15–25%

Mild to moderate intensity; rare suicide

Mild intellectual changes may coexist

Inconsistently related to

  severity of PD

  age

  sex

  medication

---

with changes in appetite, sleep and concentration, and accompanied by psycho-motor retardation; dysthymic disorder: a similar but intermittent mood disturbance with periods of relatively normal mood (8,21). In all patients with depression, a reduction in the cerebrospinal fluid (CSF) content of the metabolite of serotonin, 5-hydroxyindoleacetic acid (5-HIAA) was observed. However, the greatest reduction in CSF 5-HIAA was in those patients with major depression syndrome. This observation has important implications because it has been suggested that serotonin has a major role in the regulation of mood (22), and it has been observed that persistent disorders of serotonin metabolism can predispose to depression (22–26). This is obviously relevant to Parkinson's disease because Hornykiewicz (27) and others (28–31) have found the brain content of serotonin reduced at postmortem in some parkinsonians. Decarboxylation of amino acids in the raphe nuclei, the site of serotonin production, is also diminished in Parkinson's disease and in depressives (32,33).

Some evidence suggests that depressed parkinsonian patients represent a unique subgroup of Parkinson's disease; there is a greater frequency of psychopathology in their families (34), and they may be younger at the onset of motor disability (35). A more benign course as well as a family history of parkinsonism has also been described (35).

Criteria for the diagnosis of depression in Parkinson's disease should include those for major depression and dysthymic disorder syndromes listed in the third edition of the *Diagnostic and Statistical Manual of Mental Disorders* (*DSM-III*) (36). An abbreviated version of these criteria is listed in Table 2. Many patients experience symptoms of depression at times during the illness, but diagnosis and treatment should be guided by *DSM-III* criteria because of the overlap with other symptoms and signs commonly encountered in Parkinson's disease.

The diagnosis of depression in patients with Parkinson's disease can be difficult because of the physical signs of bradykinesia and hypomimia. Some vegetative signs, such as fatigue, insomnia, anorexia, diminished concentration, and loss of interest can also occur in parkinsonian patients who are not depressed. For these reasons, the diagnostic criteria are extremely useful as guidelines for the clinician.

Mania and Bipolar Illness

Neither of these two syndromes has been described in patients with Parkinson's disease. In a study (21) of 49 consecutively encountered parkinsonian patients only one met criteria for a manic episode (personal communication) and that was at least 20 years prior to the onset of motor signs of Parkinson's disease. There are a few reports in the literature of parkinsonian patients with a schizophrenic-like illness accompanied by depression (37). These patients could have had an unrecognized bipolar syndrome but little evidence supports that assumption. A single patient with bipolar affective disorder with mostly mania is known

TABLE 2 Criteria for Diagnosis of Depression

Major depression

Dysphoric mood or loss of interest or pleasure in all or almost all usual activities and pasttimes. May be characterized by descriptions of mood such as: depressed, sad, blue, hopeless, low, down-in-the-dumps.

At least four of the following symptoms should be present every day for at least 2 weeks:

Change in weight or appetite;

Insomnia or hypersomnia

Psychomotor agitation or retardation

Loss of interest

Fatigue

Guilt

Difficulty concentrating

Suicidal thoughts or ideas

Dysthymic disorder

Symptoms of depression for at least 2 years

"Normal" mood intermittant

Depressive periods with symptoms such as feeling blue, sad, etc.

At least three of the following symptoms:

Change in sleep

Change in appetite or weight

Fatigue

Loss of self-esteem

Diminished concentration

Social withdrawal

Loss of interest

Irritability

Inactivity

Tearful

Pessimism

Loss of pleasure

Recurrent thoughts of death or suicide

to this author. She developed Parkinson's disease several years after the onset of her psychiatric disorder, at age 25. Treatment has been difficult because dopamine agonists exacerbate her mania and lithium increases the motor disability from parkinsonism. Such a rare psychiatric disorder in Parkinson's disease suggests that it may be coincidental. Criteria for bipolar disorder and mania should be those suggested by *DSM-III* (36).

Anxiety Disorders

This is also an uncommon psychiatric occurrence in idiopathic Parkinson's disease. However, since this group of disorders occurs in 2-4% of the general population, it can be anticipated in Parkinson's disease as well.

Phobic Disorders

These symptoms are characterized by an irrational fear. Certainly parkinsonian patients experience fear of falling, fear of crowds, as well as other social phobias. These disorders are rare prior to the onset of Parkinson's disease, which suggests that they are secondary or reactive psychiatric disabilities. Typically, phobic disorders begin in the late teens and twenties, and can last a lifetime. Diagnostic criteria for phobic disorders exclude patients with depression; Parkinson's disease can coexist and this combination may be encountered. *DSM-III* criteria (36) for social phobia should be utilized for diagnosis in Parkinson's disease.

Anxiety Neurosis

This disorder is also common and may occur in patients with Parkinson's disease. However, there is no increased risk for this syndrome with Parkinson's disease. Generalized fear, motor tension, and autonomic hyperactivity can be observed in anxiety neurosis and are often present in Parkinson's disease. These symptoms may also be exacerbated by the use of dopamine agonists, particularly during episodes of drug-induced hyperkinesis (38). Criteria for the diagnosis of anxiety neurosis, not related to drugs, should be those in *DSM-III* (36).

Psychosis

Typically, hallucinations or delusions are drug-induced or are toxic manifestations of the therapy of Parkinson's disease. Mjones (39) and others (37) have described patients with Parkinson's disease who developed an idiopathic schizophrenia-like illness. Since no criteria for the diagnosis of schizophrenia are used in either report, the diagnoses could be questioned and others have not confirmed this association (3,40-42). In spite of this problem, the possible coexistence of these two disorders is of great interest because of the dopamine hypothesis of schizophrenia; increased dopamine has been implicated as a cause of schizophrenia. The diagnosis of an organic psychosis (hallucinations or de-

TABLE 3 Diagnostic Criteria for Organic Hallucinations or Delusions

Persistent or recurrent perceptual disturbance is the predominent clinical feature

No impairment of consciousness and no evidence of delirium, dementia, or depression.

lusions) in Parkinson's disease requires the absence of delirium or dementia and some proof that the cause is related to Parkinson's disease and not its treatment (36).

Premorbid Personality

Many studies attempt to identify a premorbid personality type in Parkinson's disease (43-47). All are retrospective and therefore subject to criticism, but there is a great deal of agreement. The parkinsonian patient is usually depicted as diffident, introspective, passive, and lacking emotional and moral flexibility. Several investigations have found depression to occur in at least 25% of patients before overt signs of parkinsonism are present (6,39). It is difficult to generalize from these studies and, to paraphrase Todes and Lees (47), it remains unclear whether these behavioral traits are relevant causative factors or prodromal symptoms in Parkinson's disease.

Drug-Related Disorders

Nearly every medication used in the treatment of Parkinson's disease, including anticholinergics, amantadine, levodopa, and more recent dopamine agonists, such as pergolide, is known to cause some type of psychiatric disorder (3,48-53). These toxic manifestations can range from simple confusional states to complex hallucinations. Parkinsonian patients with preexisting intellectual impairment seem to be at greater risk for this complication of therapy (54).

Delirium

This is usually characterized by an abrupt onset of clouding of consciousness, disorientation, and memory loss (see Table 4). Hallucinations, confusion (inability to maintain a coherent train of thought), agitation or apathy, and altered sleep-wake cycle (55) are also present in some patients. This problem is so common in parkinsonian patients that it is often difficult to implicate any one particular medication. The majority of patients developing this complication are demented (56-58), slightly older than the typical patient (56-58), and may have had similar problems with other classes of medication used in the treatment of Parkinson's disease (53).

Postmortem studies in Parkinson's disease indicate a reduction in biochemical and morphologic markers of cholinergic metabolism in some parkinsonian pa-

TABLE 4 Diagnostic Criteria for Delirium

Impaired consciousness
At least two of the following:
Illusions, hallucinations
Incoherent speech
Disturbed sleep–wake cycle
Increased or decreased psychomotor activity
Disorientation (memory impairment)
Rapid onset and evaluation: may fluctuate

Source: Modified from *DSM-III*.

tients that may explain why anticholinergics are so frequently the cause of this problem (56). However, delirium and confusion can also occur in younger patients who are not demented and who are not using anticholinergics (56). In this group, the prevalence of delirium increases linearly with duration of dopamine agonist therapy. Generally, discontinuation of the medication results in improvement, but this is not always true; delusions can remain persistent.

"Benign Hallucinations"

A few parkinsonian patients will experience vivid visual hallucinations during treatment with any antiparkinson agent without meeting criteria for delirium or dementia. Insight is usually preserved. A reduction in dosage of the offending agent may improve the clinical situation. No published criteria for this diagnosis are present, but it closely resembles organic hallucinosis (36) if the cause is found to be the drug in question.

Sexual Disorders

A number of investigators have noted increased libido in parkinsonian patients while on levodopa (49,57). An improvement in sexual function may be the result of improved physical activity, but hypersexuality has also been described. Increased sexual behavior usually occurs in the presence of delirium, and in some instances a relationship between peak levels of levodopa and hypersexuality has been observed (60,61). No specific psychosexual disorder (see *DSM-III*) has been related to levodopa; disinhibition of sexual impulses is most often described. There are no specific criteria for this disorder unless it occurs as a manifestation of delirium (36).

Depression

While levodopa (3,59) and other dopamine agonists (62) are occasionally useful as antidepressants, more often there is little to no improvement in depression

(63). Levodopa may exacerbate a premorbid depression (64) and was implicated in a suicide (65).

DEMENTIA AND INTELLECTUAL IMPAIRMENT

Dementia is probably the most controversial aspect of mental changes in Parkinson's disease. The literature in this area suffers from a lack of consistency in clinical diagnosis and all of the postmortem studies are retrospective. Nevertheless, dementia is probably the most frequent reason dopamine agonists are discontinued (66). Parkinsonian patients who become demented are unique because they are usually older at the onset of Parkinson's disease and have a more rapid course with an unpredictable response to levodopa (58,67).

The prevalence of dementia is difficult to estimate since uniform criteria have not been used; many epidemiologic studies did not include dementia as a manifestation of Parkinson's disease. However, an estimate can be obtained from three independent studies (3,67,68) in which similar clinical rating scales were used to judge dementia; 35-40% of nearly 1,000 parkinsonian patients were considered significantly impaired. These patients would probably meet current *DSM-III* criteria for primary degenerative dementia (36). An additional 10-15% were somewhat less impaired (3). These studies led Lieberman et al. (67) to propose that the risk for dementia was increased by 10 in Parkinson's disease. However, Brow and Marsden (69) and others (70-72) believe that this figure is inflated. Recent prospective studies indicate that only 8-10% of patients may actually meet criteria for primary degenerative dementia (70,72). The prevalence of dementia, even with these strict criteria, may still be greater in parkinsonian patients than that expected for a similar aged population (73).

Primary Degenerative Dementia

At present, the frequency of this syndrome can only be estimated because few studies have included appropriate criteria for this diagnosis. *DSM-III* criteria for primary degenerative dementia (36) are listed in a modified fashion in Table 5. Clinical studies of neuropsychologic function in demented parkinsonian patients indicate both a recent and retrograde memory disorder (74-78). The pattern of impairment is similar to that observed in equally demented patients with probable Alzheimer's disease (79), but in that study only 38.6% (22/57) of parkinsonian patients met *DSM-III* criteria for dementia (36).

Some biochemical and pathologic studies suggest that demented parkinsonian patients may have coexistent Alzheimer's disease. Cortical neuronal degeneration and "Alzheimer-type tangles" are seen in postmortem brain of patients with Parkinson's disease (58,80-85), and these patients are usually demented (58). In three different investigations (83-85), a morphology similar to that in

TABLE 5   Criteria for Dementia

Loss of intellectual skill sufficient to impair social or occupational function
Memory impairment
At least two of the following:
Impaired abstraction
Impaired judgment
Aphasia
Apraxia
Agnosia
Constructional difficulty
Personality change
No impairment of consciousness

Alzheimer's disease was noted and included senile plaques, neurofibrillary tangles, and granulovacular degeneration in greater quantity in parkinsonian brains than in those of age-matched controls. However, a correlation between severity of dementia and the intensity of the senile changes was present only in a few patients (58). In some demented parkinsonian patients choline acetyl-transferase activity (CAT) is reduced (86,87) and there is also a reduction in the number of cells in the cholinergic nuclei of the basal forebrain (85). However, Perry et al. (87) have noted that CAT may be reduced without morphologic evidence of Alzheimer's disease; this implies that the cholinergic deficit might be a primary biochemical abnormality in Parkinson's disease and not evidence of co-existent Alzheimer's disease. Norepinephrine, serotonin, and somatostatin concentrations are also reduced in the brains of demented patients with Parkinson's disease (88,89), but these data were also collected retrospectively and were not always specific to dementia. A prospective study of primary degenerative dementia in patients with Parkinson's disease will be required before conclusions regarding the frequency and the cause of this problem can be clarified.

Bradyphrenia

This disorder of intellectual function is difficult to distinguish from dementia. It is characterized by a slowing of thought processes, diminished concentration, and inattention. Birkmayer et al. (38) suggest that bradyphrenia only gives a superficial impression of dementia, and that it is the psychological equivalent of akinesia. In their experience general intellectual functions, such as judgment or concept formation, are unchanged. Attention and concentration could be impaired in a patient with primary degenerative dementia, but memory and overall

TABLE 6   Suggested Criteria for Diagnosis of Bradyphrenia

Persistent impairment of attention and vigilance

No evidence of impaired consciousness, associated with dimentia, or depression

Insidious onset with little daily fluctuation

intelligence should remain intact in patients with bradyphrenia, thus allowing the differentiation.

In a prospective investigation in which bradyphrenia was measured by reaction time and accuracy in a continuous performance task, nondemented patients with Parkinson's disease performed similar to patients with Alzheimer's disease and controls. However, demented parkinsonians had slower reaction times and were less vigilant than equally demented patients with Alzheimer's disease. CSF concentration of 3-methoxy-4-hydroxyphenylglycol (MHPG), the major metabolite of norepinephrine, increased as performance on these tasks of vigilance and attention worsened (91). A similar relationship has been observed by Mann et al. (92) relative to recent memory and digit span. The reason for this paradoxical increase in a metabolite is unclear because blockade of the post-synaptic noradrenergic receptor will increase the concentration of the metabolite, as will increased turnover and reduced clearance. Degeneration of the locus ceruleus, the brain stem site of norepinephrine production, undergoes degeneration in Parkinson's disease. This may result in bradyphrenia or mental slowing in Parkinson's disease (93) since the ceruleocortical pathways into the cortex are critical for the maintenance of attention and vigilance (94). Diagnostic criteria are not established for bradyphrenia; a suggested outline for the diagnosis is offered in Table 6.

Executive Function

This heterogenous group of disorders includes perceptual, motor, and visuospatial impairment. These may not be specifically mentioned by the patient or family. However, these problems may underlie frequent falls, difficulty driving an automobile, and other tasks that require coordination of mental and motor functions. It has been suggested that a disturbance in the frontal lobe-basal ganglia connections are responsible for the perceptual, spatial, and motor behavior deficits seen in Parkinson's disease (95–97). Defective performance in tasks such as block design, drawing and construction tasks, tracing, judgment of visual/vertical, prism adaptation, and route or map walking has been demonstrated (98–108). Flowers (102) and Stern et al. (107,108) believe the basis of these visuospatial disorders to be a defect in predictive and sequential voluntary movements. There is evidence suggesting that this problem parallels disease severity (109) and increases in frequency with duration of illness (110). Obviously, visuospatial deficits increase with dementia, but are apparent in nondemented parkinsonian patients as well (107,108). Clinically, patients might misjudge steps or the distance required for a turn while walking. These "everyday" motor skills require perceptual input, and perhaps the use and formation of motor programs to carry out such tasks (111). In Parkinson's disease, this visuospatial deficit may be caused by the degenerative process in the basal ganglia or, as suggested by Javoy-Agid and Agid (112), loss of dopamine in the frontal cortex. The loss of dopamine results in bradykinesia and many of the other motor manifestations of Parkinson's disease. Correlations observed between bradykinesia and intellectual impairment could similarly implicate the dopamine system as a cause of mental decline (76,77,90).

There are no specific criteria for the diagnosis of visuospatial disorders in Parkinson's disease. The prevalence of these problems is probably quite high, and may be the earliest cognitive disorders in the parkinsonian patient (113). Pirozzolo et al. (76) found that performance on the digit symbol subtest of the Wechsler Adult Intelligence scale measuring visuospatial skills, was impaired in 79% of patients with Parkinson's disease.

Language Disorders

A variety of speech disorders are seen in Parkinson's disease including motor dysarthria, hypophonia, tachyphemia, palilalia, and mutism (114). Language function remains intact, however. In some patients a word production anomia occurs, termed "tip-of-the-tongue" anomia (115). Parkinsonian patients with this syndrome cannot generate words without a phonemic cue, whereas visual naming ability remains relatively spared. Patients may report this as a poor memory, but that function is usually intact. Anomia can also occur in association with dementia in Parkinson's disease (116).

COMMENTS

In this brief review, a number of psychiatric syndromes and intellectual deficits have been described. However, from the current literature it is difficult to determine the exact prevalence or the expected incidence of these problems in patients with Parkinson's disease. Are mental changes inherent to Parkinson's disease? The answer to this question is most definitely yes. A review of three distinct syndromes support this view.

1. MPTP-induced parkinsonism represents a pure dopamine deficiency syndrome, and it appears that no other neurotransmitter system is involved (117). Stern and Langston (118) found visuospatial skills and executive functions impaired in these patients compared to age-matched controls, which suggest that dopamine reduction was responsible, at least in part, for some of the intellectual changes noted in idiopathic Parkinson's disease.

2. Depression in some patients without Parkinson's disease is linked to a defect in the serotonergic system. Serotonin content in the brain is reduced in some parkinsonian patients and Mayeux et al. (21) have observed a relationship between a CSF measure of serotonin and depression in Parkinson's disease. This implies that all patients with Parkinson's disease will be at greater risk for depression than the general population.

3. Primary degenerative dementia is likely the result of a disorder of cholinergic metabolism. Perry et al. (87) offer convincing evidence that a primary cholinergic deficit can be present in some parkinsonian patients with this diagnosis.

These three examples illustrate the advances recently made that improve our understanding of Parkinson's disease and indicate the need to broaden our definition of the syndrome of parkinsonism to include the mental changes. Parkinson has been maligned for not including mental changes in his description of the "shaking palsy." Perhaps we should now adopt his final comments:

> Before concluding these pages, it may be proper to observe once more, that an important object proposed to be obtained by them is, the leading of the attention of those who humanely employ anatomical examination in detecting the causes and nature of diseases, particularly to this [Parkinson's disease] malady. By their benevolent labors its real nature may be ascertained, and appropriate modes of relief, or even of cure, be pointed out (119).

ACKNOWLEDGMENT

This work was supported in part by a grant from the National Institutes of Health (AG-02802) and the Parkinson's Disease Foundation.

REFERENCES

1. Warburton JW. (1967). Depressive symptoms in parkinson patients referred for thalamotomy. *J Neurol Neurosurg Psychiatry* 30: 368–70.
2. Brown GL. (1972). Parkinsonism and depression. *South Med J* 65: 540–5.
3. Celesia GG, Wanamaker WM. (1972). Psychiatric disturbances in Parkinson's disease. *Dis Nerv Syst* 33: 577–83.
4. Horn S. (1974). Some psychological factors in parkinsonism. *J Neurol Neurosurg Psychiatry* 37: 27–31.
5. Robins AH. (1976). Depression in patients with parkinsonism. *Br J Psychiatry* 128: 141–145.
6. Mayeux R, Stern Y, Rosen J, Leventhal J. (1981). Depression, intellectual impairment and Parkinson's disease. *Neurology* 31: 645–650.
7. Mayeux R. (1982). Depression and dementia in Parkinson's disease. In: Marsden CD, Fahn S, eds., *Movement Disorders*, London: Butterworth, 75–95.

8. Mayeux R, Williams JBW, Stern Y, Cote L. Depression and Parkinson's disease. *Adv Neurol* 40: 241–50.

9. DePaulo JR, Folstein MF. (1978). Psychiatric disturbances in neurological patients: detection, recognition and hospital course. *Ann Neurol* 4: 225–228.

10. Kathol RG, Petty F. (1981). Relationship of depression to medical illness. *J Affect Dis* 3: 111–21.

11. Mindham RHS, Marsden CD, Parkes JD. (1976). Psychiatric symptoms during L-dopa therapy for Parkinson's disease and their relationship to physical disability. *Psychiatr Med* 6: 23–33.

12. Serby M. (1980). Psychiatric issues in Parkinson's disease. *Comp Psychiatry* 21: 317–321.

13. Hamilton M. (1960). A rating scale for depression. *J Neurol Neurosurg Psychiatry* 23: 56–62.

14. Strang RR. (1965). Imipramine in the treatment of parkinsonism: a double-blind placebo study. *Br J Med* 2: 33–34.

15. Laitinen L. (1969). Desipramine in the treatment of Parkinson's disease. *Acta Neurol Scand* 45: 109–113.

16. Marsh GG, Markham CH. (1973). Does levodopa alter depression and psychopathology in parkinsonism patients? *J Neurol Neurosurg Psychiatry* 36: 925–935.

17. Lebensohn Z, Jenkins RB. (1975). Improvement of parkinsonism in depressed patients with ECT. *Am J Psychiatry* 132: 283–285.

18. Asnis G. (1977). Parkinson's disease, depression and ECT: a review and case study. *Am J Psychiatry* 134: 191–195.

19. Yudofsky SC. (1979). Parkinson's disease, depression and electroconvulsive therapy: a clinical and neurobiologic synthesis. *Comp Psychiatry* 20: 579–581.

20. Anderson J, Aabro E, Gulman N, Hjelmsted A, Pedersen HE. (1980). Antidepressant treatment of Parkinson's disease. *Acta Neurol Scand* 62: 210–219.

21. Mayeux R, Stern Y, Cote L, Williams JBW. (1984). Altered serotonin metabolism in depressed patients with Parkinson's disease. *Neurology* 34: 642–6.

22. van Praag HM. (1982). Depression. *Lancet* 2: 1259–64.

23. van Praag HH. (1982). Serotonin precursors in the treatment of depression. In: Ho BT, Schoolar JC, Usdin E (Eds.), *Serotonin in Biological Psychiatry*. New York, Raven Press.

24. Coppen A, Wood K. (1982). 5-Hydroxytryptamine in the pathogenesis of affective disorders. In: Ho BT, Schoolar JC, Usdin E (Eds.), *Serotonin in Biological Psychiatry*. New York, Raven Press.

25. van Praag HM, de Haan S. (1979). Central serotonin metabolism and frequency of depression. *Psychiatr Res* 1: 219–24.

26. Asberg M, Traskman L. (1981). Studies of CSF 5-HIAA in depression and suicidal behavior. In: Haber B, Gabay S, Issidovides MR, Alivisatos SGA (Eds.), *Serotonin*. New York, Plenum Press.

27. Hornykiewicz O. (1982). Brain neurotransmitter changes in Parkinson's disease. In: Marsden CD, Fahn S (Eds.), *Movement Disorders*. London, Butterworth.

28. Bernheimer H, Birkmayer W, Hornykiewicz O. (1963). Zur Biochemie des Parkinson-syndroms des menschen: Einfluss der monoaminoxydase-hemmer-therapie auf die konzentration des dopamins, nornadrenalins and 5 hydroxytryptamine in gehivn. *Wien Klin Wochenschr* 41: 465–469.

29. Bernheimer H, Hornykiewicz O. (1964). Das verhalten des dopamin-metaoliten homovanillin saure in gehivn von normalen und parkinson-kranken menschen, *Arch Exp Path Pharmacol* 247: 305–306.

30. Bernheimer H, Hornykiewicz O. (1965). Herabgesetzte konzentration der homovanillinsaure im gehirv von parkinsonkranken menschen als ausdruck der storung de zentralen dopaminstoffwechsels. *Wien Klin Wochenschr* 43: 711–715.

31. Fahn S, Libsch LR, Cutler RW. (1971). Monoamines in the human neo-striatum: Topographic distribution in normals and in Parkinson's disease and their rate in akinesia, rigidity, chorea and tremor. *J Neurol Sci* 14: 427–455.

32. Lloyd KJ, Farley IJ, Deck JHN, Hornykiewicz O. (1974). Serotonin and 5-hydroxyindoleacetic acid in discrete areas of the brainstem in suicidal victims and control patients. *Adv Biochem Psychopharmacol* 11: 387–397.

33. Birkmayer W, Riederer P. (1975). Biochemical postmortem findings in depressed patients. *J Neurol Transm* 37: 95–109.

34. Winokur A, Dugan J, Mendels J, Hurtig HI. (1978). Psychiatric illness in relatives of patients with Parkinson's disease: an expanded survey. *Am J Psychiatry* 135: 854–5.

35. Santamaria J, Tolosa E, Valles A. Parkinson's disease with depression: a possible subgroup of idiopathic parkinsonism. *Neurology* 36: 1130–33.

36. American Psychiatric Association. (1980). *Diagnostic and Statistical Manual of Mental Disorders*, Third Edition. Washington, D.C.

37. Crow JJ, Johnstone ED, McClelland HA. (1976). The coincidence of schizophrenia and parkinsonism: some neurochemical implications. *Psychol Med* 6: 227–33.

38. Birkmayer W, Danielczyk W, Riederer P. (1983). Symptoms and side effects in the course of Parkinson's disease. *J Neurol Trans* 19: 185–199.

39. Mjones SH. (1949). Paralysis agitans: clinical and genetic study. *Acta Psychiatr Neurol Suppl* 54: 1–195.

40. Patrick HT, Levy DM. (1922). Parkinson's disease. A clinical study of 146 cases. *Arch Neurol Psychiatry* 7: 711–720.

41. Mindham RHS. (1970). Psychiatric syndromes in parkinsonism. *J Neurol Neurosurg Psychiatry* 30: 188–91.

42. Mindham RHS. (1974). Psychiatric aspects of Parkinson's disease. *Br J Hosp Med* II: 411–414.

43. Sands JJ. (1942). The type of personality susceptible to Parkinson's disease. *J Mt. Sinai Hosp* 9: 792–801.

44. Machover S. (1957). Rorschach study on the nature and origin of common factors in the personalities of parkinsonians. *Psychosom Med* 19: 33.
45. Ogawa T. (1981). Personality characteristics of Parkinson's disease. *Percept Motor Skills* 52: 375–8.
46. Poewe W, Gerstenbrand F, Ransmayr G, Plorer S. (1983). Premorbid personality in Parkinson patients. *J Neurol Trans* 19: 215–224.
47. Todes CJ, Lees AJ. (1985). The premorbid personality of patients with Parkinson's disease. *J Neurol Neurosurg Psychiatry* 48: 97–100.
48. Celesia GG, Barr AN. (1970). Psychosis and other psychiatric manifestations of levodopa therapy. *Arch Neurol* 23: 193–200.
49. Goodwin FK. (1971). Psychiatric side effects of levodopa in man. *JAMA* 218: 1915–20.
50. Sweet RD, McDowell FH, Feigenson JS, Lormanger AW, Goodell H. (1976). Mental symptoms in Parkinson's disease during chronic treatment with levodopa. *Neurology* 26: 305–310.
51. Serby M, Angrist B, Lieberman A. (1978). Mental disturbances during bromocriptine and lergotrile treatment of Parkinson's disease. *Am J Psychiatry* 135: 1227–29.
52. Tanner CM, Vogel C, Goetz CG, Klawans HL. (1983). Hallucinations in Parkinson's disease: a population study. *Ann Neurol* 14: 136.
53. Stern Y, Mayeux R, Ilson J, Fahn S, Cote L. (1984). Pergolide treatment of Parkinson's disease: neurobehavioral changes. *Neurology* 34: 201–203.
54. Sacks OW, Krohl MS, Messeloff CR, Schwartz WF. (1972). Effects of levodopa in parkinsonian patients with dementia. *Neurology* 22: 615–619.
55. Nausieda PA, Glantz R, Weber S, Baum R, Klawans HL. (1984). Psychiatric complications of levodopa therapy of Parkinson's disease. In: Hassler RG, Christ JF (Eds.), *Parkinson-specific Motor and Mental Disorders*. New York, Raven Press.
56. Desmet Y, Ruberg M, Serdara M, Dubois B, Lhermitte F, Agid Y. (1982). Confusion, dementia and anticholinergics in Parkinson's disease. *J Neurol Neurosurg Psychiatry* 45: 1161–1164.
57. Boller F. (1980). Mental status of patients with Parkinson's disease. *J Clin Neuropsychiatry* 2: 157–72.
58. Boller F, Mizutani T, Roessmann U, Gambetti P. (1980). Parkinson's disease, dementia and Alzheimer's disease: clinicopathological correlations. *Ann Neurol* 1: 329–335.
59. Barbeau A. (1969). L-dopa therapy in Parkinson's disease: a critical review of nine years experience. *J Can Med Assoc* 101: 791–800.
60. O'Brien C, DiGiacomo JN, Fahn S, Schwartz GA. (1971). Mental effects of high dosage levodopa. *Arch Gen Psychiatry* 24: 61–64.
61. Quinn NP, Toone B, Lang AE. (1983). Dopa dose-dependent sexual deviation. *Br J Psychiatry* 142: 296–298.
62. Waehrens J, Gerlach J. (1981). Bromocriptine and imipramine in endogenous depression. *J Affect Dis* 3: 193–202.
63. Damasio AR, Lobo-Antunes J, Macedo C. (1981). Psychiatric aspects in parkinsonism treated with L-dopa. *J Neurol Neurosurg Psychiatry* 34: 502–507.

64. Marsh GG, Markham CH. (1973). Does levodopa alter depression and psychopathology in parkinsonian patients? *J Neurol Neurosurg Psychiatry* 36: 925–935.

65. Raft D, Newman M, Spencer R. (1972). Suicide on L-dopa. *South Med J* 65: 312.

66. Lesser RP, Fahn S, Snider SR, Cote LJ, Isgreen WP, Barrett RE. (1979). Analysis of the clinical problems in parkinsonism and the complications of long-term levodopa therapy. *Neurology* 29: 1253–60.

67. Lieberman A, Dziatolowski M, Kupersmith M, Cerb M, Goodgold A, Lorein J, Goldstein M. (1979). Dementia in Parkinson's disease. *Ann Neurol* 6: 355–9.

68. Marttila RJ, Rinne UK. (1976). Dementia in Parkinson's disease. *Acta Neurol Scand* 54: 431–41.

69. Brown RG, Marsden CD. (1984). How common is dementia in Parkinson's disease? *Lancet* 1: 1262–5.

70. Rajput AH, Offord K, Beard CM, Kurland LT. (1984). Epidemiological survey of dementia in parkinsonism and control population. In: Hassler RG, Christ JF (Eds.), *Parkinson-Specific Motor and Mental Disorders*. New York, Raven Press.

71. Lees AJ. (1985). Parkinson's disease and dementia. *Lancet* 1: 43–4.

72. Taylor A, Saint-Cyr JA, Lang AE. (1985). Dementia prevalence in Parkinson's disease. *Lancet* 1: 1037.

73. Mindham RH, Ahmed SWA, Clough CG. (1982). A controlled study of dementia in Parkinson's disease. *J Neurol Neurosurg Psychiatry* 45: 969–974.

74. Halgin R, Riklan M, Misiak H. (1977). Levodopa, parkinsonism and recent memory. *J Nerv Ment Dis* 164: 268–272.

75. Wilson RS, Kaszniak AW, Klawans HL, Garron DC. (1980). High speed memory scanning in parkinsonism. *Cortex* 16: 67–72.

76. Pirozzolo FJ, Hansch EC, Mortimer JA, Webster DD, Kuskowski MA. (1982). Dementia in Parkinson's disease: a neuropsychological analysis. *Brain Cognition* 1: 71–83.

77. Mayeux R, Stern Y. (1983). Intellectual dysfunction and dementia in Parkinson's disease. In: Mayeux R, Rosen W (Eds.), *The Dementias*. New York, Raven Press.

78. Freedman M, Rivdira P, Butters N, Sax DS, Feldman RG. (1984). Retrograde amnesia in Parkinson's disease. *Can J Neurol Sci* 11: 297–301.

79. Mayeux R, Stern Y, Rosen J, Benson DF. (1983). Is "subcortical dementia" a recognizable clinical entity? *Ann Neurol* 14: 278–283.

80. Alvord EC. (1965). The pathology of parkinsonism: etiologic, pathogenetic and prognostic implications. *Trans Am Neurol Assoc* 90: 167–8.

81. Alvord EC, Forno LS, Kusske JA, Kauffman RJ, Rhodes JS, Goetowski CR. (1975). The pathology of Parkinsonism: A comparison of degenerations in cerebral cortex and brainstem. *Adv Neurol* 5: 175–93.

82. Hakim AM, Mathieson G. (1978). Basis of dementia in Parkinson's disease. *Lancet* 2: 729.

83. Hakim AM, Mathieson G. (1979). Dementia in Parkinson's disease: a neuropathologic study. *Neurology* 29: 1209–14.

84. Forno LS. (1982). Pathology of Parkinson's disease. In: Marsden CD, Fahn S. (Eds.), *Movement Disorders*. London, Butterworth.

85. Whitehouse P, Hedreen JC, White C, DeLong M, Price DL. (1983). Basal forebrain neurons in dementia of Parkinson's disease. *Ann Neurol* 13: 243–248.

86. Rubert M, Ploska A, Javoy-Agid F, Agid Y. (1982). Muscarinic binding and choline acetyltransferase activity in parkinsonian subjects with reference for dementia. *Brain Res* 232: 129–33.

87. Perry RH, Tomlinson BE, Candy JM, Blessed G, Foster JF, Blaxham CA, Perry E. (1983). Cortical cholinergic deficit in mentally impaired parkinsonian patients. *Lancet* 309: 789–90.

88. Epelbaum J, Ruberg M, Moyse E, Javoy-Agid F, Dubois B, Agid Y. (1983). Somatostatin and dementia in Parkinson's disease. *Brain Res* 278: 376–379.

89. Gray F, Gaspar P, Ruberg M, Dubois B, Agid F, Escourolle R, Agid Y. Neuropathology and biochemistry of demented and non demented parkinsonian subjects. *Acta Neuropathol*.

90. Stern Y, Mayeux R, Cote L. (1984). Reaction time and vigilance in Parkinson's disease: Possible role of altered norepinephrine metabolism. *Arch Neurol* 41: 1086–1089.

91. Mayeux R, Stern Y, Sano M, Cote L. Bradyphrenia in Parkinson's disease: clinical features and biochemistry. *Neurology*, (in press).

92. Mann JJ, Stanley M, Kaplan RD, Sweeny J, Neophytides A. (1983). Central catecholamine metabolism *in vivo* and the cognitive and motor deficits in Parkinson's disease. *J Neurol Neurosurg Psychiatry* 46: 905–10.

93. Gaspar P, Gray F. (1984). Dementia in idiopathic Parkinson's disease. *Acta Neuropathol* 64: 43–52.

94. Mason ST, Fibiger HC. (1979). Noradrenaline and selective attention. *Life Sci* 25: 1949–56.

95. Divac I. (1972). Neostriatum and functions of the prefrontal cortex. *Acta Neurobiol Exp* 32: 461–77.

96. Brozoski TJ, Brown RM, Rosvold HE, Goldman PS. (1979). Cognitive deficit caused by regional depletion of dopamine in prefrontal cortex of rhesus monkey. *Science* 205: 929–32.

97. Stern Y. (1983). Behavior and the basal ganglia. *Adv Neurol* 38: 195–209.

98. Bowen FP, Hoehn MM, Yahr MD. (1972). Parkinsonism: alterations in spatial orientation as determined by a route-walking test. *Neuropsychologia* 10: 355–361.

99. Bowen FP, Hoehn MM, Yahr MD. (1972). Cerebral dominance in relation to tracking and tapping performance in patients with parkinsonism. *Neurology* 22: 32–39.

100. Bowen FP. (1975). Behavioral alterations in patients with basal ganglia lesions. In: Yahr MD (Ed.), *The Basal Ganglia*. New York, Raven Press.

101. Flowers K. (1978). Lack of prediction in the motor behavior of parkinsonism. *Brain* 101: 35–52.
102. Flowers K. (1978). Some frequency response characteristics of parkinsonism on pursuit tracking. *Brain* 101: 19–34.
103. Cooke JD, Brown JD, Brecks VB. (1978). Increased dependence on visual information for movement control in patients with Parkinson's disease. *Can J Neurol Sci* 5: 413–15.
104. Aldridge JW, Anderson RJ, Murphy JT. (1980). The role of the basal ganglia in controlling a movement initiated by a visually presented cue. *Brain Res* 192: 3–16.
105. Danta G, Hilton RC. (1981). Judgment of visual vertical and horizontal in patients with parkinsonism. *Neurology* 25: 43–7.
106. Boller F, Passafiume D, Rogers K, Morrow L, Kim Y. (1982). Visuospatial impairment in Parkinson's disease: role of perceptual and motor factors and of disease stage. *Neurology* 32: 189.
107. Stern Y, Mayeux R, Rosen J, Ilson J. (1983). Perceptual motor dysfunction in Parkinson's disease: A deficit in sequential and predictive movement. *J Neurol Neurosurg Psychiatry* 46: 145–51.
108. Stern Y, Mayeux R, Rosen J. (1984). Contribution of perceptual motor dysfunction to construction and tracing disturbances in Parkinson's disease. *J Neurol Neurosurg Psychiatry* 47: 983–9.
109. Matthews CG, Haaland KY. (1979). The effect of symptom duration on cognitive and motor performance in parkinsonism. *Neurology* 29: 951–956.
110. Mortimer JA, Pirozzolo FJ, Hamsch E, Webster DD. (1982). Relationship of motor symptoms to intellectual deficits in Parkinson's disease. *Neurology* 32: 133–7.
111. Marsden CD. (1982). The mysterious motor function of the basal ganglia: The Robert Wartenberg Lecture. *Neurology* 32: 514–39.
112. Javoy-Agid F, Agid Y. (1980). Is the mesocortical dopaminergic system involved in Parkinson's disease? *Neurology* 30: 1326–30.
113. Lees AJ, Smith E. (1983). Cognitive deficits in the early stages of Parkinson's disease. *Brain* 106: 257–70.
114. Darley FL, Aronson AE, Brown JR. (1975). Hypokinetic dysarthria. In: Darley FL, Aronson AE, Brown JR (Eds.), *Motor Speech Disorders*. Philadelphia, WB Saunders.
115. Matison R, Mayeux R, Rosen J, Fahn S. (1982). "Tip-of-the-tongue" phenomenon in Parkinson's disease. *Neurology* 32: 567–70.
116. Rosen WG. (1980). Verbal fluency in aging and dementia. *J Clin Neuropsychol* 2: 135–46.
117. Burns RS, LeWitt PA, Ebert MH, Pakkenberg H, Kopin I. (1985). The clinical syndrome of striatal dopamine deficiency: parkinsonism induced by 1-methyl-4-phenyl-1,2,3,6, tetrahydropyridine (MPTP). *N Engl J Med* 312: 1418–1421.
118. Stern Y, Langston W. (1985). Intellectual changes in patients with MPTP-induced parkinsonism. *Neurology* 35: 1506–1509.
119. Parkinson J. (1938). An essay on the shaking palsy, 1817. *Med Classics* 2: 964–997.

7
Autonomic Nervous System Disorders

CAROLINE M. TANNER
Rush–Presbyterian St. Luke's Medical Center, Chicago, Illinois

CHRISTOPHER G. GOETZ
Rush Medical College, Rush-Presbyterian St. Luke's Medical Center, Chicago, Illinois

HAROLD L. KLAWANS
Rush Medical College, Chicago, Illinois

Patients with idiopathic Parkinson's disease often show signs and symptoms of autonomic nervous system dysfunction. These problems have received relatively little attention, and most investigators have focused on the more disabling autonomic difficulties of patients with multiple system atrophy (MSA), variously using Parkinson's disease patients as additional study patients or patient controls. Although the clinical distinction between Parkinson's disease and MSA is sometimes difficult, these entities are pathologically distinct. This chapter will focus entirely on disorders of the autonomic nervous system in patients with Parkinson's disease. A number of excellent works already describe dysautonomia in MSA (1,2). This chapter is divided into sections that reflect various subdivisions of the autonomic nervous system. Each section will review the relevant anatomy, describe the clinical signs and symptoms of autonomic dysfunction, and discuss therapy in the context of Parkinson's disease. The effects of antiparkinson agents on autonomic function will also be discussed.

CARDIOVASCULAR ABNORMALITIES

Although a variety of cardiovascular abnormalities have been reported in laboratory studies of Parkinson's disease patients, few patients are disabled by these signs. The evaluation of cardiovascular function in Parkinson's disease patients has been performed by many groups, all using slightly different methods. An understanding of the study of the cardiovascular manifestations of Parkinson's disease is dependent on an understanding of the relevant neuroanatomy and clinical neurophysiology.

The reflex control of arterial blood pressure and cardiac function is directly modulated by the central nervous system. Arterial baroreceptors, peripheral chemoreceptors, and cardiac mechanoreceptors all send afferent inputs to the medullary nucleus tractus solitarius (NTS), which projects to the dorsal motor nucleus of the vagus, nucleus ambiguus, raphe nuclei, medullary reticular formation, and intermediolateral column of the spinal cord. Also projecting to the NTS are cortical and hypothalamic projections. Intermediolateral cells receive suprasegmental inputs from the hypothalamus and A5 noradrenergic neurons as well as from NTS. This complex series of anatomical interconnections provides central modulation of the primary neural effectors of cardiovascular reflexes (the preganglionic sympathetic neurons) that originate in the intermediolateral cell columns of the spinal cord and the preganglionic parasympathetic neurons originating chiefly in the dorsal motor nucleus of the vagus and the nucleus ambiguus (3).

Ablation of the NTS in rats produces hypertension as the result of disinhibited sympathetic activity, while NTS stimulation produces hypotension; this suggests that this area is critical to blood pressure homeostasis. Anterior hypothalamic or preoptic area stimulation produces bradycardia, hypotension, and inhibition of baroreceptor reflexes, while bilateral destruction enhances baroreceptor reflex responses (4). Hypothalamic stimulation may also produce electrocardiographic changes suggestive of myocardial ischemia, coronary vasoconstriction, increased myocardial oxygen demand, and tachycardia (3). Central neurons important in these effects are primarily noradrenergic or adrenergic (4). These central influences modulate sympathetic and parasympathetic neurons that control arterial blood pressure by modifying peripheral resistance and venous return (largely sympathetic) as well as heart rate (slowed by vagal parasympathetic and increased by sympathetic neurons) (5).

Assessment of cardiovascular reflexes can help to localize the site of anatomical dysfunction responsible for autonomic signs. If only the afferent input to NTS is lesioned, reflex increases in pulse and blood pressure from stressful stimuli not dependent on this pathway (mental arithmetic, thermal stress) should be preserved. An intact efferent system will demonstrate the expected tachycardia and increase in blood pressure after the Valsalva maneuver (6).

Orthostatic Hypotension

Many groups have attempted to localize the anatomical site of dysfunction in Parkinson's disease patients with orthostatic hypotension (OH) using clinical tests of cardiovascular reflexes, but unfortunately no two groups have reported identical findings. If the lesion was confined to the afferent system, patients should have a normal blood pressure increase in response to stress. This response, however, has been found to be impaired in Parkinson's disease patients compared to age-matched controls (7), indicating a lesion of efferent fibers. If an efferent lesion is present, the patency of the afferent system cannot be demonstrated by this method. An intact sympathetic efferent system would be characterized by a normal tachycardia and blood pressure overshoot with the Valsalva maneuver. Although two groups reported normal Valsalva responses (8,9), two others found abnormalities (7,10). Such disparate findings in Parkinson's disease patients with OH are not easily explained by a single site of dysfunction.

Symptoms of OH occur in only a subgroup of parkinsonian patients, but laboratory evidence of dysfunction may be detected in many more. Although not all groups have described orthostatic hypotension in Parkinson's disease (8, 10), several have found a significantly different orthostatic blood pressure response when Parkinson's disease patients were compared to age-matched controls (7,9). A low resting blood pressure has also been described in some groups of Parkinson's disease patients (11,12). In most patients, however, changes in blood pressure are not accompanied by syncope, and are rarely disabling. When symptoms are present, patients may at first describe only an intermittent sense of visual blurring, the sensation of looking through a fog, grey vision, or loss of color vision. Symptoms may occur after exercise, prolonged standing, or after a meal (when blood is diverted to the splanchnic bed), as well as after a sudden postural change. Patients may have nonspecific complaints of malaise or extreme fatigue, or describe nausea or headache.

Abnormalities of renin may contribute to hypotension in parkinsonism. Barbeau et al. (13) found low plasma renin and a low rate of aldosterone secretion in 31 Parkinson's disease patients compared to normotensive controls, and low rates of aldosterone production in a smaller group. Sodium homeostasis was normal in this group, suggesting a peripheral sympathetic deficit. Aminoff and Wilcox similarly found normal sodium homeostasis in Parkinson's disease but not MSA patients (14).

Others have attempted to demonstrate the site of anatomic dysfunction by the use of intravenous infusions of biogenic amines and pressor agents. Wilcox and Aminoff (8,15) demonstrated increased pressor responses to norepinephrine in Parkinson's disease patients compared to controls, although these responses were less marked than those observed in patients with Shy-Drager syndrome (MSA). They postulated a defective "set" of central regulatory centers, with a consequent "reduction in impulse traffic at sympathetic nerve terminals," which then explains the enhanced response to infused norepinephrine. This is similar to the response reported by Polinsky and colleagues (16) in patients with MSA, suggesting primarily a central abnormality of blood pressure control, rather than denervation supersensitivity.

The contradictory results of autonomic testing are of interest in view of the distribution of Lewy bodies and neuronal degeneration in Parkinson's disease. Rajput and Rozdilsky (17) observed a direct correlation between orthostatic hypotension and cell loss and Lewy body formation in sympathetic ganglia. Further support for sympathetic neuronal dysfunction is provided by the observation of Emile and colleagues (18) that Parkinson's disease patients are significantly more likely to have antibodies to sympathetic neurons compared to controls, although direct correlation of antibody titers with orthostatic hypotension was not possible. However, Parkinson's disease patients have also been reported to have pathologic abnormalities in other areas of the neuraxis involved in autonomic regulation, particularly the hypothalamus (19,20). Since experimental studies in animals suggest that single central nervous system (CNS) lesions are not likely to result in orthostatic hypotension (3), the concept of a generalized sympathetic system degeneration proposed by Langston and Forno seems more appropriate.

When levodopa was first used to treat Parkinson's disease, OH was considered to be a major side effect (21). Subsequently, it was recognized that hypotension was a transient event of early therapy for many, and intermittent but asymptomatic in others. A small group of patients had sustained symptomatic orthostatic hypotension that responded only to a decrease in levodopa therapy (22). Ballantyne (23) evaluated patients before levodopa, and after 1 and 6 months of therapy, and found no change in the prevalence or severity of postural hypotension after treatment. The combination of a peripherally acting aromatic amino acid decarboxylase inhibitor (DCI) with levodopa may lessen the incidence of OH. Calne and colleagues found that carbidopa did not block the drop in supine blood pressure that followed levodopa administration, but did block the levodopa-induced impairment of baroreceptors (24). They determined from this that the drop in supine pressure is centrally mediated, while the baroreceptor abnormality is peripheral. These data suggest that patients receiving carbidopa with levodopa should have less OH. More recently, increased blood pressure has been described in fluctuating carbidopa/levodopa-treated Parkinson's disease patients while "off," while similarly treated patients without motor fluctuations did not have fluctuating blood pressures (25).

The dopamine receptor agonists bromocriptine and pergolide also cause orthostatic hypotension during the first weeks of therapy, which may be symptomatic, but OH is only rarely dose-limiting (26,27). Montastruc and colleagues gave bromocriptine (mean dose, 56 mg/day) alone or with carbidopa/levodopa to five Parkinson's disease patients with mild uncomplicated primary hypertension (stage II), and observed sustained reduction of systolic and diastolic blood pressure for 12 months. This effect was not blocked by the peripheral dopamine receptor agonist domperidone, suggesting to the investigators that a central mechanism was responsible for the reduction in blood pressure (28). Quinn and colleagues (29) had similar results when treating only with bromocriptine and domperidone. Goetz and colleagues (7), studying autonomic responses in patients treated for years with multiple antiparkinson agents (levodopa/carbidopa, anticholinergics, amantadine, dopamine receptor agonists, and bupropion), found that OH was similar before and after antiparkinson therapy was given.

Patients with significant orthostatic hypotension coupled with significant parkinsonian disability present a therapeutic dilemma. In evaluating these patients, it is important to try to distinguish between the subjective "dizziness" when standing or changing position described by patients with parkinsonian postural reflex impairment and the symptoms of syncope. Observant patients, when challenged with a postural threat, will be able to identify the resultant sensation of imbalance as the source of their "dizziness." In the practical assessment of Parkinson's disease patients with significant OH, whether or not the hypotension is actually aggravated by levodopa must be determined. Since most patients develop significant symptoms after years of levodopa therapy, hospitalization will be required for withdrawal of levodopa. Levodopa withdrawal can cause a dramatic deterioration in motor function, however, which requires meticulous medical care (30). Moreover, the sedentary state and prolonged bedrest may aggravate the blood pressure abnormality. To minimize this, patients should be actively involved in physical therapy. Head elevation of 14 degrees has been reported to minimize orthostatic hypotension caused by prolonged bedrest (31). After blood pressure responses have been determined for 24 hr without levodopa, response to the drug should be assessed. This is best performed several hours after rising, to avoid the OH induced by the supine posture, and not after a large meal. If the orthostatic hypotension is clearly worsened by levodopa, but the patient requires levodopa to treat his motor disability, specific therapy may be needed to treat the orthostatic hypotension.

The nonpharmacologic treatments of OH include a high-sodium diet and maintenance of the head at 14 degrees at night, the latter to increase sodium reabsorption, possibly through an increase in renin release (31). Elasticized garments for the lower body decrease the available area for blood pooling by compression, but also depress the remaining physiological muscular contraction of vascular smooth muscle, further endangering the patient when the garment is removed (32). Patients with diurnal patterns of hypotension may change their daily habits and minimize symptoms. Thus, a patient with significant postprandial hypotension (resulting from shunting of blood to the splanchnic bed) may benefit from frequent small meals. Patients with symptoms only after standing for long times (as in a grocery store line) or in excessively warm environments should avoid such situations. Patients who develop hypotension only when mildly hypovolemic should be given a strict schedule for fluid intake. Patients intermittently given diuretics for "swollen ankles" should avoid these agents.

If the above measures are not effective, pharmacologic intervention may be required. Most patients currently treated with levodopa receive a fixed combination of levodopa and a dopa decarboxylase inhibitor (DCI) such as carbidopa or benserazide. In some cases, the fixed ratio may not supply enough DCI to permit effective peripheral blockade of dopa decarboxylation, and supplemental DCI may decrease OH (24). Fludrocortisone acetate has been demonstrated to treat OH in levodopa-treated Parkinson's disease, probably both by its ability to enhance the responsiveness of vascular smooth muscle to epinephrine and its sodium-retaining properties, with consequent increased intravascular volume (33). In patients with cardiac disease, careful attention to the possibility of developing congestive failure is needed. In some patients taking fludrocortisone, potassium supplementation may be required. Indomethacin (50 mg three times daily) or ibuprofen (400 mg four times daily), both prostaglandin inhibitors, are also sometimes effective. The mechanism of this effect is not known, but inhibition of potent vasodilating prostaglandins or prostaglandin-mediated sympathetic inhibition have been postulated (34). In patients with significant postprandial blood pressure drops, administration of a prostaglandin inhibitor 1 hr before eating may be helpful. The precursor of norepinephrine, D,L,-3,4-threo-dihydroxyphenylserine, has been reported to ameliorate OH in L-dopa-treated parkinsonian patients (35), but this drug is not now commercially available. Dihydroergotamine has diminished OH in MSA patients, often requiring large doses of 20 mg/day or more. Other pressor regimens, including hydroxy-amphetamine, methylphenidate, combined tyramine and monoamine oxidase inhibitors, and ephedrine have been used in MSA with varying success (32). The investigational agent midodrine, an alpha-adrenergic agonist, has also been reported to benefit patients with orthostatic hypotension, although none of these had Parkinson's disease (36). Similarly, caffeine has been of long-term benefit in OH, but has not been studied in Parkinson's disease patients (37). Propranolol, an antihypertensive, has been suggested as a treatment of OH, its proposed mechanism being a relative shift of sympathetic tone to alpha-adrenergic predominance, since it acts as a beta-adrenergic blocker (38). However, since patients with OH may be hypersensitive to drugs with either hypo- or hypertensive actions (39), use of this agent seems especially risky.

Hypertension

Arterial hypertension is not a common problem in Parkinson's disease. Experimental lesions of the NTS, A1 noradrenergic medullary neurons, and hypothalamus all result in hypertension or labile blood pressures in animals (3), but clinical correlates of these lesions have not been described in Parkinson's disease. Occasionally, normotensive patients treated with levodopa may have transient elevations of blood pressure (40), but these are almost always short-lived, have no adverse effect, and do not require treatment.

   The more common setting in which hypertension may be observed is in the patient with significant OH requiring drug therapy. Recumbent hypertension is a common dose-limiting side effect of treatment with both pressor agents and volume expanders. In some cases, recumbent hypertension is the result of too vigorous use of sodium supplementation and fludrocortisone, but in most it likely reflects the diffuse autonomic lesion. Fluctuations in blood pressure in patients with MSA are common, and have been observed to occur without appreciable change in intravascular volume (32). A similar phenomenon is probably at work in Parkinson's disease patients with these signs. Although attempts to limit therapy to day time only are of benefit in some patients, in many cases upright normotension often occurs only at the expense of supine hypertension.

Cardiac Arrhythmias

Since the population of Parkinson's disease patients is also the age group at the greatest risk for heart disease, the discussion of cardiac abnormalities in Parkinson's disease has always been confusing. Experimental studies clearly demonstrate that cardiac arrhythmias may be mediated by central sympathetic structures, including hypothalamus (3), but the occurrence of arrhythmias in humans is generally limited to acute brain lesions, rather than chronic degenerative processes. Patients with severe impairment of cardiovascular reflexes may have a fixed pulse rate, so that the expected physiological tachycardia to heat-tilt or cold-pressor is lost. No other abnormality of cardiac rhythm has been definitely associated with Parkinson's disease or MSA (6).

The relationship of antiparkinson drugs to arrhythmias has, on the other hand, been fraught with controversy. Levodopa, via its effects on peripheral beta-adrenergic receptors, increases cardiac contractility, produces sinus tachycardia, increases atrioventricular (A-V) conduction, and precipitates ventricular arrhythmias in animal studies (41). When levodopa was first used in the treatment of Parkinson's disease, a number of investigators reported associated atrial and ventricular arrhythmias (42–44) and advised against using levodopa in Parkinson's disease patients with heart disease. A large group of patients were thus denied the potentially dramatic benefits of levodopa.

These reports were soon followed by several studies specifically addressing the possible cardiac toxicity of levodopa in patients with heart disease, in which specific toxicity could not be demonstrated (45,46). Since nonambulatory patients are at less risk for arrhythmia than those able to exercise, some of the abnormalities attributed to a specific effect of levodopa on the heart may have been related to increased activity in treated patients. Also, a number of descriptions of tremor artifact on electrocardiogram that had been misdiagnosed as "atrial flutter" questioned the accuracy of previous descriptions of arrhythmia in Parkinson's disease patients (47–49). The subsequent addition of carbidopa to levodopa was reported to diminish any arrhythmogenic potential that might be attributed to levodopa alone (50,51). More recently, the observation that oral levodopa may have a beneficial effect in congestive heart failure by increasing cardiac output has resulted in the suggestion that Parkinson's disease patients with coexisting congestive heart failure might actually benefit from treatment with levodopa without decarboxylase inhibitor (52).

Similar reports of cardiac toxicity have accompanied almost all new anti-parkinson therapies. In each case, definitive attribution of the observed cardiac abnormality to the treatment has been impossible, and subsequent more careful-ly designed studies have not substantiated definite cardiac toxicity as the result of any antiparkinson agent (53–56). For most patients, the risk imposed by failure to treat the parkinsonism is greater than any potential drug-related cardiotoxicity.

GASTROINTESTINAL DISORDERS

Gastrointestinal (GI) disorders in Parkinson's disease are of three general types: disorders of motility, sialorrhea, and disorders of appetite. Nausea and vomiting are not typical complaints in untreated Parkinson's disease patients, but are common enough in patients receiving antiparkinsonian medications to warrant discussion. Of these, disorders of motility provide the most frequent clinical complaints. GI motility abnormalities in Parkinson's disease are principally of three types: dysphagia, disordered gastric emptying, and constipation. Both sympathetic and parasympathetic nerves supply the GI tract, but parasympa-thetic input is of greater physiological significance (57). Sympathetic fibers, supplied from superior and inferior cervical ganglia, splanchnic nerve, and the celiac and mesenteric plexi, decrease bowel motility by inhibition of acetyl-choline release as well as direct inhibition of smooth muscle, and produce con-traction of the internal anal sphincter (58). Parasympathetic innervation to the oral pharynx is supplied by the glossopharyngeal nerve, while the remaining pharynx, esophagus, stomach, and small bowel are completely, and the large bowel partially, innervated by the vagus nerve (57). The role of central areas other than brain stem centers in mediating GI motility is not well understood.

Swallowing

Swallowing is mediated by three separate neural control systems. The first, voluntary, phase involves buccopharyngeal striated muscles which are innervated by motor neurons from trigeminal, facial, hypoglossal, and ambiguus nuclei. In this phase, food is propelled from the mouth to the pharynx. The second and third phases of swallowing involve smooth muscles of the esophagus and the gastroesophageal junction and are mediated by fibers originating in the dorsal motor nucleus of the vagus. The second phase quickly propels food through the esophagus via a complex reflex mechanism, while the third permits passage of food into the stomach (59).

Dysphagia was first described in Parkinson's disease by James Parkinson (60). His patient was typical, experiencing more difficulty with solid than liquid foods, living on milk alone, and suffering significant weight loss. Dysphagia generally occurs in patients with more severe Parkinson's disease, and roughly parallels the severity of motor impairment. If patients have dysphagia out of proportion to their other Parkinson's disease symptoms, another cause for the dysphagia or a different neurologic diagnosis should be considered. Initially, parkinsonian patients may report only prolonged mealtimes, difficulty chewing food, or difficulty moving the food to the back of the mouth to initiate swallowing. Patients complain of the sensation of food or liquid sticking to the back of the throat. Later, choking may occur despite a soft diet, and significant weight loss may result from decreased caloric intake. Eating is accomplished only very slowly, and is accompanied by great anxiety. Aspiration with subsequent pulmonary infection is a dreaded accompaniment of severe dysphagia.

The character of the disturbance underlying dysphagia has remained controversial. Early investigations reported defective esophageal peristalsis, with segmental esophageal spasm (61). Other studies described limited defects, involving only defective tongue movements (62) or hypopharyngeal neuromuscular incoordination ("cricopharyngeal achalasia") (63). More recent investigations have observed some abnormality of swallowing in 50% of Parkinson's disease patients (64), emphasizing that patient complaints, which are less frequent, are not a good measure of the prevalence of impaired swallowing. Studies using modern investigative techniques have demonstrated specific abnormalities in all stages of swallowing. First, passage of food to the back of the mouth by tongue movement is slowed, usually beginning rather early in the course of Parkinson's disease and worsening as the disease progresses. Next, transit through the pharynx is slowed, with vallecular stasis. Peristalsis is reduced, especially in the lower third of the esophagus, with tertiary waves and esophageal reflux in some cases. Infusion of dopamine has been found to relax the gastroesophageal sphincter further (65). The occurrence of esophageal reflux, coupled with the common finding of hiatal hernia (61), probably accounts for the common complaint of heartburn in Parkinson's disease (66).

Treatment of dysphagia in Parkinson's disease is difficult. Patients should be advised to eat soft foods, and, if there is difficulty swallowing medications, these may be crushed and mixed with jam, pudding, or a food of similar consistency. A dietitian should assist in the development of a balanced diet, and dietary supplements should be prescribed if there is significant weight loss. Dopamine is believed to increase esophageal contractions and relax the lower esophageal sphincter (67). These effects, as well as the expected beneficial effects on striated muscle function, suggest that levodopa therapy should relieve dysphagia in Parkinson's disease. Anecdotal reports have attributed dramatic improvement in dysphagia to levodopa treatment (40), and most clinicians attempt to adjust drug dose in dysphagic patients so that meals are taken at the time of maximum drug effect. However, these maneuvers are rarely completely successful, and the nature of any improvement has not been defined. Calne and colleagues (62) did not demonstrate improved swallowing after levodopa in a cinefluoroscopic study. Finally, patients who cannot maintain their weight through oral nutrition, or those who suffer from aspiration and pulmonary infections, should be considered for gastrostomy or jejunostomy (68). By permitting medication and food administration through the stoma, adequate nutrition can be maintained, and the risk of aspiration, as well as the ordeal of constant choking while trying to eat, can be greatly decreased.

In contrast to levodopa, which may be of benefit to Parkinson's disease patients with dysphagia, Bramble and colleagues (67) found that an anticholinergic agent caused a significant increase in nonperistaltic swallows in Parkinson's disease. Although no one has systematically studied the effects of any medications on swallowing in Parkinson's disease, this study suggests that anticholinergic drugs may aggravate swallowing difficulties.

Gastric Emptying

The proximal stomach functions as a reservoir, while the antral area churns the stomach contents and expels them through the pylorus. Loss of vagal innervation results in a decreased reservoir, as well as delayed emptying of solids, with enhanced emptying of liquids (65). This suggests that these functions are normally vagus mediated, although the reestablishment of normal emptying patterns after a recovery period implicates a second important role for intrinsic enteric neurons. In vivo infusion studies have demonstrated delayed gastric emptying after dopamine infusion. The mechanism of this levodopa-related antral slowing is uncertain. A physiological role for dopamine in the stomach has not been established, and dopamine-containing intrinsic neurons have not been demonstrated (69). Others have found that the addition of a peripheral decarboxylase inhibitor does not diminish the levodopa-induced slowing (70).

Gastric emptying time is delayed in Parkinson's disease (70). Thus, many patients complain of epigastric discomfort or fullness, early satiety, and postprandial distress. These symptoms are further aggravated by levodopa, which relaxes the lower esophageal sphincter (67) and further prolongs gastric emptying (70). This slowed gastric emptying is significant not only for the gastroenteric discomfort caused but, since levodopa is absorbed primarily from the duodenum, delivery of levodopa to the plasma can be impaired (71), with consequent motor deterioration (72).

Some patients experience relief from epigastric fullness with standard antacid and antiflatulent therapy, but many do not. In these patients, treatment with domperidone, a dopamine receptor antagonist that does not cross the blood-brain barrier, is often helpful (73). Domperidone, which causes increased lower esophageal sphincter pressure, and increases antral peristalsis, gastric emptying, and intestinal transit, is currently available in Europe, and is investigational in the United States. Generally, doses of 60–80 mg daily are adequate. Significant side effects have not been reported.

Intestinal Motility

Passage of contents through the small and large bowel is mediated by local mechanical and chemical reflexes initiated distal to the bolus in transit. These reflexes are finally expressed through the intrinsic enteric neurons, but parasympathetic afferent and efferent fibers mediate both excitatory and inhibitory reflexes, while sympathetic fibers also act to inhibit small bowel motility (74). In general, propulsion is accomplished by sequential contraction of circular muscles in the intestinal wall. Excessive haustral contractions in the large bowel impede motility and dehydrate stool, resulting in constipation (75). Constipation is the result of impaired colonic transit time or outlet obstruction produced by rectosigmoid spasm (76). The specific role of individual neuronal systems in constipation are not well defined.

Constipation is another common problem in Parkinson's disease. Over half of parkinsonian patients in one study failed to defecate daily, while this was true of only 12% of age-matched controls (66). Constipation in Parkinson's disease most likely is the result of many different factors, including decreased activity, decreased forcefulness of abdominal muscle contractions, and decreased intake of food and water. Although specific abnormalities of intestinal motility are assumed, these have not been conclusively demonstrated. Both anticholinergic drugs and dopaminergic agents may further interfere with lower bowel motility and increase constipation.

Megacolon with associated pseudoobstruction or true sigmoid volvulus is a more serious disorder of the lower bowel that may occur in parkinsonian patients with severe constipation (77). In some cases, megacolon may be present without clinical signs, but in others several days of progressive abdominal distention, usually with obstipation but rarely with diarrhea, accompany a tympanitic abdomen with hypoactive bowel sounds (78). The distinction between megacolon with pseudoobstruction and acute intestinal obstruction cannot be made clinically, and patients may develop an associated volvulus of the sigmoid colon with true mechanical obstruction. Acute pseudoobstruction alone may be associated with perforation and peritonitis.

Treatment of constipation in Parkinson's disease is difficult. As a first step, at least 64 oz water or other noncaffeinated beverage should be taken daily, in addition to the liquids taken with meals. This may be supplemented with increased dietary bulk, such as bran and whole grains, and fresh fruits and vegetables. A daily exercise regimen within the capabilities of the patient should also be prescribed. If this is ineffective, a bulk-forming laxative such as psyllium, or a combination stool softener and intestinal stimulant, may be added. Finally, patients may intermittently require a cathartic or enema, but use of these preparations should be kept to a minimum to avoid dependency.

When Parkinson's disease patients present with the picture of acute or subacute intestinal obstruction, abdominal plain films and, if necessary, barium enema will confirm the diagnosis, although barium should be avoided when mechanical obstruction is not a question since this may increase the risk of perforation (77). Patients should fast, and all anticholinergic medications should be discontinued. Decompression with rectal tubes should be attempted, although colonoscopic decompression may be more successful. Use of a cholinesterase inhibitor such as neostigmine may increase bowel motility. If cecal distention is progressive despite vigorous medical management, or if perforation has occurred, patients should undergo decompression with tube cecostomy.

Salivation

Salivation is also predominantly a parasympathetic phenomenon, with superior and inferior salivatory nuclei supplying preganglionic cholinergic fibers. Sympathetic innervation originates in the upper thoracic cord (57). Drooling is a common complaint in Parkinson's disease, and this has been attributed to an overproduction of saliva (79). An alternative explanation is provided by Parkinson's original description of a patient whose "saliva was continually trickling out of his mouth, and he had neither the power of retaining it, nor of spitting it out freely" (60), suggesting an abnormality of deglutition. Current investigations support this, although whether the drooling reflects an inability to initiate voluntary movement or the loss of unconscious movement (analogous to decreased associated movements while walking) is not known. Although discontinuation of anticholinergic drugs may cause transient hypersalivation (80), probably reflecting the proliferation of muscarinic cholinergic receptors associated with chronic receptor blockade (81), both untreated Parkinson's disease patients and those on chronic stable doses of antiparkinson anticholinergic drugs have been found to have saliva production within the normal range (82,83).

Since drooling can result in significant social embarrassment, patients often desire treatment of this bothersome complaint. In some cases, adjustment of the antiparkinson medications to decrease oropharyngeal akinesia is adequate to control drooling. Others, however, have persistent complaints. Despite the observation that patients taking anticholinergic drugs have normal saliva production, many patients experience relief of drooling when a peripherally acting anticholinergic drug (such as propantheline, 15–45 mg/day, in divided doses) is added to their regimes. The apparently greater efficacy of peripherally acting antimuscarinic agents may be artifactual, actually reflecting the toxicity of centrally acting agents, which limits their administration to doses insufficient to decrease salivation. When peripherally acting anticholinergic drugs are used, their potential for producing unwanted parasympathetic blockade causing symptoms in other organ systems must be considered.

Nausea and Vomiting

Vomiting requires the patterned participation of gastrointestinal and somatic muscles. This complex reflex is coordinated by the vomiting center in the medulla, located near to the nucleus solitarius. Vomiting is normally preceded by the sensation of nausea. Nausea and vomiting can be produced by a variety of peripheral and central stimuli, including distention of stomach and duodenal mucosa, and noxious substances in stomach, duodenum, or blood. The latter are identified by medullary neurons in the chemoreceptor trigger zone (CRTZ), which are physiologically outside of the blood–brain barrier. During nausea, there is a transient relaxation of the small bowel mediated by vagal parasympathetic inhibitory neurons and enteric inhibitory neurons. This is followed by sequential anal to oral contraction beginning in the lower ileum, which is mediated by vagal parasympathetic excitatory fibers and enteric excitatory neurons (74). The CRTZ is sensitive to dopamine and dopamine agonists.

Although nausea and vomiting are not symptoms of Parkinson's disease per se, most Parkinson's disease patients require therapy with dopaminergic agents, which activate the medullary vomiting center via the CRTZ. When levodopa is given alone, nausea and vomiting constitute major limitations to the dose (40). To avoid severe nausea and vomiting, treatment with levodopa must be gradually introduced, generally in combination with a peripherally active DCI. The DCI prevents the peripheral decarboxylation of levodopa to dopamine, but does not cross the blood–brain barrier. Thus, stimulation of the chemoreceptor trigger zone is prevented. In the United States, the fixed combination of levodopa 100 mg/carbidopa 25 mg is the best initial therapy to avoid GI upset. Medication may be taken with small amounts of food or milk, although large high-protein meals may impair drug absorption (84). Nonetheless if patients suffer from severe nausea, postprandial administration of levodopa may be necessary to control symptoms. Complete decarboxylase inhibition can require 200 mg or more of carbidopa daily, so that some patients may require supplemental carbidopa therapy. Levodopa-treated patients with chronic nausea, decreased appetite, or weight loss may also benefit significantly from increased carbidopa. If these treatments are ineffective, a peripheral dopamine receptor blocker such as domperidone (77) may help symptoms without worsening the Parkinson's disease. Dopamine-blocking agents with central effects (including compazine, chlorpromazine, and metoclopramide) should be avoided, however, since these drugs worsen Parkinson's disease and block the efficacy of dopaminergic drugs. In some cases without diagnosable depression, the use of a single low dose of a tricyclic antidepressant with appetite-stimulating properties (amitriptyline or doxepin 10-25 mg at bedtime) has been effective.

Appetite

Appetite is normally mediated by a complex and poorly understood interplay of central systems. Studies involving lesions of experimental animals have implicated both lateral and medial hypothalamic areas, with lateral lesions yielding aphagia and medial lesions producing hyperphagia. Subsequent studies have shown that the aphagia produced by lateral hypothalamic lesions is partially the result of lesioning dopaminergic fibers passing from the substantia nigra to the striatum (85). Although extrapolations from animal studies to humans are difficult, these observations suggest that loss of nigrostriatal dopamine fibers, as well as, possibly, intrinsic hypothalamic neurons, may underlie disorders of appetite in Parkinson's disease.

In the clinical setting, the assessment of appetite and weight control in an individual Parkinson's disease patient is complex. Clearly, patients with impaired deglutition will be more likely to lose weight, and to lose interest in food as a result of the difficulty imposed by eating. Depression is a frequent finding in Parkinson's disease (86), and in some cases change in appetite may reflect a mood disorder. Finally, many parkinsonian patients are treated with dopaminergic agents, which can cause nausea and may result in a decreased appetite. Despite this, there is some evidence that a primary central disorder of appetite does occur in Parkinson's disease.

In one study, 182 patients with Parkinson's disease were compared to 31 with progressive supranuclear palsy (PSP) (87). Both groups of patients were receiving long-term levodopa–carbidopa therapy, and their motor disabilities and disease durations were similar. Nonetheless, the Parkinson's disease patients had a significantly lower body weight than the PSP patients. These investigators hypothesized a lateral hypothalamic syndrome in Parkinson's disease.

Another group published a seemingly contradictory report of 5 Parkinson's disease patients with bulimia. In this paper "bulimia" refers to an insatiable appetite with continuous eating sustained for days or weeks. The bulimia abated after levodopa therapy was initiated (88). This, too, was proposed as evidence of hypothalamic involvement in Parkinson's disease. Although the hypothalamic control of appetite is not clearly understood, dopaminergic systems appear to participate. In an entirely different clinical setting, anorexia nervosa and true bulimia are thought to be symptoms of the same disorder. By extrapolation, these apparently contradictory findings in Parkinson's disease may reflect similar, but less dramatic, dysfunction of the same central systems.

Treatment of weight loss in Parkinson's disease requires a careful differentiation of the possible contributing factors. Patients with other GI disturbance should be specifically treated for that problem. Consultation with a dietitian, accurate calorie counts, and documentation of weight loss permit appropriate dietary recommendations. In many cases, the use of high-calorie concentrated dietary supplements help patients to maintain weight. In some cases without diagnosable depression, the use of a single low dose of a tricyclic antidepressant with appetite-stimulating properties (doxepin or amitriptyline 10–25 mg at bedtime) has been effective. There is little experience with the treatment of the much less common problem of excessive eating in Parkinson's disease. The report cited above suggests that dopaminergic therapy is of benefit in patients with this problem.

BLADDER DYSFUNCTION

Signs and symptoms of bladder dysfunction are common in Parkinson's disease. Although the exact central nervous system site underlying bladder dysfunction is not definite, both basal ganglia and hypothalamic influences alter the closed loop pathway connecting the detrusor motor area in the frontal lobes with the detrusor motor area in the pontomesencephalic–reticular formation (89). Basal ganglia input to this loop depresses detrusor reflex contraction, while hypothalamic output facilitates the detrusor reflex. These varying effects of hypothalamic and basal ganglia structures on central mechanisms of detrusor control correlate with the clinical observation that detrusor dysfunction is the predominant abnormality of bladder function in Parkinson's disease, although the more peripheral parasympathetic neuron systems providing motor innervation to the muscle are intact (90–94). Moreover, although methods of bladder evaluation vary, all reports describe detrusor hyperactivity in the majority of Parkinson's disease patients (15,90–95), while a smaller group experiences detrusor hypoactivity. Electromyographic studies have been performed in a smaller group of patients, and have demonstrated sphincter abnormalities to be uncommon (90). Urinary complaints do not differ in frequency between the sexes, do not correlate with any particular parkinsonian sign, and may present early in the course of the illness, or even precede the motor signs of Parkinson's disease (90,93).

The most common symptoms of bladder dysfunction in Parkinson's disease reflect an underlying increase in detrusor tone ("spasticity on filling" or "uninhibited detrusor contraction"). Early in the course, patients may complain of nocturia, often urinating more than three times a night. Later, frequency and urgency occur during the day. In severe cases, waking urge incontinence and nocturnal enuresis occur. Aranda and colleagues (90) correlated symptoms with urodynamic studies in 63 parkinsonian patients, and found symptoms of urgency in 74%, of whom 87% had detrusor hyperactivity. Difficulty initiating urination, weak urinary stream, and difficulty completely emptying the bladder were present in 59% of the same group. When present in isolation, these signs correlated directly with a hypoactive detrusor. Mixtures of urgency and difficulty voiding always reflected detrusor abnormalities, but either hypo- or hyperactivity could be present.

Various antiparkinson therapies have been reported to affect bladder dysfunction in Parkinson's disease, beginning with thalamotomy, a now abandoned surgical technique reported to improve (91) or produce (92) bladder dysfunction in different studies. Similarly, patients with predominantly hypoactive detrusor muscles may suffer from an exacerbation of symptoms after taking antimuscarinic cholinergic agents for their Parkinson's disease, since these drugs decrease detrusor contraction and may cause urinary retention in this clinical setting (96). Finally, levodopa (90,97-99) has been reported to decrease detrusor tone and produce bladder neck obstruction. Although these observations require further verification, such actions could also aggravate symptoms in patients with already hypotonic bladders.

Before initiating therapy for complaints of incontinence in Parkinson's disease, a careful history and, in most cases, evaluation by a urologic specialist who can exclude nonneurologic disease and determine the type of neurogenic bladder dysfunction is essential. The clinical history can often determine if complaints of incontinence are referable to true bladder disease, or to "pseudo-incontinence," reflecting only somatic akinesia. In the latter setting, akinetic patients, or ambulatory patients who are not receiving antiparkinson therapy at night, urinate because they are unable to walk to the bathroom, rather than as the result of true urologic disease. Persons with both akinesia and urinary urgency, of course, are more likely to lose control of bladder function because they have more difficulty getting to the bathroom.

The treatment of bladder disorders in Parkinson's disease is controversial (89), largely because most agents have inconsistent clinical results. Some clinicians have suggested avoiding pharmacotherapy in less severely affected persons (90). Before treatment is initiated, careful characterization of the underlying disorder with urodynamic studies is critical. If the predominant abnormality is detrusor hyperreflexia, treatment may be attempted with antimuscarinic cholinergic agents: either those with predominantly peripheral actions (oxybutynin dicyclomide, glycopyrrolate, and others) or those centrally active compounds used to treat the motor symptoms of Parkinson's disease. As discussed under sialorrhea above, centrally active compounds may produce side effects before the desired clinical effect, and predominantly peripherally acting compounds are often preferable. These drugs block transmission in pelvic nerves and the detrusor muscle itself, with resultant relaxation of uninhibited contractions. Unfortunately, if there is an associated component of detrusor damage from overdistention or infection, weakness may result, with subsequent urinary retention from poor contractile strength. Imipramine is a tricyclic antidepressant that inhibits detrusor contractility and may have fewer adverse effects than antimuscarinic agents (90,96). Finally, in some cases treatment of the Parkinson's disease with dopaminergic agents may have a beneficial effect on urinary symptoms (40,90).

The treatment of a hypoactive detrusor presents a different clinical problem, since the desired result is increased detrusor activity. In this case, agents that increase cholinergic activity would be expected to ameliorate bladder function, but the same drugs, if centrally active, should aggravate Parkinson's disease. Moreover, the actual efficacy of both cholinergic agonists (89) and peripherally active cholinesterase inhibitors (90) is uncertain. Some patients may benefit by alpha-adrenergic receptor blocking agents such as prazosin or phenoxybenzamine, which decrease tone in the bladder neck (89,90). However, these agents may cause postural hypotension or cardiac arrhythmias, and must be used with caution in these patients.

THERMOREGULATORY ABNORMALITIES

The anatomical localization of human thermoregulation continues to be poorly characterized (100). Neurons of the preoptic area and anterior and posterior hypothalamus appear to play an important role in most animal species, but thermosensitive neurons are also present in cerebral cortex, thalamus, all brain stem areas, and spinal cord. The noradrenergic, cholinergic, and serotonergic neurotransmitter systems have traditionally been implicated in central thermoregulatory mechanisms, although different animal species may have opposite responses to manipulation of a specific transmitter. Recently, a growing body of laboratory evidence has also implicated central dopaminergic systems in physiological thermoregulation, possibly in the control of pathways that mediate peripheral vasomotor tone (101). These central areas control peripheral autonomic nervous system responses such as sweating (mediated by efferent cholinergic sympathetic fibers) and vasodilation (57). The observation of pathologic abnormalities in several areas of Parkinson's disease brains (17,19) known to regulate thermoregulation in animals has led to the theory that dysfunction in these areas (particularly the hypothalamus) may also underlie thermoregulatory abnormalities in Parkinson's disease.

Abnormal sensations of heat or cold and bursts of perspiration were described in the earliest reports of Parkinson's disease and were attributed by Gowers to either vasomotor abnormalities or changes in the sensory centers of the brain (102). Disordered thermoregulatory responses in Parkinson's disease can include impairment of heat dissipation and sweating, severe hyperpyrexia after levodopa withdrawal, and accidental hypothermia.

Impaired sweating responses are the most common thermoregulatory abnormalities in Parkinson's disease. The descriptions by Gowers and Charcot of profuse sweating in Parkinson's disease patients suggest that this symptom is part of the disease in some patients. A recent study further supports this (103). Forty-eight percent of patients had episodes of excessive sweating without apparent precipitant, and in 41% of these patients, the episodes were sometimes so severe that a change in clothing was necessary. Although the majority of the affected patients had fluctuating motor responses to levodopa therapy that included episodes of chorea, 68% associated their bouts of sweating with severe akinesia, when physical exertion was at a minimum. In a subsequent study, the response of Parkinson's disease patients to an external heat source was assessed before and after treatment with their usual dopaminergic agent (7). After exposure to environmental heat, untreated patients had excessive head and neck sweating compared to controls, with associated impaired heat dissipation through peripheral vasodilatation. Similar sweating abnormalities were observed in untreated patients studied by Appenzeller and Goss (10). Elliott et al. (104) similarly observed abnormalities of hand heat elimination in Parkinson's disease patients, but response to levodopa therapy was assessed in only three and no change was noted.

Recently, several studies have reported cases of Parkinson's disease patients who developed severe fever, tachypnea, tachycardia, sweating, creatine kinase (CK) elevations, and mental status changes a few days after dopaminergic therapy was discontinued (105-107). In no case could another explanation for the fever be identified. In several cases, the syndrome was fatal. In another patient, hyperthermia, CK elevation, and obtundation occurred repeatedly in association with motor fluctuations ("off" episodes) without levodopa withdrawal, eventually resulting in death (108). The strong resemblance of the symptom complex in these Parkinson's disease patients to the neuroleptic malignant syndrome (109), an idiosyncratic reaction to agents that block central dopamine receptors, has led to the postulate that these disorders both reflect abnormalities of central dopaminergic thermoregulatory systems.

Finally, Parkinson's disease patients are described as being unusually tolerant to cold, but to occasionally suffer accidental hypothermia, the result of low environmental temperatures (79).

The role of antiparkinson agents in these various clinical states is not well established. In the case of excessive sweating, most evidence suggests that treating Parkinson's disease will partially alleviate this symptom. After levodopa therapy, both sweating and heat dissipation were normalized, and patients' values did not significantly differ from controls (7). In another study, the addition of the dopamine receptor agonist pergolide resulted in decreased sweating in a number of patients with severe end-of-dose akinesia (26), a response we have also observed with bromocriptine therapy. These effects are consistent with the observed hypothermic effects of levodopa in most animal species (101). The response of those patients with hyperthermia after withdrawal is also consistent with a hypothermic role for dopamine, although it is probable that the true action of central dopaminergic systems in thermoregulation is not so simplistic.

Since both excessive sweating and levodopa withdrawal hyperthermia respond to levodopa, treatment with dopaminergic agents should be the first response. In patients with paroxysmal sweating episodes, anticholinergic agents do not clearly help or aggravate symptoms. In some cases of severe paroxysmal sweating, propranolol can partially diminish the frequency and intensity of sweating episodes (103).

PUPILLARY ABNORMALITIES

Pupillary constriction in response to light and subsequent accommodation are mediated by parasympathetic fibers arising in the midbrain Edinger-Westphal nucleus and travel with the third cranial nerve. Descending cortical and hypothalamic sympathetic fibers synapse on the intermediolateral gray cell column of the thoracic spinal cord. Preganglionic fibers synapse in the superior cervical ganglion with postganglionic sympathetic neurons whose axons travel through the carotid plexus to join the first division of the fifth cranial nerve. Sympathetic fibers mediate pupillary dilation in response to such stimuli as fright, pain, joy, fear, and vestibular stimulation. The location of a lesion of these systems may be determined by the application to the eyes of agents with known pharmacologic effects. Lesions of the parasympathetic system produce large pupils at rest which react more briskly than normal to drugs that increase cholinergic activity. This is thought to be the result of denervation hypersensitivity. The expected dilation does not follow the application of an anticholinergic drug if a parasympathetic lesion is present. Postganglionic sympathetic lesions produce small resting pupils that dilate more briskly than normal after epinephrine (denervation hypersensitivity), but do not dilate after cocaine, which blocks the reuptake of norepinephrine (5).

Only a few studies of pupillary function in untreated Parkinson's disease patients have been reported. Martignoni and colleagues (110) reported abnormal reflex responses to light and nociceptive stimuli which suggested impairment of integrative pupillomotor pathways. Korczyn and colleagues (111) found normal responses to local cocaine, phenylephrine (an alpha-1-adrenergic agonist), and pilocarpine (a cholinergic agonist). Pupillary diameters at rest were normal, but response to light was less in Parkinson's disease patients than in controls. Patients with unilateral Parkinson's disease had only ipsilateral pupillary dysfunction. These data are also consistent with a central dysfunction with intact peripheral autonomic pathways. This dysfunction was localized by the investigators of the Edinger–Westphal nucleus. Specific correlation of these experimental abnormalities with clinical symptoms has not been reported.

The pharmacotherapy of Parkinson's disease can be accompanied by symptoms of visual dysfunction. Patients being treated with antimuscarinic anticholinergic agents have a pharmacologic parasympathetic blockade which results in pupillary dilation, impaired pupillary constriction to light, or convergence and paralysis of accommodation. Impaired convergence is also a common ocular motility disorder in untreated Parkinson's disease, and this may be worsened by anticholinergic drugs. Patients may complain of photophobia, blurring of near vision, or micropsia. Patients with narrow-angle glaucoma may experience a precipitous rise in intraocular pressure due to obstructed drainage of the aqueous humor as extreme mydriasis forces the iris into the angle of the anterior chamber. Anticholinergic drugs should not be used in the latter setting (112). If visual symptoms are disabling and anticholinergic therapy sufficiently beneficial to prohibit its withdrawal, these visual side effects can be controlled by the use of miotic eye drops such as pilocarpine (113).

The effect of levodopa on pupillary function is less certain and its clinical significance is not known. Levodopa, when given orally in large doses or topically, causes pupillary dilation, either by metabolism to norepinephrine or by enhancing norepinephrine release (114). This effect does not occur in the presence of postganglionic sympathetic injury; however, the possible additional role of central pupillary control centers has not been excluded (115). Miosis has been described after several weeks of levodopa therapy (without DCI) by one group, who postulate depletion of norepinephrine by dopamine (116), while persistent mydriasis after an equivalent duration of therapy has been described by others (115).

REFERENCES

1. Bannister R, Oppenheimer DR. (1972). Degenerative diseases of the nervous system associated with autonomic failure. *Brain* 95: 457–474.
2. Polinsky RJ. (1984). Multiple system atrophy: Clinical aspects, pathophysiology and treatment. In: Jankovic J (Ed.), *Neurologic Clinics*. Philadelphia, W.B. Saunders.
3. Talman WT. (1985). Cardiovascular regulation and lesions of the central nervous system. *Ann Neurol* 1–12.
4. Reid JL. (1983). Central and peripheral autonomic control mechanisms. In: Bannister R (Ed.), *Autonomic Failure: A Textbook of Clinical Disorders of the Autonomic System*, Oxford University Press.
5. Johnson RH, Spaulding JMK. (1974). *Disorders of the Autonomic System*. Philadelphia, F.A. Davis.
6. Bannister R. (1983). Testing autonomic reflexes. In: Bannister R (Ed.), *Autonomic Failure: A Textbook of Clinical Disorders of the Autonomic System*. Oxford University Press.

7. Goetz CG, Lutge W, Tanner CM. (1986). Autonomic dysfunction in Parkinson's disease. *Neurology* 36: 73–75.
8. Wilcox CS, Aminoff MJ. (1976). Blood pressure responses to noradrenaline and dopamine infusions in Parkinson's disease and the Shy-Drager syndrome. *Br J Clin Pharmacol* 3: 207–214.
9. Gross M, Bannister R, Godwin-Austen R. (1972). Orthostatic hypotension in Parkinson's disease. *Lancet* 1: 174–176.
10. Appenzeller O, Goss JE. (1971). Autonomic deficits in Parkinson's syndrome. *Arch Neurol* 24: 50–57.
11. Aminoff MJ, Wilcox CS. (1972). Control of blood pressure in parkinsonism. *Proc R Soc Med* 65: 944–946.
12. Barbeau A, Gillo-Joffroy L, Brossard Y. (1970). Renin, Dopamine and Parkinson Disease. In: Barbeau A, McDowell JH (Eds.), *L-Dopa and Parkinsonism*. Philadelphia, F.A. Davis.
13. Barbeau A, Gillo-Joffroy L, Boucher R, Nowaczynski W, Genest J. (1969). Renin–aldosterone system in Parkinson's disease. *Science* 18: 291–292.
14. Wilcox CS, Aminoff MJ, Slater JDH. (1977). Sodium homeostasis in patients with autonomic failure. *Clin Sci Mol Med* 53: 321–328.
15. Aminoff MJ, Wilcox MJ. (1971). Assessment of autonomic function in patients with a parkinsonian syndrome. *Br Med J* 4: 80–84.
16. Polinsky RJ, Kopin IJ, Ebert MH, Weise V. (1981). Pharmacologic distinction of different orthostatic hypotension syndromes. *Neurology* 31: 1–7.
17. Rajput AH, Rozdilsky B. (1976). Dysautonomia in parkinsonism: a clinicopathological study. *J Neurol Neurosurg Psychiatry* 39: 1092–1100.
18. Emile J, Pouplard A, Bossu Van Nieuwenhuyse C, Bernat-Viallet C. (1980). Maladie de Parkinson, dysautonomie et autoanticorps dirigés contre les neurones sympathiques. *Rev Neurol (Paris)* 136(3): 221–233.
19. Langston JW, Forno LS. (1978). The hypothalamus in Parkinson disease. *Ann Neurol* 3: 129–133.
20. Javoy-Agid F, Ruberg M, Pique L, Bertagna X, Taquet H, Studler JM, Cesselin F, Epelbaum J, Agid Y. (1984). Biochemistry of the hypothalamus in Parkinson's disease. *Neurology* 34: 672–675.
21. Calne DB, Brennan AS, Spiers D, Stern GM. (1970). Hypotension caused by l-dopa. *Br Med J* 1: 474–475.
22. Keenan RE. (1970). The Eaton collaborative study of levodopa therapy in parkinsonism: A summary. *Neurology* 20: 46–59.
23. Ballantyne JP. (1973). Early and late effects of levodopa on the cardiovascular system in Parkinson's disease: a paired study. *J Neurol Sci* 19: 97–103.
24. Calne DB, Reid JL, Vakil SD, George CF, Rao S. (1973). Effects of carbidopa-levodopa on blood pressure. In: MD Yahr (Ed.), *Treatment of Parkinsonism–The Role of Dopa Decarboxylase Inhibitors, Advances in Neurology*, Vol. 2. Amsterdam, North Holland.
25. Baratti M, Calzetti S. (1984). Fluctuation of arterial blood pressure during end-of-dose akinesia in Parkinson's disease. *J Neurol Neurosurg Psychiatry* 47: 1241–1243.

26. Tanner CM, Goetz CG, Glantz RH, Glatt SL, Klawans HL. (1982). Pergolide mesylate and idiopathic Parkinson disease. *Neurology* 32: 1175–1179.

27. LeWitt PA, Ward CD, Larsen TA, Raphaelson MI, New RP, Foster N, Dambrosia JM, Calne DB. (1983). Comparison of pergolide and bromocriptine therapy in parkinsonism. *Neurology* 33: 1009–1014.

28. Montastruc JL, Chamontin B, Rascol A. (1985). Parkinson's disease and hypertension: Chronic bromocriptine treatment. *Neurology* 35: 1644–1647.

29. Quinn N, Illas A, Lhermitte F, Agid Y. (1981). Bromocriptine in Parkinson's disease: a study of cardiovascular effects. *J Neurol Neurosurg Psychiatry* 44: 426–429.

30. Goetz CG, Tanner CM, Klawans HL. (1982). Drug holiday in the management of Parkinson disease. *Clin Neuropharmacol* 5: 351–364.

31. Mills IH. (1970). Regulation of sodium excretion: intra- and extra-venal mechanisms. *J R Coll Physicians* 4: 335–350.

32. Bannister R. (1983). Treatment of progressive autonomic failure. In: Bannister R (Ed.), *Autonomic Failure: A Textbook of Clinical Disorders of the Autonomic System*. Oxford University Press.

33. Hoehn MM. (1975). Levodopa-induced postural hypotension. *Arch Neurol* 32: 50–51.

34. Abate G, Polimeni RM, Cuccurullo F, Puddu P, Lenzi S. (1979). Effects of indomethacin on postural hypotension in parkinsonism. *Br Med J* 2: 1466–1468.

35. Birkmayer W, Birkmayer G, Lechner H, Riederer P. (1983). L-3,4-threo-DOPS in Parkinson's disease: effects on orthostatic hypotension and dizziness. *J Neural Transm* 58: 305–313.

36. Schirger A, Sheps SG, Thomas JE, Fealey RD. (1981). Midodrine: a new agent in the management of idiopathic orthostatic hypotension and Shy-Drager syndrome. *Mayo Clin Proc* 56: 429–433.

37. Onrot J, Goldberg MR, Biaggioni I, Hollister AS, Kincaid D, Robertson D. (1985). Hemodynamic and humoral effects of caffeine in autonomic failure. *N Engl J Med* 313: 549–554.

38. Breretti G, Chiariello M, Carrechia G, Rengo F. (1979). Propranolol in the treatment of orthostatic blood pressure increase. *Br Heart J* 41: 245.

39. Polinsky RJ. (1983). Pharmacological responses and biochemical changes in progressive autonomic failure. In: Bannister R (Ed.), *Autonomic Failure: A Textbook of Clinical Disorders of the Autonomic System*. Oxford University Press.

40. Cotzias GC, Papvasiliou PS, Gellene R. (1969). Modification of parkinsonism—chronic treatment with l-dopa. *N Engl J Med* 280: 337–344.

41. Goldberg LI, Whitsett TL. (1971). Cardiovascular effects of levodopa. *Clin Pharmacol Ther* 12: 376–382.

42. Labram C, Picard JJ, Jacques G. (1972). Levodopa et torsades de pointes. *Nouv Presse Med* 1(3): 2402 (letter).

43. Barbeau A. (1969). L-dopa therapy in Parkinson's disease: nine years experience. *Can Med Assoc J* 101: 791–796.

44. McDowell FH, Lee JE, Swift T, Sweet RD, Ogsburg JS, Kessler JT. (1970). Treatment of Parkinson's syndrome with L-dihydroxyphenlalanine (levodopa). *Ann Intern Med* 72: 29–35.

45. Jenkins RB, Mendelson SH, Lamid S, Klawans HL. (1972). Levodopa therapy of patients with parkinsonism and heart disease. *Br Med J* 3: 512–514.

46. Hunter KR, Hollman A, Laurence DR, Stern GM. (1971). Levodopa in parkinsonian patients with heart-disease. *Lancet* 1: 932–934.

47. Freemon FR. (1971). Parkinsonism and cardiac arrhythmias. *Lancet* 2: 83–84.

48. Pallis CA, Calne DB. (1970). Describe a case of "atrial flutter" due to tremor artifacts. *Lancet* 2: 1313 (letter).

49. Saint-Pierre A. (1973). ECG artifacts simulating atrial flutter. *JAMA* 224: 1534 (letter).

50. Mars H, Krall J. (1971). L-dopa and cardiac arrhythmias. *N Engl J Med* 285(2): 1437 (letter).

51. Desjacques P, Moret P, Gauthier G. (1973). Effet cardiovasculaires de la L-dopa et de l'inhibiteur de la décarboxylase chez les malades atteints de la maladie de Parkinson. *Schweiz Med Wochenschr* 103: 1783–1785.

52. Leibowitz M, Lieberman A. (1984). C.O. and carbidopa. *N Engl J Med* 311: 671 (letter).

53. Parkes JD, Marsden CD, Price P. (1977). Amantadine-induced heart failure. *Lancet* 1: 904 (letter).

54. Calne DB, Eisler T, Gopinathan G, Williams A. (1980). Progress in pharmacotherapy of parkinsonism. In: M Goldstein et al. (Eds.), *Ergot Compounds and Brain Function: Neuroendocrine and Neuropsychiatric Aspects*. New York, Raven Press.

55. Lieberman AN, Goldstein M, Gopinathan G, et al. (1982). Further studies with pergolide in Parkinson disease. *Neurology* 32: 1181–1184.

56. Tanner CM, Chhablani R, Goetz CG, Klawans HL. (1985). Pergolide mesylate: lack of cardiac toxicity in patients with cardiac disease. *Neurology* 35: 918–921.

57. Spalding JMK, Nelson E. (1985). The autonomic nervous system. In: AB Baker, LH Baker (Eds.), *Clinical Neurology*. Philadelphia, Harper & Row.

58. Baumgarten HG. (19xx). Morphological basis of gastrointestinal motility: structure and innervation of gastrointestinal tract. In: Born GVR, Farah A, Herken H, Welch AD (Eds.), *Handbook of Experimental Pharmacology*, Vol. 59/I.

59. Patel GK, Diner WC, Texter EC. (1983). Swallowing and pharyngoesophageal function in the aging patient. In: Clinton Texter E (Ed.), *The Aging Gut: Pathophysiology, Diagnosis and Management*. New York, Masson.

60. Parkinson J. (1817). An essay on the shaking palsy. In: *Medical Classics*. London, Whittingham and Rowland.

61. Eadie MJ, Tyrer JH. (1965). Radiological abnormalities of the upper part of the alimentary tract in parkinsonism. *Australas Ann Med* 14: 23–27.

62. Calne DB, Shaw DG, Spiers ASD, Stern GM. (1970). Swallowing in parkinsonism. *Br J Radiol* 43: 456–457.

63. Palmer ED. (1974). Dysphagia in parkinsonism. *JAMA* 229(10): 1349.

64. Logemann JA, Blonsky ER, Boshes B. (1975). Dysphagia in parkinsonism. *JAMA* 231(1): 69–70.

65. Roman C. (19xx). Nervous control of esophageal and gastric motility. In: Born GVR, Farah A, Herken H, Welch AD (Eds.), *Handbook of Experimental Pharmacology*, Vol. 59/I.

66. Pallis CA. (1971). Parkinsonism: natural history and clinical features. *Br Med J* 3: 683–690.

67. Bramble MG, Cunliffe J, Dellipiani W. (1978). Evidence for a change in neurotransmitter affecting oesophageal motility in Parkinson's disease. *J Neurol Neurosurg Psychiatry* 41: 709–712.

68. Lieberman AN, Horowitz L, Redmond P, Pachter L, Lieberman, Leibowitz M. (1980). Dysphagia in Parkinson's disease. *Am J Gastroenterol* 74: 157–160.

69. Daniel EE. (1982). Pharmacology of adrenergic, cholinergic, and drugs acting on other receptors in gastrointestinal muscle. In: Bertaccini G (Ed.), *Mediators and Drugs in Gastrointestinal Motility II*.

70. Remer S, Morgenstern E, Mendoza M, Lowe YH, Yahr MD. (1985). Gastric emptying and Parkinson's disease. Presented at the VIIIth International Symposium on Parkinson's Disease, New York.

71. Mearrick PT, Wade DN, Birkett DJ, Morris J. (1974). Metoclopramide, gastric emptying and L-dopa absorption. *Aust NZ J Med* 3: 144–148.

72. Kurlan R, Rubin AJ, Miller C, Rivera-Calimlim L, Shoulson I. (1985). Continuous intraduodenal infusion of levodopa for resistant on-off fluctuations in parkinsonism. *Ann Neurol* 18(1): 139.

73. Paulseth JE, Jensen JJ, Klawans HL. (1985). Domperidone therapy in patients with Parkinson's disease with levodopa–carbidopa-related gastrointestinal complaints. *Ann Neurol* 18(1): 127.

74. Costa M, Burness JB. (19xx). Nervous control of intestinal motility. In: Born GVR, Farah A, Herken H, Welch AD (Eds.), *Handbook of Experimental Pharmacology*, Vol. 59/I.

75. Schuster MM. (1983). Colonic motor dysfunction and incontinence in the aging patient. In: Clinton Texter E (Ed.), *The Aging Gut*. New York, Masson.

76. Schuster MM. (1983). Fiber deficiency in gastrointestinal disease. In: Clinton Texter E (Ed.), *The Aging Gut*. New York, Masson.

77. Anuras S, Shirazi SS. (1984). Colonic pseudoobstruction. *Am J Gastroenterol* 79(7): 525–532.

78. Caplan LH, Jacobson HG, Rubinstein BM, Rotman MZ. (1965). Megacolon and volvulus in Parkinson's disease. *Radiology* 85: 73–79.

79. Appenzeller O. (1982). *The Autonomic Nervous System*. Amsterdam, Elsevier Biomedical Press.

80. Hughes RC, Polgar JG, Weightman D, Walton JN. (1971). Levodopa in Parkinsonism: The effects of withdrawal of anticholinergic drugs. *Br Med J* 29: 487–491.

81. Hedlund B, Abens J, Bartfai T. (1983). Vasoactive intestinal polypeptide and muscarinic receptors: supersensitivity induced by long-term atropine treatment. *Science* 220: 519–521.

82. Cros P, Parret J, Peyrin J, Freidel M, Dumas P. (1979). Sialorrhées. *Rev Stomatol Chir Maxillofac* 6: 319–324.

83. Bateson MC, Gibberd FB, Wilson RSE. (1973). Salivary symptoms in Parkinson disease. *Arch Neurol* 29: 274–275.

84. Nutt JG, Woodward WR, Hammerstad JP, et al. (1984). The "on-off" phenomenon in Parkinson's disease. Relation to levodopa absorption and transport. *N Engl J Med* 310(8): 483–488.

85. Kupferman I. (1981). Motivation. In: Kandell ER, Schwartz JH (Eds.), *Principles of Neural Science*. New York, Elsevier/North Holland.

86. Mayeux R, Stern Y, Rosen J, Leventhal J. (1981). Depression, intellectual impairment, and Parkinson disease. *Neurology* 31: 645–650.

87. van der Linden C, Jankovic J, Jansson B. (1985). Lateral hypothalamic dysfunction in Parkinson's disease. *Ann Neurol* 18(1): 137.

88. Rosenberg P, Herishanu Y, Beilin B. (1977). Increased appetite (bulimia) in Parkinson's disease. *J Am Geriat Soc* 25(6): 177–278.

89. Bradley WE, Sundin T. (1982). The physiology and pharmacology of urinary tract dysfunction. *Clin Neuropharmacol* 5(2): 131–158.

90. Aranda B, Perrigot M, Mazieres L, Pierrot-Deseilligny E. (1983). Les troubles vésico-sphinctériens de la maladie de Parkinson. *Rev Neurol* 139(4): 283–288.

91. Porter RW, Bors E. (1971). Neurogenic bladder in parkinsonism: effect of thalamotomy. *J Neurosurg* 34: 27–34.

92. Murnaghan GF. (1961). Neurogenic disorder of the bladder in parkinsonism. *Br J Urol* 33: 403–409.

93. Langworthy OR. (1938). Vesical abnormalities associated with the Parkinsonian syndrome. *Arch Neurol Psychiatry* 40: 44–57.

94. Andersen JT, Hebjorn S, Frimodt-Møller, Walter S, Worm-Petersen J. (1976). Disturbances of micturition in Parkinson's disease. *Acta Neurol Scand* 53: 161–170.

95. Hattori T. (1983). Bladder function in autonomic failure. In: Bannister R (Ed.), Oxford University Press.

96. McGuire EJ. (1984). Clinical evaluation and treatment of neurogenic vesical dysfunction. In: JA Libertino (Ed.), *International Perspectives in Urology*. Baltimore, Williams and Wilkins.

97. Murdock MI, Olsson CA, Sax DS, Krane RJ. (1975). Effects of levodopa on the bladder outlet. *J Urol* 113: 803–805.

98. Benson GS, Raezer DM, Anderson JR, Saunders CD, Corriere JN. (1976). Effect of levodopa on urinary bladder. *Urology* 7(1): 24–28.

99. Sillén U, Rubenson A, Hjalmás K. (1979). Evidence for a central monoaminergic influence on urinary bladder control mechanism. *Scand J Urol Nephrol* 13: 265–268.

100. Reaves TA, Hayward JN. (1979). Hypothalamic and extrahypothalamic thermoregulatory centers. In: Lomax P, Schonbaum E (Eds.), *Body Temperature*. New York, Marcel Dekker.

101. Cox B. (1979). Dopamine. In: Lomax P, Schonbaum E (Eds.), *Body Temperature*. New York, Marcel Dekker.

102. Gowers WR. (1893). *Diseases of the Nervous System*. Philadelphia, Blakiston.

103. Tanner CM, Goetz CG, Klawans HL. (1982). Paroxysmal drenching sweats in idiopathic parkinsonism: response to propranolol. *Neurology* 32(2): A162.

104. Elliott K, Côté LJ, Frewin DB, Downey JA. (1974). Vascular responses in the hands of Parkinson's disease patients. *Neurology* 24: 857–862.

105. Toru M, Matsuda O, Makiguchi K, Sugano K. (1981). Neuroleptic malignant syndrome-like state following a withdrawal of antiparkinsonian drugs. *J Nerv Ment Dis* 169(5): 324–327.

106. Friedman JH, Feinberg SS, Feldman RG. (1984). A neuroleptic malignant-like syndrome due to l-dopa withdrawal. *Ann Neurol* 16(1): 126.

107. Sechi GP, Tanda F, Mutani R. (1984). Fatal hyperpyrexia after withdrawal of levodopa. *Neurology* 34: 249–251.

108. Pfeiffer RF, Sucha EL. (1985). On-off induced malignant hyperthermia. *Ann Neurol* 18(1): 138.

109. Kurlan R, Hamill R, Shoulson I. (1984). Neuroleptic malignant syndrome. *Clin Neuropharmacol* 7(2): 109–120.

110. Martignoni E, Micieli G, Magri M, Pacchetti C, Cavallini A, Sances G, Nappi G. (1985). Autonomic failure in Parkinson's disease. Presented at the VIIIth International Symposium on Parkinson's Disease.

111. Korczyn AD, Rubenstein AE, Yahr MD. (1985). The pupil in Parkinson's disease. Presented at the VIIIth International Symposium on Parkinson's Disease.

112. Weiner N. (1985). Atropine, scopolamine, and related antimuscarinic drugs. In: Goodman, Gillman (Eds.), *The Pharmacological Basis of Therapeutics*, 7th Ed. New York, Macmillan Publishing.

113. Taylor P. (1985). Cholinergic agonists. In: Goodman, Gillman (Eds.), *The Pharmacological Basis of Therapeutics*, 7th Ed. New York, Macmillan Publishing.

114. Spiers ASD, Calne DB. (1969). Action of dopamine on the human iris. *Br Med J* 4: 333–335.

115. Weintraub MI, Gaasterland D, Van Woert MH. (1970). Pupillary effects of levodopa therapy. *N Engl J Med* 283(3): 120–123.

116. Spiers ASD, Calne DB, Fayers PM. (1970). Miosis during l-dopa therapy. *Br Med J* 2: 639–640.

8
Sensory Dysfunction

STUART R. SNIDER and R. SANDYK
University of Arizona, Tucson, Arizona

Parkinson's disease is considered by most physicians to be a disorder of movement that spares the senses and intellect (1). While it is undeniably true that the major *signs* are motor signs, it has long been appreciated that some individuals with the disease experience distressing but ill-defined and intermittent sensory *symptoms* (pain, tingling, numbness, disagreeable heat or coldness) often in the limb or body region most affected with motor signs (2-4). Perhaps because sensory signs are infrequent on clinical examinations, such complaints have been underemphasized by writers of medical textbooks in the last half century.

In the last several years abnormalities of sensation in parkinsonism patients have again become an area of interest and a subject for clinical investigation (5). The first of the recent publications to attempt to characterize and define subjective sensory complaints clinically appears to be that of Sigwald and coworkers (6,7) in French, followed by Zsiboy-Gisinger (8) in German, and Snider and colleagues (9) in English.

In this chapter we have divided sensory symptoms into two categories based on their presumed origins: those caused by an abnormality within peripheral nerves, sensory tracts, and other parts of the nervous system, called "primary," and those arising outside the nervous system, called "secondary." Each may have distinctive clinical characteristics. For example, the secondary sensory symptom, hip or knee pain caused by arthritis, is worse with movement, localized to the area of the joint, and responsive to anti-inflammatory drugs. A similar sensation in the proximal leg that is not movement related, localized to the knee or hip, or diminished by anti-inflammatory agents may be neurogenic, that is, primary, in parkinsonian patients.

The clinical distinction of primary and secondary symptoms is the main focus of this chapter. Recognition of primary symptoms can prevent unnecessary diagnostic tests and inappropriate drug treatment. It may allow earlier diagnosis of Parkinson's disease; sensory complaints herald the disease in about 10% of patients (1,2-4,6-12).

PRIMARY SENSORY SYMPTOMS: CLINICAL CHARACTERISTICS

The percentage of Parkinson's disease patients with primary sensory symptoms is about 40% (4,6,8-11). Lower percentages have been obtained in surveys that include sensory complaints as one topic in a list of questions. For example, Lesser et al. (13) reported that 18% of 131 patients had "intractable" sensory symptoms; they evaluated more than 40 variables. Higher figures have been published by authors who included some complaints that were probably musculoskeletal in origin, such as the 63% reported by Zsiboy-Gisinger (8).

The character of the primary disagreeable sensation varies widely, perhaps beyond the limits of the average patient's ability to describe it in some instances. Mendel (4) listed the following descriptions: "rheumatic pain, neuralgia, lightning pain, tormenting paresthesias, . . . burning 'like there was a fire inside', . . . formication, itching, . . . 'legs wrapped with wire', . . . 'like being pricked with a needle.' " Other sensations such as numbness and coldness may occur but because they are often less unpleasant may be underreported. The broad categories of sensations are aching pain, numbness (including tingling numbness), and thermal paresthesias (coldness and burning).

Severity and frequency of occurrence are variable. It is rare for the paresthesia to be so severe as to require in-hospital treatment, but several examples have been reported in the literature (6,7,9,14). However, in-hospital diagnostic studies to rule out thrombophlebitis, angina pectoris, etc. are not uncommon. The majority of paresthesias tend to be mild, inconstant, and to diminish with either advanced disease (4) or successful treatment of the motor symptoms (6, 8-15). The median frequency of the episodes in a stable, optimally treated patient is about four per week, and the duration of an episode about 2 hr (9). However, before diagnosis or in complicated cases, symptoms may be almost constant (10,11,14,15).

RELATIONSHIP OF SENSORY SYMPTOMS TO NEUROLOGIC SIGNS AND TREATMENT

Patients with postencephalitic parkinsonism (9) or Shy-Drager syndrome early in the course (16) may have a higher prevalence of sensory symptoms than patients with idiopathic parkinsonism. In contrast, patients with essential tremor (10) are little different from a control population (9,10).

By definition, primary sensory symptoms are not caused by the motor deficit, nor does antiparkinson medication appear to be associated with an increase or decrease in the overall prevalence of sensory symptoms (6,9-12,14).

Pain is the most common primary sensory complaint, experienced by at least 10% of patients (9-12). It is usually described as intermittent, hard to localize, and cramplike or aching. If in the limbs, it is experienced more often proximal to the foot or hand on the side of initial or greater motor deficit. In some patients, the pain correlates with "off" periods and is diminished by optimal levodopa therapy. On the other hand, burning sensations are occasionally related to antiparkinsonian therapy. In about half of all cases, levodopa may produce or aggravate episodic burning sensations. Tingling and numbness are experienced more often in the distal extremities, and can coexist with pain. Although often aggravated by immobility of the involved limbs, there is no consistent relationship with bradykinesia in the majority of patients.

Pain symptoms are often of both central and somatic origins in patients with clinical fluctuations. These have been classified as follows: (1) pain predating other symptoms, (2) "off" period pain, (3) beginning-of-dose pain, (4) diphasic pain, (5) early morning pain *secondary to* dystonia, and (6) "off" period pain *secondary to* dystonia (15; W. Koller, personal communication). Pain is less severe and frequent during "on" periods.

Parkinsonian patients with primary sensory symptoms have few objective sensory abnormalities (4,5,9-12). A slight decrease in superficial pain perception and touch sensibility is found in about 15% of cases. These objective sensory abnormalities are usually found ipsilateral to the motor deficit in the limbs (but not face) and may vary from examination to examination (9,17). In about 10% of cases, there is nonspecific loss of vibration sense in the legs. Most of the parkinsonian patients who experience sensory symptoms have normal findings on sensory examination.

Sensory symptoms that fluctuate with motor disorder are usually improved with its successful therapy (6-12,14,15). The response to the various drugs is not always predictable. With levodopa, bromocriptine, and tricyclic antidepressants some patients' sensory symptoms improve, but other patients experience exacerbation. Anticholinergics may occasionally bring out paresthesias, although some patients improved with orphenadrine treatment (6,7). Neuroleptics are not recommended in the treatment of these sensations because they may aggravate the motor disability and cause sensory symptoms similar to those found in patients with primary parkinsonism (6,7). Anti-inflammatory drugs are seldom specifically beneficial (11), although narcotic analgesics have provided relief (11,14). Heat, massage, movement, and elevation of the limbs are of limited value (9). Electroconvulsive therapy and thalamotomy were found to decrease sensory complaints in small numbers of patients (8,9). While no single agent appears uniquely effective for severe sensory symptoms, the above observations provide a basis for an approach to management.

Parkinsonian patients with primary sensory symptoms seldom have significant abnormalities in primary or cortical sensation. More sophisticated examination techniques have revealed evidence suggestive of a deficit in sensory information processing, including delayed evoked responses, distortion of body image, abnormal visual and spatial orientation (5,12,17,18), and other perceptual deficits. Sensory deficits were often lateralized to the side of worse motor involvement, but not necessarily quantitatively related (9,10,18).

SECONDARY SENSORY SYMPTOMS

Secondary sensory symptoms are commonly caused by temporary peripheral nerve dysfunction due to pressure, dependent edema, abnormal vascular control mechanisms, and immobility, and by painful arthritis, dystonia, muscle cramps, and strains.

Sensory symptoms of neurogenic (primary) origin may coexist with pain and paresthesias of uncertain or mixed as well as somatic origins. An example of paresthesia of uncertain origin is the restless leg syndrome (RLS), specifically defined as a disagreeable crawling or aching sensation beneath the skin of the legs that is relieved by walking. The incidence of RLS in parkinsonian patients may be higher than in the general population (9,19). The use of opiates such as D-propoxyphene may ameliorate this symptom.

Parkinsonian patients with primary sensory symptoms may undergo diagnostic evaluation for a variety of somatic diseases, particularly angina pectoris, arthritis, and other musculoskeletal disorders. In many cases a careful critical history or a therapeutic trial (with antiparkinsonian or antiarthritic drugs) would establish the diagnosis.

PATHOGENESIS OF SENSORY DYSFUNCTION

Sensory complaints can be categorized physiologically as: (a) sensations generated by abnormal nerves or neurons and unrelated to events at peripheral sensory organs (primary paresthesias); (b) normal sensations from skin, muscles, etc., unrelated to the motor or other disorder but distorted in their conduction from the periphery to the cerebrum (dysesthesias); or (c) normal sensations related to the motor or other disorder. The assumption that the third mechanism explains most sensory complaints may be based on the occasionally dramatic correlation of sensory and motor symptoms and the coexistence of two or more types of sensory complaints. A sensation of large muscle stiffness, vague aching, and tingling-plus-numbness may occur during bradykinetic periods in patients. This sensation is similar to the discomfort experienced by someone without parkinsonism who has a several-hour period of reduced mobility, such as in plane travel. A temporal correlation of paresthesia and bradykinesia is present in some patients but in only a minority of patients is there a severity correlation, and mobilization alone does not consistently relieve the sensation (9). The coincidence of mobilization, disappearance of the "off" motor symptoms (with or without dyskinesia), and decrease in the disagreeable sensations (15) could be explained by parallel biochemical changes, for example, increased central nervous system catecholamine turnover (9).

Another explanation occasionally given for sensory complaints in parkinsonism is that a patient who is depressed and suffering from marked fatigue is more likely to be bothered by aches and pains, which are normally largely subconscious (19). In our opinion, this may be valid for those sensations of somatic or visceral origin that, however exaggerated, are clearly clinically characterized, such as the pain of arthritis or other localized musculoskeletal disorder. These secondary sensory symptoms may occur in parkinsonian patients, be relayed as a complaint to the physician during periods of depression or fatigue, and can co-exist with primary sensory symptoms. The latter are distinguished by their lack of respect for anatomical boundaries and lack of responses to movement, pressure, and anti-inflammatory drugs. In our experience, distortion of the character (quality and extent) of sensory symptoms rarely occurs in the depression of parkinsonism unless overt psychosis, causalgia, or other severe neuropathy is present.

Primary sensory symptoms may be caused by dysfunction at the level of the peripheral nervous system (e.g., peripheral nerves, autonomic nervous system) or at the level of the central nervous system (basal ganglia, cortex). There is no specific pathology of peripheral sensory nerves in idiopathic parkinsonism (20,21) but pathologic and functional abnormalities of the autonomic nervous system, which influence sensory thresholds (22), are common in parkinsonism (23,24).

In postencephalitic and vascular parkinsonism, sensory pathways in the midbrain may be affected by encephalitis and compromise of blood supply shared with the substantia nigra. There is no structural pathology of central sensory pathways in idiopathic parkinsonism (Parkinson's disease) (20). However, substantia nigra, locus ceruleus, and other catecholaminergic nuclei are potential sources of sensory dysfunction via their ascending, descending, and spinal connections. Reduced modulation by substantia nigra (9) and/or basal ganglia (10) of thalamic nuclei and their cerebral sensory projections has been suggested as a cause for sensory symptoms. The contribution of substantia nigra to the sensory abnormalities in Parkinson's disease requires further clarification. However, it is likely that the sensory abnormalities experienced by most patients result from functional abnormalities at several sites: dorsal roots, sympathetic ganglia, sensory nuclei in brainstem, periaqueductal grey.

One mechanism likely to be important in the pathogenesis of sensory symptoms in Parkinson's disease is alteration of neurotransmitter functions.

Catecholamine projections are found in many sensory areas of the central nervous system (CNS) and their loss could trigger the sensory abnormalities observed in these patients (9). Attention has also been focused on the endogenous opioids (11). Enkephalin-containing neurons have been demonstrated in the dorsal horn, where they are thought to participate in the regulation of incoming nociceptive sensory information. High concentrations of opioids and their receptors have also been found in the striatum and opioids have been shown to modulate the activity of striatal dopamine. Since opioid-containing neurons in the striatum may degenerate in Parkinson's disease, an imbalance in dopamine-opioid transmission could cause some abnormal sensory phenomena. It is of theoretical as well as practical importance that both levodopa and opiates have been reported to ameliorate some of the severe sensory disturbances that are not affected by nonnarcotic analgesics (11,14).

PATHOPHYSIOLOGICAL SIGNIFICANCE OF PRIMARY SENSORY SYMPTOMS

In addition to diagnostic and therapeutic difficulties caused by paresthesias, these symptoms may provide clues to the pathogenesis of the motor disorder if not the disease itself. Dopamine-blocking drugs may produce sensory symptoms that are bilateral but otherwise similar in character to those that occur in early idiopathic parkinsonism (6,7).

In the first months of treatment, such sensory symptoms in individuals treated with neuroleptics may correlate approximately with bradykinesia (6,7). It is possible that agents that reversibly block dopamine receptors produce paresthesias as a signal or symptom of this effect in predisposed individuals. It is also possible that some endogenous agent that blocks dopamine receptors accounts for paresthesias in treated idiopathic parkinsonism. Indeed, many patients with paresthesias seem to have clinical fluctuations and a higher incidence of treatment-related problems (9-15).

Both sensory and parkinsonian motor symptoms due to dopamine-blocking drugs usually diminish and disappear when the drug is discontinued, and there is no convincing evidence that individuals experiencing this drug-induced syndrome are more likely to develop Parkinson's disease. However, at least 10% of patients with Parkinson's disease, not exposed to dopaminolytic medications, report that paresthesias preceded the motor symptoms by months or years (2-4,6-12). One patient we treated reported that several-hour episodes of vague but disagreeable tingling ache deep in the middle and proximal left extremities occurred every few weeks for 10 years before obvious left-sided tremor and bradykinesia were present. In this situation the sensory symptoms may represent an active pathologic process that damages systems and destroys dopamine neurons in the brain, a kind of "central pain" that may in some patients precede dopamine depletion severe enough to cause motor signs. This speculation is supported by the observations of Nashold (25) that stimulation of the midbrain just dorsal to the nigrostriatal tract in humans caused disagreeable and poorly localized sensations similar, if not identical, to those that may precede idiopathic parkinsonism (9,26).

If sensory symptoms are an early indication of an intermittent or progressive disease process damaging dopaminergic neurons, therapeutic intervention may prevent progression and appearance of the motor manifestations of the disease. Identification of preclinical parkinsonism is an important research priority since pharmacologic agents that might slow or prevent progression (e.g., monoamine oxidase inhibitors) are currently being evaluated. Individuals with the syndrome of intermittent hemiparesthesias, decreased initiative and productivity, fatigue, and depression, may represent a subgroup at risk.

MANAGEMENT OF PAIN AND PARESTHESIA

The first step in management of disagreeable sensory symptoms in a patient with Parkinson's disease is to establish the possible origins of the symptoms. The most difficult situations diagnostically are when pain is the presenting symptom preceding tremor or other motor signs, and when the sensory complaints are poorly described by the patient because of dementia or some other problem in communication. In the former situation, there is no substitute for a high index of suspicion. Patients approximately 50 years of age presenting with a sensory complaint in the proximal part of the limbs of one side, and which is unrelated to movement and not reproduced by palpation, should be candidates for therapeutic trials of either mild antiparkinson drugs such as amantadine hydrochloride or nonsteroidal anti-inflammatory drugs.

In the case of patients with established parkinsonism from whom a satisfactory description of the sensory complaint cannot be obtained, it may be necessary to rule out certain potentially serious and treatable conditions such as cardiac ischemia and thrombophlebitis using specific tests. A trial of antiparkinson drugs or a change of these drugs might be indicated when more serious diseases have been ruled out with reasonable certainty.

The majority of parkinsonian patients with primary sensory symptoms have relatively mild and transient symptoms that do not require treatment separate from that of the movement disorder. When painful or disagreeable sensations occur coincident with "off" periods, they more frequently than not respond to change in antiparkinson medication, resulting in more predictable therapeutic response and longer "on" time. Likewise, cramplike sensations in the proximal extremities not associated with palpable increased muscle contraction may respond to longer-duration dopamine agonists such as bromocriptine. As noted above, the coincidence of response of motor and sensory symptoms does not indicate that the former causes the latter but can be a reflection of parallel events corrected by increasing brain dopamine levels and turnover.

In a small proportion of parkinsonian patients pain, burning, formication, and occasionally other paresthesias may require a specific therapeutic effort. Sensory complaints in this group of patients are generally not time-locked with the motor disorder, including dyskinesia, or with drug administration. Such patients often have other nonmotoric symptoms such as restlessness (akathisia) and mental or sleep disturbance. When the pain or paresthesia is obviously precipitated by the introduction or an increase in the dosage of a medication for parkinsonism, this medication can be reduced or deleted. Discomfort of the aching type can be precipitated by anticholinergic drugs and low-dosage dopamine agonists but is more often diminished than exacerbated by high-dosage levodopa and related drugs.

Nonaching paresthesias such as burning may correlate with an increase in dopaminergic therapy. Since levodopa remains the most consistently effective drug, this circumstance often creates a therapeutic problem. Nutt and Carter (14) found that in two patients this type of paresthesia was worsened during an infusion of leucine and improved during a steady infusion of levodopa in one patient. This suggested that very careful titration of oral levodopa and competitive dietary influences might reduce such sensations. Alternatively, a longer-acting dopamine agonist drug could serve the same purpose.

Other drugs for resistant paresthesias have been recommended. These include orphenadrine, diphenhydramine, and antidepressants, with their potential for accentuating synaptic affects of monoamines (9–11). However, these adjunctive drugs seldom alleviate the most distressing paresthesias.

The restless leg syndrome and similar paresthesias can be treated with diazepam or clonazepam but these agents may not be well tolerated by some parkinsonian patients. Some patients with nighttime and immobility-related extremity symptoms may benefit from nonpharmacologic therapies such as light elasticized or flannel stockings. Similarly, TENS units have been used, although with inconsistent benefit.

In extreme cases, it may be necessary to hospitalize the patient for sequential trials of medications as listed above. Electroconvulsive treatment was effective in one patient (9) and may be considered when all reasonable medication trials are ineffective. It is of interest that painful sensory symptoms have been ameliorated by thalamotomy (8). This approach to therapy cannot be recommended over the multiple medication options currently available because of the bilaterality of symptoms in more advanced idiopathic parkinsonism.

Finally, it should be mentioned that the usual approaches to pain control, including nonnarcotic and narcotic analgesics, may be variably effective in patients with primary sensory symptoms. Generally, however, aspirin and the spectrum of nonsteroidal anti-inflammatory agents, as well as acetaminophen and related drugs, are not beneficial in patients with severe symptoms. On the other hand, narcotic analgesics are often effective, and may have a specific action in some situations, for example, severe restless leg syndrome. Use of narcotics carries a real risk of addiction because of the chronic course of paresthesias severe enough to warrant their use. If narcotics are required, consideration should be given to coadministration of potentiating drugs, for example hydroxyzine, diphenhydramine, amitriptyline or in the case of restless-leg-like symptoms of the extremities, a benzodiazepine.

REFERENCES

1. Parkinson J. (1817). *An Essay on the Shaking Palsy*. London, Sherwood, Nelly and Jones.
2. Charcot JM. (1877). *Lectures on Diseases of the Nervous System*. Translated by Sigerson G. London, The New Sydenham Society.
3. Gowers WR. (1903). *A Manual of Diseases of the Nervous System*, Ed 2. Philadelphia, P Blakiston's Sons.
4. Mendel K. (1911). *Die Paralysis Agitans*. Berlin, Karger.
5. Proctor F, Riklan M, Cooper IS, et al. (1963). Somatosensory status of parkinsonian patients before and after chemothalamotomy. *Neurology* 13: 906–912.
6. (1960). Parkinson et paresthesies provoquées par les neuroleptiques. *Semin Hop Paris* 44: 2222–2225.
7. Sigwald J, Ramondeaud C. (1968). Les reactions désagréables ou douloureuses de la maladie de Parkinson et de la thérapeutique neuroleptique (paresthesies, impatiences, crampes, akathisie). Leur amelioration par l'alimenazine. *Semin Hop Paris* 44: 2897–2899.
8. Zsiboy-Gisinger M. (1970). Pain in Parkinson's syndrome. *Neurochir* 13: 165–169.
9. Snider SR, Fahn S, Isgreen WP, Cote LJ. (1976). Primary sensory symptoms in parkinsonism. *Neurology* 26: 423–429.
10. Koller WC. (1984). Sensory symptoms in Parkinson's disease. *Neurology* 34: 957–959.
11. Sandyk R. (1982). Backache as an early symptom in Parkinson's disease. *S Afr Med J* 61: 3–9.
12. Yahr MD. (1982). Parkinson's disease. In: Yahr MD (Ed.), *Seminars in Neurology* 2: 343–351. New York, Grune and Stratton.
13. Lesser RP, Fahn S, Snider SR, Cote LJ, Isgreen WP, Barrett RE. (1979). Analysis of the clinical problems in parkinsonism and the complications of long-term levodopa therapy. *Neurology* 29: 1253–1260.
14. Nutt JG, Carter JH. (1984). Sensory symptoms in parkinsonism related to central dopaminergic function. *Lancet* 2: 456–457.
15. Goetz CG, Tanner CM, Levy M, Wilson RS, Garron DG (1985). Pain in idiopathic Parkinson's disease. *Neurology* 35 (Suppl 1): 200.

16. Schwartz G. (1967). The orthostatic hypotension syndrome of Shy-Drager. *Arch Neurol* 16: 123–139.

17. Bowen F, Hoehn M, Yahr M. (1972). Cerebral dominance in relation to tracking and tapping performance in patients with parkinsonism. *Neurology* 22: 32–39.

18. Bodis-Wollner I, Yahr MD, Mylin LH. (1984). Nonmotor functions of the basal ganglia. *Adv Neurol* 40: 289–298.

19. Birkmayer W. (1976). In discussion of: Snider SR, Fahn S, Cote LJ, Isgreen WP: Primary sensory symptoms in Parkinson's disease. In: Birkmayer W, Hornykiewicz O. (Eds.), *Advances in Parkinsonism*. Basel, Editiones Roche.

20. McMenemey W, Meyer A, et al. (ed.) (1963). *Greenfield's Neuropathology*. London, Edward Arnold Limited.

21. Minckler J. (ed.) (1968). *Pathology of the Nervous System*. New York, McGraw-Hill Book Company.

22. Schiff J. (1974). Rose of the sympathetic innervation of the Pacinian corpuscle. *J Gen Physiol* 63: 601–608.

23. Appenzeller O, Goss J. (1971). Autonomic deficits in Parkinson's syndrome. *Arch Neurol* 24: 50–57.

24. Aminoff M, Wilcox C. (1971). Assessment of autonomic function in patients with a parkinsonian syndrome. *Br Med J* 4: 80–84.

25. Nashold B, Wilson W, Slaughter D. (1969). Sensations evoked by stimulation in the midbrain of man. *J Neurosurg* 30: 14–24.

26. Cooper IS. (1965). Clinical and physiologic implications of thalamic surgery for disorders of sensory communication. *J Neurol Sci* 2: 493–519.

9

Diagnosis and Treatment of Parkinsonian Dysarthria

ANTHONY G. MLCOCH
Edward Hines, Jr. Veterans Administration Hospital, Hines, Illinois

The patient with Parkinson's disease presents a myriad of medical and medically related problems. These include gait and mobility problems, the complete or partial inability to perform activities of daily living, tremor, psychosocial adjustment difficulties, and occasionally problems of orientation and cognition (Scott et al., 1985). One of the most common signs, which can have a devastating effect on the patient's personal and interpersonal relationships, is the presence of a speech disturbance. In an early prevalence study, Atarachi and Uchida (1959) found that 73% of all parkinsonian patients they observed had some form of a dysarthric speech disturbance. Oxtoby (1982), in a review of 261 cases of parkinsonism, found that 49% demonstrated significant speaking difficulties. At present, it is generally accepted that approximately half of all parkinsonian patients exhibit a speech disorder. It is also accepted that as the disease progresses, toward its later stages, the prevalence of a speech disturbance increases (Uziel et al., 1975).

This chapter aims to assist the general practitioner, internist, neurologist, speech pathologist, and other paramedical professionals in the diagnosis and treatment of the speech disorder associated with Parkinson's disease. The signs and symptoms of the disorder as well as the perceptual, acoustic, and physiological investigations supporting their presence will be reviewed. In addition, the pharmacologic and behavioral management regimens that appear to have a salutary effect on parkinsonian speech will be examined.

DESCRIPTION AND DIAGNOSIS

The classification and differential diagnosis of the speech disturbance associated with Parkinson's disease is essentially based on the perceptual characteristics exhibited by the patient. In their classic investigation of the dysarthrias, Darley and co-workers (1969a,b; 1975) tape recorded connected speech samples from 32 patients whose sole neurologic disorder was Parkinson's disease. Each sample was played to three judges who, using a seven-point equal-appearing interval scale, rated the degree to which 38 speech dimensions were present. These included dimensions pertaining to vocal pitch (4), vocal loudness (5), vocal quality (9), respiration (3), prosody (10), articulation (5), and overall impression (2) (intelligibility and bizarreness).

Using the above methodology, Darley and associates found that patients with Parkinson's disease produce a distinct constellation of features which they collectively called "hypokinetic dysarthria." Table 1 shows those dimensions found to be the most deviant and characteristic of this dysarthria. The pattern that emerges shows that the Parkinsonian patient demonstrates (a) deviations of phonation in that his or her voice is produced with monotony of pitch, monotony of loudness, and with a breathy or mildly harsh quality; (b) a prosodic disturbance, showing that hypokinetic dysarthric patients' rate of speech may be slow or extremely fast and that arrests of speech might occur aperiodically resulting in inappropriate silences and/or repetition of sounds and syllables, giving the examiner the impression of stuttering behavior (see Koller, 1983 for discussion); and (c) an articulatory disorder demonstrating that

TABLE 1 Most Deviant Speech Dimensions Observed in 32 Patients with Parkinson's Disease

Rank	Dimension	Mean scale value
1	Monopitch	4.64
2	Reduced stress	4.46
3	Monoloudness	4.26
4	Imprecise consonants	3.59
5	Inappropriate silences	2.40
6	Short rushes	2.22
7	Harsh voice quality	2.08
8	Breathy voice (continuous)	2.04
9	Pitch level	1.76
10	Variable rate	1.74

Source: From Darley et al., 1975.

patients with Parkinson's disease often distort the sounds of speech. In addition, the overall loudness and decay of the voice should be mentioned as features of hypokinetic speech. Even though the mean rating of these dimensions was not within the deviant range, reduction of vocal intensity is common and often the only speech symptom exhibited by the parkinsonian patient.

Perceptual–Acoustic–Physiological Correlates

From Darley et al.'s (1969a,b; 1975) investigation, it should become clear that the hypokinetic dysarthric disturbance exhibited by the parkinsonian patient is usually not manifested in only one subsystem of speech. The respiratory, phonatory, and articulatory components are all involved to some extent while the presence and the severity of each is dependent on the stage of the disease (Logemann and Fisher, 1981). The existence of these signs and symptoms has been studied acoustically and physiologically. The following is a review of those investigations.

Respiratory

The perceptual characteristics of diminished vocal loudness, short phrases, variable speech rate, and sporadic arrests of speech exhibited by parkinsonian patients suggest that their respiratory as well as their phonatory musculature may be limited in range and/or that there is a lack of coordination with the speech act. Schilling (1925, as reviewed by Grewel, 1957), found the negative breathing and respiratory patterns for speech of eight parkinsonian subjects to be irregular in amplitude from cycle to cycle and wider in extent than normal. He also described hesitations or abnormally long pauses between inhalatory and exhalatory cycles as well as the absence of regular undulations during resting tidal breathing. Cramer (1940, as reviewed by Grewel, 1957) reported that six patients with postencephalitic Parkinson's disease showed significantly reduced vital capacity (i.e., below 1.5 L). Tidal volume was reduced and was observed to be unchanged by forced breathing. Rapid tidal breathing, at times twice the normal rate, was observed as well. In addition, Cramer found that the expiratory cycle during her patients' oral reading was often interrupted by small inhalations.

Laszewski (1956) also reported a marked decrease of vital capacity in most cases of parkinsonism along with an extremely limited thoracic excursion during both respiratory cycles. She attributed this to overall rigidity of the intercostal muscles.

In looking at the respiratory functions of 12 patients with parkinsonism, De la Torre and colleagues (1960) found that vital capacity varied from patient to patient. Nearly two-thirds of their patients' vital capacities were between 90 and 120% of the expected values while one-third produced vital capacities below the 80% level. Tidal volume was within normal limits for all patients. However, their resting breathing pattern was marked by irregularities of rate and amplitude.

The investigators attributed this to a lack of coordination and synergism between the agonist and antagonist respiratory muscles.

In contrast, Ewanowski (1964; as reported by Darley et al., 1975) in one of the few extensive dissertations on parkinsonian speech behavior, found no significant difference between the tidal respiratory patterns of a group of female parkinsonian subjects and a normal control group matched for age. The only significant finding was that the rate of quiet breathing was positively related to the degree of neurologic impairment. The more severe the parkinsonian symptoms, the faster the respiratory rates.

Using an ink recording respirometer and a pneumatic mask, Kim (1968) observed the respiratory patterns of nine parkinsonian patients. He found that all patients demonstrated rapid resting respiratory rates compared to normals. However, unlike previous research scientists who found the cycles of quiet respiration to be irregular, Kim found more regularity than the norm. The mean deviation for the parkinsonian patients was 5.6% with a range of 4.3–11.6%, while the control subjects showed a 12.3% mean deviation with a spread of 9.8–14.2 percent. Kim also found that the oral reading and recitations were often interrupted by numerous breaths, which is in agreement with Schilling and Cramer's observations. Kim interpreted this to mean that parkinsonian patients have difficulty modulating automatic respiration during rest to a mode of respiration for speech.

The investigators reviewed above were essentially interested in respiratory patterns during quiet breathing. A small but significant group of investigations have emerged, aimed at determining whether "respiratory support for speech" was disturbed for the parkinsonian patient. The method used by these studies involved having the patient sustain a vowel to determine (a) the amount of time the patient could sustain vowel prolongation and (b) the latency between the time the expiratory cycle begins and the initiation of phonation.

Canter (1965a) showed that, as a group, his 17 Parkinson's disease patients were not able to sustain the vowel "a" as long as a control group matched for age (medians of 9.5 and 20.6 secs, respectively). Boshes (1966) also reported durations less than normal. Mean durations of 11.7 and 25.1 sec were recorded for his group of parkinsonian patients and matched control group, respectively. On the other hand, Ewanowski (1964; as reviewed by Darley et al., 1975) reported that even though his control subjects as a group could sustain vowels longer than parkinsonian subjects (25.9 and 21.4 sec, respectively), these differences were not significant. However, these vowel prolongations were elicited under the condition of verbal reinforcement (i.e., examiner encouraging the patient to continue phonating). Similarly, Kruel (1972) found that his 23 parkinsonian patients (mean age, 55 years) could sustain the vowels "a" and "o" (20.5 and 22.2 sec, respectively) longer than 10 younger (mean age, 21.3

years) normal controls (18.2 and 18.5 sec, respectively). These disparate findings are obviously due to differences in task requirements and subject selection.

The relatively short phonation times demonstrated by parkinsonian patients would appear, at first glance, to be due to poor respiratory support for speech, considering that, as a group, they have diminished vital capacity. However, a second possibility exists: these shortened durations might be due to poor laryngeal valving, that is, the partial inability to adduct or approximate the vocal cords for phonation due to neurologic deficit or structural anomaly. Mueller (1971), in an attempt to resolve this issue, measured the amount of air expelled during the sustained phonation of the vowel "a" using a face mask and pneumo-tachometer. As expected, the parkinsonian subjects' (five male and five female) sustained phonations were shorter than those of a matched control group (11.43 and 10.60 sec for the male and female parkinsonian patients and 13.05 and 15.43 sec for the male and female control subjects). At the same time, the total amount of air used during sustained phonation was also less for the parkinsonian patients. Mean values were 2.35 and 0.49 L for the male and female controls while the male and female parkinsonian patients achieved values of 1.72 and 0.24 L of expelled air. Rate of oral airflow between the two groups was not found to be significantly different. Mueller believed that this indicated that shortened phonation time associated with parkinsonian speakers was due to the "overall decrement of respiratory air supply" for speaking purposes. He also believed this may account for the "vague and thin vowel production" (reduced vocal intensity) often observed in speakers with Parkinson's disease.

However, in a recent investigation, Hanson et al. (1984), using telescopic cinelaryngoscopy, examined the larynges of 32 unselected patients with confirmed diagnosis of Parkinson's disease. Thirty of the 32 patients exhibited some degree of vocal cord bowing when approximation was made for phonation. All of the patients demonstrated and complained of vocal weakness, breathiness, and poor intensity. Thus, while reduced vital capacity or respiratory support for speech does appear to be related to the hypokinetic speech characteristics of diminished vocal loudness, and the use of short phrases, structural anomalies of the vocal cords also appear to play a role. Air wastage through the glottis due to inadequate vocal cord closure can give the listener the same perceptual impression. Most likely, these effects are a combined result of diminished respiratory support and laryngeal dysfunction. On the other hand, the aperiodic arrests of speech exhibited by some parkinsonian patients do not appear to be due to structural problems of the vocal cords. This characteristic is most likely due to the dyssynchrony between the inhalatory and exhalatory cycles as well as the parkinsonian patients' need for numerous inhalations during speaking, which has been documented by meany of the investigators reviewed here.

Phonatory

The presence of some type of laryngeal dysfunction is a common feature exhibited by the parkinsonian patient with hypokinetic dysarthria. Logemann and associates (1978) found that 80% of 200 parkinsonian patients studied demonstrated some type of voice disorder.

This included primarily voice quality disorders such as vocal breathiness, hoarseness, roughness, and tremulousness. Of the 55 patients observed by Scott and Caird (1983) all presented a prosodic disorder (i.e., disturbed melody or intonation of speech) while only one subject exhibited disordered articulation. Six of the ten most deviant speech dimensions (Table 1) identified by Darley et al. (1975) involved signs and symptoms of laryngeal dysfunction. These included the features of monopitch, monoloudness, the use of an inappropriate pitch level, harsh and breathy voice quality, and reduced stress. Darley and colleagues stated that the presence of these dimensions indicates that the laryngeal musculature of the parkinsonian patient has a "limited range of motion" and lacks the "vigor of movement."

VOCAL PITCH   In a study of the vocal characteristics of 17 Parkinson's disease patients, Canter (1963) showed that parkinsonian patients as a group produce a higher fundamental vocal pitch level than normal. Oscillographic analysis of a select portion of each subject's oral readings of the "Rainbow Passage" revealed that the patients spoke at a median fundamental vocal frequency of 129 cps while an age-matched control group spoke at a fundamental frequency of 106 cps. In addition, Canter found that his patients used a restricted pitch range in oral reading. Eleven of the 17 patients exhibited pitch ranges less than those used by the control subjects. None of the patients had a range of more than an octave while eight normal speakers had ranges of an octave or more.

In a subsequent investigation using the same 17 parkinsonian patients, Canter (1965a) determined each patient's overall vocal pitch range by having him sing the syllable "no" up and down the musical scale. As would be expected, the patients' ranges were restricted in comparison to the controls. Parkinson's disease patients had an average pitch range of 1.25 octaves while the control subjects produced a range of 1.84 octaves.

Ludlow and Bassich (1984) also found that parkinsonian patients with hypokinetic dysarthria demonstrate a higher fundamental vocal frequency than normal. The mean fundamental frequency for a series of sentences imitated by their Parkinson's disease patients was 165.80 cps while a group of age- and sex-matched controls achieved a fundamental frequency of 143.20. Eleven of the patients also had vocal frequencies higher than the controls. Also in agreement with Canter's findings, vocal pitch range was found to be reduced in the majority of the patients used by Ludlow and Bassich. Seventy-five percent of their patients demonstrated a fundamental vocal frequency range restricted to a greater degree than 90% of the normal population. In addition, a significant correlation ($r = -0.65$; $p < 0.01$) between vocal frequency range and perceptual ratings of monopitch was disclosed. This, along with Canter's data, indicates that the parkinsonian patient is more apt (when hypokinetic dysarthria is present) to produce a voice with a higher than normal pitch for age and sex and with a restricted range that may be perceived as monotony of pitch.

VOCAL LOUDNESS   Using a high-speed level recorder, Canter (1963) derived measurements of vocal intensity from the oral reading samples of his 17 Parkinson's disease patients. Mean peak sound pressure levels of the patients did not differ significantly from those of a matched control group. Ranges of vocal intensity levels within the speech samples were not found to distinguish the two groups as well. However, when the patients were asked to produce the syllable "no" at four different levels (i.e., quiet, average, loud and shouted), marked differences were discovered. While the vocal intensity levels for the "quiet" and "average" loudness conditions were essentially the same for both groups, the parkinsonian patients averaged 4.4 dB and 12.2 dB less than the control group for the "loud" and "shouted" condition, respectively. Parkinson's disease patients do appear to have an overall restricted vocal intensity range.

In contrast, Ludlow and Bassich (1984) showed that the overall vocal intensity level and range was highly variable in their group of patients. Five of their 12 parkinsonian patients obtained average intensity levels in sentences below that of 80% of the normals while the remainder performed at or above the normal level. Likewise, 7 of the 12 patients demonstrated a range of vocal intensity below that of 90% of the normals. It was also found that the degree of restriction was significantly correlated ($r = -0.67$; $p < 0.01$) with the perception of monoloudness. Thus, while parkinsonian patients may demonstrate an overall reduction of vocal loudness and monotony of loudness, they are just as likely to show no deviation of these speech dimensions. Most likely, their presence or absence will depend on the degree of severity of the disease.

PROSODY   The disturbance of prosody (i.e., the melodic and intonational patterns of speech) is often a sign or symptom of neurologic disease. Monrad-Krohn (1947, 1963) recognized this when he described three different forms of prosodic disturbances: hyperprosody, dysprosody, and aprosody. Hyperprosody is a condition characterized by fluent-exaggerated patterns of intonation frequently exhibited by patients in maniacal states or suffering from a sensory or Wernicke's type of aphasia. Dysprosody, on the other hand, is marked by a dysfluent speech pattern in which the patient speaks in a syllable-by-syllable fashion (i.e., scanning speech). The use of uneven stress is characteristic of this condition as well. This type of prosodic disturbance is associated with ataxic dysarthria and patients who are recovering from Broca's aphasia with apraxia of speech. Aprosody, the last condition Monrad-Krohn described and the one that this chapter is concerned with, refers to the patient whose overall speech prosody is substantially attenuated. As shown by the literature reviewed in the last two sections, the Parkinson's disease patient best fits this condition since the hypokinetic dysarthria speech he or she exhibits is marked by monopitch and monoloudness, indicating that the range of vocal pitch and intensity is significantly reduced. The reduced loudness and a lack of stress contrasts also add to the listener's impression of an aprosodic condition.

Considering that aprosodia may be a sign of Parkinson's disease, it is unfortunate that only two investigations have been designed to examine this feature more closely. By employing spectrographic analysis, Kent and Rosenbek (1982) compared the prosodic patterns of parkinsonian patients and normals. In general, they found that parkinsonian speech is marked by "a reduction of acoustic contrast or detail." This was manifested in two ways. First, on inspection of their spectrograms (see Fig. 1) it can be noted that the parkinsonian patients failed to produce the pauses or stop gaps normally found between words in connected speech and within words for the acoustic production of stop-plosive consonants. Instead, these gaps were "replaced by low-intensity frication giving the listener the impression of continuous uninterrupted speech." Second, patterns of acoustic energy (i.e., formant patterns) were not as clearly marked (see Fig. 2). While consonant–vowel and vowel–consonant transitions were easily discernible for the normal speakers, these transitions were severely reduced from the Parkinson's disease patients, resulting in the perception of murmured or rushed speech. Continuous voicing was also observed to be characteristic of parkinsonian speech, adding to the impression of reduced acoustic contrast.

Ludlow and Bassich (1984), in a unique investigation, attempted to determine whether parkinsonian speech contained the necessary acoustic features to distinguish compound nouns. Twelve patients with Parkinson's disease imitated the following six sentences:

It was a blue bell.
It was a bluebell.
They will sail boats.
They were sailboats.
She said a cross word.
She said a crossword.

Each of the imitated sentences was spectrographically analyzed to determine the patient's ability to produce adequate frequency (pitch), intensity (loudness), and durational (syllable, word, and interword) cues to differentiate the compound nouns (blue bell and bluebell, sail boat and sailboat, and cross word and crossword). From this analysis, Ludlow and Bassich found that while differences were found for each of the acoustic features, these differences were not

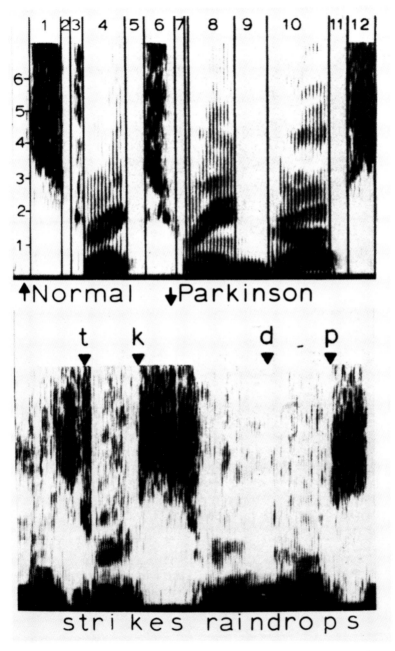

FIGURE 1 Wide-band spectrograms of a normal speaker and a parkinsonian speaker saying the words "strikes raindrops." (From Kent and Rosenbek, 1982).

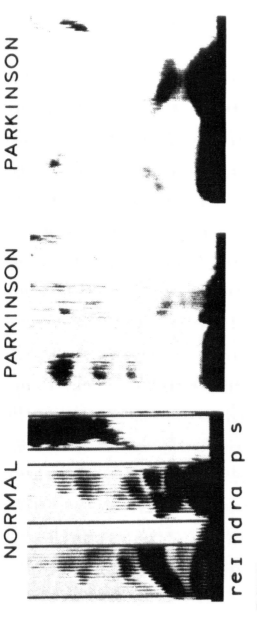

FIGURE 2 Wide-band spectrograms of the word "raindrops" produced by a normal speaker and two parkinsonian speakers. (From Kent and Rosenbek, 1982.)

consistent across all patients. Five patients were unable to use fundamental frequency to contrast compound nouns. Parkinson's disease patients were also unsuccessful in using vocal intensity. Seven of the 12 patients were found to be monoloud. Likewise, seven of the patients had reduced differences in word boundary durations that were significantly less than those found for an age-matched control group. However, this difference was not due to reduced word lengths but to the time interval between words. In fact, a significant correlation ($r = -0.75$, $p < 0.01$) was found between interword interval length and the perception of equal stress. In other words, the less likely the patient was to use the time interval between words to differentiate compound nouns, the more likely his or her production of syllables and words in connected speech would be perceived as stressed equally, creating another form of reduced acoustic contrast and detail.

Articulatory

The articulation of the parkinsonian dysarthric speaker has been described in many ways. These range from descriptions pertaining to articulatory precision such as vague, soft, indistinct, thick, slurred, and imprecise to words depicting the rate of articulation such as variable, slow, hypokinetic, festinated, murmured, blurred, and accelerated (see Grewel, 1957 for review of these terms). They all refer to the diminished or disturbed valving action of the tongue, lips, mandible, and soft palate for the production of vowels and consonants in connected discourse.

ARTICULATION Canter (1965b), finding that parkinsonian patients perform normally on standard single-word articulation tests, evaluated the articulation of his 17 patients in the context of connected speech (i.e., oral reading). He found that the most frequent errors involved plosive sounds (i.e., "p," "b," "t," "d," "k," and "g"). Fricative noise often accompanied the production of these sounds, while sound spectrograms revealed that the stop gaps (the time interval between the release of the tongue or lips and initiation of phonation of the following vowel) were frequently absent. Continuous phonation or voicing during normally silent periods of connected discourse was also noted. Canter concluded that ". . . the primary articulatory deviations noted in this group of patients were those due to inadequate articulatory valving during the production of plosives and those due to breakdowns in the coordination of laryngeal and oral activity" (p. 221).

In a comprehensive study, Logemann and Fisher (1981) investigated the articulation of 200 patients with idiopathic or postencephalitic Parkinsonism. Using the sentence version of the *Fisher-Logemann Test of Articulation Competence* (1971), 90 (45%) of the 200 patients exhibited misarticulations. The speech sounds produced in error most often were stop consonants and fricatives. In descending rank order, the stop-plosives "k" and "g" showed the highest incidence of misarticulation (all 90 patients misarticulated these sounds) followed by the fricatives "s" and "z" (63) and "sh" and "dz" (43), the affricates "ch" and "j" (39), and the stop consonants "p" and "b" (29) and "t" and "d" (18). The consistency with which each of these misarticulated sounds was made within and across patients was also high, 98 and 97%, respectively. That is, once a sound was produced in error, the likelihood was excellent it would be misarticulated again in a different context or word position.

When the type of articulation error was examined, Logemann and Fisher found that manner errors (i.e., the way in which the exhalatory air stream is impounded or directed by the articulator) were most characteristic of their patients. Stop consonants and affricates were changed to a fricative production while, perceptually, the articulation of fricative consonants was less sharp. The type of error produced in both instances indicates that the articulators were not achieving adequate constriction. That is, "analysis of the articulatory deficit reveals inadequate tongue elevation to achieve complete closure on stop-plosives and affricates, and close constriction of the airway in lingual fricatives" (p. 351). The investigators concluded that this diminished valving was not due to weakness but to the overall rigidity of the speech musculature.

Using a storage oscilloscope, Weismer (1984) compared the articulatory valving of a group of eight Parkinson's disease patients (ranging in age from 51 to 83) with a group of five young adults (21–27 years) and a group of eight geriatric adults (65–82 years). Specifically, this investigation was designed to determine whether spirantization (i.e., the presence of high-frequency frication) and/or continuous voicing is commonly found within the stop gaps of plosive consonants produced by these groups. It was assumed that the presence of either feature indicated reduced articulatory valving.

Spirantized stop-plosive consonants were found in each group of subjects. However, the phenomenon of spirantization was much more typical for the Parkinson's disease patient than either the young or geriatric subjects. In addition, spirantization appeared to be specific to certain phonemes and phonemic environments for the two control groups while this characteristic was produced by the parkinsonian speaker in all contexts and phonemes. This supports Logemann and Fisher's assertion that the constriction of the tongue and lips for stop-plosive consonants is significantly reduced for these patients.

The presence of "continuous voicing" (i.e., for more than 20 sec), during the stop-gaps of voiceless plosives was less clear. The young adults infrequently exhibited voicing during the production of voiceless stops while "continuous voicing" was commonly found for both groups of older subjects. The Parkinson's disease group showed a slight tendency to produce more "partially and fully voiced" voiceless stop-gaps than the geriatric group. However, these differences were minimal and it is unclear whether continuous voicing is characteristic of parkinsonian speech or is age-related.

The studies reviewed so far indicate that the parkinsonian patient with hypo-kinetic dysarthria produces misarticulations indicating that the contact between the lips, tongue, teeth, and roof of the mouth is reduced or less constricted than normally observed. Unfortunately, the methodology employed by these investi-gators (perceptual and spectrographic) are indirect and can only provide inferences as to why these patients exhibit poor articulation, that is, whether diminished articulatory valving is due to muscular weakness and/or rigidity. In an attempt to answer this question, Leanderson and co-workers (1970) em-ploying electromyography (EMG), compared the labial activity associated with parkinsonian speech and that of normal speakers. Three differences were ob-served: (a) the Parkinson's disease patients exhibited a greater degree of overall muscular tone (hypertonia); (b) the normal reciprocal activity between the agonist and antagonist muscle groups was disturbed; both groups tended to func-tion simultaneously for the parkinsonian patients; and (c) the EMG activity preceding the production of a sound was longer, often interfering with or pre-venting the parkinsonian patient from producing a particular sound. In addition, a relationship between EMG activity and the severity of dysarthria was ob-served. Patients who exhibited severe dysarthria were also those whose muscular hypertonia was more apparent. Thus, according to these results, muscular rigidity is the best explanation for the parkinsonian patient's diminished articu-latory valving.

Hunker et al. (1982) examined directly the degree of labial muscular rigidity of four parkinsonian patients with dysarthria (age range, 60–76 years) and four neurologically intact subjects (age range, 65–71 years). In this investigation, muscle rigidity was measured by applying a known force to the lips (via a cantilever strain gauge force transducer) and observing the degree of displace-ment. When displacement is plotted as a function of force, those muscles demon-strating a greater stiffness will have steeper slopes. In other words, the assump-tion is that rigid muscles will require greater force to be moved or displaced while complaint muscles will need less force to be moved the same distance.

Using this reasoning, the investigators found that all four parkinsonian sub-jects demonstrated a significantly greater lower lip stiffness than the controls. On the other hand, the findings for the upper lip were variable. Two of the parkinsonian patients exhibited increased stiffness of the upper lip while the values for the remaining two patients were within the normal range.

In a second part of their investigation, Hunker and associates had each pa-tient and control say the sentence, "Buy Bobby a poppy," three times with an intraincisal bite block in place to eliminate mandibular movement. A head-mounted lip and jaw movement transduction system recorded the bilabial move-ments while EMG signals were recorded from the orbicularis oris superior and inferior and the mentalis muscles. Consistent with the stiffness observations, two parkinsonian patients showed significantly less range of bilabial movement for the production of the sentence while two patients exhibited differences between the upper and lower lip movements. Upper lip displacements for these patients were normal whereas lower lip displacements were significantly reduced. The EMG recordings mirrored these findings as well. The recordings for the two patients with upper and lower lip stiffness were marked by a high degree of tonic EMG background activity and ". . . bursts of EMG antagonist to labial opening movements." By contrast, the two patients demonstrating only lower lip rigidity exhibited EMG patterns normal for the upper lip and marked by tonic EMG activity for the lower lip. These results are in agreement with Leanderson et al. (1970) that the reduced articulatory valving exhibited by the parkinsonian patient with dysarthria, perceptually and acoustically, is most likely due to overall rigidity of the speech musculature. However, Hunker and colleagues' findings also indicate that hypertonia may be present in different muscles or speech motor subsystems depending on the patient, that is, muscle rigidity may affect each Parkinson's disease patient differentially.

Employing the same four parkinsonian patients, Abbs and colleagues (1983) examined this hypothesis more closely. Using a set of three force transducers, they determined whether their patients could produce prespecified levels of steady force with their lips, tongue, and mandible. The investigators found that the stability of force generation varied from articulator to articulator for each patient. In one patient, for example, the low level forces of the tongue were marked by ". . . large fluctuations and general instability" while ". . . the lips and jaw were generally stable." Thus, the presence of rigidity (as well as its degree) may vary from one speech motor subsystem to another.

Logemann et al. (1978) also found that the speech motor subsystems were differentially affected when they observed the phonatory, articulatory, and resonatory behavior of 200 Parkinson's disease patients (see review of Logemann and Fisher, 1981 in this section). They found that their patients could be classified into five groups according to their symptom complex. Group 1, consisting of 45% of the patients, exhibited laryngeal dysfunction (e.g., breathy, hoarse, rough, and/or tremulous voice quality) as their only symptom; Group 2 (13.5%) consisted of patients with laryngeal and back-tongue involvement (i.e., difficulty producing the phonemes "k" and "g"); Group 3 (17%) presented with laryngeal, back-tongue, and tongue-blade dysfunction (i.e., misarticulation of "sz," "sh," "j," "ch," and "dz"); Group 4 (5.5%) included patients demonstrating laryngeal dysfunction, back-tongue, tongue-blade, and labial misarticulations (i.e., "p" and "b"); and Group 5 (9%) exhibited all the speech and voice symptoms of Group 4 patients with the addition of tongue tip misarticulations (i.e., "t" and "d"). While dysfluencies and hypernasality were noted, they were not prevalent nor did they follow any systematic pattern of occurrence. Thus, the clusters of symptoms of each group could ". . . represent a progression in dysfunction, beginning with laryngeal changes and increasing to include other areas of neuromuscular control of their vocal tract, for example, the lips and tongue" (p. 56). In this way, the differential effects noted by Hunker et al. and Abbs et al. could be explained. Studies pertaining to the longitudinal effects of Parkinson's disease on speech are needed.

RATE OF SPEECH The rate at which the Parkinson's disease patient speaks has been characterized by Darley and associates (1975) as variable. Some patients demonstrate an abnormally slow rate of speech which is "in tune" with the label of hypokinetic dysarthria while others appear to talk extremely fast, to the point where their speech becomes blurred or murmured. Still others may exhibit normal rates or alternate between these two abnormal speaking rates. At best, these disparate characteristics are probably due to different neurogenic causes.

Canter (1965b) found that the median oral reading rate of his 17 parkinsonian patients was not statistically different from his control group (172.6 words per min and 177.6 wpm, respectively). However, deviations from the norm were noted. Two patients had reading rates half of the norm, whereas one read at a rate of 249.6 wpm, over 40% faster than normal. Canter concluded that patients with Parkinson's disease could exhibit reduced or accelerated speech and that this ". . . may represent an important aspect of the speech disturbance."

Canter (1965b) also investigated his patients' ability to repeat rapidly the syllables "ba," "da," "ga," and "ha" over a 30-sec period. Measurements of diadochokinetic rate (i.e., alternate motion rate) proved to be difficult since, instead of producing a distinct string of syllables, a number of patients produced repetitions blurred beyond recognition, perceptually or on graphic level tracings. When this pattern was observed over the total 30-sec period, it was labeled "complete freezing"; when it was produced only part of the time, it was labeled "partial freezing."

With the inclusion of these individuals Canter showed that the diadochokinetic rate of his parkinsonian patients was significantly slower than his age-matched control group regardless of the syllable repeated. When the type of syllable was considered, the parkinsonian patients were able to produce the syllable "ba" faster than the syllable "da." This showed that tongue-tip movements were slower than the rapid repetitive movements of the lips.

Likewise, Mueller (1971) observed that the diadochokinetic rate of his 10 parkinsonian speakers was significantly slower than an age- and sex-matched control group. Repeating the syllable "sa" over a 7-sec period, he found that his male and female parkinsonian patients produced 26.9 and 20.20 syllables during this period while the male and female controls produced 32.6 and 39.30, respectively. Intraoral pressure was also found to be less for the parkinsonian group, indicating that the slow rate of syllabic repetition may be due to diminished respiratory support as well as reduced articulatory valving of the tongue.

Kruel (1972) investigated the Parkinson's disease patients' ability to repeat the vowel "ee" and the vowel sequence "oo-ee." The parkinsonian group produced significantly slower rates on both measures than either a young or a geriatric control group. The patients were unable to produce diadochokinetic rates within the normal limits regardless of whether the activity involved oral–articulatory or laryngeal valving.

The slow rate of articulation exhibited by most Parkinson's disease speakers is most logically due to the overall rigidity of the speech musculature. The paradoxical phenomenon of fast, festinated, or accelerated speech exhibited by some patients with this disease is not as easily explained. The question arises as to whether this characteristic is a true phenomenon of deviant neuromuscular control or is perceptually induced by articulatory undershoot, that is, due to diminished articulatory valving giving the listener the impression of accelerated speech. In an attempt to answer this question Netsell and co-workers (1975) studying 11 parkinsonian patients demonstrating "short rushes of speech" made simultaneous recordings of the EMG activity of the orbicularis oris superior and the degree of intraoral and intranasal pressure during their repetition of the syllable "pa" and the phrase "Papa pops." In each case, an increase of intraoral pressure during the production of the consonant "p" was absent, indicating that lip contact was not made. However, from the EMG recordings it was evident that discrete upper lip movements were made toward closure and that the rate of these excusions exceeded ". . . the upper limit for voluntary control of repetition rates . . . ." Thus while articulatory undershoot certainly influenced the perception of accelerated speech, this manifestation is physiologically real representing aberrant neuromuscular control.

In support, Netsell and associates also discovered that by speaking louder, one patient could obtain some control over his accelerated speech. They found that "the muscle action potential bursts preceeding each lip contact are of greater amplitude and longer duration . . ." than if the patients spoke at a normal loudness level. In Netsell et al.'s opinion, "An increase in physiologic effort associated with increased loudness may somehow override or suppress a neural feedback circuit that is involved in the acceleration behavior" (p. 173).

As reviewed by Netsell et al. (1975) and Kent and Rosenbek (1982), one explanation of the neurogenic basis of the abnormally slow and the extremely fast rates of movement exhibited by some parkinsonian patients is offered by Hassler (1966). In his explanation, two distinct neural feedback circuits between the cerebral cortex and thalamic and other subcortical nuclei and the cerebellum are proposed: an anterior loop formed by Brodmann's area (supplementary motor area of the cerebral cortex), globus pallidus, and the anterior ventrolateral thalamic nucleus, and a posterior loop formed by Brodmann's area 4 (precentral gyrus), pontine nucleus, cerebellum, red nucleus, and the posterior ventrolateral nucleus. Under Hassler's schema, slow speech exhibited by the Parkinson's disease patient should be associated with greater involvement of the anterior circuit, since stimulation of the anterior ventrolateral nucleus results in slowed or blocked speech while ablation of this area relieves overall muscular rigidity. In contrast, accelerated speech should be associated with involvement of the posterior circuit since stimulation of the posterior ventrolateral circuit directly results in festinated speech while relief from tremor and ataxia is associated with ablation. Of course, the fact that many parkinsonian patients exhibit both slow and accelerated speech argues for involvement of both circuits or the ventrolateral nucleus of the thalamus as a whole.

In a unique study, Hunker and Abbs (1984) showed that the rate of repetitive labial movement is related to the force tremor frequency of the lips. Using a headmounted strain gauge transduction system, the movements of the upper and lower lips of eight patients with Parkinson's disease were observed while each patient was maintaining a target force level by compressing his lips against a bilabial force transducer. Overall, the labial force tremor exhibited by the parkinsonian patients during this isometric task was found to be slower than that of an age-matched control group. The control subjects showed a dominant spectral peak of 8.5 Hz (i.e., the number of oscillatory labial tremor movements produced/sec), while the parkinsonian labial oscillations ranged from 4.0 to 5.0 Hz. The EMG activity of the lip musculature appeared to be related to the isometric postural tremor. Prominent action potentials of the superior and inferior orbicularis oris, levator labii superior, and the depressor labii inferior were observed at roughly the same frequency as the labial force tremor, indicating that these seemingly independent measures probably have a common neurogenic basis. However, more importantly, a relationship was found between the volitional movement rate of the lips and the force tremor frequency demonstrated by each of the patients. When asked to repeat the syllable "pa" as rapidly but as accurately as possible, the patients always selected a diadochokinetic rate of less than 5.0 Hz, a finding which has been replicated by other researchers (Hirose et al., 1981). On the other hand, when instructed to produce rates faster than 5.0 Hz, the range of movement of the upper and lower lips and the jaw became markedly reduced and an acceleration of speech was noted. According to Hunker and Abbs,

These findings suggest that controlled movements cannot exceed the 4.0 to 5.0 Hz limit as predicted from the force tremor spectra and that the phenomenon of acceleration might be related to an aberrant neuromotor system "resonance" at this dominant force tremor frequency. Seemingly, the neural pathways responsible for the isometric force tremors are also implicated in the aberrant movements observed in the parkinsonian population (p. 85).

Summary

This review of the literature should provide the reader with the impression that the hypokinetic dysarthric speech exhibited by the Parkinson's disease patient is primarily characterized by diminished functioning of all subsystems serving speech. From a phonatory standpoint, the patient's speech is marked by reduced vocal intensity and by a breathy or hoarse voice quality. Prosody or the melody of speech is affected as well since the patient's voice is often described as being monotonous (i.e., combination of monoloudness and monopitch). While the reason for these phonatory difficulties could be due to poor respiratory support for speech (considering that the vital capacity for many parkinsonian patients is significantly reduced), it also could be due to structural or mechanical changes of the larynx such as vocal cord bowing or overall muscular rigidity. Most likely, the phonatory dysfunction in Parkinson's disease is due to a combination of these factors.

The articulation of the Parkinson's disease patient is affected as well. The valving action of the tongue and the lips necessary to produce oral sounds is less constricted, resulting in diminished intraoral pressure and giving the listener the impression of slurred speech or overall articulatory imprecision. Movement and EMG studies indicate that these errors are due to muscular rigidity. The presence of certain articulation errors may also provide the clinician with some clues as to the progression of the disease. Patients in the initial stages of the disease may exhibit laryngeal dysfunction only, followed by the addition of errors pertaining to back tongue, tongue blade, labial, and finally tongue-tip movement as the severity of the disease process increases.

The rate at which the Parkinson's disease patient speaks may be slow, accelerated, normal, or, in some cases, a combination of these conditions. The paradoxical condition of accelerated speech appears to be due both to articulatory undershoot and diminished oral valving, giving the impression of murmured speech, and to aberrant neuromuscular control. Whether a particular patient demonstrates slow or accelerated speech is probably dependent on differential neurogenic involvement.

TREATMENT

Treatments of the hypokinetic speech disturbance demonstrated by the Parkinson's disease patient can be divided into two categories: those which use pharmacologic agents and those that provide behavioral management to help the patient compensate for a speech handicap. In either case, the goal is to reduce, eliminate, or overcome the rigidity of the musculature responsible for symptoms such as diminished vital capacity, variable rate, aprosodia, reduced vocal volume, and articulatory imprecision. As will be reviewed, the treatment of first choice is probably pharmacologic since L-dopa, an agent known to stimulate dopamine production, often has a dramatic effect on specific speech symptoms as well as on the patient's overall speech intelligibility. Behavioral management or speech therapy, on the other hand, has been less effective because it is difficult for the parkinsonian patient to monitor his or her speech and to apply the necessary corrections or compensations learned in the clinic to everyday speaking situations. However, recent technologic advances have given the patient the means by which to monitor speech continuously, thereby enhancing the chances of therapeutic carry-over. The investigations pertaining to these advances will also be reviewed.

Pharmacologic

One of the first investigations specifically designed to determine the effects of L-dopa on parkinsonian speech was conducted by Rigrodsky and Morrison (1970). In this study, speech recordings of 21 patients with Parkinson's disease were made at three different times during drug therapy: (a) before the initiation of L-dopa therapy; (b) during an intermediate dosage of L-dopa; and (c) after a maximal dosage (4–8 g daily). Each speech sample was rated for the relative normality of four speech characteristics including overall adequacy, clarity of articulation, nasal resonance, and the time factor in speaking. Of these four, only the factor of time during speaking was significantly better during the maximal dosage of L-dopa. While the remaining three factors were rated higher, they did not reach statistical significance. In addition, a greater number of patients exhibited a mild speech impairment at the time of maximal dosage than was found initially. That is, L-dopa had a salutary effect not only on the speed at which the parkinsonian patient spoke but also on the perceived severity of the speech disorder.

Similarly, Mawdsley and Gamsu (1971) also found that the timing aspects of parkinsonian speech are affected by L-dopa therapy. They found that when a group of 20 parkinsonian patients were asked to count from 1 to 10, the duration as well as the variability of phonation time for each single digit diminished significantly after L-dopa treatment. The timing of parkinsonian speech became more periodic and regular. One interesting side light is that while all 20 patients derived benefit from L-dopa in their overall functional capacity and mobility, 6 showed no speech improvement. Of these, four had post-encephalitic parkinsonism and two patients had undergone bilateral thalamotomies; this suggests that the speech deficits of these type of patients may be resistive to L-dopa therapy.

L-Dopa has also been shown to have an effect on the EMG activity of the speech musculature. In a subsequent investigation (see Leanderson et al., 1970) to their study of EMG activity of parkinsonian labial movements, Leanderson and co-workers (1971) showed that after L-dopa treatment, the tonic muscular hyperactivity usually found was reduced and the reciprocal activity between agonist and antagonist labial muscle groups was reestablished. Six of 7 parkinsonian patients showed overall speech improvement accompanied by either complete or partial normalization of their EMG articulatory pattern. Likewise, Nakano and colleagues (1973) found that a significant increase in speech intelligibility was associated with L-dopa when compared to the effects of placebo and procyclidine hydrochloride. When labial activity was examined, tonic hyperactivity diminished as each parkinsonian patient went from placebo to procyclidine and finally to L-dopa. The findings from both of the above studies suggest that the severity of the hypokinetic dysarthria is highly correlated with the muscular hyperactivity exhibited by the parkinsonian patient. L-Dopa obviously diminishes this activity.

Using 17 Parkinson's disease patients Wolf et al. (1975) attempted to determine not only the treatment effects of L-dopa on hypokinetic dysarthria but also whether these effects are influenced by the age of the patient, the duration of the disease, the degree of initial impairment, and the changes in physical findings. As would be expected, L-dopa therapy markedly improved the patients' speech. However, this improvement was selective. The patients' voice quality, pitch variation, and articulation changed significantly whereas the rate at which they spoke before and after treatment was not found to be different.

When the relationship between the amount of physical improvement and the degree of speech improvement was examined, a significant correlation coefficient of 0.62 was obtained. Interestingly, a low nonsignificant correlation ($r=0.09$) was obtained for these factors before treatment, suggesting that physical status concurrently improves with improvement in speech. In contrast, the factors of the patients' age and their durations of disease were not correlated with speech changes, since some patients over 70 years of age or with Parkinson's disease for 15 years or longer demonstrated more than 20% improvement.

One caveat should be made to the uninitiated clinician about the use of L-dopa. While L-dopa has a beneficial effect on the speech of these patients, its long-term use can be deleterious. Marsden and Parkes (1976) reported that after 1-3 years of L-dopa treatment, some patients may experience an orofacial dyskinesia, at times accompanied by oromandibular dystonia and/or a respiratory dyskinesia. This type of behavior is called "peak-dose dyskinesia" and often disappears when the dosage of L-dopa is reduced. In an interesting case study, Critchley (1976) describes a 52-year-old man who, after being successfully maintained on a 3-g daily dosage of L-dopa for 6 years, developed a dysphonia. To make himself more intelligible during a clinic visit, the patient purposely left off his morning dosage. Unfortunately, the patient arrived ". . . rigid in a typical parkinsonian state, barely able to totter into the room." Thus, it is apparent that long-term use of L-dopa should be monitored closely.

Recently, clonazepam therapy has been shown to have a beneficial effect on the parkinsonian patient's hypokinetic dysarthria. Biary and Pimental (1985) found that the speech of 10 of 11 parkinsonian patients significantly improved with clonazepam treatment. Optimal improvement occurred with dosages of 0.25 mg and 0.50 mg while deterioration of speech was associated with higher dosages (1 mg). The speech features showing the most improvement were short rushes, variable speaking rate, the production of imprecise consonants, and inappropriate silences. Low pitch level and breathy voice quality were not affected. The mechanism by which clonazepam acts on Parkinson's disease is not known and deserves further research.

Behavioral

For the most part, speech therapy has not been shown to be an effective means by which to change the hypokinetic speech patterns of the Parkinson's disease patient. Sarno (1968), in retrospect, found that none of the 300 patients seen at her clinic over a 15-year period benefited from speech therapy, regardless of the techniques employed. These ranged from "exercises" aimed at maintaining or controlling vocal volume and increasing the range, speed and precision of the speech musculature, to "mirror and tape recorder practice" whereby the patient could monitor his or her articulatory movements. At best, Sarno found that her patients "impressively improved" during the speech therapy session ". . . only to revert to the pathologic patterns immediately after . . ." even though they were aware of their condition and highly motivated. Sarno concluded ". . . that [speech] therapeutic efforts are probably of greatest benefit to the patient's psyche rather than to his ability to speak" (p. 274).

However, recent investigations have shown that speech therapy can be of functional benefit to the parkinsonian patient, especially if it is aimed at improving his or her prosodic output. Scott and Caird (1981) evaluated the effectiveness of two forms of speech therapy on the dysarthric speech exhibited by nine patients with Parkinson's disease: (a) intonational exercises aimed at improving the patient's recognition and production of pitch, volume, and durational contours associated with speech, using a Vocalite (a voice-operated light source); and (b) proprioceptive neuromuscular facilitation consisting of motor exercises aimed at enhancing the intensity of the multisensory information and proprioceptive feedback the patient receives during speaking. When specific aspects of the patients' speech were rated before and after treatment, only their breath control and ability to initiate speech failed to improve. On the other hand, the patients' ability to vary their voice intensity did improve with intonational therapy but not with proprioceptive facilitation. Prosodic abnormality, surprisingly, was significantly better using either type of treatment. More importantly, 6 months after treatment was terminated, the patients' prosodic abnormality had increased but was still markedly less than the pretreatment level, suggesting that the changes in prosodic output achieved in speech therapy may be resistive to regression.

In a subsequent study, Scott and Caird (1983) examined the question of whether prosodic therapy is as effective with or without the use of a visual reinforcement device. Two independent groups of 13 parkinsonian patients with hypokinetic dysarthria were employed. The first group received 10 1-hr speech therapy sessions over a 2-week period consisting of prosodic exercises with the assistance of a Vocalite. The second group also received prosodic therapy over the same period of time but without the Vocalite. Significant differences were revealed for both groups when the pre- and posttreatment ratings of their aprosodic output was compared. That is, the patients' prosodic outputs improved regardless of whether a visual reinforcement device such as a Vocalite was employed. Similar to their previous investigation, Scott and Caird also found the speech deficit of both groups of patients worsened 3 months after therapy was discontinued. However, neither group regressed to their pretreatment levels, indicating that some carryover of the effects of prosodic therapy is maintained.

Electroprosthetic management, the use of external feedback devices that enable the parkinsonian patient to monitor and thereby change or self-correct particular parameters of disordered speech, has only recently been investigated (Berry, 1983). To determine the effects of delayed auditory feedback (DAF), Hanson and Metter (1983) had two parkinsonian patients with hypokinetic dysarthria use a miniature, portable, solid-state, battery-powered unit that functioned to feed patients' speech back to them, via headphones, at a time delay selected by the clinician. Without the unit, the speech of both patients was marked by diminished vocal intensity and an "excessively rapid speaking rate" that significantly impaired their overall speech intelligibility. With the DAF unit in operation, each patient demonstrated pronounced changes in their speaking rate, vocal intensity, and vocal pitch. Their rate of word production decreased, their vocal intensity increased, and their vocal pitch levels increased with the imposition of DAF. Concurrently, the speech intelligibility ratings had also improved significantly.

Unfortunately, these changes only occurred with DAF device in use. "Daily use of DAF . . . did not result in any noticeable carry-over of the reduction of speech rate when DAF was not used." This indicates that DAF does not reduce muscular rigidity as pharmacologic or speech therapy purports but essentially forces the parkinsonian patient to modify his or her speaking style. The investigators suggest that this modification is an increase of "physiological effort" on the part of the patient, considering that enhanced vocal intensity and pitch are signs of such effort. The use of the DAF device merely forces the parkinsonian patient into this mode of speaking. Similar findings were obtained by Hanson and Metter (1980) for a 59-year-old man with progressive supranuclear palsy and hypokinetic dysarthria, which also suggests that DAF does not change the disease process. In any case, the portable DAF device used in these studies may be a viable alternative for Parkinson's disease patients, enabling them to decrease their speaking rate, thereby enhancing overall speech intelligibility in everyday situations.

In an attempt to determine whether parkinsonian patients would benefit from continuous self-monitoring of their vocal intensity, Rubow and Swift (1985) devised a microcomputer-based wearable biofeedback device designed to (a) continuously sample the intensity of the patient's voice from a throat microphone; (b) determine whether the patient's vocal intensity was below a defined level; (c) deliver a feedback alarm (i.e., a 1,000 Hz tone) to the patient (via an earphone) indicating that the voice was below this level; and (d) collect and store data on the frequency with which the patient needed to be reminded to raise the voice. The subject employed was a 67-year-old man with Parkinson's disease whose speech was characterized by a breathy voice quality, mild imprecise articulation, and a marked reduction in loudness. Treatment was divided into two phases. Phase 1 consisted of 18 sessions during which the patient received feedback cues from the device while undergoing speech therapy aimed at improving his expiratory airflow, vocal intensity, and articulation for connected speech. The device was also worn outside of the clinic during this phase. However, the microcomputer only collected data during this time and did not provide feedback cues. Phase 2 consisted of 26 speech therapy sessions similar to those given in Phase 1 except for one major difference. The microcomputer delivered intensity cues to the patient outside as well as inside the clinic.

The results of this study show that the use of a vocal intensity biofeedback device has a significant effect on their patients' overall speech pattern and ability to monitor the loudness of voice. Nine of 12 dimensions found to be abnormal before Phase 1 had improved significantly after Phase 2 therapy. The patients' vocal loudness, monopitch, monoloudness, rate, stress patterning, vowel production, bizarreness, and the presence of irregular articulatory breakdowns had all improved with biofeedback treatment. In addition, this speech improvement was maintained 10 and 20 weeks after treatment was terminated, indicating that the use of the biofeedback device promoted therapeutic carryover. More importantly, when the interval of time between feedback alarms received by the patient within the clinic was considered, the average interval was longer for Phase 2 than for Phase 1 (14.2 sec and 2.6 sec respectively). When the average alarm interval for outside the clinic during Phase 2 was considered, much of the increase was maintained (11.3 seconds). That is, as the biofeedback treatment progressed, patients' need for reminders to increase the volume of the voice diminished, especially when provided during daily living activities as well as within the clinic setting.

The use of biofeedback devices such as that developed by Rubow and Swift may prove to be indispensable to the clinician treating hypokinetic dysarthria. Traditional speech therapy has not been effective since most parkinsonian patients cannot sufficiently monitor their ongoing speech in daily living, thereby preventing them from using the compensations they have learned in the treatment room. The use of the Vocalite, DAF, or some type of biofeedback device allows patients to make such applications in and out of the clinic. These devices as well as those yet to be invented will be commonly used by the clinician to treat the parkinsonian speaker in the future.

CONCLUSIONS

Parkinson's disease patients with hypokinetic dysarthria exhibit a constellation of symptoms that span all motor speech subsystems. Respiratory dysfunction is indicated by patients' reduced vital capacity as well as diminished vocal intensity. Phonatory dysfunction is represented primarily by breathy/hoarse voice quality and pitch, and temporal variations during connected discourse (i.e., prosodic insufficiency). The general imprecision in which most speech sounds are produced and the variable rate at which they are elicited by the parkinsonian speaker also suggests that his articulatory system is not functioning optimally. The presence or absence of these systemic speech deficits is due to the severity of the Parkinson's disease. In any case, it is generally accepted that these symptoms are due to the rigidity of the respiratory, phonatory, and articulatory musculature. The diagnosis of parkinsonian hypokinetic dysarthria entails a detailed evaluation of each of these speech subsystems.

The primary treatment of parkinsonian dysarthria is pharmacologic. L-Dopa has been shown to reduce the overall hypertonicity of the speech musculature resulting in marked improvement of particular speech symptoms as well as the patients' overall speech intelligibility. Behavioral management or speech therapy has been less effective. However, recent developments have suggested that speech therapy can benefit the Parkinson's disease patient if the aim is either to improve prosodic output or provide a biofeedback device that allows the patient to monitor his or her speech on a continuous basis. The clinician who treats the patient with Parkinson's disease should be aware of the relative strength and weakness of these therapeutic regimens.

REFERENCES

Abbs JH, Hunker CJ, Barlow SM. (1983). Differential speech motor subsystem impairments with suprabulbar lesions: neurophysiological framework. In: WR Perry (Ed.), *Clinical Dysarthria*. San Diego, College-Hill Press.

Atarashi J, Uchida E. (1959). A clinical study of parkinsonism. *Recent Adv Res Nerv Syst* 3: 871–882.

Berry WR. (1983). Treatment of hypokinetic dysarthria. In: WH Perkins (Ed.), *Dysarthria and Apraxia*. New York, Thieme-Stratton.

Biary N, Pimental PA. (1985). A double-blind trial of clonazepam in parkinsonian hypokinetic dysarthria. Paper presented to the Convention of the American Academy of Neurology, Dallas, Texas.

Boshes B. (1966). Voice changes in parkinsonism. *J Neurosurg* 24: 286–288.

Canter GJ. (1963). Speech characteristics of patients with Parkinson's disease: I. intensity, pitch, and duration. *J Speech Hear Res* 28: 221–229.

Canter GJ. (1965a). Speech characteristics of patients with Parkinson's disease: II. physiological support for speech. *J Speech Hear Res* 30: 44–49.

Canter GJ. (1965b). Speech characteristics of patients with Parkinson's disease: III. articulation, diadochokinesis, and overall speech adequacy. *J Speech Hear Res* 30: 217–224.

Cramer W. (1940). De spraak bij patienten met Parkinsonisme. 22: 17–23.

Critchley EMR. (1976). Peak-dose dysphonia in parkinsonism. *Lancet* 1: 544.

Darley FL, Aronson AE, Brown JR. (1969a). Clusters of deviant speech dimensions in the dysarthrias. *J Speech Hear Res* 12: 462–496.

Darley FL, Aronson AE, Brown JR. (1969b). Differential diagnostic patterns of dysarthria. *J Speech Hear Res* 12: 246–269.

Darley FL, Aronson AE, Brown JR. (1975). *Motor Speech Disorders*. Philadelphia, W.B. Saunders.

de la Torre R, Mier M, Boshes B. (1960). Studies in parkinsonism: Evaluation of respiratory function—preliminary observations. *Q Bull Northwestern Univ Med School* 34: 232–236.

Ewanowski SJ. (1964). Selected motor-speech behavior of patients with parkinsonism. Ph.D. dissertation, University of Wisconsin.

Fisher HB, Logemann JA. (1971). *The Fisher-Logemann Test of Articulation Competence*. Boston, Houghton-Mifflin.

Gawel MJ. (1981). The effects of various drugs on speech. *Br J Dis Commun* 16: 51–57.

Grewel F. (1957). Dysarthria in post-encephalitic parkinsonism. *Acta Psychiatr Neurol Scand* 32: 440–449.

Hanson DG, Gerratt BR, Ward PH. (1984). Cinegraphic observations of laryngeal function in Parkinson's disease. *Laryngoscope* 94: 348–353.

Hanson WR, Metter EJ. (1983). DAF speech rate modification in Parkinson's disease: a report of two cases. In: Berry WR (Ed.), *Clinical Dysarthria*. San Diego, College-Hill Press.

Hassler R. (1966). Thalamic regulation of muscle tone and the speed of movements. In: Purpura D, Yahr M (Eds.), *The Thalamus*. New York, Columbia University Press.

Hirose H, Kirtani S, Ushijima T, Yoshioka H, Sawashima M. (1981). Patterns of dysarthric movements in patients with parkinsonism. Folia Phoniatr 33: 204–215.

Hunker CJ, Abbs JH, Barlow SM. (1982). The relationship between parkinsonian rigidity and hypokinesia in the orofacial system: a quantitative analysis. *Neurology* 32: 749–754.

Hunker CJ, Abbs JH. (1984). Physiological analysis of parkinsonian tremors in the orofacial system. In: McNeil MR, Rosenbek JC, Aronson AE (Eds.), *The Dysarthrias: Physiology, Acoustics, Perception, Management.* San Diego, College-Hill.

Kent RD, Rosenbek JC. (1982). Prosodic disturbance and neurologic lesion. *Brain Lang* 15: 259–291.

Kim R. (1968). The chronic residual respiratory disorder in post-encephalitic parkinsonism. *J Neurol Neurosurg Psychiatry* 31: 393–398.

Koller WC. (1983). Dysfluency (stuttering) in extrapyramidal disease. *Arch Neurol* 40: 175–177.

Kreul JE. (1972). Neuromuscular control examination (NMC) for parkinsonism: vowel prolongations and didochokinetic and reading rates. *J Speech Hear Res* 15: 72–83.

Laszewski Z. (1956). Role of the department of rehabilitation in preoperative evaluation of parkinsonian patients. *J Am Geriatr Soc* 4: 1280–1284.

Leanderson R, Meyerson BA, Person A. (1971). Effect of L-dopa on speech in function of the facial muscles in dysarthria. *Acta Otolaryngol Suppl.* 263: 89–94.

Leanderson R, Meyerson BA, Person A. (1971). Effect of L-dopa on speech in parkinsonism: An EMG study of labial articulatory function. *J Neurol Neurosurg Psychiatry* 34: 679–681.

Logemann JA, Fisher HB, Boshes B, Bbnsk ER. (1978). Frequency and occurrence of vocal tract dysfunctions in the speech of a large sample of parkinsonian patients. *J Speech Hear Dis* 43: 47–57.

Logemann JA, Fisher HB. (1981). Focal tract control in Parkinson's disease: phonetic feature analysis of misarticulations. *J Speech Hear Dis* 46: 348–352.

Ludlow CL, Bassich CJ. (1984). Relationships between perceptual ratings and acoustic measures of hypokinetic speech. In: McNeil MR, Rosenbek JC, Aronson AE (Eds.), *The Dysarthrias: Physiology, Acoustics, Perception, Management.* San Diego, College-Hill Press.

Marsden CD, Parkes JD. (1976). On-off effects in patients with Parkinson's disease on chronic levodopa therapy. *Lancet* 1.

Mawdsley C, Gamsu CV. (1971). Periodicity of speech in parkinsonism. *Nature* 231: 315–316.

Monrad-Krohn GH. (1947). Dysprosody or altered "melody of language." *Brain* 70: 405–415.

Monrad-Krohn GH. (1963). The third element of speech: prosody and its disorders. In: Halpern L (Ed.), *Problems of Dynamic Neurology.* Jerusalem, Hebrew University Press.

Mueller PB. (1971). Parkinson's disease: motor speech behavior in a selected group of patients. *Folia Phoniatr* 23: 333–346.

Nakano KM, Zubick H, Tyler H. (1973). Speech defects of parkinsonian patients: Effects of levodopa therapy on speech intelligibility. *Neurology* 23: 865–870.

Netsell R, Daniel B, Celesia G. (1975). Acceleration and weakness in parkinsonian dysarthria. *J Speech Hear Dis* 40: 170–178.

Oxtoby M. (1982). *Parkinson's Disease, Patients and Their Social Needs*. London, Parkinson's Disease Society.

Rigrodsky S, Morrison EB. (1970). Speech changes in parkinsonism during L-dopa therapy: preliminary findings. *J Am Geriatr Soc* 18: 142–151.

Rubow R, Swift E. (1985). A microcomputer-based wearable biofeedback device to improve transfer of treatment in parkinsonian dysarthria. *J Speech Hear Dis* 50: 178–185.

Sarno MT. (1968). Speech impairment in Parkinson's disease. *Arch Phys Med Rehab* 49: 269–275.

Schilling R. (1925). Experimental phonetische utersuchungen bei erkrankungen des extraphyramidalen systens. *Arch Psychiatry Nervenkr* 17: 419–471.

Scott S, Caird FI. (1981). Speech therapy for patients with Parkinson disease. *Br Med J* 283: 1088.

Scott S, Caird FI. (1983). Speech therapy for Parkinson's disease. *J Neurol Neurosurg Psychiatry* 46: 140–144.

Scott S, Caird FI, Williams BO. (1985). *Communication in Parkinson's Disease*. Rockville, Maryland, Aspen.

Uziel A, Bohe M, Cadilhac J, Passouant P. (1975). Les troubles de la voix et de la parole dans le syndrome Parkinsonien. *Folia Phoniatr* 27: 166–176.

Weismer G. (1984). Articulatory characteristics of parkinsonian dysarthria: segmental and phrase-level timing, spirantization, and lottal–supraglottal corrdination. In: McNeil MR, Rosenbek JC, Aronson AE (Eds.), *The Dysarthrias: Physiology, Acoustics, Perception, Management*. San Diego, College-Hill Press.

Wolf VI, Garvin JS, Bacon M, Waldrop W. (1975). Speech changes in Parkinson's disease during treatment with L-dopa. *J Commun Disord* 8: 271–279.

10
Pathology

ELLSWORTH C. ALVORD, JR.
University of Washington School of Medicine, Seattle, Washington

LYSIA S. FORNO
Veterans Administration Medical Center, Palo Alto, and Stanford University, Stanford, California

PERSPECTIVE

Contemplating the history of the pathology of parkinsonism (Table 1; Lewy, 1940a; Forno, 1986b) has led to two opposing thoughts.

The first is that the exponential increase in information indicates that "the end" is in sight. Of course, science is never-ending since each answer provokes at least one more question, but soon we will know the genetic codes for the proteins involved in the production of Lewy bodies and Alzheimer neurofibrillary tangles. Then we will learn what the normal functions and precursors of these proteins are and how they become distorted by posttranslational phosphorylations, sulfations, or other reactions. The reasons will soon become clear why, from relatively large pools of subclinically affected individuals, some of us develop accelerating degenerations of one or the other type affecting one or more places in the nervous system so that we manifest various degrees of parkinsonism, dementia, and/or other disorders. Table 2 summarizes the clinical syndromes related to the types of degenerations of nerve cells that are the subject of this chapter.

The second is that the problem has become increasingly complex. We began by recognizing the classic idiopathic (Lewy body) and postencephalitic (Alzheimer neurofibrillary tangle) types of parkinsonism which we discussed in our earlier reviews (Alvord, 1959, 1968; Forno, 1966). Then we were forced in subsequent reviews (Forno, 1969, 1977, 1982, 1986a; Forno and Alvord, 1971; Alvord, 1971; Alvord et al., 1974) to recognize subclinical forms and at least two types (Lewy body and Alzheimer neurofibrillary tangle) of idiopathic parkinsonism frequently accompanied by dementia. The lesions related to this

TABLE 1 Milestones in the History of the Pathology of Parkinsonism

1817	Parkinson: clinical description of the shaking palsy (paralysis agitans, idiopathic parkinsonism)
1907	Alzheimer: neurofibrillary tangles in dementia
1912	Lewy: Lewy bodies in parkinsonism
1919	Trétiakoff: substantia nigra in parkinsonism
1921	Souques: clinical descriptions of encephalitic and postencephalitic parkinsonism
1931	Critchley: clinical description of arteriosclerotic parkinsonism and other syndromes of old age
1935	Hallervorden: neurofibrillary tangles in postencephalitic parkinsonism
1938	Hassler: subdivisions of substantia nigra affected in idiopathic vs. postencephalitic parkinsonism
1952	Beheim-Schwarzbach: Lewy bodies and neurofibrillary tangles in locus ceruleus in idiopathic vs. postencephalitic parkinsonism
1953	Greenfield and Bosanquet: Lewy bodies and neurofibrillary tangles in idiopathic vs. postencephalitic parkinsonism
1960	Bethlem and Jager: protein in Lewy bodies
1961	Okazaki et al.: Lewy body dementia
1961	Hirano et al.: clinicopathologic definition of parkinsonism, dementia, and amyotrophic lateral sclerosis in Guam
1963	Terry: electron microscopy reveals 10–20 nm twisted neurotubules in neurofibrillary tangles
1964	Kidd: electron microscopy reveals paired helical filaments in neurofibrillary tangles
1965	Duffy and Tennyson: electron microscopy of Lewy bodies
1966	Pollock and Hornabrook: dementia in parkinsonism
1969	Jager: sphingomyelin in Lewy bodies
1978	Forno et al.: intraneuritic vs. perikaryal Lewy bodies
1983	Kimula et al.: Lewy bodies contain calcium, sulfur and phosphate
1983	Goldman et al.: Lewy bodies react with antibodies to neurofilaments
1983	Forno et al.: Lewy bodies and neurofibrillary tangles react with antibodies to neurofilaments
1985	Sternberger et al.: neurofibrillary tangles react with antibodies to phosphorylated neurofilaments
1986	Forno et al.: Lewy bodies react with antibodies to phosphorylated neurofilaments

TABLE 2 A Comparison of Clinical Syndromes Associated with Specific Types of Neuronal Degeneration[a]

Clinical syndrome	Lewy body degeneration	Alzheimer neurofibrillary tangle degeneration	Pick body degeneration
Subclinical	% = 1/3 of age > 50 years	SN % = 1/3 of age > 50 years LC % = 4/3 of age > 30 years	?
Parkinsonism	Idiopathic 15% of Alzheimer's disease	Postencephalitic Idiopathic Guam: PD-ALS	?
Dementia	Lewy body dementia	Alzheimer's disease presenile senile	Pick's disease
Other	20% of Shy–Drager syndrome	Progressive supranuclear palsy?[b]	Familial ALS?[c]

[a]SN, substantia nigra; LC, locus ceruleus; PD-ALS, parkinsonism, dementia, and ALS; ALS, amyotrophic lateral sclerosis.
[b]Some tangles consist of straight tubules, not paired helical filaments.
[c]Argentophilic Lewy-like bodies in spinal cord (Hirano et al., 1967).

dementia appeared to be different from those described by Hirano et al. (1961) in the complex of parkinsonism, dementia, and amyotrophic lateral sclerosis in Guam. The increasing complexity of the problem appears to represent the same kind of escalating frustration that Lewy (1940b) expressed 45 years ago, 20 years before we began our own studies:

> When I had investigated my first two dozen cases of Parkinson (sic), I was convinced that I knew where the cause of tremor and rigidity was located. When I had examined pathologically the seventh dozen of Parkinson brains, I was completely confused because you seemed to be able to prove just as well one theory as the contrary one.

From these two opposing thoughts the caution expressed by Santayana (1905) began to emerge ever more clearly: "Those who cannot remember the past are condemned to repeat it." How ironic, however, that history has revealed itself to us so slowly on the one hand, while progressing so increasingly rapidly on the other.

GENERAL SUMMARY

The lesions in parkinsonism are multifocal, those in the substantia nigra generally correlating with the signs of parkinsonism and those in the cerebral cortex, substantia innominata, and locus ceruleus generally correlating with the signs of dementia. Many other sites are also affected, but their clinical correlations are not so precise, perhaps because the cell losses are rarely so severe as in the substantia nigra and the cerebral cortex, substantia innominata, and locus ceruleus. Two examples may suffice: the locus ceruleus has also been implicated in the delayed reaction time and diminished vigilance of parkinsonian patients and related to a decrease in norepinephrine (Stern et al., 1984). The ventral tegmental area has been implicated in depression and bradyphrenia (Agid et al., 1984).

In the substantia nigra the changes consist of gross depigmentation and microscopic depigmentation of neurons, loss of neurons, extracellular melanin, "tombstone" formation (foci of macrophages containing the rather indigestible melanin pigment), and accumulation of either Lewy bodies or Alzheimer neurofibrillary tangles in some of the remaining neurons. In idiopathic parkinsonism, although the depigmentation of neurons is questionable (Forno and Alvord, 1974), the loss of neurons occurs in a reasonably stereotyped pattern, with the medial cell groups being relatively preserved. Lewy bodies (but, in some of the older patients, only Alzheimer neurofibrillary tangles) tend to occur in some of the remaining neurons. By contrast, in postencephalitic parkinsonism the loss of neurons is usually more severe and more randomly scattered, the medial cell groups tending to be especially destroyed. Alzheimer neurofibrillary tangles tend to occur in some of the remaining neurons.

In the cerebral cortex, substantia innominata, and locus ceruleus the changes consist of those usually associated with "ordinary" aging and the milder forms of Alzheimer's disease (presenile and senile dementia): Alzheimer neurofibrillary tangles are found in the hippocampus, neocortex, substantia innominata, and locus ceruleus; Marinesco senile plaques in the hippocampus and neocortex; Simchowicz granulovacuolar change in the hippocampus; and neuronal loss in the hippocampus, neocortex, substantia innominata, and locus ceruleus. Amyloid occurs as part of the senile plaques and perhaps also as a congophilic angiopathy affecting leptomeningeal and parenchymal vessels.

For the record it should be noted that there have always been "unitarians," people who have believed that all cases of "idiopathic" parkinsonism are due to encephalitis (Poskanzer and Schwab, 1963) or exogenous toxins (Calne and Langston, 1983). In addition there have been "disunitarians," people who have doubted that any significant lesions of parkinsonism have been discovered (Meyers, 1963; Mettler, 1964; Spiegel, 1965). Time, however, has ways of resolving these issues, as well as other more specific ones, such as the importance of the basal ganglia in parkinsonism. After all, parkinsonism is still one of the classic and major "basal ganglionic" diseases, but Pakkenberg and Bottcher (1974) have shown that the volumes of the caudate, putamen, and globus pallidus are the same in idiopathic parkinsonism (paralysis agitans) as in age-matched controls. Thus, no matter what some anatomists might say, we conclude that the substantia nigra must be included among the basal ganglia or deep cerebral nuclei, even though it is of mesencephalic origin.

LEWY BODY DEGENERATION

What are Lewy Bodies?

Lewy bodies are found within nerve cells, either near the nucleus (perikaryal) or within dendrites (intraneuritic). Perikaryal Lewy bodies are found typically in the dopaminergic substantia nigra and the noradrenergic locus ceruleus. They are frequently seen in the cholinergic substantia innominata (nucleus basalis of Meynert) and the raphé nuclei and occasionally in the cerebral cortex. They are easily seen by light microscopic examination of ordinary chromatically stained sections (e.g., hematoxylin and eosin, trichrome) as intracytoplasmic, single or multiple, spherical, acidophilic, or polychromatophilic masses possessing a dense core and a peripheral halo (Fig. 1). By electron microscopy (Duffy and Tennyson, 1965) the pattern resembles a sunflower (Fig. 2): the core is extremely dense and either amorphous or composed of circular profiles while the

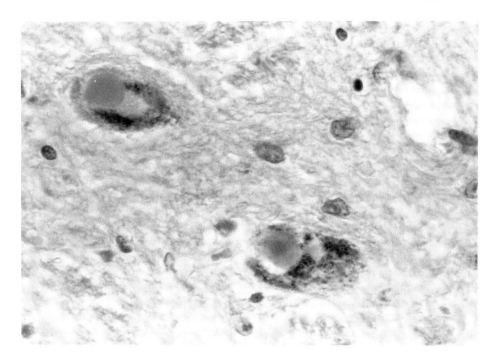

FIGURE 1   Two Lewy bodies in pigmented nerve cells in the substantia nigra. (Hematoxylin and eosin stain, x 550.)

peripheral halo is composed of radiating filaments that end without a membrane among the neuromelanin granules of the pigmented neurons. Tomonaga (1981) has found paired helical filaments of Alzheimer neurofibrillary tangles among the filaments of some Lewy bodies. Histochemical analyses reveal protein (Bethlem and Jager, 1960)—especially in the core, which is rich in basic amino acids (Issidorides et al., 1978)—and sphingomyelin (Jager, 1969) but no carbohydrate.

Intraneuritic Lewy bodies are most often found within dendrites of neurons in other sites, especially where melanin pigment is sparse or absent. Lewy (1912, 1923) originally described them in parkinsonian patients in the dorsal motor nucleus of the vagus and in the substantia innominata as spherical, elongated, or serpiginous. Similar bodies also occur in many other sites: commonly in the ventral tegmental area, hypothalamus (especially the posterior and lateral portions), and sympathetic ganglia; less commonly in the amygdala and spinal cord; rarely in the basal ganglia; and never in the dorsal root ganglia. By electron microscopy (Forno and Neville, 1976) intraneuritic Lewy bodies are much more variable than the perikaryal ones, containing amorphous or granular material,

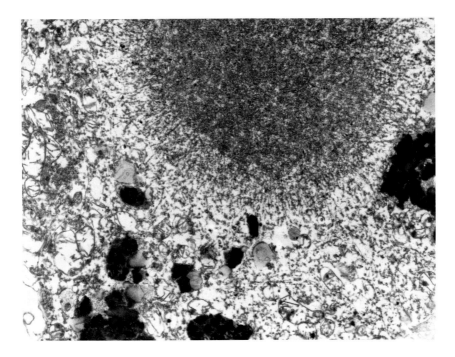

FIGURE 2 Electron micrograph of a perikaryal Lewy body in the substantia nigra, showing the typical sunflower appearance produced by the dense core and the halo composed of radiating filaments ending among the neuromelanin and lipofuscin granules.

filaments, dense core vesicles, multivesicular bodies, and various entrapped organelles.

The filaments of Lewy bodies have been related to neurofilaments because they react with antibodies directed against neurofilaments (Goldman et al., 1983; Forno et al., 1986b). However, they differ in other ways that may be at least as important: they are more variable in diameter (7–8 or even 20 nm rather than the 10–20 nm straight filaments of Pick bodies or the 20 nm paired helical filaments of Alzheimer neurofibrillary tangles) and they do not stain with the silver reagents that characteristically stain axons, neurofilaments, neurofibrillary tangles, and Pick bodies.

The early stage of Lewy bodies remains enigmatic, represented by pale areas devoid of most organelles, Nissl bodies, and neuromelanin (Alvord, 1959; Forno, 1986a,b). These pale areas may relate to some abnormal accumulations of protein without halos described by Issidorides et al. (1978) and to the "cytoplasmic inclusions without separation into core and halo" described by Kahn et al. (1985) as reacting with antineurofilament antibodies.

In Whom do Lewy Bodies Occur?

Nonparkinsonian Patients

Lewy bodies occur in the substantia nigra and locus ceruleus in about 10% of nonparkinsonian individuals coming to autopsy after age 60 years (Forno and Alvord, 1971; Alvord et al., 1974). Based on the data of Forno and Alvord (1971), one can estimate the percentage of cases in which either of these nuclei is affected as one-third of the age above 50 years: age – 50 divided by 3.

The inclusions are rare in younger persons but, as reviewed by Forno (1986a), they have been reported down to age 17 years in patients with a wide variety of diseases, such as neuroaxonal dystrophy, Hallervorden-Spatz disease, ataxia telangiectasia, subacute sclerosing panencephalitis, spinocerebellar degeneration, striatonigral degeneration (see below), progressive supranuclear palsy, and Alzheimer's disease (presenile and senile dementia). While degeneration of the substantia nigra and parkinsonism occasionally occurs in these diseases, Lewy bodies usually do not occur. In some of these diseases Alzheimer neurofibrillary tangles are the rule: Alzheimer's disease, progressive supranuclear palsy, and subacute sclerosing panencephalitis (especially in cases of long duration).

Idiopathic Parkinsonism

In idiopathic parkinsonism Lewy bodies in the substantia nigra and elsewhere are the rule and the severity of the loss of neurons in the substantia nigra (Figs. 3 and 4) correlates well with the severity of the parkinsonism (Alvord et al., 1974).

From these observations the concept has been developed that there is a large pool of individuals (about 10% of those over age 60 years) who have "Lewy body disease" with subclinical parkinsonism. From this pool, for reasons that remain undefined, various rates of degeneration of the dopaminergic neurons in the substantia nigra occur in different individuals, leading to loss of these cells and the development of various degrees of severity of parkinsonism (Forno, 1969, 1982, 1986a,b; Forno and Alvord, 1971; Alvord, 1971; Alvord et al., 1974).

Many other nuclei contain Lewy bodies (Bethlem and Jager, 1960; Jager and Bethlem, 1960), including the nuclei of Edinger-Westphal and Darkschewitz (Hunter, 1985). As Gaspar and Gray (1984) said, "The lesions in the different neuronal systems do not seem to evolve in parallel, but may be additive or potentiate one another in terms of functional expression." Therefore, other signs may develop, especially dementia. Gaspar and Gray (1984) correlate dementia in parkinsonism with increased neuronal loss and Lewy bodies in the basal nucleus of Meynert and locus ceruleus and, to a lesser extent, with senile plaques and neurofibrillary tangles in the cerebral cortex. By contrast, these latter changes, as well as other changes that we usually relate to mild forms of Alzheimer's disease, have been emphasized by Alvord et al. (1974), Hakim and

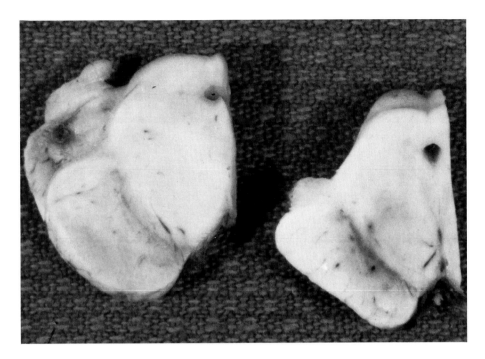

FIGURE 3 Depigmented substantia nigra typical of idiopathic parkinsonism contrasted with the normally pigmented substantia nigra of nonparkinsonian patient.

Mathieson (1979), and Jellinger and Riederer (1984). The dementia may occasionally take the form of Lewy body dementia (Okazaki et al., 1961; Forno et al., 1978; Kosaka et al., 1984; Yoshimura, 1983). One wonders whether the appearance of cortical Lewy bodies is real, possibly related to exogenous toxins, or merely the result of more careful attention to small lesions. Yoshimura (1983) reports a spectrum of cases, ranging from simple parkinsonism without dementia or cortical Lewy bodies and with senile changes corresponding to the age of the patient, through cases of parkinsonism with dementia and some cortical Lewy bodies to cases with severe dementia and many cortical Lewy bodies.

Shy-Drager Syndrome

Lewy bodies also occur in about 20% of patients with progressive autonomic failure, a syndrome originally described by Shy and Drager (1960). Oppenheimer (1983) has tabulated 51 cases and has divided them into two groups. About 20% of the cases have Lewy bodies in the brain stem and autonomic ganglia. About

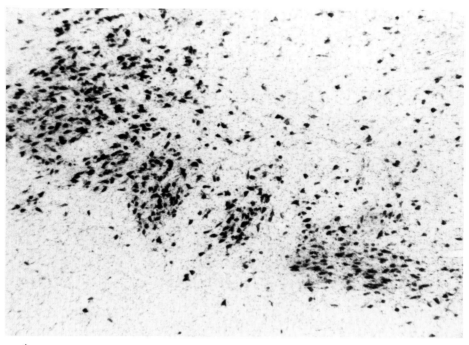

A

FIGURE 4 Nissl-stained sections of the medial to middle thirds of the substantia nigra (A) in a nonparkinsonian patient and (B) in a patient with idiopathic parkinsonism.

half of these have clinical parkinsonism but no other neurologic deficits are
present. Ages at death have varied from 66 to 83 years (average, 72 years). The
more common other cases have more diffuse degenerative changes with a variety
of neurologic deficits, that may or may not include parkinsonism. These cases
are now classified as multiple system atrophy (MSA) and include many cases
previously classified as striatonigral degeneration (see below) or olivopontocerebellar atrophy. In 2 of 41 cases Lewy bodies occurred, but "the lesions in
the striatum, olives, and cerebellum make it plain that the condition was of MSA
rather than of Parkinson's disease." In both groups the autonomic failure is attributed to a decrease in number of neurons in the lateral horns of the thoracic
spinal cord.

Although Oppenheimer (1983) did not mention dementia in his review, and
although Bannister and Oppenheimer (1972) stated that "dementia—one of the

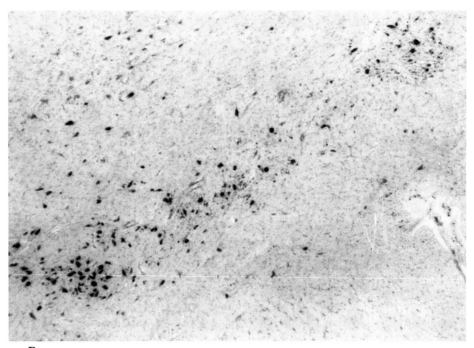

B

commonest results of severe cerebral ischaemia–is rarely a feature of the condiition," Alvord (unpublished data) has observed at least two cases, both men, aged 66 and 81 years, of Shy-Drager syndrome with Lewy bodies and severe dementia but with little or no parkinsonism (one patient had a masklike facies but no other symptoms). The cerebral cortical changes were relatively mild, hardly more than would be expected due to age alone.

The question naturally arises as to whether the Lewy bodies are really related to the Shy-Drager syndrome or are merely present by chance. From the ages given in the 51 cases summarized by Oppenheimer (1983), one can calculate that only about 4% might have had Lewy bodies by chance, whereas the actual incidence was about 25%. The association seems, therefore, to be real and not fortuitous. Whether Parkinson's disease is associated with subclinical orthostatic hypotension is an interesting question but in a small number of cases the lateral horns of parkinsonians without autonomic insufficiency appeared normal (Oppenheimer, 1983).

ALZHEIMER NEUROFIBRILLARY TANGLE DEGENERATION

What are Alzheimer Neurofibrillary Tangles?

Neurofibrillary tangles were first described by Alzheimer (1907a,b) in cases of presenile and senile dementia. There are at least two types of Alzheimer neuro-fibrillary tangles: those composed of paired helical filaments and those com-posed of straight tubules. Most are argyrophilic but some are not. The classic Alzheimer neurofibrillary tangles are seen in patients with Alzheimer's disease in the perikaryon of large neurons in the hippocampus and neocortex. Here they are most easily seen by light microscopy of silver-stained sections as thick, parallel, curvilinear fibers resembling sumi paintings, calligraphic streaks, or swirls. In the substantia nigra and locus ceruleus, however, they are rarely argyrophilic and are most easily seen in ordinary chromatic sections as un-stained, roughly spherical whorls of slightly refractile fibrils displacing the neuro-melanin pigment. Neurofibrillary tangles stain with congo red and thioflavin S or T, which render them brightly fluorescent under ultraviolet light.

The relationship of neurofibrillary tangles to normal neurofilaments has been a problem that has not been simplified by electron microscopy but is apparent-ly being unraveled by immunocytochemistry. Terry (1963, 1971) differentiated normal and abnormal neurofilaments (both 10 nm in diameter with a poorly de-fined lumen) from neurofibrillary tangles ("twisted neurotubules," 20 nm in diameter with periodic narrowings to 10 nm every 80 nm). Almost simultaneous-ly, however, Kidd (1964) showed that the tangles, which "could be mistaken for irregular filaments or even tubules," were really "two-stranded, antiparallel right-handed helices," each strand being 10 nm in diameter and each helix making a full turn in 160 nm.

Since neurofibrillary tangles react with antibodies to neurofilaments, it is necessary to review briefly what neurofilaments are. Neurofilaments consist of three major proteins with molecular weights of about 200, 145, and 68 kilo-daltons. The smallest forms the core or backbone and the largest forms cross-bridges helically wrapped around the core so as to appear periodically arranged at 100 nm intervals (Hirokawa et al., 1984; Sharp et al., 1982). The cross-bridges are long in axonal neurofilaments and short in dendritic ones (Hirokawa et al., 1984). The two smaller proteins contain three and nine phosphorylation sites, respectively, but the largest contains many more: 22 (Julien and Mushynski, 1983). With immunologic reagents phosphorylated neurofilaments are detected normally only in axons and nonphosphorylated neurofilaments in both axons and perikarya (Sternberger and Sternberger, 1983). However, perikaryal neuro-fibrillary tangles have phosphorylated neurofilamentous material both in Alzheimer's disease (Sternberger et al., 1985; Cork et al., 1985, 1986; Forno et al., 1983, 1986b) and in experimental aluminum intoxication (Troncoso et al.,

1986). The tangles react minimally—never in the hippocampus (Forno et al., 1986b)—with antibodies to nonphosphorylated neurofilaments. These latter antibodies react with widely distributed neurons and axons in the rat (Sternberger and Sternberger, 1983) but with much greater selectivity in the human: many large neurons (e.g., Betz cells, cranial motor neurons, sympathetic, and dorsal root ganglia) but not with the large pyramidal cells of the hippocampus (Forno et al., 1986b).

Table 3 summarizes the similarities and differences between Lewy bodies and Alzheimer neurofibrillary tangles, and also compares these with Pick bodies and normal neurofilaments. As Rasool and Selkoe (1985b) pointed out, it appears that some inclusions contain normal neurofilament antigens, some partially or completely denatured antigens, and some have acquired new antigens. These differences appear to correlate reasonably well with the degree of aggregation of proteins: those in the core of Lewy bodies are so greatly denatured that the neurofibrillary antigens are masked and new antigenic determinants appear. Those in the halo of Lewy bodies and those in the helically twisted neurofibrillary tangles—which may be due to increased phosphorylation of neurofilaments—are less severely denatured, so that their phosphorylated sites can be detected even while new antigenic determinants are produced. Figures 5 and 6 illustrate the staining of a Lewy body and an Alzheimer neurofibrillary tangle by immunoreactions with antibodies to phosphorylated neurofilaments.

In Whom do Alzheimer Neurofibrillary Tangles Occur?

Nonparkinsonian Patients

Alzheimer neurofibrillary tangles occur in the substantia nigra of nonparkinsonian patients with about the same frequency as do Lewy bodies. In the locus ceruleus, however, they occur much more commonly: beginning about age 30 years, they increase linearly, affecting about 90% of individuals coming to autopsy after age 90 years (Forno and Alvord, 1971; Alvord et al., 1974). From the data of Forno and Alvord (1971) one can estimate the percentage of individuals affected as four-thirds of the age above 30 years: age - 30 times 4/3. It is interesting that dementia appears at about the same age (Alvord et al., 1974). Alzheimer neurofibrillary tangles also occur commonly in the hippocampus and parahippocampus, beginning about age 50 years and progressively increasing in severity more rapidly than in any other site (Alvord et al., 1974; Ball, 1976).

Neurofibrillary tangles occur in other sites (Hirano and Zimmerman, 1962; Forno, unpublished data), such as the glomeruli of the parahippocampus, amygdala, nucleus basalis, lateral and posterior hypothalamic nuclei, reticular nucleus of the thalamus, periaqueductal gray, and midline reticular formation (raphe nuclei) of the brain stem. Other moderately susceptible neurons include those in the limbic cortex, insula, claustrum, anterior and posterior perforated

TABLE 3 Differential Reactivities of Specific Inclusion Bodies

Stain	Lewy body		Neurofibrillary tangle	Neurofilaments	Pick body
	Core	Halo			
H & E et al.	+	0	0-±	0	±
Silver (axons)	0	0	+	+	+
Antibodies to					
Neurofilaments[a,f]	0	+	0	+	0
Nonphosphorylated neurofilaments[b]	0	0-+	0-±	+[c]	
Phosphorylated neurofilaments[b]	0	+	+	+[d]	+
neurofibrillary tangles[e,f]	0	0	+	0	+
tyrosine hydroxylase[g,h]	0-±	+	0-±	0	
Lewy bodies[i]	+	0		0	

[a] Goldman et al., 1983
[b] Forno et al., 1983, 1986b
[c] Many axons and neuron types in the rat but very selective in the human: many large cells (but not hippocampus)[b]
[d] Axons[b]
[e] Rasool and Selkoe, 1985a,b
[f] Kahn et al., 1985
[g] Nakashima and Ikuta, 1984: only Lewy bodies in melanin-containing neurons, not those in substantia innominata, raphe nuclei, or spinal cord
[h] Nakashima and Ikuta, 1985: cytoplasm of cells containing neurofibrillary tangles is positive
[i] Hirsch et al., 1985.

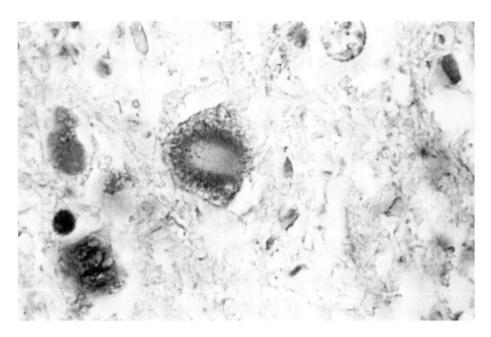

FIGURE 5 The halo of this substantia nigra Lewy body from a case of Lewy body dementia is revealed by immunoreaction with antibody (07–5) directed against phosphorylated neurofilaments. The nuclei are stained with hematoxylin.

substances, and only rarely in the nucleus ambiguus and oculomotor and hypoglossal nuclei (but never in other cranial or spinal motor neurons).

In the cerebral cortex Alzheimer neurofibrillary tangles are characteristically found in patients with Alzheimer's disease, in individuals over age 35 years with Down's syndrome, and in Guamanians with the complex of parkinsonism, dementia, and amyotrophic lateral sclerosis.

In the brain stem, tangles characterize individuals with postencephalitic parkinsonism, cases of idiopathic Alzheimer tangle parkinsonism, Down's syndrome patients over the age of 35, some cases of chronic encephalitis without parkinsonism, pugilistic encephalopathy, and the complex of parkinsonism, dementia, and amyotrophic lateral sclerosis in Guam. It should be noted that in progressive supranuclear palsy (Steele et al., 1964), in which tangles occur diffusely, some of the tangles have a different morphology being composed of straight tubules rather than paired helical filaments.

Postencephalitic Parkinsonism

Ever since Hallervorden (1935) called attention to them, Alzheimer neurofibrillary tangles in the substantia nigra have been considered the hallmark of post-

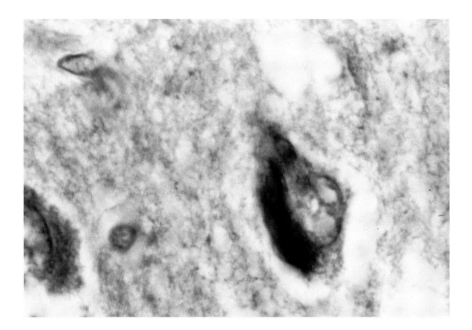

FIGURE 6 This Alzheimer neurofibrillary tangle in the hippocampus is revealed by the same immunoreaction as in Figure 5.

encephalitic parkinsonism. Such cases tend to have severe loss of neurons in the substantia nigra (Fig. 7), correlating well with the severe degree of parkinsonism seen clinically (Alvord et al., 1974). There are no Lewy bodies but moderate to large numbers of Alzheimer tangles (Forno and Alvord, 1971). Cases of post-encephalitic parkinsonism have virtually disappeared by now.

Idiopathic Parkinsonism

Other relatively rare cases of parkinsonism without a history of encephalitis may also have only Alzheimer tangles in some of the remaining neurons of the substantia nigra. These tend to occur in persons coming to autopsy after age 80 years and probably represent a variant of Alzheimer's disease (Forno and Alvord, 1971; Alvord, 1971; Alvord et al., 1974; Forno, 1982). These parkinsonians with idiopathic Alzheimer tangle tend to have mild to severe loss of neurons in the substantia nigra, no Lewy bodies, and moderate to large numbers of Alzheimer tangles (Forno and Alvord, 1971). The correlation between the severity of parkinsonism and the degree of neuron loss is especially poor for those patients with only moderate (definite but not severe) parkinsonism

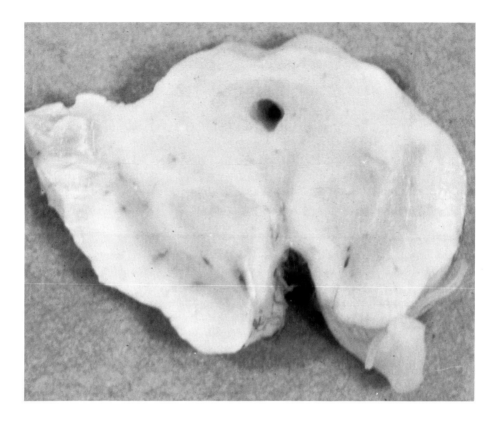

FIGURE 7   Completely depigmented substantia nigra in a case of postencephalitic parkinsonism.

(Alvord et al., 1974), an indication that the disease is more diffuse than that in the usual parkinsonian patient.

The marked difference between the slopes of the lines representing the age-related incidence and severity of Alzheimer neurofibrillary tangles in the locus ceruleus and in the substantia nigra is quite unlike the parallel lines for Lewy bodies in these two nuclei. Can one, nevertheless, by analogy with the concept of "Lewy body disease," postulate an "Alzheimer neurofibrillary tangle disease?" If so, one has to be at least somewhat cautious and not overemphasize the tangles occurring in the locus ceruleus or hippocampus, since they can be found in practically every aged individual. Especially when making the diagnosis of idiopathic Alzheimer tangle parkinsonism, one should pay attention only to the tangles in the substantia nigra.

Complex of Parkinsonism, Dementia,
and Amyotrophic Lateral Sclerosis

The parkinsonism–dementia complex was first recognized in the Chamorro
Indians on the island of Guam and was then found to be frequently associated
with amyotrophic lateral sclerosis (Koerner, 1952; Kurland and Mulder, 1954;
Hirano et al., 1961a,b, 1966; Elizan et al., 1966a,b). Autopsies provided the
clues to understanding the complex: about one-sixth of the patients had typical
amyotrophic lateral sclerosis clinically and pathologically but at autopsy also
had Alzheimer neurofibrillary tangles in many neurons, especially in the substantia nigra. The other patients had relatively pure parkinsonism and dementia
although some had additional clinical signs of upper motor neuron involvement;
at autopsy all had even more widespread neurofibrillary tangles. In addition
there was gross atrophy of the frontal lobes and depigmentation of the substantia nigra and locus ceruleus as well as microscopic evidence of atrophy of the
temporal lobes, globus pallidus and thalamus. No senile plaques were found but
Simchowicz granulovacuolar inclusions were present in the hippocampus and
elsewhere. Lewy bodies were found in about 10% of the cases. In addition to
these clinically obvious cases, about 20% of the Chamorros dying without
clinical evidence of parkinsonism, dementia, or amyotrophic lateral sclerosis had
histologic evidence of the neurofibrillary tangle disease at autopsy. This is a
statistical pattern very similar to those of "Lewy body disease" and "Alzheimer
neurofibrillary tangle disease" described above.

Two other foci of high incidence of motor neuron disease have been recognized in the Kii peninsula of Japan (Shiraki and Yase, 1975; Uebayashi, 1980)
and in West New Guinea (Gajdusek and Salazar, 1982).

Less than 20 years after the discovery of the disease complex it was recognized that the high incidence of this complex was decreasing (Reed et al., 1966;
Brody and Chen, 1966) and by now it has virtually disappeared (Garruto et al.,
1985). The suggestion has been made that nutritional deficiencies of calcium and
magnesium in garden soil and drinking water may have led to "subtle" defects
in calcium and vitamin D metabolism (Yanagihara et al., 1984), with secondary
hyperparathyroidism causing deposition of calcium and aluminum in neurons
(Perl et al., 1982; Garruto et al., 1984). The hypothesis suffers from the fact
that the metabolic defects were mild and discoverable in only a minority of patients but, whatever the explanation, the disease has apparently disappeared,
perhaps as the population has become less isolated and has accepted "changes in
dietary habits and local water supplies and much less dependence on locally
grown food" (Garruto et al., 1985).

The aluminum has been demonstrated in neuronal nuclei and cytoplasm,
associated with ribosomal RNA- and DNA-containing chromatins but not in
the tangles, at least in experimental rabbits (Wen and Wisniewski, 1985). One
should note, however, that the hypothesis that aluminum plays a role in the

development of Alzheimer neurofibrillary tangles in humans is still controversial (Crapper et al., 1976; Markesbery et al., 1981). The most bothersome aspect of the controversy, aside from the possible artifactual contamination of fixative solutions with aluminum, is that the experimental aluminum-induced neurofibrillary tangles consist of 10 nm neurofilaments, not paired helical filaments (Wisniewski et al., 1970; Terry, 1971).

Combination of Lewy Body and Alzheimer Neurofibrillary Tangle Degeneration

From the discussion above, it should be obvious that the combination of Lewy bodies and Alzheimer neurofibrillary tangles should be relatively common just by chance in individuals coming to autopsy after age 60 years. Considering only the substantia nigra, if each change occurs in about 10% of such nonparkinsonians, the combination should occur in about 1%. However, considering also the locus ceruleus (and hippocampus), where the incidence of Alzheimer tangles rises rapidly with age to affect at least 90% of the nonparkinsonian population, the combination should occur by chance alone in about 4–9% of persons over age 60 years.

A number of studies (Woodard, 1962; Forno, 1982; Jellinger and Riederer, 1984; Leverenz and Sumi, 1986) indicate that 10–35% of patients with Alzheimer's disease (senile and presenile dementia) have Lewy bodies in the substantia nigra. The average incidence is about 15%, or about twice that we would expect by chance alone. Many of these patients have clinical evidence of possible or definite parkinsonism, usually with rigidity more than tremor. Some doubt is cast on the significance of these observations by Woodard's finding of the same percentage of Lewy bodies in cases of organic dementia and others without the morphologic evidence of Alzheimer's disease as in cases with Alzheimer's disease. Perhaps the problem is that the more one looks, the more one finds. On the other hand, perhaps some of the factors that cause one process to accelerate also cause the other degenerative process to accelerate. Or, perhaps, the immunocytochemical similarities between Lewy bodies and Alzheimer neurofibrillary tangles are more significant, indicating that the degenerative processes are essentially the same, even though the morphologic appearances are different.

DRUG-INDUCED PARKINSONISM

Several decades of morphologic studies of iatrogenic parkinsonism and similar movement disorders following the administration of various psychotropic drugs yielded virtually nothing but frustration (Hunter et al., 1968; Christensen et al., 1970) until the accidental introduction to street-drug abusers of 1-methyl-4-phenyl-1,2,3,6-tetrahydropyridine (MPTP), a product of meperidine analogue synthesis (Davis et al., 1979; Langston et al., 1983). The striking clinical and neuropathologic features immediately suggested the possibility of exogenous toxins as the cause of idiopathic parkinsonism (Calne and Langston, 1983). The similarities between the experimental lesions and those of idiopathic parkinsonism have even led Forno (1986a) to pursue the electron microscopic sunflower analogy by stating that "we are still waiting for Lewy bodies to bloom in the MPTP-induced experimental parkinsonism in the monkey."

However, parkinsonism undoubtedly existed long before Parkinson defined it, long before such exotic toxins were synthesized. Perhaps more to the point, Forno et al. (1986a) admit that there are differences between the human and experimental parkinsonians: the experimental lesions are remarkably restricted to the substantia nigra, the medial portion of which is not spared. In addition there is some disparity between the severity of the parkinsonism and the severity of the lesions: one monkey "seemed to have recovered completely from its parkinsonian state" in spite of "almost complete nerve cell loss" in the middle and lateral portions of the substantia nigra after 15 months survival, while five monkeys with parkinsonism "had only questionable nerve cell loss" in contrast to the six other parkinsonian monkeys who had severe cell loss. Such a dissociation between clinical and pathologic signs, seen in about half of the affected monkeys, could be accepted as suggesting that the metabolic effects of MPTP are more severe than the morphologic effects, as is commonly the case with toxins. However, the dissociation is more reminiscent of some human cases without Lewy bodies than of cases with Lewy bodies (Alvord et al., 1974).

OTHER CAUSES OF PARKINSONISM

Striatonigral Degeneration

Striatonigral degeneration (Adams, 1968; Jellinger and Danielczyk, 1968) is a rare disorder characterized by multifocal degeneration of the striatal neurons (especially in the putamen) upon which the dopaminergic nigral afferents end synaptically. Thus, unlike the common Lewy body and Alzheimer neurofibrillary tangle cases of parkinsonism, in which replacement of the neurotransmitter dopamine is of therapeutic value, there are no neurons for the dopamine to act upon and there is little or no therapeutic response (Andrews et al., 1970). As noted above, many of the cases of striatonigral degeneration have autonomic insufficiency and are being reclassified as examples of the Shy-Drager syndrome due to multiple system atrophy.

Arteriosclerotic Parkinsonism

Arteriosclerotic parkinsonism is a surprisingly rare condition, but not so rare as its denial in previous reviews (Alvord, 1959, 1968, 1971). Its clinical features, as well as those of other neurologic syndromes in the elderly, were described

beautifully by Critchley (1931). Denny-Brown (1962), who undoubtedly over-
emphasized the importance of the globus pallidus in parkinsonism, did provide
pathologic confirmation, describing seven cases of "arteriosclerotic lacunar
lesions" or "état criblé" of the putamen, to which he attributed "every conceivable proportion of tremor to rigidity." In the experience of Forno (1977)
such small cystic infarcts or lacunae in the basal ganglia produce atypical or mild
parkinsonism, usually with rigidity more than tremor. Having seen more cases,
Alvord can now agree with Forno (1982): "pathological processes in the
striatum can give rise to parkinsonian symptoms."

Other Diseases

As reviewed by Alvord (1971), a wide variety of other diseases may occasionally
cause parkinsonism: carbon monoxide or manganese intoxication, Wilson's
disease, various viral infections, trauma, neoplasm, syringomesencephalia, spinocerebellar degenerations, and other diseases. Such variety does not so much cast
doubt upon the significance of the sites affected in ordinary parkinsonism (e.g.,
the substantia nigra) but emphasizes the difficulty of analyzing cases with
diffuse lesions or effects.

CONCLUSIONS

This review of the pathology of parkinsonism has concentrated on four areas:
Lewy body degeneration, Alzheimer neurofibrillary tangle degeneration, drug-
induced parkinsonism, and other causes of parkinsonism. The importance of the
substantia nigra in relation to all forms of parkinsonism is emphasized. All of
these forms of parkinsonism may also be associated with dementia, which can
be related to various types of lesions, including Lewy body degeneration and
Alzheimer neurofibrillary tangle degeneration, in the cerebral cortex, nucleus
basalis, and locus ceruleus. The concept is presented of "Lewy body disease"
and "Alzheimer neurofibrillary tangle disease" as including relatively large pools
of susceptible (subclinical) individuals.

Why do some individuals appear to respond to as-yet-unknown accelerating
factors by developing more rapid degeneration of the substantia nigra which
produces clinically apparent parkinsonism of appropriate severity at ages determined by the rate of neuronal degeneration? Whatever the answer, a similar
pattern of subclinical microscopic changes and clinical diseases of varying
severity can be seen in the complex of parkinsonism, dementia, and amyotrophic
lateral sclerosis reported in Guam and a few other isolated geographic foci. The
good news is that environmental factors appear to have changed sufficiently in
the last two decades practically to have eliminated this complex. Whether similar
environmental factors will be found to eliminate the worldwide degenerations of

Lewy body and Alzheimer neurofibrillary tangle parkinsonism and dementia remains to be discovered.

REFERENCES

Adams RD. (1968). The striatonigral degenerations. In: Vinken PJ, Bruyn GW (Eds.), *Handbook of Clinical Neurology*, Vol. 6. Amsterdam, North Holland Publ. Co.

Agid Y, Ruberg M, Dubois B, Javoy-Agid F. (1984). Biochemical substrates of mental disturbances in Parkinson's disease. *Adv Neurol* 40: 211–218.

Alvord EC Jr. (1959). Pathology of parkinsonism. In: Fields WS (Ed.), *Pathogenesis and Treatment of Parkinsonism*. Springfield, Charles C. Thomas.

Alvord EC Jr. (1968). The pathology of parkinsonism. In: Minckler J (Ed.), *Pathology of the Nervous System*, Vol. 1. New York, McGraw-Hill.

Alvord EC Jr. (1971). The pathology of parkinsonism. Part II. An interpretation with special reference to other changes in the aging brain. *Contemp Neurol* 8: 131–161.

Alvord EC Jr, Forno LS, Kusske JA, Kauffman RJ, Rhodes JS, Goetowski CR. (1974). The pathology of parkinsonism: a comparison of degenerations in cerebral cortex and brainstem. *Adv Neurol* 5: 175–193.

Alzheimer A. (1907a). Ueber eine eigenartige Erkrankung der Hirnrinde. *Allg. Zeits Psych.* 64: 146–148.

Alzheimer A. (1907b). Ueber eine eigenartige Erkrankung der Hirnrinde. *Zentralbl Ges Neurol Psych* 18: 177–179.

Andrews JM, Terry RD, Spataro J. (1970). Striatonigral degeneration: clinical-pathological correlations and response to sterotaxic sugery. *Arch Neurol* 23: 319–329.

Ball MJ. (1976). Neuronal loss, neurofibrillary tangles and granulovacuolar degeneration in the hippocampus with ageing and dementia; a quantitative study. *Acta Neuropathol* 37: 111–118.

Bannister R, Oppenheimer D. (1972). Degenerative diseases of the nervous system associated with autonomic failure. *Brain* 95: 457–474.

Beheim-Schwarzbach D. (1952). Uber Zelleib-Veränderungen im Nucleus Coeruleus bei Parkinson-Symptomen. *J Nerv Ment Dis* 116: 619–632.

Bethlem J, Jager WAdH. (1960). The incidence and characteristics of Lewy bodies in idiopathic paralysis agitans (Parkinson's disease). *J Neurol Neurosurg Psychiatry* 23: 74–80.

Brody JA, Chen K. (1969). Changing epidemiologic patterns of amyotrophic lateral sclerosis and parkinsonism-dementia on Guam. In: Norris FH Jr, Kurland LT (Eds.), *Motor Neuron Diseases: Research on Amyotrophic Lateral Sclerosis and Related Disorders*, vol 2. New York, Grune and Stratton.

Calne DB, Langston JW. (1983). Aetiology of Parkinson's disease. *Lancet* 2: 1457–1459.

Christensen E, Moller JE, Faurbye A. (1970). Neuropathological investigation of 28 brains from patients with dyskinesia. *Acta Psychiatr Scand* 46: 14–23.

Cork LC, Altschuler RJ, Struble RG, Casanova MF, Price DL, Sternberger N, Sternberger L. (1985). Changes in the distribution of phosphorylated neurofilaments in Alzheimer's disease. *J Neuropathol Exp Neurol* 44: 368.

Cork LC, Sternberger NH, Sternberger LA, Casanova MF, Struble RG, Price DL. (1986). Phosphorylated neurofilament antigens in neurofibrillary tangles in Alzheimer's disease. *J Neuropathol Exp Neurol* 45: 56–64.

Crapper DR, Krishnan SS, Quittkat S. (1976). Aluminum, neurofibrillary degeneration and Alzheimer's disease. *Brain* 99: 67–80.

Critchley M. (1931). The neurology of old age. *Lancet* 220: 1119–1127.

Davis GC, Williams AC, Markey SP, Ebert MH, Caine ED, Reichert CM, Kopin IJ. (1979). Chronic parkinsonism secondary to intravenous injection of meperidine analogues. *Psychiatr Res* 1: 249–254.

Denny-Brown D. (1962). *The Basal Ganglia and Their Relation to Disorders of Movement*. London, Oxford University Press.

Duffy PE, Tennyson VM. (1965). Phase and electron microscopic observations of Lewy bodies and melanin granules in the substantia nigra and locus caeruleus in Parkinson's disease. *J Neuropathol Exp Neurol* 24: 398–414.

Elizan TA, Chen K-M, Mathai KV, Dunn D, Kurland LT. (1966a). Amyotrophic lateral sclerosis and parkinsonism-dementia complex, a study in non-Chamorros of the Mariana and Caroline islands. *Arch Neurol* 14: 347–355.

Elizan TS, Hirano A, Abrams BM, Need RL, Van Nuis C, Kurland LT. (1966b). Amyotrophic lateral sclerosis and parkinsonism–dementia complex of Guam, neurological reevaluation. *Arch Neurol* 14: 356–368.

Forno LS. (1966). Pathology of parkinsonism. A preliminary report of 24 cases. *J Neurosurg* 24: 266–271.

Forno LS. (1969). Concentric hyalin intraneuronal inclusions of Lewy type in the brains of elderly persons (50 incidental cases): relationship to parkinsonism. *J Am Geriatr Soc* 17: 557–575.

Forno LS. (1977). Pathology of parkinsonism: nigro-striatal relationships; extranigral lesions; review. In: Worm-Peterson J, Bottcher J (Eds.), *Proceedings of a Symposium on Parkinsonism*, Denmark, Merck, Sharp and Dohme.

Forno LS. (1982). Pathology of Parkinson's disease. In: Marsden CD, Fahn S (Eds.), *Movement Disorders*. London, Butterworth Scientific.

Forno LS. (1986a). The Lewy body in Parkinson's disease. In: Yahr M (Ed.), *Proceedings of the VIII International Symposium on Parkinson's Disease*. New York, Raven Press.

Forno LS. (1986b). Pathology of Parkinson's disease. The importance of the substantia nigra and the Lewy bodies. In: Stern G (Ed.), *Parkinson's Disease*. London, Chapman and Hall.

Forno LS, Alvord EC Jr. (1971). The pathology of parkinsonism, Part I. Some new observations and correlations. *Contemp Neurol* 8: 120–130.

Forno LS, Alvord EC Jr. (1974). Depigmentation in the nerve cells of the substantia nigra and locus ceruleus in Parkinsonism. *Adv Neurol* 5: 195–202.

Forno LS, Norville RL. (1976). Ultrastructure of Lewy bodies in the stellate ganglion. *Acta Neuropathol* (Berlin) 34: 183–197.

Forno LS, Barbour PJ, Norville RL. (1978). Presenile dementia with Lewy bodies and neurofibrillary tangles. *Arch Neurol* 35: 818–822.

Forno LS, Strefling AM, Sternberger LA, Sternberger NH, Eng LF. (1983). Immunocytochemical staining of neurofibrillary tangles and of the periphery of Lewy bodies with a monoclonal antibody to neurofilaments. *J Neuropathol Exp, Neurol* 42: 342.

Forno LS, DeLanney LE, Irwin I, Langston JW. (1986a). Neuropathology of MPTP-treated monkeys: comparison with the neuropathology of human idiopathic Parkinson's disease. In: Markey SP, Castagnoli N Jr., Trevor AJ, and Kopin IJ (Eds.), *MPTP, a Neurotoxin Producing a Parkinsonian Syndrome.* New York, Academic Press.

Forno LS, Sternberger LA, Sternberger NH, Strefling AM, Swanson K, Eng LF. (1986b). Reaction of Lewy bodies with antibodies to phosphorylated and non-phosphorylated neurofilaments. *Neurosci Lett* 64: 253–258.

Gajdusek DC, Salazar AM. (1982). Amyotrophic lateral sclerosis and parkinsonian syndromes in high incidence among the Auyu and Jakai people of West New Guinea. *Neurology* 32: 107–126.

Garruto RM, Fukatsu R, Yanagihara R, Gajdusek DC, Hook G, Fiori CE. (1984). Imaging of calcium and aluminum in neurofibrillary tangle-bearing neurons in parkinsonism-dementia of Guam. *Proc. Natl. Acad Sci USA* 81: 875–879.

Garruto RM, Yanagihara R, Gajdusek DC. (1985). Disappearance of high-incidence amyotrophic lateral sclerosis and parkinsonism-dementia on Guam. *Neurology* 35: 193–198.

Gaspar P, Gray F. (1984). Dementia in idiopathic Parkinson's disease. A neuropathological study of 32 cases. *Acta Neuropathol* (Berlin) 64: 43–52.

Goldman JE, Yen S-H, Chiu FC, Peress NS. (1983). Lewy bodies of Parkinson's disease contain neurofilament antigen. *Science* 221: 1082–1084.

Greenfield JG, Bosanquet FD. (1953). The brain-stem lesions in parkinsonism. *J Neurol Neurosurg Psychiatry* 16: 213–226.

Hakim AM, Mathieson G. (1979). Dementia in Parkinson disease: a neuropathologic study. *Neurology* 29: 1209–1214.

Hallervorden J. (1935). Anatomische Untersuchungen zur Pathogenese des postencephalitischen Parkinsonismus. *Dtsch. Nervenheilkd* 136: 68–77.

Hassler R. (1938). Zur Pathologie der Paralysis agitans und des postenzephalitischen Parkinsonismus. *J. Psychol. Neurol* 48: 387–476.

Hirano A, Zimmerman HM. (1962). Alzheimer's neurofibrillary changes, a topographic study. *Arch Neurol* 7: 227–242.

Hirano A, Kurland LT, Krooth RS, Lessell S. (1961a). Parkinsonism-dementia complex, an endemic disease on the island of Guam. I. Clinical features. *Brain* 84: 642–661.

Hirano A, Malamud N, Kurland LT. (1961b). Parkinsonism-dementia complex, an endemic disease on the island of Guam. II. Pathologic features. *Brain* 84: 662–679.

Hirano A, Malamud N, Elizan TS, Kurland LT. (1966). Amyotrophic lateral sclerosis and parkinsonism-dementia complex on Guam, further pathologic studies. *Arch Neurol* 15: 35–51.

Hirano A, Kurland LT, Sayre GP. (1967). Familial amyotrophic lateral sclerosis, a subgroup characterized by posterior and spinocerebellar tract involvement and hyaline inclusions in the anterior horn cells. *Arch Neurol* 16: 232–243.

Hirokawa N, Glicksman MA, Willard MB. (1984). Organization of mammalian neurofilament polypeptides within the neuronal cytoskeleton. *J Cell Biol* 98: 1523–1536.

Hirsch E, Ruberg M, Dardenne M, Portier M-M, Javoy-Agid F, Bach J-F, Agid Y. (1985). Monoclonal antibodies raised against Lewy bodies in brains from subjects with Parkinson's disease. *Brain Res* 345: 374–378.

Hunter R, Blackwood W, Smith MC, Cumings JN. (1968). Neuropathological findings in three cases of persistent dyskinesia following phenothiazine medication. *J Neurol Sci* 7: 263–273.

Hunter S. (1985). The rostral mesencephalon in Parkinson's disease and Alzheimer's disease. *Acta Neuropathol* (Berlin) 68: 53–58.

Issidorides MR, Mytilineou C, Whetsell WO Jr, Yahr MD. (1978). Protein-rich cytoplasmic bodies of substantia nigra and locus ceruleus–a comparative study in parkinsonian and normal brain. *Arch Neurol* 35: 633–637.

Jager WAdH. (1969). Sphingomyelin in Lewy inclusion bodies in Parkinson's disease. *Arch Neurol* 21: 615–619.

Jager WAdH, Bethlem J. (1960). The distribution of Lewy bodies in the central and autonomic nervous systems in idiopathic paralysis agitans. *J. Neurol. Neurosurg. Psychiatry* 23: 283–290.

Jellinger K, Danielczyk W. (1968). Striato-nigral degeneration. *Acta Neuropathol* 10: 242–257.

Jellinger K, Riederer P. (1984). Dementia in Parkinson's disease and (pre) senile dementia of Alzheimer type: morphological aspects and changes in the intracerebral MAO activity. *Adv Neurol* 40: 199–210.

Julien J-P, Mushynski WE. (1983). The distribution of phosphorylation sites among identified proteolytic fragments of mammalian neurofilaments. *J Biol Chem* 258: 4019–4025.

Kahn J, Anderton BH, Gibb WRG, Lees AJ, Wells FR, Marsden CD. (1985). Neuronal filaments in Alzheimer's, Pick's, and Parkinson's diseases. *N Engl J Med* 313: 520–521.

Kidd M. (1964). Alzheimer's disease–an electron microscopic study. *Brain* 87: 307–320.

Kimula Y, Utsuyama M, Yoshimura M, Tomonaga M. (1983). Element analysis of Lewy and adrenal bodies in Parkinson's disease by electron probe microanalysis. *Acta Neuropathol* 59: 233–236.

Koerner DR. (1952). Amyotrophic lateral sclerosis on Guam: a clinical study and review of the literature. *Ann Intern Med* 37: 1204–1220.

Kosaka K, Yoshimura M, Ikeda K, Budka H. (1984). Diffuse type of Lewy body disease: progressive dementia with abundant cortical Lewy bodies and senile changes of varying degree–a new disease? *Clin Neuropathol* 3: 185–192.

Kurland LT, Mulder DW. (1954). Epidemiologic investigations of amyotrophic lateral sclerosis. I. Preliminary report on geographic distribution, with special reference to the Mariana Islands, including clinical and pathological observations. *Neurology* 4: 355–378.

Langston JW, Ballard P, Tetrud JW, Irwin I. (1983). Chronic parkinsonism in humans due to a product of meperidine-analog synthesis. *Science* 219: 979–980.

Leverenz J, Sumi SM. (1986). Parkinson's disease in patients with Alzheimer's disease. *Arch Neurol* 43: 662–664.

Lewy FH. (1912). Paralysis agitans. I. Pathologische Anatomie. In: Lewandowski M (Ed.), *Handbuch der Neurologie*. Berlin, Springer.

Lewy FH. (1923). *Die Lehre vom Tonus und der Bewegung zugleich systematische Untersuchungen zur Klinik, Physiologie, Pathologie und Pathogenese der Paralysis Agitans*. Berlin, Springer Verlag.

Lewy FH. (1940a). Historical introduction: the basal ganglia and their diseases. *Proc Assoc Res Nerv Ment Dis* 21: 1–20.

Lewy FH. (1940b). Discussion. *Proc Assoc Res. Nerv Ment Dis* 21: 487.

Markesbery WR, Ehmann WD, Hossain TIM, Alauddin M, Goodin DT. (1981). Instrumental neutron activation analysis of brain aluminum in Alzheimer disease and aging. *Ann Neurol* 10: 511–516.

Mettler FA. (1964). Substantia nigra and parkinsonism. *Arch Neurol* 11: 529–542.

Meyers R. (1963). Pathogenetic theories of hyperkinesia. The importance of the negative case. *Trans Am Neurol Assoc* 88: 84–90.

Nakashima S, Ikuta F. (1984). Tyrosine hydroxylase protein in Lewy bodies of parkinsonian and senile brains. *J Neurol Sci* 66: 91–96.

Nakashima S, Ikuta F. (1985). Catecholamine neurons with Alzheimer's neurofibrillary changes and alteration of tyrosine hydroxylase. Immunohistochemical investigation of tyrosine hydroxylase. *Acta Neuropathol* (Berlin) 66: 37–41.

Okazaki H, Lipkin LE, Aronson SM. (1961). Diffuse intracytoplasmic ganglionic inclusions (Lewy type) associated with progressive dementia and quadriparesis in flexion. *J Neuropathol Exp Neurol* 20: 237–244.

Oppenheimer D. (1983). Neuropathology of progressive autonomic failure. In: Bannister R (Ed.), *Autonomic Failure: Textbook of Clinical Disorders of the Autonomic Nervous System*. New York, Oxford University Press.

Pakkenberg H, Bottcher J. (1974). Corpus striatum in paralysis agitans and in perphenazine-injected rats. *Adv Neurol* 5: 203–206.

Parkinson J. (1817). *An Essay on the Shaking Palsy*. London, Whittingham and Rowland. Reprinted in Critchley M (Ed.), *James Parkinson*. London, Macmillan.

Perl DP, Gajdusek DC, Garruto RM, Yanagihara RT, Gibbs CJ Jr. (1982). Intraneuronal aluminum accumulation in amyotrophic lateral sclerosis and parkinsonism-dementia of Guam. *Science* 217: 1053–1055.

Pollock M, Hornabrook RW. (1966). The prevalence, natural history and dementia of Parkinson's disease. *Brain* 89: 429–448.

Poskanzer DC, Schwab RS. (1963). Cohort analysis of Parkinson's syndrome. Evidence for a single etiology related to subclinical infection about 1920. *J Chron Dis* 16: 961–973.

Rasool CG, Selkoe DJ. (1985a). Sharing of specific antigens by degenerating neurons in Pick's disease and Alzheimer's disease. *N Engl J Med* 312: 700–705.

Rasool CG, Selkoe DJ. (1985b). Response. *N Engl J Med* 313: 521.

Reed D, Plato C, Elizan T, Kurland LT. (1966). The amyotrophic lateral sclerosis/parkinsonism-dementia complex: a ten-year follow-up on Guam. I Epidemiological studies. *Am J Epidemial* 83: 54–73.

Santayana G. (1905). *The Life of Reason, Reason in Common Sense*. New York, C. Scribner's Sons, p. 284.

Sharp GA, Shaw G, Weber K. (1982). Immunoelectronmicroscopical localization of the three neurofilament triplet proteins along neurofilaments of cultured dorsal root ganglion neurons. *Exp Cell Res* 137: 403–413.

Shiraki H, Yase Y. (1975). Amyotrophic lateral sclerosis in Japan. In: Vinken PJ, Bruyn GW (Eds.), *Handbook of Clinical Neurology*, vol. 22. New York, Elsevier.

Shy GM, Drager GA. (1960). A neurological syndrome associated with orthostatic hypotension. *Arch Neurol* 2: 511–527.

Souques A. (1921). Rapport sur les syndromes parkinsoniens. *Rev Neurol* 37: 534–573.

Spiegel EA. (1965). Is pathological study the ultimate solution in Parkinson's disease. In: Barbeau A, Doshay LJ, Spiegel EA (Eds.), *Parkinson's Disease, Trends in Research and Treatment*. New York, Grune and Stratton.

Steele JC, Richardson JC, Olzewski J. (1964). Progressive supranuclear palsy. A heterogeneous degeneration involving the brain stem, basal ganglia and cerebellum, with vertical gaze and pseudobulbar palsy, nuchal dystonia and dementia. *Arch Neurol* 10: 333–359.

Stein Y, Mayeux R, Cote L. (1984). Reaction time and vigilance in Parkinson's disease. Possible role of altered norepinephrine metabolism. *Arch Neurol* 41: 1086–1089.

Sternberger LA, Sternberger MH. (1983). Monoclonal antibodies distinguish phosphorylated and nonphosphorylated forms of neurofilaments in situ. *Proc Natl Acad Sci USA* 80: 6126–6130.

Sternberger NH, Sternberger LA, Ulrich J. (1985). Aberrant neurofilament phosphorylation in Alzheimer's disease. *Proc Natl Acad Sci USA* 82: 4274–4276.

Terry RD. (1963). The fine structure of neurofibrillary tangles in Alzheimer's disease. *J Neuropathol Exp Neurol* 22: 629–642.

Terry RD. (1971). Presidential address. Neuronal fibrous protein in human pathology. *J Neuropathol Exp Neurol* 30: 8–19.

Tomonaga M. (1981). Neurofibrillary tangles and Lewy bodies in the locus ceruleus neurons of the aged brain. *Acta Neuropathol* (Berlin) 53: 165–168.

Trétiakoff C. (1919). *Contribution à l'Étude de l'Anatomie Pathologique du Locus Niger de Soemmering avec Quelques Déductions Relatives à la Pathogénie des Troubles du Tonus Musculaire et de la Maladie de Parkinson*. Thèse de Paris.

Troncoso JC, Sternberger NH, Sternberger LA, Hoffman PN, Price DL. (1986).

Immunocytochemical studies of neurofilament antigens in the neurofibrillary pathology induced by aluminum. *Brain Res* 364: 295–300.

Uebayashi Y. (1980). Epidemiological investigation of motor neuron disease in the Kii peninsula, Japan, and on Guam: the significance of long survival cases. *Wakayama Med Rep* 23: 13–27.

Wen GY, Wisniewski HM. (1985). Histochemical localization of aluminum in the rabbit CNS. *Acta Neuropathol* (Berlin) 68: 175–184.

Wisniewski H, Terry RD, Hirano A. (1970). Neurofibrillary pathology. *J Neuropathol Exp Neurol* 29: 163–176.

Woodard JS. (1962). Concentric hyaline inclusion body formation in mental disease, analysis of twenty-seven cases. *J Neuropathol Exp Neurol* 21: 442–449.

Yanagihara R, Garruto RM, Gajdusek DC, Tomita A, Uchikawa T, Konagaya Y, Chen K-M, Sobue I, Plato CC, Gibbs CJ Jr. (1984). Calcium and vitamin D metabolism in Guamanian Chamorros with amyotrophic lateral sclerosis and parkinsonism-ementia. *Ann Neurol* 15: 42–48.

Yoshimura M. (1983). Cortical changes in the parkinsonian brain: a contribution to the delineation of "diffuse Lewy body disease." *J Neurol* 229: 17–32.

11
Neurochemistry

G. FREDERICK WOOTEN
University of Virginia Medical School, Charlottesville, Virginia

INTRODUCTION

It is now well-established that the motor signs and symptoms of Parkinson's disease result primarily from dysfunction of the basal ganglia. In the past 20 years much progress has been made in identifying the anatomical connections and characterizing the regional neurochemistry of the basal ganglia. The major intrinsic and extrinsic connections of the several cell groups of which the basal ganglia is composed together with identified neurotransmitters for each pathway are summarized in Figure 1. Probably the earliest findings to support the relationship between Parkinson's disease and the basal ganglia were the early clinical–pathological correlations of S.A.K. Wilson (1), coupled with the observations by neuropathologists of neuronal loss and depigmentation of the substantia nigra in brains of patients with Parkinson's disease (2). The subsequent discovery of profound reductions in concentration of the monoamine neurotransmitter dopamine in the striatum of patients with Parkinson's disease (3) and the recognition that pigmented neurons of the substantia nigra project to the striatum and provide the dopaminergic input to that structure further strengthened the evidence that Parkinson's disease is primarily a disease of the basal ganglia (4). The recent observations that the neurotoxic opiate derivative MPTP produces parkinsonism in humans and other primates, with resultant neuropathologic changes restricted primarily to the substantia nigra and large decrements in the striatal concentration of dopamine, provide further substantiation for the pathophysiological basis of Parkinson's disease (5).

For purposes of definition the following structures are considered to comprise the basal ganglia: putamen, caudate, globus pallidus (external and

237

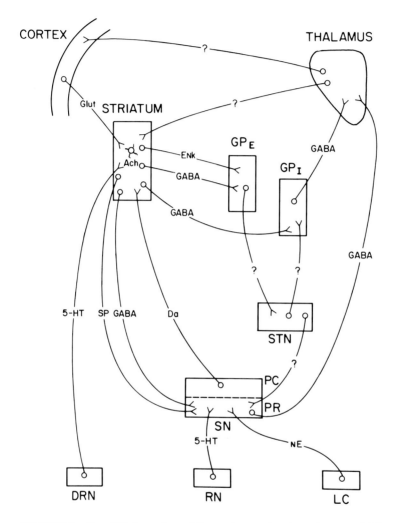

FIGURE 1 Simplified version of the major anatomic pathways within the basal ganglia including identification of known neurotransmitters, where such information is available. Large case names and initials identify anatomically distinct nuclear groups within the basal ganglia; small case abbreviations and contractions denote neurotransmitters. GP_E, globus pallidus external segment; GP_I, globus pallidus internal segment; STN, subthalamic nucleus; SN, substantia nigra (PC, pars compacta; PR, pars reticulata); DRN, dorsal raphe nucleus; RN, raphe nuclei; LC, locus ceruleus; Glut, glutamate; ACh, acetylcholine; Enk, enkephalin; GABA, gamma amino butyric acid; SP, substance P; 5-HT, serotonin; NE, norepinephrine.

internal segments), subthalamic nucleus, and substantia nigra (pars reticulata and pars compacta). The major sources of afferents to basal ganglia structures arising from extrinsic neuronal groups include neocortex to caudate and putamen (collectively referred to as striatum); nonspecific nuclei of thalamus to striatum; locus ceruleus to substantia nigra; and raphe nuclei to substantia nigra and striatum. The major efferent pathways from basal ganglia structures to extrinsic neuronal groups include substantia nigra pars reticulata and globus pallidus internal segment to thalamus, and substantia nigra pars reticulata to deep layers of superior colliculus, brain stem reticular formation, and spinal cord. The various nuclear groups of the basal ganglia are intimately interconnected anatomically. The striatum and substantia nigra have prominent reciprocal connections. The striatum also projects to both segments of the globus pallidus. The subthalamic nucleus receives afferents from the external segment of the globus pallidus and projects to both the substantia nigra pars reticulata and the internal segment of the globus pallidus. In addition, the striatum contains numerous interneurons that do not project outside the striatum. For an extensive review of basal ganglia anatomy see reference 6. The neurotransmitters that have been identified for each projection pathway are depicted in Figure 1. It should be stressed, however, that the transmitters depicted may not represent the entirety of a particular projection. For example, there is good evidence that glutamate is utilized by neurons projecting from neocortex to striatum but other, as yet unidentified, transmitters may also be active in this extensive projection. The neurotransmitters employed by many of the basal ganglia projection pathways are known; this provides the potential for selective modification of activity in specific basal ganglia circuits by drugs.

DOPAMINE

General Metabolism

Dopamine is synthesized in the brain from the amino acid L-tyrosine via the intermediate compound, L-3,4-dihydroxyphenylalanine (L-dopa). Tyrosine hydroxylase, the enzyme that catalyzes the conversion of L-tyrosine to L-dopa, is the rate-limiting step in dopamine synthesis. Because tyrosine hydroxylase is highly localized in catecholamine neurons, it is often utilized by investigators as a specific marker for dopamine neurons. L-Aromatic amino acid decarboxylase (L-AAAD), the enzyme that catalyzes the conversion of L-dopa to dopamine, has a relatively low substrate specificity and is thought to be present not only in dopamine neurons but also in other cells not specialized to synthesize catecholamines. Once synthesized, dopamine is concentrated in storage vesicles. The membranes of these cytoplasmic organelles contain a high-affinity, energy-dependent, carrier-mediated transport system that concentrates dopamine within the vesicle against a concentration gradient.

Under physiologic conditions dopamine is released by a calcium-dependent process from dopaminergic neurons. Dopamine thus released into the synaptic cleft is inactivated primarily by a high-affinity, stereospecific, carrier-mediated reuptake process back into dopamine neuronal terminals where it may be sequestered again in storage vesicles for reuse. Newly released dopamine in the synaptic cleft may bind to specific cell surface dopamine receptors on the same neuron from which it is released (autoreceptor) or on another neuron (postsynaptic receptor). Some dopamine receptors are positively linked to a dopamine-sensitive adenylate cyclase enzyme. When dopamine occupies this receptor, the rate of synthesis of cyclic AMP is increased. Other cell surface dopamine receptors appear to be negatively linked to adenylate cyclase. When these receptors are occupied by dopamine, there is a reduction in the rate of cyclic AMP synthesis (7).

Dopamine is enzymatically inactivated by the action of both monoamine oxidase (MAO), an enzyme associated with mitochondria, and catechol-O-methyltransferase (COMT), an enzyme localized primarily in glial cells in the brain. The resultant deamination and 3-O-methylation of dopamine produces homovanillic acid, the principal metabolite of dopamine.

Disposition of Dopamine Neurons in Brain

There are several identified dopaminergic neuronal cell groups in the central nervous system (8). The most prominent group is the mesotelencephalic group. This group is composed of the nigrostriatal system, with cell bodies in the substantia nigra pars compacta that project primarily to the striatum, and the mesocortical system, with cell bodies in the ventral tegmental area that project to the mesial frontal, anterior cingulate, and entorhinal cortices and the olfactory bulb, anterior olfactory nucleus, olfactory tubercle, piriform cortex, nucleus accumbens, and amygdaloid complex. The tuberohypophysial system projects from the arcuate and periventricular hypothalamic nuclei to the intermediate lobe of the pituitary gland and the median eminence. The incertohypothalamic system projects from the zona incerta and posterior hypothalamus to the dorsal hypothalamic area and septum. Finally, the periventricular system contains cell bodies in the periventricular region of the medulla that project to the periventricular and periaqueductal gray, tegmentum, tectum, thalamus, and hypothalamus.

Parkinson's Disease

The first findings to suggest a role for dopamine in Parkinson's disease were the observations that reserpine treatment produced both the clinical picture of parkinsonism and a depletion of striatal dopamine (9). Carlsson and his colleagues subsequently showed in laboratory animals that treatment with the dopamine precursor, L-dopa, reversed the behavioral effects of reserpine and partially restored brain dopamine levels. These observations in laboratory animals, coupled with early histofluorescence data showing very high concentrations of dopamine in the striatum, led Hornykiewicz and colleagues to study the concentration of dopamine in postmortem brain material from patients who had died with Parkinson's disease (3).

Their finding of marked reductions in the concentration of dopamine and homovanillic acid in the caudate, putamen, and substantia nigra of patients with Parkinson's disease opened the door to a new era in the diagnosis and treatment of brain disease (Table 1). These workers further demonstrated a strong positive correlation between the severity of the premorbid parkinsonian clinical syndrome and the degree of dopamine depletion in the striatum. The data summarized in Table 1 show a reduction in dopamine concentration not only in

TABLE 1 Dopamine (DA) and Homovanillic Acid (HVA) Concentrations in Discrete Brain Regions from Controls and Parkinson's Disease Patients

Brain region	DA (μg/g wet wt)	HVA (μg/g wet wt)	DA/HVA
Putamen[a]			
Control	5.06±0.39 (17)	4.92±0.32 (16)	1.03
Parkinsonian	0.14±0.13 (3)	0.54±0.13 (3)	0.26
Caudate nucleus[a]			
Control	4.06±0.47 (18)	2.92±0.37 (19)	1.39
Parkinsonian	0.20±0.19 (3)	1.19±0.10 (3)	0.17
Substantia nigra			
Control	0.46 (13)[b]	2.32 (7)[c]	0.20
Parkinsonian	0.07 (10)[b]	0.41 (9)[c]	0.17
Nucleus accumbens[d]			
Control	3.79±0.82 (8)	4.38±0.64 (8)	0.86
Parkinsonian	1.61±0.28 (4)	3.13±0.13 (3)	0.51
Lateral hypothalamus[d]			
Control	0.51±0.08 (4)	1.96±0.28 (3)	0.26
Parkinsonian	<0.03 (2)	1.03±0.23 (3)	—
Parolfactory gyrus[d]			
Control	0.35±0.09 (4)	0.98 (2)	0.35
Parkinsonian	0.03 (2)	—	—

Results are expressed as mean±S.E.M. Numbers of cases are in parentheses.
[a]Reference 10; [b]reference 3; [c]reference 11; [d]reference 12.

TABLE 2 Activities of Tyrosine Hydroxylase (TOH), L-Aromatic Amino Acid Decarboxylase (L-AAAD), Catechol-O-methyltransferase (COMT), and Monoamine Oxidase (MAO) in Discrete Brain Regions from Controls and Parkinson's Disease Patients

Brain region	TOH (nmol CO_2/ 30 min/100 mg protein)	L-AAAD (nmol CO_2/ 2 hr/100 mg protein)	COMT (nmol NMN/ hr/100 mg protein)	MAO (nmol PPA/ 30 min/100 mg protein)
Putamen				
Control	17.4±2.4 (3)	432±109 (18)	24.1±2.5 (11)	1520±127 (11)
Parkinsonian	3.1±1.2 (3)[a]	32±7 (13)[b]	19.8±3.7 (9)	1648±128 (10)
Caudate nucleus				
Control	18.7±2.0 (3)	364±95 (19)	25.4±2.8 (10)	1726±149 (10)
Parkinsonian	3.2±0.5 (2)[a]	54±14 (13)[b]	17.8±3.8 (9)	1742±197 (10)
Substantia nigra				
Control	17.4 (1)	549±294 (15)	26.4±4.7 (5)	1828±200 (5)
Parkinsonian	6.1±1.5 (3)	21±6 (10)	21.7±10.2 (9)	1477±284 (4)
Hypothalamus				
Control	4.4 (2)	149±53 (9)	29.4±4.5 (3)	—
Parkinsonian	2.7 (2)	63±17 (5)	—	—
Frontal cortex				
Control	3.7 (2)	32±4 (6)	24.1±4.4 (9)	—
Parkinsonian	2.5±0.2 (3)	10±2 (3)[a]	28.7±4.1 (7)	—

Results are expressed as mean ± S.E.M. Numbers of cases are shown in parentheses.
[a]Differs from control p < 0.02
[b]Differs from control p < 0.01
Source: Data derived from reference 10.

basal ganglia structures (i.e., caudate, putamen, and substantia nigra), but also in several forebrain limbic structures innervated by dopamine neurons in the more medially located ventral tegmental area of the midbrain (i.e., nucleus accumbens, lateral hypothalamus, and parolfactory gyrus).

It is interesting to note that the degree of reduction in dopamine concentration is much greater than the reduction in homovanillic acid (HVA) concentration in brains of patients with Parkinson's disease. Thus, the ratio of dopamine to HVA is much lower in these brains than in controls. Similar changes in the dopamine to HVA ratio have been noted following partial lesions of the nigrostriatal pathway in experimental animals, and also as a consequence of treatment with dopamine antagonist drugs. These probably reflect both an increase in the metabolic activity of the few remaining dopamine neurons and a reduced capacity for reuptake and storage of released dopamine (13).

Subsequent postmortem studies have focused on enzymatic markers of dopamine neurons and dopamine metabolism (Table 2). These studies revealed marked reductions in the activities of tyrosine hydroxylase and L-AAAD in the caudate, putamen, and substantia nigra of patients with Parkinson's disease, but no changes were found in the levels of activity of MAO and COMT. These results reflect the high degree of localization of tyrosine hydroxylase and L-AAAD in dopamine neurons in the striatum compared to the more general distribution of MAO and nonneuronal distribution of COMT activities.

Recently, tritium-labeled cocaine has been used as a ligand marker for the neuronal membrane transport site responsible for the reuptake of catecholamines into catecholaminergic neurons. The binding of $[^3H]$ cocaine to striatal membranes prepared from patients who died with Parkinson's disease was greatly reduced compared to controls (14). These results further document a large reduction in the number of dopaminergic neuronal terminals in the striata of patients with Parkinson's disease.

Thus, there is clear evidence for a large reduction in all measurable neuronal markers for nigrostriatal dopaminergic neurons in the brains of patients with Parkinson's disease.

NOREPINEPHRINE

The principal source of noradrenergic afferents to the forebrain is the locus ceruleus (15). As discussed in the previous chapter, the locus ceruleus is one of the pigmented brain stem nuclei characteristically abnormal in the brains of patients with Parkinson's disease. Specifically, these brains show depigmentation and loss of neurons, with Lewy bodies in the locus ceruleus. Several investigators have described reductions of norepinephrine concentration and dopamine-β-hydroxylase activity (a specific enzymatic marker of noradrenergic neurons) in forebrain regions (16,17). Data are conflicting as to whether norepinephrine levels are affected in the hypothalamus of patients with Parkinson's disease (16, 18). Recent studies of dopamine-β-hydroxylase activity in the A1 and A2 noradrenergic areas of the brainstem of patients with Parkinson's disease fail to reveal any changes suggesting that these nuclear groups, which also have rostral projections, are spared in Parkinson's disease (19). Since levels of norepinephrine are rarely below 50% of control in the brains of patients with Parkinson's disease and because certain noradrenergic cell groups of the lower brain stem are apparently completely spared, it is unlikely that Parkinson's disease is associated with a generalized central catecholaminergic deficiency. The consequences of reduced norepinephrine levels in the adult brain are not clear, although evidence for both motor and cognitive functions of noradrenergic systems has been presented (15).

SEROTONIN

The principal locations of cell bodies of serotonergic neurons are the raphe nuclei of the brainstem. There is no neuropathologic evidence to suggest that these cell groups are specifically affected in Parkinson's disease. Nevertheless, serotonin levels are reduced throughout the forebrain in patients with Parkinson's disease, particularly in the striatum, substantia nigra, and hippocampus (17,20). The mechanism and significance of the reduction in brain serotonin levels are not known. A likely speculation would be that reduced serotonin levels represent regulation of serotonergic neuronal activity in response to reduced activity of dopaminergic and/or noradrenergic neurons.

GAMMA AMINO BUTYRIC ACID

Gamma amino butyric acid (GABA) is a neurotransmitter found in several prominent basal ganglia projection pathways. There are probably GABA-releasing interneurons in the striatum as well as GABA-ergic striatopallidal, striatonigral, nigrocollicular, and pallidothalamic projections (6). There is no evidence to suggest that these neurons are affected primarily by the pathologic process in Parkinson's disease. It would not be unlikely, however, that up- or down-regulation of GABA activity might occur as a consequence of dopamine depletion in the striatum.

Two specific markers for GABA-ergic neurons have been studied in postmortem brains from patients with Parkinson's disease. These include direct measurement of brain GABA levels and assay of activity of glutamic acid decarboxylase (GAD), the enzyme that catalyzes the conversion of glutamic acid to GABA. Perry et al. found that GABA levels were significantly elevated in the putamen of patients with Parkinson's disease (21), while Laaksonen et al. found reduced GABA levels in cerebral and cerebellar cortices, but no change in GABA levels in any other brain region (22). Lloyd and Hornykiewicz found reduced GAD activity (approximately 50% of control) in striatum, globus pallidus, and substantia nigra (23), a finding confirmed by Laaksonen (22). Perry et al. more recently reported, however, that GAD activity in the putamen of patients with Parkinson's disease does not differ from that in controls (21).

Thus, there is controversy as to whether GAD activity is altered in the brains of patients with Parkinson's disease. Nevertheless, the critical issue is whether GABA turnover is altered, and if so, in which neuronal groups. The recent development of pharmacologic means to manipulate GABA neurotransmission is a potential avenue for new therapeutic strategies in the management of Parkinson's disease.

ACETYLCHOLINE

The principal site of action of cholinergic neurons in basal ganglia circuitry is thought to be the numerous cholinergic interneurons identified in the striatum (6). Measurement of the activity of choline acetyltransferase (ChAT), the enzyme that catalyzes the one-step synthesis of acetylcholine, is the most frequently utilized marker for the cholinergic neurons. Lloyd et al. have reported a significant reduction in ChAT activity in the putamen, caudate nucleus, globus pallidus, and substantia nigra of brains of patients with Parkinson's disease (24). These changes in activity again probably reflect regulation in response to reduced dopamine levels rather than primary pathologic involvement. Ruberg et al. have found reduced ChAT activity in cerebral cortex and hippocampus in brains of patients with Parkinson's disease, which perhaps relates to the dementing process in these patients (25).

NEUROPEPTIDES

Several of the neuropeptides that are putative neurotransmitters or neuro-modulators are present in high concentrations in some nuclear groups of the basal ganglia. Their distribution has been mapped by immunocytochemical techniques, and radioimmunoassays (RIAs) have been employed to quantify regional concentrations of various peptides.

With the use of RIA techniques, substance P levels were reported to be reduced in the substantia nigra, putamen, and globus pallidus external segment (26). Immunocytochemical studies of patients with Parkinson's disease, however, failed to confirm any change in the substance P concentration in any basal ganglia area (27).

Methionine–enkephalin concentration documented by RIA was found to be diminished in the substantia nigra and ventral tegmental area (28). In addition, RIA studies showed reductions in both leucine– and methionine–enkephalin in the putamen and pallidum (28). In contrast, immunocytochemical studies did not confirm any changes in enkephalin levels in the globus pallidus (27). The discrepant findings using RIA and immunocytochemical techniques remain to be explained.

Cholecystokinin-8 (CCK-8) has been suggested by some investigators to co-exist with dopamine in dopaminergic neurons (29). With the use of RIA methods, CCK-8 levels were found to be reduced in the substantia nigra but not in striatal or corticolimbic areas innervated by dopaminergic neurons (30). These results from postmortem brains of patients with Parkinson's disease cast doubt on the coexistence of dopamine and CCK-8 in nigral neurons.

Somatostatin levels in the basal ganglia of nondemented patients with Parkinson's disease do not differ from those in controls (31). Somatostatin levels in the frontal cortex, hippocampus, and entorhinal cortex of demented patients with Parkinson's disease are reduced compared to levels in nondemented patients with Parkinson's disease (31).

As more information is accumulated about the cellular localization and physiologic function of neuropeptides, the significance of these various changes in Parkinson's disease may be appreciated. Currently it appears that these changes represent secondary consequences of striatal dopamine depletion.

ENDOGENOUS FREE RADICAL SCAVENGERS

Studies aimed at elucidating the mechanism of MPTP-induced neuronal toxicity have focused much attention on the possibility that the oxidative metabolism of MPTP generates cytotoxic free radical species. Cohen has speculated that the generation of free radical species by monoamine oxidase activity may contribute to dopaminergic neuronal death in Parkinson's disease (32). In primates, the dopaminergic nigrostriatal neurons contain high concentrations of the pigment neuromelanin. Graham has argued that Parkinson's disease may result from cyto-toxicity of the products of catecholamine and melanin oxidation (33). Thus, several levels of investigation implicate free radicals in the premature death of dopamine neurons.

Free radicals are constantly being generated in all living tissue. When their intracellular concentrations become too high, damage to cellular elements (lipid, protein, DNA, etc.) may occur. Such damage is minimized by endogenous agents such as glutathione, ascorbate, β-carotene, and tocopherol (34). Also, enzymatic defenses exist that scavenge free radicals; these enzyme activities include super-oxide dismutase, catalase, and glutathione peroxidase (which requires reduced glutathione) (34). Perry and co-workers recently reported that reduced glutathione levels were significantly lower in substantia nigra than in any other human brain region; and that reduced glutathione levels were virtually absent from the substantia nigra of patients dying with Parkinson's disease (35). Be-cause reduced glutathione is an important endogenous antioxidant as well as a cofactor for the free-radical-scavenging enzyme, glutathione peroxidase, it is interesting to speculate that the substantia nigra may be that region of the brain most susceptible to the toxic effects of free radicals. This line of work has raised the question of whether patients with early symptoms of Parkinson's disease should be treated with monoamine oxidase inhibitors and free radical scavengers such as vitamin E and ascorbic acid in an attempt to arrest the progression of nigral cell death.

REGIONAL CEREBRAL GLUCOSE UTILIZATION

Using fluorine-18-labeled fluorodeoxyglucose and positron emission tomographic (PET) imaging techniques, it has been possible in recent years to estimate in vivo the regional rate of glucose utilization in brains of patients with Parkinson's disease. Because glucose is a primary substrate for brain energy production and because the major expenditure of energy in the brain is for pumping ions across membranes, estimates of regional brain glucose utilization represent an estimate of regional brain physiologic activity.

In studies to date of patients with both unilateral and bilateral parkinsonism, strikingly little change in glucose has been measured in cortical areas or in the caudate–putamen region of the basal ganglia (36–38). Increased glucose utilization in the inferomedial portion of the basal ganglia, probably corresponding to the globus pallidus, in patients with Parkinson's disease was found by Martin and colleagues (38). Similar changes have also been reported using oxygen-15 imaging with PET techniques in patients with Parkinson's disease (39). Such an increase in glucose utilization in the globus pallidus of experimental animals with lesions of the substantia nigra has been reported and may represent increased physiologic activity in striatal efferents to the globus pallidus as a consequence of reduced dopamine neurotransmission in the striatum (40).

Another recent advance in the field of in vivo neurochemistry using PET technology has been the development (41) of a method to image dopamine neurons using $[^{18}F]$ 6-fluoro-L-dopa. Garnett et al. have reported that fluorine-18 accumulation is reduced in the striatum contralateral to the side of involvement in patients with unilateral parkinsonism, particularly in the putamen (42). Further development of quantitative methods for estimating brain dopamine concentration in vivo should greatly facilitate research directed at the development of therapeutic strategies to reduce the rate of progression of Parkinson's disease.

NEUROCHEMICAL ANALYSIS OF LEWY BODIES

Lewy bodies are a histologic hallmark of Parkinson's disease. These intraneuronal cytoplasmic inclusions were first described in neurons of the substantia innominata and dorsal motor nucleus of the vagus (43). Subsequently, Lewy bodies were described in pigmented cells of the substantia nigra as well as in the hypothalamus, locus ceruleus, raphe nuclei of the midbrain and rostral pons, sympathetic ganglia, and spinal cord (44). Current evidence would suggest that the Lewy body is a highly specific marker of neuronal degeneration in Parkinson's disease (44).

Despite the apparently unique appearance of Lewy bodies in degenerating neurons in the brains of patients with Parkinson's disease, very little is known about their biochemical composition and nothing is known of their genesis. Histologic reactions suggest that Lewy bodies have a proteinaceous nature (45, 46). The dense core of Lewy bodies is composed of tightly packed aggregates of filaments, vesicular profiles, and other granular material. At the periphery, filamentous structures emerge radially and are mixed with granular and vesicular material. Recent immunocytochemical studies using polyclonal antibodies to neurofilament polypeptides have demonstrated specific staining of Lewy bodies (47). These data suggest that abnormal organization of the neuronal cytoskeleton may be a pathologic feature of Parkinson's disease. Further biochemical characterization of the composition of Lewy bodies may provide new insights into the mechanism(s) of neuronal degeneration in Parkinson's disease. It must be noted, however, that Lewy bodies may simply represent a cellular response to some other primary insult.

SIGNIFICANCE OF NEUROCHEMICAL STUDIES OF PARKINSON'S DISEASE

Selective degeneration of the dopaminergic nigrostriatal pathway is the central pathologic process in Parkinson's disease. The resulting reduction in striatal dopamine concentration is a sufficient condition for the emergence of the signs and symptoms of parkinsonism. The development of levodopa therapy as well as newer direct-acting dopamine agonists in the treatment of Parkinson's disease grew out of the recognition of this relationship between dopamine deficiency and parkinsonian symptoms.

The changes in levels of other neurotransmitters, in neuronal markers, and in regional brain metabolism probably represent regulatory responses to the decrement in striatal dopamine neurotransmission. Future neurochemical studies holding the greatest promise for benefit to patients with Parkinson's disease may be divided into two categories: (a) studies aimed at understanding the effects of dopamine depletion on other neurons and neurotransmitter systems that allow the symptoms of parkinsonism to emerge may form the basis for new therapeutic strategies to supplement dopamine replacement; and (b) studies aimed at identifying the source of the selective vulnerability of dopamine neurons in patients with Parkinson's disease could result in therapeutic strategies to arrest the progression of or actually prevent Parkinson's disease.

REFERENCES

1. Wilson SAK. (1912). Progressive lenticular degeneration: a familial nervous disease associated with cirrhosis of the liver. *Brain* 34: 295–489.
2. Hassler R. (1938). Zur pathologie der paralysis agitans und des postenzephalitischen Parkinsonismus. *J Psychol Neurol* 48: 387–476.
3. Hornykiewicz O. (1963). Die Topische Lokalisation und das Verhalten von Noradrenalin und Dopamin (3-Hydroxytyramin) in der Substantia nigra des normalen und Parkinsonkranken Menschen. *Wien Klin Wochenschr* 75: 309–312.
4. Hornykiewicz O. (1966). Dopamine (3-hydroxytyramine) and brain function. *Pharmacol Rev* 18: 925–962.
5. Langston JW, Ballard P, Tetrud JW, Irwin I. (1983). Chronic parkinsonism in humans due to a product of meperidine-analog synthesis. *Science* 291: 979–980.
6. Carpenter MB. (1981). Anatomy of the striatum and brainstem integrating systems. In *Handbook of Physiology*. Bethesda, Maryland, American Physiological Society.
7. Stoof JC, Kebabian JW. (1984). Two dopamine receptors: biochemistry, physiology and pharmacology. *Life Sci* 35: 2281–2296.
8. Moore RY, Bloom FE. (1978). Central catecholamine neuron systems: Anatomy and physiology of the dopamine systems. *Annu Rev Neurosci* 1: 129–169.
9. Carlsson A, Lindquist M, Magnusson T. (1957). 3,4-Dihydroxyphenylalanine and 5-hydroxytryptophan as reserpine antagonists. *Nature* 180: 1200–1201.
10. Lloyd KG, Davidson L, Hornykiewicz O. (1975). The neurochemistry of Parkinson's disease: effect of L-dopa therapy. *J Pharmacol Exp Ther* 195: 453–464.
11. Bernheimer H, Hornykiewicz O. (1965). Herabgesetzte Konzentration der Homovanillinsäure im Gehirn von Parkinsonkranken Menschen als Ausdruck der Störung des zentralen Dopaminstoffwechsels. *Klin Wochenschr* 43: 711–715.
12. Price KS, Farley IJ, Hornykiewicz O. (1978). Neurochemistry of Parkinson's disease: relation between striatal and limbic dopamine. *Adv Biochem Psychopharmacol* 19: 293–300.
13. Zigmond MJ, Stricker EM. (1984). Parkinson's disease: studies with an animal model. *Life Sci* 35: 5–18.
14. Pimoule C, Schoemaker H, Javoy-Agid F, Scatton B, Agid Y, Langer SZ. (1983). Decrease in [^{3}H] cocaine binding to the dopamine transporter in Parkinson's disease. *Eur J Pharmacol* 95: 145–146.
15. Moore RY, Bloom FE. (1979). Central catecholamine neuron systems: anatomy and physiology of the norepinephrine and epinephrine systems. *Annu Rev Neurosci* 2: 113–168.
16. Farley IJ, Hornykiewicz O. (1976). Noradrenaline in subcortical brain regions of patients with Parkinson's disease and control subjects. In: Birkmayer W, Hornykiewicz O. (Eds.), *Advances in Parkinsonism*. Basel, Editiones Roche.

17. Scatton B, Javoy-Agid F, Rouquier L, Dubois L, Agid Y. (1983). Reduction of cortical dopamine, noradrenaline, serotonin, and their metabolites in Parkinson's disease. *Brain Res* 275: 321–328.

18. Javoy-Agid F, Rubert M, Taquet H, Bokobza B, Agid Y, Gaspar P, Berger B, N'Guyen-Legros J, Alvarez C, Gray F, Escourelle R, Scatton B, Rouquier L. (1984). Biochemical neuropathology of Parkinson's disease. In: Hassler RG, Christ JF. (Eds.), *Advances in Neurology*. New York, Raven Press.

19. Kopp N, Denoroy L, Thomasi M, Gay N, Chazot G, Renaud B. (1982). Increased in noradrenaline-synthesizing enzyme activity in medulla oblongata in Parkinson's disease. *Acta Neuropathol* 56: 17–21.

20. Bernheimer H, Birkmayer W, Hornykiewicz O. (1961). Verteilung des 5-hydroxytryptamins (Serotonin) in Gehirn des menschen und sein Verhalten bei Patienten mit Parkinson-Syndrom. *Klin Wochenschr* 39: 1056–1059.

21. Perry TL, Javoy-Avid F, Agid Y, Fibiger HC. (1983). Striatal gabaergic neuronal activity is not reduced in Parkinson's disease. *J Neurochem* 40: 1120–1123.

22. Laaksonen H, Rinne UK, Sonninen V, Riekkinen P. (1978). Brain GABA neurons in Parkinson's disease. *Acta Neurol Scand* (Suppl 67) 57: 282–283.

23. Lloyd KG, Hornykiewicz O. (1973). L-glutamic acid decarboxylase in Parkinson's disease: effect of L-dopa therapy. *Nature* 243: 521–523.

24. Lloyd KG, Möhler H, Hertz P, Bartholini G. (1975). Distribution of choline acetyltransferase and glutamic acid decarboxylase within the substantia nigra and other brain regions from control and parkinsonian patients. *J Neurochem* 25: 789–785.

25. Ruberg M, Ploska A, Javoy-Agid F, Agid Y. (1982). Muscarinic binding and choline acetyltransferase activity in parkinsonian subjects with reference to dementia. *Brain Res* 232: 129–139.

26. Mauborgne A, Javoy-Agid F, Legrand JC, Agid Y, Cesselin F. (1983). Decrease of substance P-like immunoreactivity in the substantia nigra and pallidum of parkinsonian brains. *Brain Res* 268: 167–170.

27. Grafe MR, Forno LS, Eng LF. (1985). Immunocytochemical studies of substance P and metenkephalin in the basal ganglia and substantia nigra in Huntington's, Parkinson's and Alzheimer's diseases. *J Neuropathol Exp Neurol* 44: 47–59.

28. Taquet H, Javoy-Agid F, Hamon H, Legrand JC, Agid Y, Cesselin F. (1983). Parkinson's disease affects differently met[5]- and leu[5] enkephalin in the human brain. *Brain Res* 280: 379–382.

29. Hökfelt T, Skirboll L, Rehfeld JF, Goldstein M, Markey K, Dann O. (1980). A subpopulation of mesencephalic dopamine neurons projecting to limbic areas contains a cholecystokinin-like peptide: evidence from immunohistochemistry combined with retrograde tracing. *Neuroscience* 5: 2093–2124.

30. Studler JM, Javoy-Agid F, Cesselin F, Legrand JC, Agid Y. (1982). CCK-8-immunoreactivity distribution in human brain: selective decrease in the substantia nigra from parkinsonian patients. *Brain Res* 243: 176–179.

31. Epelbaum J, Ruberg M, Moyse E, Javoy-Agid F, Dubois B, Agid Y. (1983). Somatostatin and dementia in Parkinson's disease. *Brain Res* 278: 376–379.

32. Cohen G. (1983). The pathobiology of Parkinson's disease: Biochemical aspects of dopamine neuron senescence. *J Neurol Trans* Suppl. 19: 89–103.

33. Graham DG. (1984). Catecholamine toxicity: a proposal for the molecular pathogenesis of manganese neurotoxicity and Parkinson's disease. *Neurotoxicology* 5: 83–96.

34. Freeman BA, Crapo JD. (1982). Biology of disease: free radicals and tissue injury. *Lab Invest* 47: 412–426.

35. Perry TL, Godin DV, Hansen S. (1982). Parkinson's disease: a disorder due to nigral glutathione deficiency? *Neurosci Letts* 33: 305–310.

36. Kuhl DE, Metter EJ, Riege WR. (1984). Patterns of local cerebral glucose utilization determined in Parkinson's disease by the [^{18}F] fluorodeoxyglucose method. *Ann Neurol* 15: 419–424.

37. Rougemont D, Baron JC, Collard P, Bustany P, Comar D, Agid Y. (1984). Local cerebral glucose utilization in treated and untreated patients with Parkinson's disease. *J Neurol Neurosurg Psychiatry* 47: 824–830.

38. Martin WRW, Beckman JH, Calne DB, Adam JM, Harrop R, Rogers JG, Ruth TJ, Sayre CI, Pate BD. (1984). Cerebral glucose metabolism in Parkinson's disease. *Can J Neurol Sci* 11 (suppl. 1): 169–173.

39. Leenders K, Wolfson L, Gibbs J, Wise R, Jones T, Legg N. (1983). Regional cerebral blood flow and oxygen metabolism in Parkinson's disease and their response to L-dopa. *J Cerebral Blood Flow Metab* 3 (suppl. 1): S488–S489.

40. Wooten GF, Collins RC. (1981). Metabolic effects of unilateral lesion of the substantia nigra. *J Neurosci* 1: 285–291.

41. Garnett ES, Firnau G, Nahmias C. (1983). Dopamine visualized in the basal ganglia of living man. *Nature* 305: 137–138.

42. Garnett ES, Nahmias C, Firnau G. (1984). Central dopaminergic pathways in hemiparkinsonism examined by positron emission tomography. *Can J Neurol Sci* 11 (suppl. 1): 174–179.

43. Lewy FH. (1912). Paralysis agitans. I. Pathologische anatomie. In: Lewandowski M (Ed.), *Handbuck der Neurologie*. Berlin, Springer.

44. Greenfield JG, Bosanquet FD. (1953). The brainstem lesion in parkinsonism. *J Neurol Neurosurg Psychiatry* 16: 213–226.

45. Bethlem J, den Hartog Jager WA. (1960). The incidence and characteristics of Lewy bodies in idiopathic paralysis agitans (Parkinson's disease). *J Neurol Neurosurg Psychiatry* 23: 74–80.

46. Issidorides MR, Mytilineou C, Whetsell WO, Yahr MD. (1978). Protein-rich cytoplasmic bodies of substantia nigra and locus ceruleus. *Arch Neurol* 35: 633–637.

47. Goldman JE, Yen S-H, Chiu F-C, Peress NS. (1983). Lewy bodies of Parkinson's disease contain neurofilament antigens. *Science* 221: 1082–1084.

12
Neurotransmitter Receptor Alterations

MARK M. VOIGT and GEORGE R. UHL
Harvard Medical School and Massachusetts General Hospital, Boston, Massachusetts

Parkinson's disease is a neurodegenerative disorder with primary clinical signs consisting of rigidity, resting tremor, and bradykinesia. Investigation of the pathophysiology of this disease has increased our knowledge of the cell groups and neurotransmitter systems at risk in Parkinson's disease. Numerous studies since the 1960s concur on the major neurochemical feature of Parkinson's disease: loss of dopamine and its metabolites in nigrostriatal pathways (1-3). These biochemical findings are correlated with a dramatic loss of melanin-containing neurons from the substantia nigra pars compacta (SNc) (4), as well as lesser degrees of loss in the adjacent ventral tegmental area (3,5). More recent studies have also demonstrated perturbations in other neurotransmitter systems in the central nervous system in Parkinson's disease, including alterations in regional noradrenergic, cholinergic, and somatostatinergic circuitry (6-9).

TECHNIQUES

Over the past decade, several techniques that enable us to detect and quantitate regional neurotransmitter receptor densities have been applied to studies of Parkinson's disease brains. Homogenate binding studies of postmortem human tissue permit good receptor quantitation with limited anatomical accuracy. In parkinsonian nigra, striatum, and cerebral cortex, these approaches have been applied to studies of several receptor subtypes. Unfortunately, these techniques lack the ability to distinguish reliably between small anatomical areas, or to provide correlations with focal pathology. In addition, they can require relatively large tissue samples and are limited by the availability of accurate premorbid information on patients' status with respect to such important variables as drug treatments.

A second approach relies on the recent development of receptor ligands labeled with positron-emitting isotopes. Using $[^{11}C]$ N-methyl spiperone or $[^{11}C]$ carfentanil, striatal dopamine and opiate receptor densities have been detected in vivo in normal volunteers and Parkinson's disease patients (11,12). These studies allow for control of drug effects and for examination of disease subtypes in a fashion not readily possible in postmortem approaches. Unfortunately, the expense and limited availability of essential equipment as well as the technique's low anatomical resolution can limit its usefulness.

The third approach to detecting neurotransmitter receptors utilizes in vitro receptor autoradiography. This method enables quantitation of receptor densities in small or complexly defined brain regions in human tissues. We and others have defined substantia nigra compacta (SNc) densities of several peptide receptors with good anatomical resolution using this technique (13). Although it is possible to measure changes in relative levels of receptors, absolute quantitation in this technique is more cumbersome than in homogenate systems. Obtaining adequate information about patients' histories is also vital in the interpretation of results.

RATIONALE FOR RECEPTOR STUDIES

These techniques have been applied to studies in Parkinson's disease tissue with several goals in mind.

Determination of the Fate of Striatal Receptors

Dopamine Receptors

At least two types of dopamine receptors are present in the striatum and are designated D_1 and D_2. These subtypes are distinguished on the basis of their distinctive pharmacologic profiles and their effects on adenylate cyclase activity. D_1 receptor activation results in an increase in cAMP generation whereas D_2 occupancy results in no change or an inhibition of cAMP production (14). Virtually all behavioral effects of dopaminergic drugs are correlated with their potencies at D_2 receptors; the physiological significance of D_1 receptor activation is currently less clear (15).

As noted earlier, the nigrostriatal pathway is a primary target in Parkinson's disease. In animal studies, lesions of this pathway produce supersensitivity of denervated striatal dopamine receptors as measured by testing of locomotor behavior (16). Receptor binding studies in rat striatal homogenates also show supersensitivity following such lesions (15,17). In rats, this sensitization can be attenuated by dopamimetic drug administration (15). Based on these animal studies, receptor supersensitivity in the denervated Parkinson's disease striatum has been hypothesized. This presumed receptor supersensitivity has been thought to be responsible for some of the beneficial effects of "drug holiday," where withdrawal of dopamine agonist therapy might allow the reappearance of increased receptor sensitivity (17,18). Receptor sensitivity alterations have also been speculated as underlying the exaggerated responses in some Parkinson's disease patients to fluctuations in plasma or brain levodopa levels, resulting in dose-related dyskinesias or even the "on-off" phenomena (18,19). Ascertainment of the state of the dopamine receptors in Parkinson's disease striatum is thus of substantial clinical importance.

Nondopamine Receptors

Numerous studies have reported that peptides (such as the enkephalins) and classic transmitters (such as serotonin, acetylcholine, and gamma-aminobutyric acid, or GABA) can alter basal- and stimulus-evoked dopamine release from striatal slices in vitro (20). These findings suggest that dopamine terminals in the striatum possess a number of presynaptic receptors, whose occupancy can modulate dopamine release from these processes. With the use of the natural lesion of Parkinson's disease, observations of changes in the striatal densities of these receptors could suggest which receptor populations are localized on these important dopamine-containing nerve terminals.

Fate of Neurotransmitter Receptors in the SNc

Nigrostriatal dopaminergic neurons play key roles in regulating motor function and may display disordered function not only in Parkinson's disease but also in Huntington's disease, progressive supranuclear palsy, and tardive dyskinesia. Studies in experimental animals suggest that a number of peptide and classic neurotransmitters may have an impact on these DA-containing cells. Immuno-histochemical studies in SNc demonstrate the presence of fibers and terminals for classic transmitters such as 5-HT, GABA, and DA as well as several peptides such as enkephalin, somatostatin, substance P/substance K, and cholecystokinin (21). Receptor autoradiographic studies reveal the presence of binding sites for GABA/benzodiazepines, neurotensin, opiates, and somatostatin in the rat SNc. Physiologic studies in animals have also provided evidence for effects of neurotensin, cholecystokinin, GABA, and opiates on DA neuronal function in the SNc (20,21).

The SNc cell loss in Parkinson's disease provides a natural lesion that may help in elucidating the normal receptor complement of these neurons in humans and in indicating potential sites for modulation of the cells' functions. Receptors lost when these cells degenerate are likely to be normally present on the affected neurons. Homogenate binding studies and receptor autoradiographic approaches have been used to demonstrate that SNc neurons normally display densities of receptors for several neurotransmitters and to indicate alterations in Parkinson's disease (13,22,23).

Neurotransmitter Receptor Changes in Other Regions

Interest in receptor levels in regions outside of nigrostriatal areas has focused chiefly on the cerebral cortex, a target for cholinergic, noradrenergic and somatostatinergic defects in Parkinson's disease (6-9). Many patients with Parkinson's disease exhibit marked deficits in mental function. These deficits may be manifested as depression and/or dementia. The dementia observed in this subpopulation of Parkinson's disease patients is similar to that observed in another dementing neurodegenerative disorder, Alzheimer's disease, and consists of memory impairment and confusion (24). In addition, Parkinson's disease patients frequently experience medication-induced confusion, hallucinations, or delirium (19,24). Since each of these clinical disorders may involve cerebral cortical mechanisms, definition of cerebral cortical receptor alterations induced by drugs or disease is also of potential importance.

RESULTS

Striatal Receptors

Dopamine Receptors

The caudate and putamen contain high concentrations of both D_1 and D_2 receptors, with lower levels found in the globus pallidus. In experimental animals subjected to lesions of the ascending dopamine system, there is an increase in D_2 receptors. This increase is ascribed to homeostatic responses to the lack of receptor stimulation by dopamine and is termed denervation supersensitivity. Such a phenomenon, if present in Parkinson's disease, might explain such clinically observed phenomena as the "on-off" and "drug-holiday" response. On the other hand, decreased receptor numbers might reflect losses of terminals or perikarya containing the receptors, since the loss of intrinsic striatal neurons has also been reported in Parkinson's disease.

D_1 dopamine receptor levels are affected in this disease. Several reports have demonstrated a decrease in caudate dopamine-sensitive adenylate cyclase activity in patients with Parkinson's disease (10,25). However, the clinical relevance of this decreased D_1 population is unclear, since correlation between D_1 receptors and specific behavioral parameters has been difficult to demonstrate.

D_2 receptor levels may also be altered in certain patients with Parkinson's disease, although results differ in various reports. Using samples from 10 medicated Parkinson's disease patients, Reisine et al. (26) reported decreased D_2 receptor numbers in the caudate but no change in either the putamen or pallidum. Lee et al. (27) reported increased D_2 binding in the putamen of six Parkinson's disease patients not treated with L-dopa but observed no change in D_2 binding in the caudates of these same individuals. Quik et al. (23) studied eight L-dopa-treated Parkinson's disease patients and Bokobza et al. (28) 21 L-dopa-treated patients. Caudate D_2 binding was normal in both of these series. However, in the last study, a small (16%) but significant increase in D_2 binding levels was observed in the putamen.

The largest study of dopamine receptor densities in Parkinson's disease is that of Rinne et al. (29). In their study of tissue from 44 patients, they reported a decreased density of D_2 receptors in the caudates or putamens of small numbers of both treated and nontreated patients. These patients were found retrospectively to have little or no response to L-dopa treatment. In a larger number of nontreated patients, an elevated level of D_2 binding was observed. In treated patients who were judged to be responsive to L-dopa therapy, levels of D_2 receptors were not different from control values.

We have recently examined this question using an in vivo estimation of D_2 receptor densities obtained by positron emission tomography (PET) (12). The PET scanning of the caudate and putamen following intravenous administration of the high-affinity positron-emitting ligand $[^{11}C]$ N-methyl-spiperone can provide a good estimate of striatal dopamine receptor densities in living patients. We have used this technique in ambulatory drug-treated Parkinson's disease patients with asymmetrical expression of this disease. In our study, striatal binding values were well within control levels. Furthermore, there was no asymmetry in receptor binding despite right/left differences in rigidity and tremor noted in these patients (Fig. 1).

In summary, the interplay of several factors could conceivably influence striatal dopamine receptor sensitivity in Parkinson's disease patients. Denervation, supersensitivity, and the neuroleptic drugs occasionally used to treat behavioral manifestations of Parkinson's disease could increase receptor densities, while dopamimetic therapy and the loss of intrinsic striatal neurons found in some parkinsonian brains could reduce the densities. The bulk of evidence obtained to date suggests that, in treated Parkinson's disease patients, striatal D_2 receptor densities are normal. This conclusion does not exclude the possibility of receptor alterations in subgroups of patients.

Nondopamine Receptors

OPIATE Opiate receptor densities have been reported to be decreased in caudate, but not in putamen, of patients with Parkinson's disease. Based on the ligands used in this study, mu sites were most probably measured (30,31). Delta-opiate receptor densities, as detected by an enkephalin analog, were unchanged in two studies of binding to Parkinson's disease caudate (22,31). Changes in opiate receptor densities may thus occur in a subtype-selective manner. Decreases in mu receptors could conceivably reflect loss of receptors normally present on processes of nigrostriatal neurons.

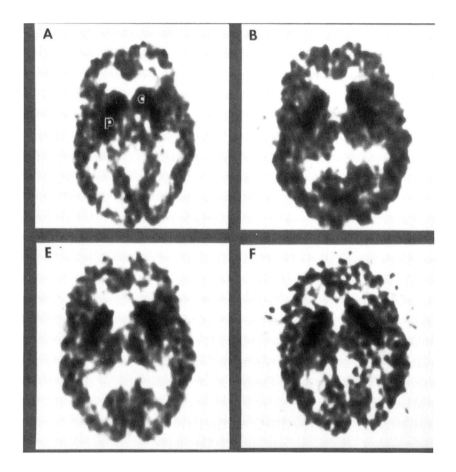

FIGURE 1 PET scans through the level of the caudate–putamen obtained from eight patients with asymmetrical Parkinson's disease. Receptor densities were labeled using ^{11}C-N-methyl-spiperone injected 10 minutes before testing.

SEROTONIN   Raphe serotonin (5-HT) neurons project to both the substantia nigra and the basal ganglia. There are at least two subtypes of 5-HT receptors in brain. 5-HT$_1$ and 5-HT$_2$ receptors are defined on the same basis as are D$_1$ and D$_2$ receptors: effects on adenylate cyclase and structure–activity profiles in binding studies and pharmacologic test systems (21). Neither subclass of 5-HT receptors appears to be affected in the Parkinson's disease caudate or globus pallidus, but 5-HT$_1$ binding is decreased in the putamen (26). 5-HT can alter the release of DA from terminals within the rat striatum (20). Conceivably, these

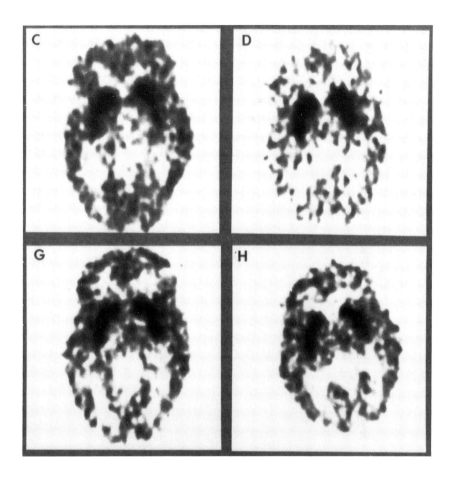

findings could reflect the presence of 5-HT receptors on striatal dopaminergic terminals.

ACETYLCHOLINE   In the striatum, acetylcholine is present chiefly in interneurons affected by dopaminergic activity. Muscarinic cholinergic receptors are reported to be increased in the parkinsonian putamen but unchanged in either the caudate or globus pallidus (26,32). However, the effects of anticholinergic Parkinson's disease therapies on regional muscarinic cholinergic receptors are not detailed in these studies.

GABA   GABA-containing striatal neurons are both local circuit and projection in nature. Striatal GABA receptor densities, as determined using [³H]-GABA and [³H] muscimol binding, are unaltered in Parkinson's disease (26,33, 34).

Substantia Nigra Receptors

Dopamine Receptors

Binding studies of dopamine receptors in the human substantia nigra have concentrated on D_2 receptors. The density of the D_2 dopamne receptor subtype is decreased in this region in both receptor homogenate and autoradiographic binding studies (13,23). This finding, together with electrophysiological and biochemical experiments in animals, supports the concept that nigral dopamine neurons express dopamine autoreceptors, and that at least some of these are of the D_2 subtype in humans.

Nondopamine Receptors

In addition to information flow from nigra to the striatum, the striatal and pallidal areas also send reciprocal striatonigral projections back to the nigra. These descending projections, which contain such transmitters as GABA, substance P/substance K, and dynorphin, impinge upon both dopamine and nondopamine neurons in the nigra. Nigral inputs also arise from other brain regions and GABAergic nigral interneurons are also present in the zone reticulata. The activity of nigrostriatal dopaminergic neurons can thus be modulated by inputs on or close to their cell bodies, as well as by synapses on their terminals in the striatum. Several receptor types are normally expressed in the substantia nigra and many of these are affected in Parkinson's disease. Autoradiographic and/or homogenate binding studies suggest that GABA, somatostatin, neurotensin, and kappa-opiate receptors are all substantially reduced in parkinsonian nigra in conjunction with disease-induced cell losses (13,21,35) (Fig. 2). Delta- and mu-opiate receptors, glycine receptors, and high-affinity benzodiazepine receptors are decreased to a lesser extent, whereas low-affinity benzodiazepine and 5-HT receptor densities are unchanged (13). These results indicate which transmitter receptors are expressed by nigral dopamine neurons, and suggest which systems might influence the activity of these important cells.

Other Regions

Several investigators have examined the parkinsonian cerebral cortex and hippocampus for changes in neurotransmitter receptors. Parkinson's disease brains display normal densities of GABA, D_2, and 5-HT_2 receptors in hippocampus and frontal cortex (23,28,33,36). In Parkinson's disease patients who are demented there are decreased densities of muscarinic cholinergic and 5-HT_1 receptors in frontal cortex (36,37). Alterations in muscarinic receptor densities in conjunction with decreases in presynaptic cerebral cortical cholinergic innervation in demented Parkinson's disease patients may explain the increased susceptibility to mental confusion induced by anticholinergics in demented Parkinson's disease patients (8,37).

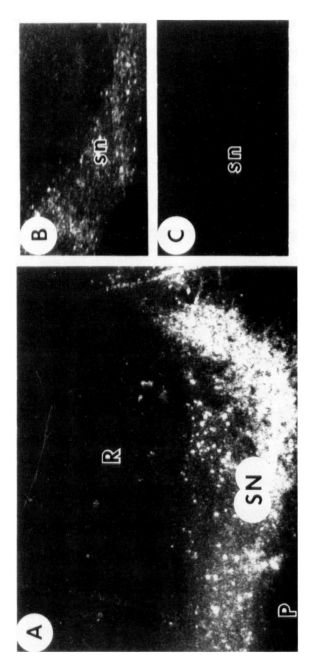

FIGURE 2 Prints of film autoradiograms of human basal midbrain receptor densities. Increased whiteness corresponds to greater receptor densities in these images. P, cerebral peduncle; R, red nucleus; SN, substantia nigra. (Original magnification, 13.5.) A. Somatostatin receptors. Autoradiogram from a control brain. B. Substantia nigra somatostatin receptor density in Parkinson's disease. C. Control "blank" substantia nigra autoradiogram, from a section adjacent to A, treated identically except that 10^{-7} M unlabeled SOM-14 was added to primary incubations.

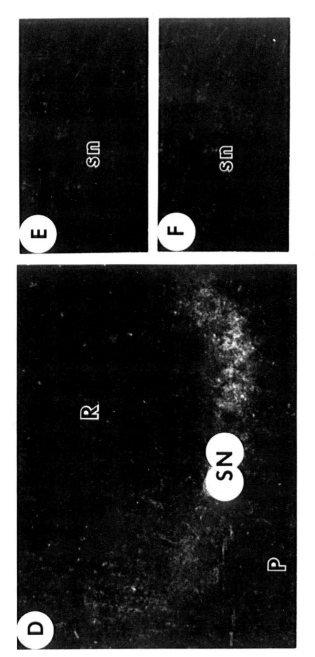

FIGURE 2 (Continued) D. Neurotensin receptors, normal distribution. [³H] neurotensin autoradiogram from control brain. E. Substantia nigra neurotensin receptor density in Parkinson's disease (³H-neurotensin autoradiogram). F. Control "blank" substantia nigra autoradiogram, from a section adjacent to D, treated identically except that 5 × 10⁻⁶M unlabeled neurotensin was added to primary incubation.

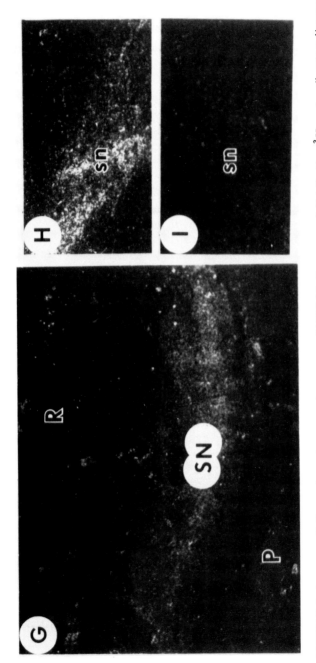

FIGURE 2 (Continued) G. Angiotensin converting enzyme (ACE) binding, normal distribution ^{3}H-captopril autoradiogram from a control brain. H. Substantia nigra ACE binding density in PD (^{3}H-captopril autoradiogram). I. Control "blank" normal distribution, from section adjacent to G, treated identically except that 1 X 10^{-6} M unlabeled captopril was added to primary incubation.

Adrenergic receptors are also affected in parkinsonian cortex (38), as levels of alpha-2 receptors are decreased. In addition, alpha-1-receptor densities appear to be increased but only in demented Parkinson's disease patients. Cortical beta-1-adrenergic receptor binding densities are increased in Parkinson's disease while beta-2-receptor levels are unchanged. The increases in beta-1-receptor levels correlate, in retrospective analyses, with the symptoms of depression shown by some Parkinson's disease patients. Conceivably, changes in adrenergic receptors could also reflect decreases in innervation of cerebral blood vessels, as a result of cell losses in the locus ceruleus.

SUMMARY

Changes in regional receptor populations do occur in Parkinson's disease. Studies of these receptor alterations can be of help in deciphering the neurotransmitter systems which are involved in the pathophysiology of Parkinson's disease. This information could subsequently help to pinpoint possible targets for improved drug treatment of this disabling disorder. The parkinsonian lesion may also help in defining the receptor complements of important human neuronal populations. Finally, receptor alterations in response to disease and treatment may provide substantial insight into the dynamic, adaptive mechanisms of the human brain.

REFERENCES

1. Ehringer H, Hornykiewicz D. (1960). Verteiling von noradrenal in and dopamin (3-hydroxytyramin) im gehirn des menschen und ihr verhalten bei erkrankungen des extrapyramidalen systems. *Lin Wochenschr* 38: 1236–1239.
2. Hornykiewicz O. (1971). Neurochemical pathology and pharmacology of brain dopamine and acetylcholine: rational basis for the current drug treatment of parkinsonism. In: McDowell FH, Markham CH (Eds.), *Recent Advances in Parkinson's Disease*. Philadelphia, F.A. Davis.
3. Javoy-Agid F, Ploska A, Agid Y. (1981). Microtopography of tyrosine hydroxylase, glutamic acid decarboxylase and choline acetyltransferase in the substantia nigra and ventral tegmental area of control and Parkinsonian brains. *J Neurochem* 37: 1218–1227.
4. Alvord EC. (1968). The pathology of parkinsonism. In: Minckler J (Ed.), *Pathology of the Nervous System*, Vol 1. New York, McGraw-Hill.
5. Uhl GR, Hedreen JC, Price DL. (1985). Parkinson's disease: loss of neurons from the ventral tegmental area contralateral to therapeutic surgical lesions. *Neurology* 35: 1215–1218.
6. Epelbaum J, Ruberg M, Moyse E, Javoy-Agid F, Dubois B, Agid Y. (1983). Somatostatin and dementia in Parkinson's disease. *Brain Res* 278: 376–379.
7. Javoy-Agid F, Ruberg M, Tacquet H, Bokobza B, Agid Y, Gaspar P, Berger B, N'Guyen-Legros J, Alvarez C, Gray F, Escourelle R, Scatton B, Rouquier

L. (1984). Biochemical neuropathology of Parkinson's disease. *Adv Neurol* 40: 189–198.

8. Perry EK, Curtis M, Dick DJ, Candy JM, Atack JR, Bloxham C, Blessed G, Fairbairn A, Tomlinson BE, Perry RH. (1985). Cholinergic correlates of cognitive impairment in Parkinson's disease: comparisons with Alzheimer's disease. *J Neurol Neurosurg Psychiatry* 48: 413–421.

9. Scatton B, Javoy-Agid F, Rouquier L, Dubois B, Agid Y. (1983). Reduction of cortical dopamine, noradrenaline, serotonin and their metabolites in Parkinson's disease. *Brain Res* 275: 321–328.

10. Shibuya M. (1979). Dopamine-sensitive adenylate cyclase activity in the striatum in Parkinson's disease. *J Neural Transm* 44: 287–295.

11. Freidman AM, DeJesus OT, Revenaugh BA, Dinerstein RJ. (1984). Measurements in vivo of parameters of the dopamine system. *Ann Neurol* 15 (Suppl.): S66–S76.

12. Frost JJ, Uhl G, Lavik P, Petronis J, Wong DF, Preziosi TJ, Dannals RF, Wilson AA, Ravert HT, Links JM, Wagner HN. (1985). Measurement of dopamine receptor binding in asymmetrically affected patients with Parkinson's disease by ^{11}C-N-methyl-spiperone and positron tomography. *Ann Neurol.* (submitted).

13. Uhl GR, Hackney GO, Torchia M, Stanov V, Tourtellotte WW, Whitehouse PJ, Tran V, Strittmatter S. (1986). Parkinson's disease: nigral receptor changes support peptidergic role in nigrostriatal modulation. *Ann Neurol* (in press).

14. Kebabian JK, Calne DB. (1979). Multiple receptors for dopamine. *Nature* 277: 92–96.

15. Seeman P. (1980). Brain dopamine receptors. *Pharmacol Rev* 32: 229–313.

16. Ungerstedt U, Ljungberg T, Steg G. (1974). Behavioral, physiological, and neurochemical changes after 6-hydroxydopamine-induced degeneration of the nigro-striatal dopamine neurons. *Adv Neurol* 5: 421–426.

17. Pycock CJ, Marsden CD. (1977). Central dopaminergic receptor supersensitivity and its relevance to Parkinson's disease. *J Neurol Sci* 31: 113–121.

18. Weiner WJ, Koller WC, Perlik S, Nausieda P, Klawans HL. (1980). Drug holiday and management of Parkinson disease. *Neurology* 30: 1257–1265.

19. Sweet RD, McDowell FH, Figneson JS, Loranger AW, Goodell H. (1976). Mental symptoms in Parkinson's disease during chronic treatment with levodopa. *Neurology* 26: 305–310.

20. Chesselet M-F. (1984). Presynaptic regulation of neurotransmitter release in the brain: fact and hypothesis. *Neuroscience* 2: 347–375.

21. Uhl GR. (1985). Neuropeptide systems in Parkinson's disease and tardive dyskinesia. In: Nemeroff CB (Ed.), *Neuropeptides in Neuropsychiatric Disorders*. New York, Raven Press.

22. Llorens-Cortes C, Javoy-Agid F, Agid Y, Tacquet H, Schwartz JC. (1984). Enkephalinergic markers in substantia nigra and caudate nucleus from Parkinsonian subjects. *J Neurochem* 43: 874–877.

23. Quik M, Spokes EG, Mackay VP, Bannister R. (1979). Alterations in ^{3}H-spiperone binding in human caudate nucleus, substantia nigra and frontal

cortex in the Shy-Drager syndrome and Parkinson's disease. *J Neurol Sci* 43: 429–437.

24. De Smet Y, Ruberg M, Serdau M, Dubois B, Lhermitte F, Agid Y. (1982). Confusion, dementia and anticholinergics in Parkinson's disease. *J Neurol Neurosurg Psychiatry* 45: 1161–1164.

25. Riederer P, Rausch W-D, Birkmayer W, Jellinger K, Danielcyzk R. (1978). Dopamine-sensitive adenylate cyclase activity in the caudate nucleus and adrenal medulla in Parkinson's disease and in liver cirrhosis. *J Neural Transm* Suppl. 14: 153–161.

26. Reisine TD, Fields JZ, Yamamura HI, Bird ED, Spokes E, Schreiner PS, Enna SJ. (1977). Neurotransmitter receptor alterations in Parkinson's disease. *Life Sci* 21: 335–344.

27. Lee T, Seeman P, Rajput A, Farley IJ, Hornykiewicz O. (1978). Receptor basis for dopaminergic supersensitivity in Parkinson's disease. *Nature* 273: 59–61.

28. Bokobza B, Ruberg M, Acatton B, Javoy-Agid F, Agid Y. (1984). ^{3}H-spiperone binding, dopamine and HVA concentrations in Parkinson's disease and supranuclear palsy. *Eur J Pharmacol* 99: 167–175.

29. Rinne UK, Lonnberg P, Koskinen V. (1981). Dopamine receptors in the Parkinsonian brain. *J Neural Transm* 51: 97–106.

30. Reisine TD, Rossoor M, Spokes LL, Yamamura HI. (1979). Alterations in brain opiate receptors in Parkinson's disease. *Brain Res* 173: 378–382.

31. Rinne UK, Rinne JO, Rinne JK, Laakso K, Laitinen A, Lonnberg P. (1983). Brain receptor changes in Parkinson's disease in relation to the disease process and treatment. *J Neural Transm* Suppl. 18: 279–286.

32. Dubois B, Ruberg M, Javoy-Agid F, Ploska A, Agid Y. (1983). A sub-cortico-cortical cholinergic system is affected in Parkinson's disease. *Brain Res* 288: 213–218.

33. Lloyd KG, Shemen L, Hornykiewicz O. (1977). Distribution of high-affinity sodium-independent ^{3}H-gamma-aminobutyric acid binding in the human brain: alterations in Parkinson's disease. *Brain Res* 127: 269–278.

34. Rinne UK, Loskinen V, Laaksonen H, Lonnberg P, Sonninen V. (1978). GABA receptor binding in the Parkinsonian brain. *Life Sci* 22: 2225–2228.

35. Sadoul JL, Checler F, Kitabgi P, Rostene W, Javoy-Agid F, Vincent JP. (1984). Loss of high affinity neurotensin receptors in substantia nigra from parkinsonian subjects. *Biochem Biophys Res Commun* 125: 395–404.

36. Perry EK, Perry RH, Candy JM, Fairbairn AF, Blessed G, Dick DJ, Tomlinson BE. (1984). Cortical serotonin-S_2 receptor binding abnormalities in patients with Alzheimer's disease: comparisons with Parkinson's disease. *Neurosci Letts* 51: 353–357.

37. Ruberg M, Ploska A, Javoy-Agid F, Agid Y. (1982). Muscarinic binding and choline acetyltransferase activity in Parkinsonian subjects with reference to dementia. *Brain Res* 232: 129–139.

38. Cash R, Ruberg M, Raisman R, Agid Y. (1984). Adrenergic receptors in Parkinson's disease. *Brain Res* 322: 269–275.

13
MPTP and Animal Models of Parkinsonism

RICHARD E. HEIKKILA, PATRICIA K. SONSALLA, M. VICTORIA KINDT, and ROGER C. DUVOISIN
University of Medicine and Dentistry of New Jersey-Robert Wood Johnson Medical School, Piscataway, New Jersey

1-Methyl-4-phenyl-1,2,3,6-tetrahydropyridine (MPTP) is a commercially available chemical intermediate used in the synthesis of more complex compounds. Varying amounts of MPTP may be formed as a byproduct, depending upon the reaction conditions, in the synthesis of the potent analgesic agent 1-methyl-4-phenyl-4-proprionoxypiperidine (MPPP), the reverse ester of meperidine. The inadvertent self-administration of relatively small amounts of MPTP by several young drug abusers who were using MPPP as an alternative to heroin resulted in a severe and permanent parkinsonian syndrome (Davis et al., 1979; Langston et al., 1983). The parkinsonism induced in these patients was very similar though not identical to idiopathic Parkinson's disease in its clinical, pathologic, and biochemical features. Moreover, patients responded favorably to drugs used to treat Parkinson patients. The intravenous injection of MPTP, but not of MPPP, to monkeys caused behavioral, biochemical, and pathologic changes in monkeys similar to those seen in parkinsonian patients (Burns et al., 1983). This finding confirmed the suspicion that the agent responsible for causing parkinsonism in the human drug abusers was MPTP.

The observation that it produces an enduring parkinsonian syndrome in humans and nonhuman primates has stimulated considerable research with MPTP in a variety of in vivo and in vitro model systems. Biochemical and pathologic manifestations of MPTP toxicity have been characterized in several species and it is hoped that animal models may be established which would be appropriate for screening new therapeutic agents and for testing drug regimens in the treatment of Parkinson's patients. A great deal of effort has also been focused on the elucidation of the mechanism by which MPTP produces its selective destruction of nigrostriatal neurons, and there has been considerable speculation that a neurotoxin like MPTP could be involved in the pathogenesis of Parkinson's disease (Langston et al., 1983; Burns et al., 1984; Snyder, 1984). This speculation is particularly interesting when one considers the low concordance rate for parkinsonism observed in monozygotic twins, which appears to rule out genetic factors as being causative (Ward et al., 1983). In this chapter we will discuss various aspects of MPTP-induced parkinsonism, describe MPTP toxicity in humans and in animals, and present current knowledge and hypotheses as well as speculations on what we believe to be the mechanisms by which MPTP produces its remarkably selective nigrostriatal toxicity. Finally, we will compare aspects of MPTP-induced parkinsonism with idiopathic parkinsonism.

MPTP TOXICITY IN HUMANS

The first documented case of MPTP poisoning in humans was a 23-year-old graduate student who inadvertently produced MPTP as a byproduct in the synthesis of the meperidine analog MPPP (Davis et al., 1979). This individual made and injected himself with MPPP for several months with no apparent ill effects, until, in November 1978, he took certain synthetic shortcuts in one preparation. These included reduction in the reaction time, running the reaction at higher temperatures, and failing to isolate and crystallize the product properly. Traces of the "sloppy batch" remaining on laboratory glassware were subsequently analyzed by Dr. S.P. Markey and colleagues at the National Institute of Mental Health and found to be a mixture of MPPP, 4-hydroxy-4-phenyl-N-methyl-piperidine, and MPTP. After several days of injection, the patient presented with severe rigidity, weakness, muteness, tremor, flat facial expression, and seborrhea. Treatment with levodopa/carbidopa or benztropine resulted in marked improvement. When treatment was discontinued, severe bradykinesia, generalized rigidity, and mild tremor developed over a 3-day period. Resumption of drug therapy resulted in rapid improvement.

While undergoing bromocriptine therapy for the next 18 months, the patient continued to abuse several drugs including cocaine, codeine, dihydromorphine, and levodopa, and, in September 1978, he died of an overdose of cocaine and codeine. Postmortem study of his brain revealed severe destruction of the pars compacta of the substantia nigra with much neuromelanin pigment present, both extracellular and within microglial cells. A single rounded eosinophilic Lewy body was noted. The locus ceruleus was essentially normal.

There have been several other reports of MPTP-induced parkinsonism among narcotic addicts in northern California who purchased MPTP-contaminated MPPP sold as new "synthetic heroin" (Langston et al., 1983; Ballard et al., 1983, 1985; Langston and Ballard, 1984). All patients became symptomatic within 1 week after the use of the new drug, the first symptoms being visual hallucinations, jerking of limbs, and stiffness. Within 2 weeks, these patients experienced general bradykinesia. Other symptoms included near total immobility, flexed posture, cogwheel rigidity, fixed stare, decreased blinking, constant drooling, facial seborrhea, and festinating gait. All patients responded to therapy with L-dopa and carbidopa. Langston and co-workers (1984) also described the early onset of "end of dose" deterioration, "peak dose" dyskinesias, and "on-off" phenomenon in several patients. Analysis of cerebrospinal fluid revealed relatively normal concentrations of 3-methoxyphenylethylene glycol (norepinephrine metabolite) and 5-hydroxyindoleacetic acid (serotonin metabolite), but very low levels of homovanillic acid (dopamine metabolite).

Parkinsonism following intranasal and cutaneous MPTP exposure in humans has also been documented. Wright and co-workers (1983) reported a case of MPTP-induced parkinsonism in a man who described "snorting" home-synthesized MPPP. Langston and Ballard (1983) reported MPTP-induced parkinsonism in a 49-year-old chemist who, while working for 8 years at a pharmaceutical firm, synthesized many compounds requiring repeated preparation of MPTP. Opportunities for cutaneous and inhalation exposure to MPTP were present.

MPTP TOXICITY IN OTHER SPECIES

Primate Models

In 1983 Burns and co-workers reported that intravenous administration of MPTP produced a parkinsonian-like syndrome in rhesus monkeys (*Mucaca mulatta*). Behavioral changes were observed after two or three doses of 0.33 mg/kg MPTP and consisted of eyelid closure, a decreased number of spontaneous movements, loss of facial expression, and postural tremor. After four or five doses, abnormal facial movements, changes in posture and muscle tone, rigidity, head extension, and drooling were observed. At a cumulative dose of 1.7 mg/kg there was persistent eyelid closure, decreased spontaneous motor activity, rigidity, postural tremor, and difficulty in swallowing. Two weeks following cessation of MPTP treatment, motor problems continued to worsen and the animals exhibited severe bradykinesia, flexed posture, loss of hand dexterity, and so-called "freezing episodes." Levodopa treatment corrected all of these above behavioral changes.

The neurochemical changes induced by MPTP treatment included transient reductions in the levels of 5-HIAA and MHPG in the cerebrospinal fluid, midbrain, putamen, and caudate nucleus. In contrast, concentrations of HVA in the cerebrospinal fluid and dopamine and HVA concentrations in the caudate and putamen were depressed for as long as 3 months after MPTP administration.

Histopathologic examination of the monkey brain at 2 months after MPTP treatment revealed that less than 10% of the normal cell population of the zona compacta of the substantia nigra was present. Dopaminergic neurons of the ventral midbrain and median eminence were normal as were noradrenergic neurons of the locus ceruleus and hypothalamus. It was later reported that the major clinical signs of the extrapyramidal syndrome, except for resting tremor, appeared only when there was greater than an 80% loss of nigrostriatal neurons (Chiueh et al., 1985).

Similar observations were made in later studies of MPTP toxicity in other primates such as the squirrel monkey, *Saimiri sciureus* (Langston et al., 1984; Langston, 1985), macaque monkey, *Macaca fascicularis* (Crossman et al., 1985), and the marmoset (Jenner et al., 1984). In summary, MPTP treatment in these primates results in a neurologic disorder similar in clinical signs (akinesia, rigidity, resting tremor, flexed posture) to that seen in MPTP-induced and idiopathic parkinsonism in humans. Strikingly, these behavioral changes are reversed by levodopa therapy. Although transient decrements in the levels of other neurotransmitters and their metabolites have been observed, only decrements in striatal dopamine and dopamine metabolite levels are chronic. Histopathologic analysis confirmed a selective loss of nigrostriatal dopaminergic neurons. It should be emphasized that the actual number of animals utilized in these studies is rather small. In most cases systematic studies and complete studies have not been carried out in monkeys and much of our body of knowledge concerning MPTP in primates is "anecdotal."

Rodent Models

After the first successful animal model with MPTP was established in the monkey, considerable efforts were expended by several groups of investigators to establish a rodent model in which to study MPTP toxicity since this would provide a less expensive, more manageable model than the monkey. Guinea pigs and rats were found, compared to primates, to be relatively resistant to MPTP-induced nigrostriatal dopaminergic toxicity (Chiueh et al., 1983, 1984; Boyce et al., 1984; Enz et al., 1984; Perry et al., 1985). It has been shown by some, however, that with rigorous injection paradigms, MPTP can work to some extent in the rat (Fuller and Hemrick-Luecke, 1985; Jarvis and Wagner, 1985).

It was subsequently discovered by several groups of investigators that the mouse was relatively sensitive to MPTP toxicity (Hallman et al., 1984; Hess et al., 1984; Heikkila et al., 1984a,b). For example, Hess and co-workers (1984) reported that 5–10 intraperitoneal injections of MPTP once a day at 30 mg/kg produced pronounced (80%) decreases in the levels of dopamine and its metabolites in the striatum while dopamine concentrations in the nucleus accumbens and hypothalamus were unaffected. Cresyl violet staining revealed that MPTP-treated mice had a marked bilateral loss of neurons in the zona compacta of the substantia nigra (A9) but there was no apparent effect on the A10 area, locus ceruleus, raphe nuclei, or hypothalamus. The reduction in the number of neurons in the substantia nigra was also demonstrated by retrograde transport of horseradish peroxidase injected unilaterally into the caudate nucleus.

In our laboratory, we have found considerable variation among individual animals and strains of mice with regard to susceptibility to MPTP-induced nigrostriatal damage. Swiss-Webster (CF-W) mice, although sensitive, are more resistant to MPTP-induced nigrostriatal damage than are C57-Bl mice; younger animals are more resistant than older animals. Because MPTP treatment can bring about marked behavioral deficits in C57-Bl mice, we have focused much of our attention on experiments in these mice. The basis for these differences is unknown and currently under intense investigation.

ROLE OF BIOCHEMICAL SYSTEMS
IN MPTP TOXICITY

The mechanism by which MPTP produces neurotoxicity is not yet fully known. However, several important steps in the neurotoxic process have been identified and are described below. Based on these findings, several hypotheses regarding the mechanism of MPTP neurotoxicity hade been proposed and are discussed.

MPTP and Monoamine Oxidase

Markey et al. (1984) first demonstrated in a fascinating series of experiments that MPTP is rapidly oxidized to 1-methyl-4-phenylpyridinium (MPP^+) in the brains of monkeys, rats, and mice following systemic administration of MPTP. They further reported that MPP^+ was the major metabolite of MPTP and that detectable levels of MPP^+ could be found in monkey brains for many days after MPTP administration. From these data, they speculated that MPP^+ itself (or the process of MPP^+ formation) was responsible for MPTP-induced toxicity. In contrast, the half-life of MPP^+ in the mouse brain was considerably shorter, being approximately 2 hr while the half-life of MPP^+ in the rat was even shorter, approximately 15 min. It follows that if MPP^+ is indeed the ultimate toxin, the rapid clearance of MPP^+ from the mouse brain may partially explain why the mouse is less susceptible than the monkey to the neurotoxic action of MPTP. Furthermore, this difference may explain why the mouse is far more sensitive to MPTP than the rat.

The role for monoamine oxidase B in the conversion of MPTP to MPP^+ was discovered by Chiba et al. (1984), who found that MPP^+ was formed in rat brain mitochondrial preparations and, more importantly, that this formation could be prevented by the presence of monoamine oxidase B (MAO-B) inhibitors in the preparation. These investigators found that deprenyl (a selective MAO-B inhibitor), but not clorgyline (a selective MAO-A inhibitor), prevented the in vitro formation of MPP$^+$ and suggested that the B form of MAO was responsible for the oxidation of MPTP to MPP$^+$. Additional studies, using purified enzymes, have confirmed these findings (Fritz et al., 1985). It was subsequently shown in vivo that MPTP-induced neurotoxicity in mice was also prevented by pretreatment of the animals with inhibitors of MAO-B, but not MAO-A (Heikkila et al., 1984c, 1985a). These findings were subsequently confirmed in monkeys (Cohen et al., 1981; Langston et al., 1984). Thus it is evident that MAO-B plays a critical role in the oxidation and bioactivation of MPTP and that MPP$^+$ formation is a critical part of the neurotoxic process.

Various in vitro techniques have been used to characterize MPTP oxidation by MAO-B. Heikkila et al. (1985b), reported that the kinetics of MPTP oxidation (K_m and V_{max} values) by mouse brain mitochondrial preparations were very similar to those for benzylamine, a typical substrate for MAO-B. They also compared the abilities of various MAO inhibitors to inhibit the oxidation of MPTP, benzylamine (a substrate for MAO-B), and tryptamine (a substrate for MAO-A) and found a highly significant correlation between the capacity of various MAO inhibitors to inhibit the oxidation of MPTP and their capacity to inhibit the oxidation of benzylamine. However, there was no correlation between the capacity of these MAO inhibitors to inhibit MPTP oxidation and their capacity to inhibit the oxidation of tryptamine, the MAO-A substrate.

Chiba et al. (1985), have done in-depth studies to characterize the oxidation of MPTP and have found the conversion of MPTP to MPP$^+$ proceeds via the formation of the intermediate 2 electron oxidative product, 1-methyl-4-phenyl-2,3-dihydropyridinium (MPDP$^+$); see Figure 1. MPDP$^+$ is then rapidly oxidized to MPP$^+$. MAO-B is required for the first step in this oxidation process; however, it is unclear what, if any, enzyme or catalyst is required for the second step in this process. We have found, in preliminary experiments, that this latter oxidation is dependent upon the superoxide radical.

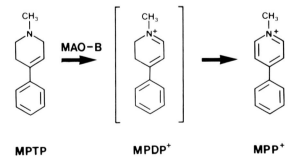

MPTP   **MPDP$^+$**   **MPP$^+$**

FIGURE 1   Reaction sequence for MPTP oxidation involves the conversion of MPTP to the dihydropyridinium intermediate, MPDP$^+$, by MAO-B and the subsequent oxidation of MPDP$^+$ to MPP$^+$.

MPP$^+$ and the Dopamine Transport System

An interesting and perplexing aspect of MPTP toxicity is the highly selective action of this neurotoxin on nigrostriatal dopaminergic neurons. Although MAO-B activity is high in the substantia nigra and caudate nucleus, MAO-B is also present in many other brain areas that are unaffected by MPTP and MPP$^+$ formation occurs ubiquitously throughout the brain (Johannessen et al., 1985). If MPP$^+$ is responsible for toxicity and if it is present in so many brain regions, why is toxicity primarily limited to the nigrostriatal dopamine neurons? Although a complete explanation is not available at this time, part of the answer certainly can be attributed to the fact that MPP$^+$ is actively transported into dopamine neurons by the dopamine transport system. This important observation was made by Javitch et al. (1985), who found that MPP$^+$, but not MPTP, is readily accumulated in striatal synaptosomes; indeed, the kinetics of MPP$^+$ uptake are very similar to those of dopamine uptake. Thus it is very likely that high concentrations of MPP$^+$ are reached within dopamine neurons. Consistent with these findings, it has been demonstrated that pretreatment of mice with compounds that block dopamine transport (e.g., mazindol or amfonelic acid) prevent MPTP-induced neurotoxicity to the nigrostriatal dopaminergic neurons (Javitch et al., 1985; Fuller and Hemrick-Luecke, 1985; Heikkila et al., 1985c). It is thus apparent that the dopamine transport system plays an important role in the neurotoxic actions of MPTP, presumably by transporting the MPP$^+$ molecule from the extracellular space into the dopamine neuron.

Based on the information thus far, the following picture emerges regarding MPTP toxicity; see Figure 2. Immunohistochemical studies have localized MAO-B to astrocytes and serotonin-containing neurons, but not to catecholaminergic neurons. Thus MPP$^+$ formation probably occurs outside dopaminergic neurons, possibly in astrocytes. It is likely that the lipophilic compound MPTP diffuses into astrocytes where it is oxidized by MAO-B to MPDP$^+$, which in turn is oxidized to MPP$^+$. It is not clear how or if MPP$^+$ (or MPDP$^+$) is released into the extracellular space. Because of its polarity, it is unlikely that MPP$^+$ would merely diffuse out of the astrocyte. One possibility is that it is not MPP$^+$, but rather MPDP, in an uncharged tautomeric form of MPDP$^+$, that diffuses from the astrocyte (Chiba et al., 1984). In the extracellular space, MPDP$^+$ could then be converted to MPP$^+$ by nonenzymatic reactions. Another possibility is that MPP$^+$ is formed within the astrocyte and causes damage to the cells; as a consequence MPP$^+$ is "leaked" into the extracellular space. However, once released, MPP$^+$ is subsequently accumulated in the dopamine neurons via the dopamine transport system. Inside the neuron, the concentration of MPP$^+$ reaches critical levels capable of producing damage. Although this hypothesis seemingly fits with much of the data available regarding MPTP toxicity, there are still many perplexing and unanswered questions. For example, why are other dopaminergic systems that possess dopamine uptake systems with reasonably high affinity and

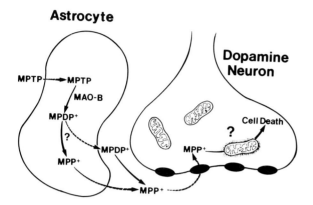

FIGURE 2 Hypothesis for the mechanism of neurotoxicity produced by MPTP on nigrostriatal dopaminergic neurons. MPTP is oxidized by MAO-B, presumably in astrocytes, to MPDP$^+$, which undergoes further oxidation either within the astrocyte or the extracellular space to MPP$^+$. The MPP$^+$ is then avidly accumulated within the dopaminergic neurons by the dopamine transport system where it eventually reaches critical concentrations capable of producing damage. It is not clear how MPP$^+$ causes cell death. MPP$^+$ inhibits mitochondrial respiration and we hypothesize that this effect of MPP$^+$ may play a prominent role in cell death.

capacity unaffected by MPTP? Why is there no apparent cytotoxicity in the adrenal gland, an organ in which MPP$^+$ reaches very high concentrations? Why are serotonergic neurons, which contain high amounts of MAO-B, relatively resistant to the toxic actions of MPTP?

Possible Mechanisms of Cell Destruction

The cellular mechanism of toxicity produced by MPTP on the nigrostriatal dopaminergic neurons is unknown. Several hypotheses have been proposed that would invoke a role for dopamine in the neurotoxic process. Castagnoli et al. (1985) proposed that MPTP may be oxidized by monoamine oxidase within the dopamine neuron to the MPDP$^+$ intermediate, which could then interact with dopamine. The net effect of this interaction would result in the reformation of MPTP and the oxidation of dopamine with the subsequent formation of quinone or oxyradicals (Castagnoli et al., 1985). However, it has recently been demonstrated that the effects of MPTP are not prevented in mice that have a greatly diminished content of neostriatal dopamine (Fuller and Hemrick-Luecke, 1985; Schmidt et al., 1985). These findings seem to rule out a critical role for dopamine in the neurotoxic actions of MPTP.

We have recently reported that MPP$^+$ inhibits NADH-linked respiration in brain mitochondria (Nicklas et al., 1985). In these experiments, it was demonstrated that MPP$^+$ is capable of inhibiting the uncoupled oxidation of NADH-linked substrates (but not succinate) by brain mitochondrial preparations. Based on these findings, we believe that MPP$^+$ may inhibit mitochondrial respiration within the dopaminergic neuron, which would clearly lead to cell death.

DISCUSSION AND CONCLUSIONS

The discovery that a compound such as MPTP can cause such a selective and destructive effect on nigrostriatal dopaminergic neurons has had an important impact on research associated with parkinsonism. Not only does the MPTP-treated animal provide us with a long-sought after model of parkinsonism, but it also opens a new area of thought regarding the cause of idiopathic parkinsonism. The potency and selectivity of MPTP in producing dopaminergic toxicity in humans and monkeys have led several investigators to suggest that endogenously formed or exogenously acquired MPTP-like compounds may be the cause of human parkinsonism. Recent studies have failed to show a concordance of parkinsonism among monozygotic twins (Ward et al., 1983), thus it does not appear there is a genetic component associated with the development of this disease. Whether or not an environmental factor contributes to the destruction of the dopaminergic neurons will require well-designed epidemiologic studies.

It should be pointed out, however, that there are differences between MPTP-induced and idiopathic parkinsonism. In Parkinson's disease, the mesocortical and mesolimbic as well as the nigrostriatal dopaminergic pathways are affected and pathologic and neurochemical changes are seen in many brain areas (e.g., substantia nigra, locus ceruleus, hypothalamus, dorsal motor vagal nucleus). In contrast, only the nigrostriatal dopaminergic pathway has, thus far, been shown to be affected by MPTP self-administration. Does this indicate that MPTP has a unique action or is it possible that longer exposure time may be required before effects on other brain areas are seen? Are the changes in other brain areas seen in parkinsonian brains secondary to the loss of nigrostriatal dopaminergic neurons, which require years to develop? Only one human patient has thus far been studied postmortem. Will more data obtained from MPTP-intoxicated individuals demonstrate a more extensive pathology? Obviously, more knowledge and long-term effects of MPTP, both in experimental animals and in humans, are required to answer such questions.

In any case, it is clear that the MPTP-treated animal as a model for parkinsonism will be invaluable in future research in Parkinson's disease. It will help define the role of dopamine deficiency in the pathophysiology of the parkinsonian state. It will now be possible to test potential therapeutic agents in a behavioral model of parkinsonism as well as to research the on–off phenomenon and dyskinesias that occur in patients being treated with L-dopa. In addition, it is likely that new approaches to drug therapy will be tested as a result of the research findings regarding the mechanism of MPTP toxicity. In summary, research conducted with MPTP has already led to some fascinating discoveries regarding its mechanism of action and the neurotoxic process. Whether a similar process is associated with the destruction of dopaminergic neurons in Parkinson's disease or some other forms of human parkinsonism remains to be determined by future research.

REFERENCES

Ballard PA, Langston JW, Tetrud JW, Burns RS. (1983). Chemically induced chronic parkinsonism in young adults: clinical and neuropharmacologic aspects. *Neurology* 33: 90.

Ballard PA, Tetrud JW, Langston, JW. (1985). Permanent human parkinsonism due to 1-methyl-4-phenyl-1,2,3,6-tetrahydropyridine (MPTP): Seven cases. *Neurology* 35: 949–946.

Boyce S, Kelly E, Reavill C, Jenner P, Marsden CD. (1984). Repeated administration of N-methyl-4-phenyl-1,2,5,6-tetrahydropyridine to rats is not toxic to striatal dopamine neurones. *Biochem Pharmacol* 33: 1747–1752.

Burns RS, Chiueh CC, Markey SP, Ebert MH, Jacobowitz DM, Kopin IJ. (1983). A primate model of parkinsonism: selective destruction of dopaminergic neurons in the pars compacta of the substantia nigra by N-methyl-4-phenyl-1,2,3,6-tetrahydropyridine. *Proc Natl Acad Sci USA* 80: 4546–4550.

Burns RS, Markey SP, Phillips JM, Chiueh CC. (1984). The neurotoxicity of 1-methyl-4-phenyl-1,2,3,6-tetrahydropyridine in the monkey and man. *Can J Neurol Sci* 11: 166–168.

Castagnoli N Jr, Chiba K, Trevor AJ. (1985). Potential bioactivation pathways for the neurotoxin 1-methyl-4-phenyl-1,2,3,6-tetrahydropyridine (MPTP). *Life Sci* 36: 225–230.

Chiba K, Trevor A, Castagnoli N Jr. (1984). Metabolism of the neurotoxic tertiary amine, MPTP, by brain monoamine oxidase. *Biochem Biophys Res Commun* 120: 574–578.

Chiba K, Peterson LA, Castagnoli KP, Trevor AJ, Castagnoli N Jr. (1985). Studies on the molecular mechanisms of bioactivation of the selective nigro-striatal toxin 1-methyl-4-phenyl-1,2,3,6-tetrahydropyridine. *Drug Metab Dispos* 13: 342–347.

Chiueh CC, Markey RS, Johannessen J, Jacobowitz DM, Kopin IJ. (1983). N-methyl-4-phenyl-1,2,3,6-tetrahydropyridine, a parkinsonian syndrome causing agent in man and monkey, produces different effects in guinea pig and rat. *Pharmacologist* 25: 131.

Chiueh CC, Markey SP, Burns RS, Johannessen JN, Pert A, Kopin IJ. (1984). Neurochemical and behavioral effects of systemic and intranigral administration of N-methyl-4-phenyl-1,2,3,6-tetrahydropyridine in the rat. *Eur J Pharmacol* 100: 189–194.

Chiueh CC, Burns RS, Markey SP, Jacobowitz DM, Kopin IJ. (1985). Primate model of parkinsonism: selective lesion of nigrostriatal neurons by 1-methyl-4-phenyl-1,2,3,6-tetrahydropyridine produces an extrapyramidal syndrome in rhesus monkeys. *Life Sci* 36: 213–218.

Cohen G, Pasik P, Cohen B, Leist A, Mytilineou C, Yahr MD. (1984). Pargyline and deprenyl prevent the neurotoxicity of 1-methyl-4-phenyl-1,2,3,6-tetrahydropyridine (MPTP) in monkeys. *Eur J Pharmacol* 106: 209–210.

Crossman AR, Mitchell IJ, Sambrook MA. (1985). Regional brain uptake of 2-deoxyglucose in N-methyl-4-phenyl-1,2,3,6-tetrahydropyridine (MPTP)-induced parkinsonism in the macaque monkey. *Neuropharmacology* 24: 587–591.

Davis GC, Williams AC, Markey SP, Ebert MH, Caine ED, Reichert CM, Kopin IJ. (1979). Chronic parkinsonism secondary to intravenous injection of meperidine analogues. *Psychiatry Res* 1: 249–254.

Enz A, Hefti F, Frick W. (1984). Acute administration of 1-methyl-4-phenyl-1,2,3,6-tetrahydropyridine (MPTP) reduces dopamine and serotonin but accelerates norepinephrine metabolism in the rat brain. Effect of chronic pretreatment with MPTP. *Eur J Pharmacol* 101: 37–44.

Fritz RR, Abell CW, Patel NT, Gessner W, Brossi A. (1985). Metabolism of the neurotoxin in MPTP by human liver monoamine oxidase B. *FEBS Lett* 186: 224–228.

Fuller RW, Hemrick-Luecke SK. (1985). Effects of amfonelic acid, α-methyl-tyrosine, Ro 4-1284 and haloperidol pretreatment on the depletion of striatal dopamine by 1-methyl-4-phenyl-1,2,3,6-tetrahydropyridine in mice. *Res Commun Chem Pathol Pharmacol* 1: 17–25.

Hallman H, Olson L, Jonsson G. (1984). Neurotoxicity of the meperidine analogue N-methyl-4-phenyl-1,2,3,6-tetrahydropyridine on brain catecholamine neurons in the mouse. *Eur J Pharmacol* 97: 133–136.

Heikkila RE, Hess A, Duvoisin RC. (1984a). Dopaminergic neurotoxicity of 1-methyl-4-phenyl-1,2,3,6-tetrahydropyridine in mice. *Science* 224: 1451–1453.

Heikkila RE, Cabbat FS, Manzino L, Duvoisin RC. (1984b). Effects of 1-methyl-4-phenyl-1,2,3,6-tetrahydropyridine on neostriatal dopamine in mice. *Neuropharmacology* 23: 711–713.

Heikkila RE, Manzino L, Cabbat FS, Duvoisin-RC. (1984c). Protection against the dopaminergic neurotoxicity of 1-methyl-4-phenyl-1,2,3,6-tetrahydropyridine by monoamine oxidase inhibitors. *Nature* 311: 467–469.

Heikkila RE, Hess A, Duvoisin RC. (1985a). Dopaminergic neurotoxicity of 1-methyl-4-phenyl-1,2,3,6-tetrahydropyridine (MPTP) in the mouse: relationships between monoamine oxidase, MPTP metabolism and neurotoxicity. *Life Sci* 36: 231–236.

Heikkila RE, Manzino L, Cabbat FS, Duvoisin RC. (1985b). Studies on the oxidation of the dopaminergic neurotoxin 1-methyl-4-phenyl-1,2,3,6-tetrahydropyridine by monoamine oxidase B. *J Neurochem* 45: 1049–1054.

Heikkila RE, Youngster SK, Manzino L, Cabbat FS, Duvoisin RC. (1985c). Effects of 1-methyl-4-phenyl-1,2,3,6-tetrahydropyridine and related compounds on the uptake of ^{3}H-3,4-dihydroxyphenylethylamine and ^{3}H-5-hydroxy-tryptamine in neostriatal synaptosomal preparations. *J Neurochem* 44: 310–313.

Hess A, Yamasaki D, Bretschneider A, Meadows I, Adamo P, Heikkila RE, Duvoisin RC. (1984). Murine model of MPTP-induced parkinsonism: histopathology. 14th Annual Meeting Soc. for Neuroscience, 10: 705.

Jarvis MF, Wagner CG. (1985). Neurochemical and functional consequences following 1-methyl-4-phenyl-1,2,3,6-tetrahydropyridine (MPTP) and methamphetamine. *Life Sci* 36: 249–254.

Javitch JA, D'Amato RJ, Strittmatter SM, Snyder SH. (1985). Parkinsonism-inducing neurotoxin, N-methyl-4-phenyl-1,2,3,6-tetrahydropyridine by dopamine neurons explains selective toxicity. *Proc Natl Acad Sci USA* 82: 2173–2177.

Jenner P, Rupniak NMJ, Rose S, Kelly E, Kilpatrick G, Lees A, Marsden CD. (1984). 1-Methyl-4-phenyl-1,2,3,6-tetrahydropyridine-induced parkinsonism in the common marmoset. *Neurosci Letts* 50: 85–90.

Johannessen JN, Kelner L, Hanselman D, Shih MC, Markey SP. (1985). In vitro oxidation of MPTP by primate neural tissue: a potential model of MPTP neurotoxicity. *Neurochem Int* 7: 169–176.

Langston JW. (1985). MPTP neurotoxicity: an overview and characterization of phases of toxicity. *Life Sci* 36: 201–206.

Langston JW, Ballard PA. (1983). Parkinson's disease in a chemist working with 1-methyl-4-phenyl-1,2,3,6-tetrahydropyridine. *N Engl J Med* 309: 310.

Langston JW, Ballard PA. (1984). Parkinsonism induced by 1-methyl-4-phenyl-1,2,3,6-tetrahydropyridine (MPTP): implications for treatment and the pathogenesis of Parkinson's disease. *Can J Neurol Sci* 11: 160–165.

Langston JW, Ballard PA, Tetrud JW, Irwin I. (1983). Chronic parkinsonism in humans due to a product of meperidine-analog synthesis. *Science* 219: 979–980.

Langston JW, Forno LS, Rebert CS, Irwin I. (1984). Selective nigral toxicity after systemic administration of 1-methyl-4-phenyl-1,2,3,6-tetrahydropyridine (MPTP) in the squirrel monkey. *Brain Res* 292: 390–394.

Markey SP, Johannessen JN, Chiueh CC, Burns RS, Herkenham MA. (1984). Intraneuronal generation of a pyridinium metabolite may cause drug-induced parkinsonism. *Nature* 311: 464–467.

Nicklas WJ, Vyas I, Heikkila RE. (1985). Inhibition of NADH-linked oxidation in brain mitochondria by 1-methyl-4-phenylpyridine, a metabolite of the neurotoxin, 1-methyl-4-phenyl-1,2,3,6-tetrahydropyridine. *Life Sci* 36: 2503–2508.

Perry TL, Yong VW, Ito M, Jones K, Wall RA, Foulks JG, Wright JM, Kish SJ. (1985). 1-Methyl-4-phenyl-1,2,3,6-tetrahydropyridine (MPTP) does not destroy nigrostriatal neurons in the scorbutic guinea pig. *Life Sci* 36: 1233–1238.

Schmidt CJ, Bruckwick E, Lovenberg W. (1985). Lack of evidence supporting a role for dopamine in 1-methyl-4-phenyl-1,2,3,6-tetrahydropyridine neurotoxicity. *Eur J Pharmacol* 113: 149–150.

Snyder SH. (1984). Parkinson's disease: clues to aetiology from a toxin. *Nature*
    311: 514.
Ward CD, Duvoisin RC, Ince SE, Nutt JG, Eldridge R, Calne DB. (1983). Parkin-
    son's disease in 65 pairs of twins and in a set of quadruplets. *Neurology* 33:
    815–825.
Wright JM, Wall RA, Perry TL, Paty DW. (1983). Chronic parkinsonism
    secondary to intranasal administration of a product of meperidine–analogue
    synthesis. *N Engl J Med* 310: 325.

14
Animal Models Used to Evaluate Potential Antiparkinsonian Drugs

JOHN H. GORDON
The Chicago Medical School, North Chicago, Illinois

WILLIAM C. KOLLER
Loyola University Stritch School of Medicine, Maywood, Illinois

It has been known for many years that the anatomical substrate for Parkinson's disease is a profound loss of neurons in the substantia nigra (1,2). The biochemical substrate for this disease however, appears to be the loss of endogenous dopamine in the basal ganglia, which results from the loss of dopamine-containing neurons in the substantia nigra, which project to the basal ganglia. Currently the most efficacious drug for the treatment of Parkinson's disease is the dopamine precursor levodopa. Levodopa has no direct effect on dopamine receptors in the basal ganglia, instead it acts indirectly by increasing the levels of endogenous dopamine. Levodopa therapy is thought to increase the levels of endogenous dopamine by being decarboxylated to dopamine in the remaining dopamine nerve terminals and/or alternative sites such as other monoamine nerve terminals, glial cells or vascular smooth muscle and endothelial cells. In addition to levodopa a variety of direct-acting dopamine agonists have been shown to alleviate the symptoms of Parkinson's disease. Thus any drug with central dopaminergic activity could have potential as an antiparkinson agent. However, the site (anatomical location) and type of dopamine receptor may vary with the animal model used to evaluate the central dopaminergic activity of drugs.

CENTRAL DOPAMINERGIC PATHWAYS

Several distinct dopaminergic neuronal systems have been described with respect to their anatomy (Table 1) and function (3). The nigrostriatal pathway is of

TABLE 1 Dopamine Neuronal Pathways

Neural system	Nucleus of origin	Site(s) of termination
Nigrostriatal	Substantia nigra	Basal ganglia
		Caudate–putamen
Mesolimbic	Substantia nigra and ventral tegmental area	Limbic forebrain
		Olfactory tubercle
		Amygdaloid complex
		Nucleus accumbens septi
		Lateral and medial septum
Mesocortical	Substantia nigra and ventral tegmental area	Cortical areas
		Prefrontal
		Entorhinal
		Perirhinal
		Piriform
		Cingulate
Tuberohypophyseal	Arcuate and periventricular nucleus	External layer of the median eminence; neural and intermediate lobe of the pituitary
Incertohypothalamic	Zona incerta and periventricular hypothalamus	Zona incerta, preoptic area and periventricular hypothalamus; septum
Periventricular	Periaqueductal gray; periventricular gray of the thalamus	Periaqueductal gray, medial thalamus, and hypothalamus
Retinal	Inner nuclear layer of the retina	Inner and outer plexiform layers of retina
Periglomerular	Periglomerular cells of the olfactory bulb	Glomeruli (mitral cells)

primary importance in Parkinson's disease as the axons for this tract arise from the substantia nigra and project to the caudate/putamen. Other dopamine systems that may be relevant during the treatment of Parkinson's disease are the mesolimbic and mesocortical dopamine systems. The mesolimbic dopamine cells originate in the substantia nigra and/or ventral tegmental area and project diffusely to the olfactory tubercle, nucleus accumbens, septum, and amygdala complex. The mesocortical dopamine system also originates in cell bodies located in the substantia nigra and/or ventral tegmental area, similar to the mesolimbic, but projects diffusely to areas of the frontal cortex. The mesolimbic and mesocortical dopamine systems are thought to be involved in the psychiatric manifestations or side effects related to chronic levodopa therapy.

DOPAMINE RECEPTORS

Current evidence suggests that there are multiple types and/or subtypes of dopamine receptors in the central nervous system. In addition to multiple dopamine receptors, there are at least five distinct anatomical sites where dopamine receptors are thought to exist (4). Classically one thinks of a neurotransmitter receptor as being located postsynaptic to the nerve terminal, and the basal ganglia is no exception: postsynaptic dopamine receptors are found on the dendrites and/or soma of interneurons and on axons (nerve terminals) of neurons projecting into the basal ganglia (i.e., cortical afferents). However dopamine receptors are located not only postsynaptic to the dopamine neuron but also on the dopamine neuron itself. These dopamine receptors have been termed autoreceptors and are found on all parts of the dopamine neuron, including cell processes within the substantia nigra (i.e., dendritic autoreceptors) and on the dopamine nerve terminals located in the basal ganglia (i.e., presynaptic autoreceptors). In addition to these four distinct anatomical sites within the nigrostriatal system, dopamine receptors are also found on presynaptic or axonal elements of the striatonigral system in the substantia nigra.

Dopamine receptors have been classified according to either the behavioral, biochemical, or electrophysiological responses that they mediate or by ligand binding studies. Unfortunately, these various methods of classification have resulted in the reporting of at least 18 different dopamine receptors and/or binding sites. Most of these putative receptors or binding sites will probably be in search of a physiological function for a very long time, if not forever. Fortunately, however, there are some aspects of the dopamine receptor nomenclature that most investigators can agree on. For example the nomenclature proposed by Kebabian and Calne (5) that divides dopamine receptors into two categories, D-1 and D-2, is generally accepted. In this classification the D-1 receptors are coupled to adenylate cyclase and increase the activity of this enzyme. A prototype of the D-1 receptor is found in the parathyroid glands where dopamine agonists stimulate cAMP synthesis and parathyroid hormone release (6). The D-2 receptors were originally classified by the process of exclusion, that is, not associated with the stimulation of adenylate cyclase activity, although recently the D-2 dopamine receptors have been postulated to be negatively linked to this enzyme (6). Even though no clear or unifying concept has been formulated with regard to the molecular events that occur following D-2 receptor activation, evidence does suggest that the antiparkinsonian effects of dopamine agonists are mediated predominantly through D-2 receptor activation (6).

Receptor binding techniques have existed for over a decade, and there are a variety of [3H] ligands available for labeling the various proposed dopamine receptors (4,6,7). Compounds can be tested for their ability to displace the various dopamine-receptor-targeted ligands and their relative potency or affinity can be estimated and compared to prototype drugs. In general there is a good correlation between agonist-induced behaviors in animals, the antiparkinsonian action in humans, and the IC_{50} value for displacing [3H] neuroleptics from striatal membranes by dopamine agonists. In addition, binding techniques offer the advantage of directly testing the potency or affinity for dopamine receptors at distinct anatomical sites (i.e., mesolimbic vs. basal ganglia, etc.). Although receptor binding techniques have several distinct advantages, the inherent problems of not distinguishing agonists from antagonists, or the possible lack of in vivo activity because of pharmacokinetic or distribution problems and the unproven predictive power, have generally placed these techniques into a confirmatory rather than discovery role in most pharmaceutical houses.

In the past, based on receptor binding techniques, all D-2 dopamine receptors were proposed to be located solely postsynaptic to the dopamine nerve terminals in the basal ganglia (4,7). The high-affinity (nM range) binding sites for [3H]-spiroperidol in striatal membranes are saturable, stereospecific, and appear to be homogeneous. Moreover, these high-affinity binding sites for [3H] spiroperidol, and other butyrophenones, have been used empirically to define the D-2 dopamine receptors (4,6,7). However the release-inhibiting, presynaptic dopamine autoreceptors also have nM affinities for the butyrophenones (8-10); thus we must either redefine the D-2 dopamine receptor or accept that the presynaptic dopamine autoreceptors are D-2 or "D-2 like" receptors, as are the dendritic/somatic dopamine autoreceptors in the substantia nigra.

In the striatum, the D-1 dopamine receptors, unlike the D-2s, appear to be entirely postsynaptic to the dopamine neurons. In the substantia nigra the D-1 dopamine receptors appear to be located presynaptically on the striatonigral axon terminals.

LOCOMOTOR AND STEREOTYPIC BEHAVIOR

A common property of dopaminergic agonists is the production of locomotor and/or stereotype responses (11,12). The specific characteristics of these behavioral changes are species and dose specific (12–15). In rats dopamine agonists will induce a syndrome of increased locomotor activity and/or stereotypic behavior consisting of repetitive movements of the head and forelegs, sniffing, licking, biting, and gnawing (14,15). In the guinea pig, the pattern of stereotypic behavior is usually less complex than that displayed by the rat, and it consists predominantly of increased locomotion and gnawing (16). Quantification of these dopamine-agonist-induced behavioral changes has generally been accomplished by assigning numeric values to specific behavior(s) and "scoring" the intensity of the stereotypic by an observer (11). One of the major drawbacks to scoring stereotypic behavior by assigning values to various patterns of behavior is that the scale may be arbitrary. Moreover, often the observer must decide whether or not to assign an animal to one group or another. Even if the observer is blinded to the treatments the assignment of a specific score to a complex behavior or group of behaviors can be arbitrary. Some investigators have attempted to circumvent this inherent problem by scoring the incidence of specific, easily defined behaviors (14,15). Using these techniques, the observers no longer need to make decisions as to what predominant behavior(s) or pattern of behaviors are being displayed by the animals, they only need to score the presence of specific, defined behaviors.

DOPAMINE AND DOPAMINE AGONISTS

The local intracerebral injection of dopamine has been shown to produce behavioral changes, such as increased locomotor activity and stereotypy behavior in several species (17). The dopamine precursor, L-dopa, when injected systemically, can also stimulate these behaviors. However the intensity of the stereotypy behavior produced by L-dopa is low relative to other dopamine agonists, unless a dopadecarboxylase inhibitor is administered concomitantly, in which case the intensity of the induced stereotypy can reach maximal levels.

Apomorphine is the prototype of the direct-acting dopamine agonists and is the drug to which most new dopamine agonists are compared. Apomorphine, and most direct-acting agonists (18,19) will induce a biphasic response in terms of locomotor activity. When low doses are administered, a decrease in locomotor activity will be apparent. This decreased locomotor response is thought to represent the "selective" activation of dopamine autoreceptors, which effectively antagonizes the endogenous dopamine activity by inhibiting its release (20).

Most investigators interpret the selective activation of the dopamine autoreceptors by low doses of apomorphine or other dopamine agonists as indicative of
a higher affinity for these receptors. Although this may be the case, this biphasic
response may only represent a distribution or access phenomenon rather than a
profound difference in affinity of the dopamine agonists for subpopulations of
dopamine receptors. At higher doses, apomorphine, and other direct-acting
agonists, still effectively antagonize the release of endogenous dopamine by activating the dopamine autoreceptors. However, at these higher doses enough of
the drug gets into the synaptic cleft to activate postsynaptic dopamine receptor
responses, such as increased locomotor responses and stereotypic behavior.

Amphetamine is considered to be the prototype indirect-acting dopamine
agonist. Amphetamine increases dopaminergic activity by increasing the amount
of dopamine released from the nerve terminals. Thus, for amphetamine to act as
a dopamine agonist, there must be adequate endogenous dopamine innervation
and presynaptic storage. Like apomorphine, amphetamine is widely used as a
neuropharmacologic research tool, and it is well established that its administration will result in a dose-dependent increase in locomotor activity and in the induction of stereotypic behavior. Although both amphetamine and apomorphine
are dopamine agonists, their patterns of behavioral activation are quite different
(14).

ANIMAL MODELS USED TO EVALUATE
DOPAMINE AGONISTS

Stereotypic Behavior

Because dopamine in the striatum appears to be involved in motor regulation,
the production of either locomotor or stereotypic behavior by dopamine
agonists can be used to evaluate potential dopamine agonists (18,19). Current
data suggest that dopaminergic mechanisms in the nucleus accumbens may be
involved in dopamine agonist-induced locomotion (21), and that stereotypy behavior appears to represent the stimulation of striatal dopamine receptors (22).
The ability of various agents to produce locomotor or stereotypic behavior is
considered a reflection of their ability to act as dopamine agonists at these
distinct anatomic locations.

If the dopamine receptors in the mesocortic and mesolimbic projection areas
are involved in the psychiatric side effects of levodopa therapy, then one would
hope to find drugs with reduced efficacy for the locomotor responses while retaining full activity in producing stereotypic behavior.

Emetic Activity

Another property of drugs that possess central dopaminergic activity is the
ability to induce vomiting in several animal species (23). Apomorphine is a po-

tent emetic in cats, dogs, and humans. The dog is relatively sensitive to the emetic effects of apomorphine and is an animal commonly used to study emesis. In addition to apomorphine, several other dopamine agonists, including levodopa and bromocriptine, are potent emetics. It is interesting that indirect-acting dopamine agonists that require an intact endogenous innervation, (i.e., amphetamine) are not potent emetic drugs. This suggests that the dopamine receptors that mediate emesis are not neurotransmitter receptors since they appear to lack endogenous dopaminergic innervation.

The site of action for apomorphine and other emetic drugs is thought to be the chemoreceptor trigger zone in the floor of the fourth ventricle in the medulla oblongata. Ablation of this area will prevent the effects of most emetic agents; thus, the ability of drugs to induce emesis is a reflection of their ability to activate dopamine receptors in the area postrema. Vomiting is a common clinical problem, and there are many studies testing the efficacy of drugs as antiemetics. Phenothiazine and butyrophenone compounds are very potent antiemetics both in animal models and in clinical practice. These drugs are generally thought to act by blocking dopamine receptors, but their antiemetic efficacy does not parallel their efficacy in blocking dopamine receptors in the extrapyramidal system. Thus there may be some hope of developing direct-acting dopamine agonists with a reduced affinity for the dopamine receptors in the area postrema, while retaining full activity at striatal receptor sites.

Thermoregulatory Effects of Dopamine Agonists

The activation of central dopamine receptors will induce thermoregulatory changes in several species (24). The systemic administration of dopamine agonists will induce hypothermia in rats and mice, while in the rabbit apomorphine causes a rise in core body temperature. This difference in response probably relates to the mechanisms used by these different species to regulate temperature, since rodents depend upon liver metabolism, while rabbits use muscle contraction to increase body temperature. However, both the hypothermic effect in rodents and the hyperthermic effect in rabbits can be blocked by dopamine-receptor-blocking agents. For example, pimozide will inhibit apomorphine-induced changes in core temperature when given either systemically or injected bilaterally into the hypothalamus. Similarly, apomorphine and dopamine injected directly into the hypothalamus will induce hypothermia in rats and mice in a dose-related manner. These and other experiments have suggested that the dopamine receptors involved in the thermoregulatory responses are those in the preoptic anterior hypothalamic areas of the brain, and it has been suggested that endogenous dopamine has a physiologic role in thermoregulation by acting to lower the temperature set-point in the hypothalamus (24).

Thermoregulatory responses can also be obtained by direct injection of apomorphine into other brain areas, including the caudate nucleus and the nucleus accumbens. Moreover, cholinergic and serotonergic mechanisms also appear to be involved in thermoregulation. Thus thermoregulation is complex and probably involves multiple brain pathways and mechanisms and so is of minimal value in screening new therapeutic agents for antiparkinsonian efficacy.

Lesion Models

In primates the most consistent observation following large substantia nigra lesions that do not affect adjoining structures is hypokinesia (25,26). Small lesions of the substantia nigra that do not reduce the endogenous levels of dopamine dramatically are generally without neurologic effects (25). Hypokinesia has also been observed in unlesioned primates following drugs that deplete catecholamines, such as reserpine and alpha-methyl-paratyrosine (27,28). Extensive lesions of the substantia nigra in primates do not lead to a typical parkinsonian tremor, unless there is a concomitant lesions of the red nucleus (25,29). Similarly, lesions of the red nucleus alone do not produce tremor unless the nigrostriatal dopamine system is compromised either by lesions or by the administration of dopamine depleting drugs (30).

In rodents, bilateral lesions of the nigrostriatal system, whether produced electrolytically or with the neurotoxin 6-hydroxydopamine, result in behavioral hyperactivity for the first few hours after lesioning (31–33). This hyperactive phase is thought to result from the release of dopamine from the degenerating terminals in the striatum. Following the hyperactive phase, a syndrome consisting of aphagia, adipsia, akinesia, and sensorimotor disintegration is observed (32,33). The administration of apomorphine or L-dopa will reverse this syndrome (34,35). Most animals will recover from this syndrome within several days to a few weeks after the lesion (32). However, the process of recovery is not uniform, and animals may show phases of hypophagia and hypodipsia. Even though these animals develop a hypersensitivity to dopamine agonists, they are not routinely used to evaluate new dopamine agonists.

When nigrostriatal 6-hydroxydopamine lesions are limited to one side, unilateral hypokinesia and sensorimotor disintegration are observed. Hypophagia and hypodipsia are also observed after unilateral lesions, but are much less pronounced than in bilaterally lesioned animals (36). Animals tend to deviate spontaneously toward the side of the lesion. The injection of dopamine agonists results in a tight head-to-tail rotation. Turning or rotational behavior is thought to result from an imbalance of striatal dopamine receptor stimulation. Following administrational apomorphine or other direct-acting dopamine agonists, lesioned animals will turn in a direction opposite to the lesion. The administration of indirect-acting agonists (i.e., amphetamine) will result in the animal turning toward the side of the lesion. The rotation model offers several advantages for evaluating potential dopamine agonists, among which are the ability to separate the pre- from the postsynaptic effects of the agonists.

PHARMACOLOGIC MODELS

Dopamine Antagonists

Various pharmacologic agents have been used to investigate basic dopaminergic and/or parkinsonian compensatory mechanisms. Reserpine, a rauwolfia alkaloid, has been used as a model of parkinsonism (37). In rats it causes a syndrome characterized by increased muscle tone, lack of spontaneous movements, hunchback posture, and ptosis. A dose of 5 mg/kg will produce maximal changes in 24 hr. Similar behavioral effects are produced by other reserpine-like drugs such as tetrabenazine, a synthetic benzoquinolizine. Patients taking reserpine for psychiatric conditions or for control of blood pressure often develop a form of drug-induced parkinsonism indistinguishable from Parkinson's disease.

Reserpine depletes dopamine in the striatum and other dopamine-containing regions of the brain by blocking the uptake and storage of monoamines into synaptic vesicles (37). The extrapyramidal syndrome induced by reserpine in humans is probably secondary to a dopamine deficiency in the basal ganglia. Reserpine also decreases the levels of norepinephrine and serotonin in the brain; however, there is a good temporal correlation between the motor disorders induced and the degree of dopamine depletion in the striata of animals. Moreover levodopa, but not serotonin precursors, will readily reverse the reserpine-induced syndrome in both animals and humans. Other dopamine agonists such as apomorphine and amphetamine will reverse the reserpine-induced syndrome. Amphetamine will reverse the reserpine-induced syndrome because it releases the newly formed or unbound dopamine stores, while reserpine depletes the bound dopamine (i.e., the dopamine contained in the storage granules).

Another drug that causes dopamine depletion is alpha-methyl paratyrosine (AMPT), which acts by inhibiting tyrosine hydroxylase, the rate-limiting enzyme in the synthesis of dopamine. Like reserpine, AMPT can worsen symptoms in parkinsonian patients. The administration of AMPT to rats (200 mg/kg) will significantly decrease striatal dopamine levels in 2 hr and induce a syndrome of hypoactivity (38). Levodopa and apomorphine will reverse this syndrome but amphetamine will not. Amphetamine releases dopamine from the unbound or newly formed dopamine stores that are sensitive to AMPT.

Reserpine and AMPT, besides being used to test for drugs with dopaminergic activity, are useful either alone or in combination in determining whether dopaminergic drugs are acting through pre- or postsynaptic mechanisms. If a drug is behaviorally active when animals are pretreated with both reserpine and AMPT, it is assumed that the agent is acting directly on postsynaptic receptors.

The neuroleptic or antipsychotic drugs, regardless of chemical classification, will decrease spontaneous motor activity and will antagonize the behavioral and neurochemical effects of dopaminergic drugs (39) and will precipitate a parkinsonianlike syndrome in humans (40). These actions are thought to be related to the ability of these drugs to block the dopamine receptors competitively. Investigations of dopamine agonists routinely test for the ability of neuroleptics to block the observed effects. Specific blockade of D-1 (SCH 23390) and D-2 (sulpiride) dopamine receptor blockers has been reported (41). Recent data also suggest that some neuroleptics may have a greater affinity for either the dopamine autoreceptors or the postsynaptic or "classic" D-2 dopamine receptors (42). Although the role, if any, for the proposed dopamine autoreceptors in the treatment of the symptoms of Parkinson's disease would appear to be negligible because of the loss of the presynaptic elements in the basal ganglia, the role of these receptors in mediating the adverse effects of levodopa therapy has not been studied.

Tremorine and Oxotremorine

Tremorine and its active metabolite oxotremorine will induce an autonomic activation and a syndrome of tremor, rigidity, and hypothermia in several animal species (43).

Tremorine produces its effects directly in the central nervous system by increasing acetylcholine. Tremorine- and oxotremorine-induced tremor is blocked by anticholinergic drugs. Anticholinergic drugs have been used in the treatment of Parkinson's disease symptoms for over a hundred years, but possess only limited efficacy. Duvoisin (44) observed that centrally active cholinergics exacerbated parkinsonism and antagonized the therapeutic effects of anticholinergics. Klawans (45) has suggested that a dopamine–acetylcholine balance exists in the striatum. Tremorine-induced tremor is not a model of parkinsonian tremor; it does, however, provide a model to test drugs for anticholinergic activity.

COMPLICATIONS OF CHRONIC THERAPY

Levodopa provides adequate therapy for the symptoms of Parkinson's disease during the initial years of treatment. Thereafter, complications including loss of efficacy, fluctuations in motor performance, and psychiatric side effects may intervene. Because of the problems with long-term levodopa therapy, other drugs have been sought that might be devoid of these complications. It has been suggested that various animal models may have value in predicting the potential of therapeutic agents for inducing these long-term side effects.

The loss of clinical efficacy observed with chronic levodopa therapy has been postulated to be due to combined progression of the underlying disease and alteration of dopamine receptor sensitivity with long-term therapy (46). Chronic levodopa treatment may induce the down-regulation of dopamine receptors. In studies with rodents, dopamine receptor supersensitivity induced by denervation or chronic neuroleptic treatment can be reversed with chronic levodopa or other dopamine agonists, such as pergolide (46–48). In animals with unilateral 6-hydroxydopamine lesions of the substantia nigra, chronic treatment with levodopa and pergolide reversed the increase in striatal [^{3}H] spiroperidol binding sites (46). In Parkinson's disease the postsynaptic dopamine receptors may become hypersensitive in an attempt to compensate for the loss of presynaptic elements, thus increasing the potency of the dopamine released from the remaining neurons (49). The density of dopamine receptors in postmortem brains from parkinsonian patients not treated with levodopa has been reported to be higher than in nonparkinsonian controls, while levodopa-treated patients have a normal or decreased density of dopamine receptors in the basal ganglia (50). Thus the dopamine-agonist-induced down-regulation of dopamine receptors may result in the loss of its therapeutic efficacy. The clinical observation that efficacy is sometimes restored after temporary drug withdrawal suggests that reversible pharmacodynamic changes of dopamine receptors may occur in Parkinson's disease (51).

The mechanisms of levodopa-induced involuntary movements and mental changes may be related to dopamine receptor hypersensitivity. In rats, the long-term administration of dopamine agonists will result in an enhancement of locomotor and stereotypic behavior (52). This behavioral supersensitivity has been observed following levodopa, bromocriptine, and pergolide (53,54) treatment, but not with the partial dopamine agonists ciladopa and quinpirole (18, 19). In this experimental paradigm the chronic administration of levodopa renders the animals hypersensitive to subsequent challenge with apomorphine. This agonist-induced hypersensitivity usually lasts several weeks after cessation of the chronic treatment. In this model, doses of agonists that would not induce behavioral changes before initiation of the chronic treatment will induce stereotypic behavior after chronic administration. Apomorphine given chronically does not produce supersensitivity, probably because of its short duration of action (55). Levodopa-induced dyskinesias and psychiatric side effects are related to the duration of therapy (56). Whether or not these effects of chronic levodopa are due to an agonist-induced receptor hypersensitivity will need the support of future studies in both animal models and Parkinson's disease. Currently the value of this model in predicting psychomotor toxicity of drugs remains unproven.

CONCLUSIONS

Several animal models are available to test for the presence of central dopaminergic activity. Prudent use of the presently available animal models can define direct or indirect, full or partial agonist properties and location and subtype(s) of dopamine receptors. In general, drugs that stimulate D-2 dopamine receptors in the central nervous system will possess some efficacy in the treatment of Parkinson's disease symptoms. However it is currently impossible to predict from animal models whether a compound will cause the long-term side effects associated with levodopa therapy. The use of animal models for the design and evaluation of drugs will become more valuable as our knowledge of the basic mechanisms involved in basal ganglia function and the pathophysiology of Parkinson's disease increases.

REFERENCES

1. Blocq P, Marinesco G. (1893). Sur un cas de tremblement parkinsonien hemiplegique. Symptomatique d'une tumeur du pedoncule cérébral. *CR Soc Biol* 5: 105–111.
2. Hassler R. (1938). Pathologie der paralysis agitans und des postenzephalitischen Parkinsonismus. *J Psychol Neurol* 48: 387–476.
3. Moore RY, Bloom FE. (1978). Central catecholamine neuron systems. *Annu Rev Neurosci* 1: 129–179.
4. Creese I. (1982). Dopamine receptors explained. *Trends Neurosci* 5: 40–43.
5. Kebabian JW, Calne DB. (1979). Multiple receptors for dopamine. *Nature* 277: 93–96.
6. Creese I, Sibley DR, Hamblin MW, Leff SE. (1983). The classification of dopamine receptors. *Annu Rev Neurosci* 6: 43–71.
7. Seeman P. (1981). Brain dopamine receptors. *Pharmacol Rev* 32: 229–313.
8. Abrilla S, Langer SZ. (1980). Stereoselectivity of presynaptic autoreceptors modulating dopamine release. *Eur J Pharmacol* 76: 345–351.
9. Starke K, Reimann W, Zumstein A, Hertting G. (1978). Effect of dopamine receptor agonists and antagonists on the release of dopamine in the rabbit caudate nucleus in vitro. *Arch Pharmacol* 302: 27–36.
10. Cebuddu LX, Hoffmann IS, James MK, Niedzwiecki DM. (1983). Changes in the sensitivity of dopamine receptors modulating dopamine and acetylcholine release after chronic treatment with bromocriptine or haloperidol. *J Pharmacol Exp Ther* 226: 680–685.
11. Ernst AM. (1967). Mode of action of apomorphine and dextroamphetamine in gnawing compulsion in rats. *Psychopharmacologia* 10: 316–323.
12. Randrup A, Munkvad I. (1968). Behavioral stereotypies induced by pharmacological agents. *Pharmacopsychiatrie* 1: 18–26.
13. Fog R. (1969). Stereotyped and non-stereotyped behavior in rats induced by various stimulant drugs. *Psychopharmacologia* 14: 299–314.
14. Fray PJ, Sahakian BJ, Robbins TW, Koob GF, Iversen SD. (1980). An observation method for quantifying the behavioral effects of dopamine agonists: contrasting effects of d-amphetamine and apomorphine. *Psychopharmacologia* 69: 253–259.
15. Gordon JH, Diamond BI. (1984). Enhancement of hypophysectomy-induced dopamine receptor hypersensitivity in male rats by chronic haloperidol administration. *J Neurochem* 42: 523–528.

16. Koller WC, Diamond BI, Nausieda PA, Weiner WJ, Klawans HL. (1980). The pharmacologic evaluation of pergolide mesilate as an antiparkinson agent. *Neuropharmacology* 19: 831–837.
17. Cools AR. (1973). Chemical and electrical stimulation of the caudate nucleus in freely moving cats: the role of dopamine. *Brain Res* 58: 437–451.
18. Koller WC, Fields JZ, Gordon JH, Perlow MJ. (1986). Evaluation of ciladopa hydrochloride as a potential anti-parkinsonism drug. *Neuropharmacology* 25: 973–981.
19. Koller WC, Herbster G, Gordon JH, Anderson D. (1987). Quinpirole, a potential anti-parkinsonism drug. *Neuropharmacology*, in press.
20. Montanaro N, Vaccheri A, Dall'Olio R, Gandolfi O. (1983). Time course of rat motility response to apomorphine: a model to study brain dopamine receptors. *Psychopharmacology* 81: 214–219.
21. Gordon JH. (1983). Hypophysectomy-induced striatal hypersensitivity and mesolimbic hyposensitivity to apomorphine. *Pharmacol Biochem Behav* 19: 807–811.
22. Pigrenberg AAJ, Honig WMM, Van Rossum JM. (1975). Antagonism of apomorphine and d-amphetamine-induced stereotypic behavior by injection of low doses of haloperidol into the caudate nucleus and the nucleus accumbens. *Psychopharmacologica* 45: 65–71.
23. Borison HL, Wang SC. (1953). Physiology and pharmacology of vomiting. *Pharmacol Rev* 5: 193–230.
24. Cox B, Lee TF. (1979). Effect of central injections of dopamine on core and thermoregulatory behavior in unrestrained rats. *Neuropharmacology* 18: 537–550.
25. Poirer LJ, Sourkes TL, Bouvier G, Boucher R, Carabin S. (1966). Striatal amines, experimental tremor and the effect of harmaline in the monkey. *Brain* 89: 37–52.
26. Viallet F, Trouche E, Beaubaton D, Nieoullon A, Legallet E. (1981). Bradykinesia following unilateral lesions restricted to the substantia nigra in the baboon. *Neurosci Letts* 24: 97–102.
27. Windle WF, Cammermayer J. (1958). Functional and structural observations in chronically reserpinised monkeys. *Science* 127: 1503.
28. Bedard P, Larochelle L, Poirer LJ, Sourkes TL. (1976). Reversible effect of L-dopa on tremor and catatonia induced by alpha-methyl-p-tyrosine. *Can J Physiol Pharmacol* 48: 82–84.
29. Velasco F, Valasco M, Romo R, Maldonado H. (1979). Production and suppression of tremor by mesencephalic tegmental lesions in monkeys. *Exp Neurol* 64: 516–527.
30. Poirer LJ, Bouvier G, Bedard P, Boucher R, Larochelle L, Olivier A, Singh P. (1969). Essai sur circuits neuronaux impliqués dans le tremblement postural et l'hypokinesie. *Rev Neurol* 120: 15–40.
31. Iversen SD. (1971). The effect of surgical lesions to frontal cortex and substantia nigra on amphetamine responses in rats. *Brain Res* 31: 295–311.

32. Ungerstedt U. (1971). Adipsia and aphagia after 6-hydroxydopamine induced degeneration of the nigrostriatal dopamine system. *Acta Physiol Scand* Suppl. 367: 95–117.

33. Fibiger HC, Lonbury B, Cooper HP, Lytle LD. (1972). Early behavioral effects of intraventricular administration of 6-hydroxydopamine in rat. *Nature New Biol* 236: 209–211.

34. Ljungberg T. (1976). Ungerstedt U: Reinstatement of eating by dopamine agonists in aphagic dopamine denervated rats. *Physiol Behav* 16: 277–283.

35. Butterworth RF, Belanger F, Barbeau A. (1978). Hypokinesia produced by anterolateral hypothalamic 6-hydroxydopamine lesions and its reversal by some antiparkinson drugs. *Pharmacol Biochem Behav* 8: 41–45.

36. Ungerstedt U. (1971). Striatal dopamine release after amphetamine or nerve degeneration revealed by rotational behaviour. *Acta Physiol Scand* Suppl 367: 49–68.

37. Roos B, Steg G. (1964). The effect of L-3,4-dihydroxyphenylalanine and dl-5-hydroxytryptophan on rigidity and tremor induced by reserpine chlorpromazine and phenoxybenzamine. *Life Sci* 3: 251–360.

38. Gordon JH, Shellenberger MK. (1974). Regional catecholamine content in the rat brain: sex differences and correlation with motor activity. *Neuropharmacology* 13: 129–137.

39. Van Rossum JM. (1960). The significance of dopamine receptor antagonism for the mechanism of action of neuroleptic drugs. *Arch Int Pharmaco Ther* 160: 492–495.

40. Baldessarini RJ. (1960). Drugs and the treatment of psychiatric disorders. In: Gilman AG, Goodman ls, Gilman A (Eds.), *The Pharmacological Basis of Therapeutics*. New York, Macmillan.

41. Arnt J, Hyttel J. (1985). Differential involvement of dopamine D-1 and D-2 receptors in rotation induced by apomorphine, SKF 38393, pergolide and LY 171555 in 6-hydroxydopamine-lesioned rats. *Psychopharmacology* 85: 346–352.

42. Clopton JK, Koller WC, Curtin JC, Gordon JH. (1985). A role for presynpatic blockade in the development of a neuroleptic-induced dopamine receptor hypersensitivity. *Soc Neurosci Abstr* 11: 924.

43. Everett GM. (1961). Tremorine. *Rev Can Biol* 20: 278–310.

44. Duvosin RC. (1967). Cholinergic-anticholinergic antagonism in parkinsonism. *Arch Neurol* 17: 124–136.

45. Klawans HL. (1968). The pharmacology of parkinsonism. *Dis Nerv Syst* 29: 805–816.

46. Reches A, Wanger HR, Jackson V, Lewis V, Yablonskaya-Adler E, Fahn S. (1984). Chronic levodopa or pergolide administration induces downregulation of dopamine receptors in denervated striatum. *Neurology* 34: 1208–1212.

47. Ezran-Waters C, Seeman P. (1978). L-dopa reversal of hyper-dopaminergic behavior. *Life Sci* 22: 1027–1032.

48. Reches A, Wagner HR, Jiang DA, Jackson V, Fahn S. (1982). The effect of chronic L-dopa administration on supersensitivity pre- and postsynaptic dopaminergic receptors in rat brain. *Life Sci* 11: 37–44.

49. Hornykiewicz O. (1979). Compensatory biochemical changes at the striatal dopamine synapse in Parkinson's disease. *Adv Neurol* 24: 275–281.
50. Rinne UK, Lomberg P, Koskinen V. (1981). Dopamine receptors in the Parkinsonian brain. *J Neurol Transm* 51: 97–109.
51. Weiner WJ, Koller WC, Perlik S, Nausieda PA, Klawans HL. (1980). The role of "drug holiday" in the management of Parkinson's disease. *Neurology* 30: 1257–1261.
52. Klawans HL, Margolin DI. (1975). Amphetamine induced dopaminergic hypersensitivity in guinea pigs. *Arch Gen. Psychiatry* 32: 725–732.
53. Nausieda PA, Weiner WJ, Kanapa DJ, Klawans HL. (1978). Bromocriptine-induced behavioral hypersensitivity: Implications for the therapy of parkinsonism. *Neurology* 28: 1183–1188.
54. Klawans HL, Goetz G, Nausieda PA, Weiner WJ. (1977). Levodopa-induced dopamine receptor hypersensitivity. *Ann Neurol* 2: 125–129.
55. Flemenbaum A. (1979). Failure of apomorphine to induce dopamine receptor hypersensitivity. *Psychopharmacology* 62: 175–179.
56. Klawans HL, Corssett P, Dana N. (1975). Effect of chronic amphetamine exposure on stereotyped behavior: implication for pathogenesis of L-dopa-induced dyskinesia. *Adv Neurol* 9: 105–112.

15
Etiology

J. WILLIAM LANGSTON
Institute for Medical Research, San Jose, California

> The etiology of Parkinson's disease is unknown at this time and there is a dearth of sound clues on which to base reasonable speculations.
>
> Roger C. Duvoisin, 1982

Because we still do not know the cause of Parkinson's disease, writing a chapter on this subject is always challenging. As highlighted in the above quotation, even identifying reasonable speculations has been a trying affair. However, during the last few years there been a true renaissance of interest in the search for an etiology of Parkinson's disease. In fact, the area is virtually bustling with new ideas. Although it remains to be determined just how close we really are to unraveling some of the basic questions, several recent observations have sharply focused attention on environmental factors that might cause Parkinson's disease. One objective in this chapter will be to explore these thoroughly. Whether history will confirm or refute some of these new hypotheses remains to be determined. But there is much that is new to report and a chance to review this topic is as welcome as it is timely.

In this discussion I will use the term Parkinson's disease to imply a specific clinicopathologic entity (Duvoisin, 1982; Forno, 1982) with the following characteristics. The disease is gradual in onset, slowly progressive, and typically begins after the age of 40. Cardinal clinical features include bradykinesia, rigidity, tremor, and postural instability. Neuropathologic confirmation of the diagnosis requires, at the very least, cell loss in the substantia nigra and the presence of round concentric inclusions known as Lewy bodies (Forno, 1982). The term "parkinsonism," on the other hand, will be used to refer to any clinical syndrome in which signs typical of Parkinson's disease are prominent, regardless of the cause of the condition or its underlying pathologic substrate (see Chap. 3). This distinction is important because a discussion of etiology of Parkinson's disease becomes unmanageably complicated unless it can be limited to a specific entity. Furthermore, if we are indeed talking about unified disease entity, the likelihood that there may be a single or at least a limited number of causes becomes more tenable and we can indeed begin to talk about *the* etiology of the disease. As pointed out by Barbeau (1984), ". . . proper investigations will only be feasible on completely homogeneous entities."

HYPOTHETICAL CRITERIA

As a guide to judging some of the ideas outlined in this chapter, I would like to suggest several requirements that any hypothesis should be able to satisfy before deserving serious consideration. An hypothesis should be able to explain: (a) the age at onset of the disease, (b) its selectivity for some individuals and not others, (c) the preferential cell death of the neurons in the substantia nigra and other pigmented nuclei in the brainstem, (d) the presence of Lewy bodies, (e) a prolonged preclinical phase, and (f) the progressive nature of the disease. I have not included any requirements about changes in incidence rate over time because of the limited number of relevant studies utilizing community survey techniques, a methodology recommended by Kurland (1958) for the study of Parkinson's disease. I will return to this issue in more detail in the section on epidemiology.

ENVIRONMENTAL FACTORS

Based on currently available evidence, one can launch a formidable argument that Parkinson's disease is due to an environmental toxin. First, the completion of a twin study of Parkinson's disease (Ward et al., 1983) has provided strong evidence against a purely genetic origin for this disease. The concordance rate among twins, in which at least one twin had typical Parkinson's disease, was very low. Further, the concordance in monozygotic twins did not exceed that seen in dizygotic twins, thus confirming the null hypothesis that Parkinson's disease is not genetic in origin. In a recent thorough review of evidence regarding heredity and Parkinson's disease, Duvoisin (1982) concluded ". . . the role of genetic factors in the etiology of Parkinson's disease is negligible and consequently, the disease is acquired." If not genetic in origin, then the disease must be due to something in the environment, but what? The two most obvious candidates are infectious agents and toxins (Duvoisin, 1982).

With regard to infectious agents, one cannot omit mention of postencephalitic parkinsonism. However, it is now widely accepted that this entity is clearly different from Parkinson's disease (Forno, 1982) and, in fact, is now rarely seen

(Rajput et al., 1984). On the other hand, it is quite unusual for chronic parkinsonism to follow other forms of encephalitis (Duvoisin, 1982). Furthermore, Parkinson's disease is virtually devoid of the neuropathologic hallmarks of an infectious process (Forno, 1982). Finally, the disease has yet to prove transmissible, even when techniques for the study of unconventional agents are employed (Gibbs and Gadjusek, 1973). To quote Duvoisin (1982) again, this time in regard to an infectious etiology for Parkinson's disease, "It must be candidly admitted that, at present, there is no positive evidence of any sort in its favor." This line of reasoning leaves us with an environmental toxin as the major remaining contender, and it is in precisely this area that we have a solid new lead.

MPTP AND PARKINSON'S DISEASE

The origin of this "new development" actually dates back to 1947 when a compound known as 1-methyl-4-phenyl-1,2,3,6-tetrahydropyridine (MPTP) was first synthesized (Ziering et al., 1947). Remarkably, MPTP underwent animal testing and clinical trials as a potential antiparkinson agent in the 1950s (Langston, et al., 1984c) and then made the rounds in the illicit drug market on a number of occasions (Davis et al. 1979; Wright et al., 1984) before the final denouement, when it was distributed on a grand scale as synthetic heroin in northern California, and its parkinsonogenic effects were finally recognized (Langston et al., 1983; Ballard et al., 1985; Langston, 1986b). A brief review of the effects of this compound will reveal why it has generated such interest as a potential etiologic agent for Parkinson's disease (see Chap. 3 for a more detailed review). Individuals who injected MPTP under the impression that it was heroin have developed virtually all of the features of Parkinson's disease and, perhaps even more remarkably, their parkinsonism was unalloyed (Ballard et al., 1985). Furthermore, they responded to therapy in an identical manner to that seen in Parkinson's disease. In fact, these patients are now experiencing all of the typical side effects of chronic L-dopa therapy, including "end-of-dose" deterioration, dyskinesias, and "on-off" effects (Langston and Ballard, 1984). Finally, the condition has proved to be permanent in our original seven cases, again similar to Parkinson's disease. Given this remarkable resemblance to the idiopathic disease, it should come as no surprise that the primary lesion in human (Davis et al., 1979) and nonhuman primates (Burns et al., 1983; Langston et al., 1984a; Jenner et al., 1984) is degeneration of the substantia nigra, quite similar to that seen in Parkinson's disease.

Interest in MPTP as a potential environmental agent was further kindled with the discovery of a chemist who had developed Parkinson's disease at the age of 38 while working with the compound for legitimate purposes. This indicates that cutaneous contact or inhalation may be adequate for MPTP to exert its parkinsonogenic effects (Langston and Ballard, 1983). Could MPTP (or a similar compound) be an actual cause of Parkinson's disease? In attempting to answer this question, we should apply the criteria outlined earlier in this chapter. I will begin with the issue of progression.

Is MPTP-induced parkinsonism a progressive disease? We now have preliminary evidence that it may be. In a preliminary study of 40 individuals exposed to MPTP who presented as asymptomatic initially, approximately one-half were found to be complaining of new or worsening symptoms; they included one patient who has experienced progressive micrographia (Langston, 1986a). However, this evidence rests primarily on historical data and we believe that a much larger cohort must be studied over time before the issue of disease progression can be firmly settled (Langston, 1986b).

In terms of neuropathology, MPTP clearly meets another of our criteria; it produces clear and selective degeneration of the substantia nigra (Burns et al., 1983; Langston et al., 1984a; Jenner et al., 1984). On the other hand, one of the major arguments against a direct link between MPTP and Parkinson's disease has been the lack of involvement of another pigmented nucleus in the brain stem, the locus ceruleus. This nucleus is typically affected in Parkinson's disease (Forno, 1982), but not in MPTP-induced parkinsonism (Davis et al., 1979; Burns et al., 1983; Langston et al., 1984a; Jenner et al., 1984). We have now seen unequivocal evidence of damage to the locus ceruleus in nine monkeys given MPTP (unpublished observations). This leaves us only with the need to produce Lewy bodies to fulfil our original neuropathologic criterion. Here there are some new observations as well, as we have recently observed intraneuronal inclusions that bear a definite resemblance to Lewy bodies in several animals (Forno et al., 1986). If these preliminary observations can be confirmed in additional animals, we will indeed be very close to Parkinson's disease.

The two remaining hypothetical criteria against which a potential environmental toxin model must be judged are those relating to aging and individual selectivity.

THE AGING NERVOUS SYSTEM

Donald Calne and I have proposed an hypothesis that could link the relatively late onset of Parkinson's disease with exposure to an environmental toxin (Calne and Langston, 1983). It is worth noting that this hypothesis does not necessarily require that the offending agent be MPTP or an MPTP-like substance, but is compatible with any type of environmental insult to the substantia nigra in early to middle adult life. If such an insult resulted in less than an 80% depletion of striatal dopamine, affected individuals would remain asymptomatic due to the large reserve capacity of this system (Riederer and Wuketich, 1976). However, if the normal age-related decline in striatal dopamine and nigral cell numbers continued (McGeer et al., 1977; Carlsson and Winblad, 1976), such individuals might be expected to become symptomatic at some time later in life (see Fig. 1). This is not really a multifactorial hypothesis, but it suggests that the seeds of the disease (an environmental insult) are sown on fertile ground (normal aging).

This hypothesis implies a prolonged "preclinical phase," and hence meets that criterion as well (see Fig. 1). In fact we have recently demonstrated, using positron emission tomography scanning techniques to assess striatal dopamine content, that such a preclinical state can exist in humans (Calne et al., 1985). This was accomplished by studying individuals known to have had an insult to the substantia nigra due to intravenous injection of MPTP, but who did not as yet have diagnosable parkinsonism (Calne et al., 1985). In these individuals, striatal dopamine levels were lower than in normal controls, but above those seen in patients with Parkinson's disease.

Another attractive feature of this hypothesis is that it has the advantage of being testable. We have now identified over 400 individuals who may have been exposed to MPTP (Ruttenbur et al., 1986). Our hypothesis predicts that many, if not all, of these young individuals will eventually show signs of Parkinson's disease. A major effort is now underway to locate and evaluate them over time. It will be most important to see what the future has in store for these asymptomatic individuals with a "preclinical striatal dopamine deficiency state."

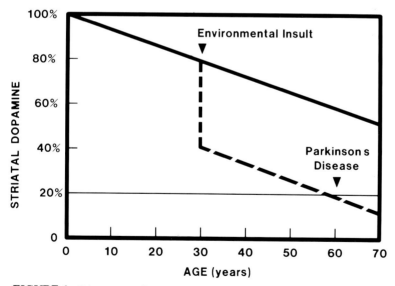

FIGURE 1 Diagrammatic representation showing how an environmental insult at age 30 might produce parkinsonism at age 60, assuming that the striatal dopamine levels continue to decline with aging and an 80% or greater dopamine depletion is required for symptoms to develop.

One could raise the issue of whether Parkinson's disease might simply be an accentuation of the normal aging process; however, there are a number of arguments against this hypothesis (Calne and Langston, 1983) including recent observations that the incidence of the disease may actually begin to decline in the later stages of aging (Koller et al., 1986).

There is a second way in which we might relate the effects of aging to an environmental toxin. Perhaps all of us are exposed to one or more exogenous agents from time to time during life, but certain nuclei become susceptible to the neurodegenerative effects of these compounds only with aging. In the case of Parkinson's disease, this hypothesis requires the existence of a compound that not only affects the substantia nigra selectively but also is age dependent in terms of toxicity. It has recently been shown that MPTP induces extensive nigral cell degeneration in older, but not young mature mice (Ricaurte et al., 1985). Hence MPTP may represent just such a compound. Understanding the mechanism of this age-dependent neuronal degeneration could shed light on the factors leading to the neuronal degeneration that occurs in the aging nervous system of patients with Parkinson's disease.

INDIVIDUAL SELECTIVITY

We are still left with the need to explain the fact that Parkinson's disease affects some individuals but not others. This "individual selectivity" may result from a complex interaction between degree of exposure to one or more toxins and variations in individual susceptibility to these toxins. One of the most striking observations in working with MPTP in primates is a profound degree of variation in the susceptibility to this compound that different animals show.

This concept leads us to another hypothesis recently put forth by Barbeau (1984), who has suggested that disease results from a combination of genetic susceptibility and one or more environmental "trigger factors." Potential trigger factors include stress and environmental toxins. The selectivity for the dopaminergic systems would be accounted for at least in part by the potential for cell damage resulting from oxidative stress resulting from increased catecholamine turnover (Barbeau, 1984; Cohen, 1983). Lewy bodies are explained on the basis of an autoimmune reaction to the damaged nervous system. The attractive element of this hypothesis is that it might explain why both classic epidemiologic and genetic techniques have individually failed to identify clear patterns or clues about the cause of the disease. Problems with the hypothesis include the difficulty in testing it, as well as the fact that there was no trace of the susceptibility factor in the twin study.

However, this same group has gone some distance from the theoretical to the practical in a recent report (Barbeau et al., in press). Struck by the similarity between the 1-methyl-4-phenylpyridinium ion (MPP+: the putative toxic

metabolite of MPTP) (Langston et al., 1984b; Markey et al., 1984) and the
herbicide paraquat, they investigated the prevalence of Parkinson's disease in
Quebec province and found a very uneven distribution of the disease with the
highest concentration in hydrographic region 3 (the province is divided into nine
such regions). It is in region 3 that the agricultural industry is concentrated.
Going a step further, these investigations found a remarkable correlation
between the sales of pesticides and the prevalence of Parkinson's disease. Having
obtained evidence of one or more environmental factors at work, they then
assessed the possibility that a defect in liver detoxifying mechanisms might
represent a potential "susceptibility factor." To do this they studied the ability
to hydroxylate debrisoquine, which involves one or more hepatic cytochromes
in the P 450 system. They found that 68% of patients with Parkinson's disease
were carriers of the gene for this hydroxylization defect, whereas only 18% of
controls were similarly affected. Thus the intriguing possibility is raised that
these individuals might be more susceptible to environmental toxins. As Eldridge
has said "on to a case controlled study!" (Eldridge and Rocca, in press).

ENVIRONMENTAL TOXINS AND THE EPIDEMIOLOGY OF PARKINSON'S DISEASE

Although epidemiologic investigations have yet to provide "any solid clues"
(Chap. 2) about the cause(s) of Parkinson's disease, the fact that the incidence
of Parkinson's disease is not changing has been used to argue against an environmental cause (Duvoisin, 1982; Eldridge and Rocca, in press; also see Chap. 2).
Although it is not clear why this necessarily follows, one presumption may be
that increased production of industrial pollutants, if they are responsible, should
be reflected in an increased incidence of the disease. Careful examination of the
epidemiologic data on which the observation of a "stable incidence" of Parkinson's disease rests is surprisingly limited. In fact, the only sequential study of the
prevalence over time using the community controlled techniques, is that from
Rochester, Minnesota (Rajput et al., 1984). However, this study spans only four
decades (1935-1979). The other report often cited comes from mortality
records from England and Wales (Duvoisin and Schweitzer, 1966), a form of
prevalence determination generally considered to be somewhat unreliable. In
the opinion of this reviewer, it is difficult to see how the apparent stability in
the prevalence of Parkinson's disease in Rochester between 1935 and 1979
argues strongly either for or against an environmental toxin as a cause of Parkinson's disease. For example, if heavy industry were contributing a toxin to the
environment, such industry may well have been stable during this period (in fact,
in many areas the concentration of heavy industry is on the decline).

One recent study, which utilized the tightest form of epidemiologic technique (i.e., door to door community survey), appears to indicate a lower inci-

dence of Parkinson's disease in China than in the United States or Europe (Schoenberg et al., 1985). It is interesting that this study was carried out to see if the prevalence rate was lower in a nonindustrialized country, which it appears to be.

HOW EARLY THE INSULT?

Two novel hypotheses have been proposed that literally take us back to the womb in our search for an environmental factor as the cause of Parkinson's disease. Eldridge and Ince (1984) have proposed that individuals destined to contract the disease may receive less of a "Parkinson's disease protective factor" for some reason during prenatal development and, therefore, start life with fewer nigral neurons, which, in turn, leads to the appearance of the disease later in life. This suggestion was put forth in part to explain the near life-long personality differences noted in the twin study (those twins destined to have Parkinson's disease tended to be more "self-controlled") (Ward et al., 1983). The major problem with this hypothesis is that it does not account for the clear neuropathologic evidence of the actual death of neurons in affected areas of the brain of patients dying with Parkinson's disease. Further, the existence of a protective factor remains, at least for the moment, in the realm of speculation. Robbins and colleagues (1985) have suggested that a somatic dominant mutation might be the cause of Parkinson's disease. Such a mutation during embryogenesis would result in inadequate repair of x-ray-type DNA damage which, in turn, would eventually lead to premature neuronal death. They have demonstrated that irradiated lymphoblastoid lines from parkinsonian patients have a shortened survival rate compared to controls. For the moment one can only say that this remains an interesting theory.

SUMMARY

This review is by no means meant to be comprehensive. Rather, I have attempted to focus on several new hypotheses. The weight of current evidence appears to favor a major role for environmental factors, although a supporting role of genetic factors has by no means been ruled out. Because MPTP represents a new lead as a potential environmental agent, new ideas generated by its discovery have been given a certain degree of emphasis. With regard to the future, there is reason to hope that the next epoch in our search for an etiology of Parkinson's disease will be a fertile time indeed. It should be most interesting to see where the new ideas reviewed in this chapter will lead us in the years ahead.

REFERENCES

Ballard PA, Tetrud JW, Langston JW. (1985). Permanent human parkinsonism due to 1-methyl-4-phenyl-1,2,3,6-tetrahydropyridine (MPTP): seven cases. *Neurology* 35: 949–956.

Barbeau A. (1984). Etiology of Parkinson's disease: a research strategy. *Can J Neurol Sci* 11: 24–28.

Barbeau A, Roy M, Cloutier T, Plasse L, Paris S. (1986). Environmental and genetic factors in the etiology of Parkinson's disease. In: Yahr, M, Bergmann K (Eds.), *Advances in Neurology*, Vol. 45, *Parkinson's Disease*. New York, Raven Press.

Burns RS, Chiueh CC, Markey SP, Ebert MH, Jacobowitz DM, Kopin IJ. (1983). A primate model of parkinsonism: selective destruction of dopaminergic neurons in the pars compacta of the substantia nigra by n-methyl-4-phenyl-1,2,3,6-tetrahydropyridine. *Proc Natl Acad Sci* 80: 4546–4550.

Calne DB, Langston JW. (1983). On the etiology of Parkinson's disease. *Lancet* 2: 1457–1459.

Calne DB, Langston JW, Martin WR, Stoessel AJ, Ruth TJ, Adam MJ, Pate BD, Schulzer M. (1985). Observations relating to the cause of Parkinson's disease: PET scans after MPTP. *Nature* 317: 246–248.

Carlsson A, Winblad B. (1976). Influence of age and time interval between death and autopsy on dopamine and 3-methoxytyramine levels in human basal ganglia. *J Neurol Transm* 38: 271–276.

Cohen G. (1983). The pathobiology of Parkinson's disease: biochemical aspects of dopamine neuron senescence. *J Neural Transm* 19: 89–103.

Davis GC, Williams AC, Markey SP, Ebert MH, Caine ED, Reichert CM, Kopin, IJ. (1979). Chronic parkinsonism secondary to intravenous injection of meperidine analogues. *Psych Res* 1: 249–254.

Duvoisin RC. (1982). On the cause of Parkinson's disease. In: Marsden CD, Fahn S (Eds.), *Movement Disorders*. London, Butterworth Scientific.

Duvoisin RC, Schweitzer MD. (1966). Paralysis agitans mortality in England and Wales, 1855–1962. *Br J Med* 20: 27–33.

Eldridge R, Ince SE. (1984). The low concordance rate for Parkinson's disease in twins: a possible explanation. *Neurology* 34: 1354–1356.

Eldridge R, Rocca WA. (1986). Parkinson disease: etiologic considerations. In: Motulsky A, Rotter J, King R (Eds.), *Genetics of Common Disease*. New York, McGraw-Hill.

Forno LS. (1982). Pathology of Parkinson's disease. In: Marsden SD, Fahn S (Eds.), *Movement Disorders*. London, Butterworth Scientific.

Forno LS, Langston JW, DeLanney LE, Irwin I, Ricaurte GA. (1986). Locus ceruleus lesions and eosinophilic inclusions in MPTP-treated monkeys. *Ann Neurol* 20: 449–455.

Gibbs CJ Jr, Gajdusek DC. (1973). Amyotrophic lateral sclerosis, Parkinson's disease, and the amyotrophic lateral sclerosis-parkinsonism-dementia complex on Guam: a review and summary of attempts to demonstrate infection as the aetiology. *J Clin Pathol* 25: 132–140.

Jenner P, Rupniak NM, Rose S, Kelly E, Kilpatrick G, Lees A, Marsden CD. (1984). 1-methyl-4-phenyl-1,2,3,6-tetrahydropyridine-induced parkinsonism in the common marmoset. *Neurosci Lett* 50: 85–90.

Koller WC, O'Hara R, Weiner WJ, Lang AA, Nutt JG, Agid Y, Bonnet AM, Jankovic J. (1986). Relationship of aging to Parkinson's disease. In: Yahr M, Bergmann K (Eds.), *Advances in Neurology*, Vol. 45, *Parkinson's Disease*. New York.

Kurland LT. (1958). Epidemiology: incidence, geographic distribution and genetic considerations. In: Fields WS (Ed.), *Pathogenesis and Treatment of Parkinsonism*. Springfield, Charles C Thomas.

Langston JW. (1986a). MPTP-induced parkinsonism: how good a model is it? In: Fahn S, Marsden CD, Teychenne PS, Jenner P (Eds.), *Recent Developments in Parkinson's Disease*. New York, Raven Press.

Langston JW. (1986b). MPTP: the promise of a new neurotoxin. In: Marsden CD, Fahn S (Eds.), *Movement Disorders 2*. London, Butterworth Scientific.

Langston JW, Ballard PA. (1983). Parkinson's disease in a chemist working with 1-methyl-4-phenyl-1,2,5,6-tetrahydropyridine (MPTP). *N Engl J Med* 309: 310.

Langston JW, Ballard PA. (1984). Parkinsonism induced by 1-methyl-4-phenyl-1,2,5,6-tetrahydropyridine: implications for treatment and the pathophysiology of Parkinson's disease. *Can J Neurol Sci* 11: 160–165.

Langston JW, Ballard PA, Tetrud JW, Irwin I. (1983). Chronic parkinsonism in humans due to a product of meperidine-analog synthesis. *Science* 219: 979–980.

Langston JW, Forno LS, Rebert CS, Irwin I. (1984a). 1-Methyl-4-phenyl-1,2,3,6-tetrahydropyridine causes selective damage to the zona compacta of the substantia nigra in the squirrel monkey. *Brain Res* 292: 390–394.

Langston JW, Irwin I, Langston EB, Forno LS. (1984b). 1-Methyl-4-phenyl-pyridinium ion (MPP+): identification of a metabolite of MPTP, a toxin selective to the substantia nigra. *Neurosci Lett* 48: 87–92.

Langston JW, Langston EB, Irwin I. (1984c). MPTP-induced parkinsonism in human and non-humans primates. *Acta Neurol Scand* 70 (Suppl 100): 49–54.

Markey SP, Johannessen JN, Chiueh CC, Burns RS, Herkenham MA. (1984). Intraneuronal generation of a pyridinium metabolite may cause drug-induced parkinsonism. *Nature* 311: 464–467.

McGeer PL, McGeer EG, Suzuki JS. (1977). Aging and extrapyramidal function. *Arch Neurol* 34: 33–35.

Rajput AH, Offord DP, Beard CM, Kurland LT. (1984). Epidemiology of parkinsonism: incidence, classification, and mortality. *Ann Neurol* 16: 278–282.

Ricaurte GA, Langston JW, Irwin I, DeLanney LE, Forno LS. (1985). The neurotoxic effect of MPTP on the dopaminergic cells of the substantia nigra in mice is age-related. *Soc Neurosci* Abst 11: 631.

Riederer P, Wuketich ST. (1976). Time course of nigrostriatal degeneration in Parkinson's disease. *J Neurol Transm* 38: 277–301.

Robbins JH, Otsuka F, Tarone RE, Polinsky RJ, Brumback RA, Nee LE. (1985). Parkinson's disease and Alzheimer's disease: hypersensitivity to x-rays in cultured cell lines. *J Neurol Neurosurg Psychiatry* 18: 916–923.

Ruttenbur AJ, Garbe PL, Kalter HD, Castro KG, Tetrud JW, Porter P, Irwin I, Langston JW. (1986). Meperidine analog exposure in California narcotics abusers: initial epidemiologic findings. In: Markey SP, Castagnoli N Jr, Trevor AJ, Kopin IJ. (Eds.), *MPTP: A Neurotoxin Producing a Parkinsonian Syndrome*. New York, Academic Press.

Schoenberg BS, Anderson DW, Haerer AF. (1985). Prevalence of Parkinson's disease in the biracial population of Copiah County, Mississippi. *Neurology* 35: 841–845.

Ward CD, Duvoisin RC, Ince SE, Nutt JG, Eldridge R, Calne DB. (1983). Parkinson's disease in 65 pairs of twins and in a set of quadruplets. *Neurology* 33: 815–824.

Wright MD, Wall RA, Perry TL, Paty DW. (1984). Chronic parkinsonism secondary to intranasal administration of a product of meperidine-analogue synthesis. *N Engl J Med* 310: 325.

Ziering A, Berger L, Heineman SD, Lee J. (1947). Piperidine derivatives. Part III. 4-Arylpiperidines. *J Org Chem* 12: 894–903.

16
Anticholinergics and Amantadine

JOSÉ A. OBESO and J.M. MARTÍNEZ-LAGE
*Clínica Universitaria, University of Navarra Medical School,
Pamplona, Spain*

The discovery of the therapeutic efficacy of anticholinergics and amantadine in the treatment of the symptoms of Parkinson's disease was, in both cases, a casual finding. Charcot included hyoscine (scopolamine) among the list of empirical remedies recommended for the treatment of disease symptoms in the 19th century (1). Robert Schwab realized in 1968 that amantadine had induced a remarkable improvement in a parkinsonian patient who was taking 100 mg twice daily to prevent the flu (2).

At present, there is unanimous agreement among doctors caring for patients with Parkinson's disease that the therapeutic activity of anticholinergics and amantadine is usually only slight or moderate. Nevertheless, in spite of the decisive impact of levodopa therapy, anticholinergics and amantadine continue to be used with frequency in clinical practice. The fundamental explanation for this is the intention of many neurologists to delay the use of levodopa therapy (3) or, at the very least, to use the lowest possible dosages of levodopa. In this chapter, the available evidence supporting the use and the clinical applications of anticholinergics and amantadine in Parkinson's disease are reviewed.

ANTICHOLINERGICS

Favorable reports in the first half of the 20th century concerning stramonium, extracted from white wine, and atropine led in the 1950s to the development of synthetic belladonna alkaloids with anticholinergic properties. Coramiphen hydrochloride (Parpanit) was the most efficient and least toxic drug among the initial group of synthetic anticholinergics (4). Over the following years a wide

range of anticholinergic drugs with variable selectivity and actions on the CNS
have been developed. Among the most frequently used anticholinergic drugs in
clinical practice are trihexyphenidyl (Artane), cycrimine (Pagitane), procyclidine (Kemadrin), biperiden (Akineton), and ethopropazine (Parridol). Diphenhydramine (Benadryl), and benztropine (Cogentin) are anticholinergic drugs
that also possess antihistaminic action.

Mechanism of Action

In the early 1960s, Barbeau (5) postulated that in Parkinson's disease the normal
equilibrium between dopamine (DA) and acetylcholine (ACh) activity in the
striatum was disrupted as a consequence of the loss of nigrostriatal dopaminergic
neurons. It was therefore assumed that the resulting functional preponderance of
the cholinergic system in conjunction with the dopaminergic hypoactivity could
be compensated for by decreasing ACh transmission with anticholinergic drugs,
or by increasing DA activity with levodopa. Although it is well established that
the dopaminergic system exerts a tonic inhibitory action on ACh striatal release
(6), it is also recognized that the neurochemical basis of basal ganglia pathophysiology is far more complex (7). In Parkinson's disease there is a reduction in
the basal ganglia of several major neurotransmitters including, in addition to DA,
norepinephrine, serotonin, substance P, and enkephalins, all of which may have
a certain role in the control of motor function (8). It is therefore unlikely that
the therapeutic action of anticholinergic drugs can be explained solely on the
basis of reestablishing DA–ACh equilibrium. In fact, some anticholinergic drugs
(particularly benztropine and trihexyphenidyl) have a definite reuptake-blocking
action on central dopaminergic neurons (9,10).

Pharmacokinetics

The peak clinical activity of most anticholinergic drugs occurs between 1 and 4
hr (11), but pharmacokinetic data are only available for trihexyphenidyl. Burke
and Fahn (12) reported that the half-life of this drug was 1.7+0.3 hr in patients
with torsion dystonia who were receiving higher daily dosages. Studies in patients with Parkinson's disease have not apparently been undertaken (13).

Clinical Efficacy

Several studies evaluating the antiparkinson activity of anticholinergics were
carried out before levodopa was introduced. Schwab and Leigh (4) found a mean
25% improvement in 62% of 50 patients they treated with Parpanit. Doshay and
Constable (14) and Corbin (15), independently, found better results with trihexyphenidyl (Artane), reporting improvement in about 77% of a large number
of patients. In general, rigidity was more reduced than tremor, while akinesia

responded poorly. However no clear evidence exists for a selective action of some anticholinergics on rigidity, tremor, or akinesia (16). Although there are different opinions about the relative antiparkinson activity of each anticholinergic drug used in clinical practice, such preference emerges mainly from personal experience. Overall, anticholinergics reduce motor disability by 10–25% when used in monotherapy (17).

It is now very common to treat parkinsonian patients with an anticholinergic drug combined with levodopa plus a decarboxylase inhibitor and/or a direct dopamine agonist. It is surprising that there are virtually no data about pharmacokinetic and pharmacodynamic interactions among these different drugs. It is known that anticholinergic drugs cause a delay in absorption of levodopa by slowing gastric mobility. This effect may produce lower peaks of plasma levodopa levels (17).

Long-term use of both levodopa and anticholinergics may be associated with cortical cholinergic hypersensitivity (13,18), which may increase the possibility of psychiatric side effects (19). Taking into consideration the lack of information about the positive or negative effects or interactions between anticholinergic drugs and dopamine agonists, the authors recommend the use of anticholinergics only in monotherapy or associated with amantadine.

Side Effects

Anticholinergic drugs can cause a number of adverse reactions due to the blockade of both peripheral and central cholinergic neurons. Common peripheral effects are dry mouth, constipation, and urinary retention. Some of these actions may have therapeutic value on occasion. Thus, anticholinergic drugs may be very effective in the treatment of sialorrhea and in some patients with urinary incontinence. On the other hand, in our experience, benzhexol has occasionally had to be discontinued because it produces impotence. Near-vision difficulties frequently interfere with daily activities in many patients. In addition, anticholinergics are contraindicated in patients with narrow-angle glaucoma.

The most important side effects caused by anticholinergic drugs are the changes in mental activity. Memory loss is very common even in patients under 50 years of age. Both short-term and long-term memory are impaired by anticholinergics. Language difficulties, already present in a significant proportion of parkinsonian patients, such as the "tip of the tongue phenomenon," may be drastically exaggerated. However, the development of a confusional state is the most striking "psychiatric" side effect of anticholinergic drugs. This occurs primarily in older patients many of whom had preexisting intellectual impairment, and is often triggered by a concomitant illness. The clinical picture is typical but not exclusive of intoxication with anticholinergic drugs. One usually finds an agitated patient, disoriented as to time and space, whose logical conversation is difficult to follow and memory loss is profound. In these instances, the patient is often dehydrated due to low ingestion of liquids and the possible presence of intercurrent hyperthermia. Upon withdrawal of anticholinergics and treatment of the general physical symptoms (if present), the confusional state improves in 2–5 days. The extreme sensitivity of patients with Parkinson's disease to mental side effects during treatment with anticholinergic drugs probably is based on the deficit of frontal cholinergic activity (19,20). Thus, although the cholinergic system is normal in the basal ganglia, there is a 50% deficit of choline acetyltransferase activity in the hippocampus and frontal cortex of parkinsonian patients (20). Such reduction is due to damage of the substantia innominata, as in Alzheimer's disease, but also to intracortical loss of cholinergic neurons (20). Agid and colleagues have proposed that use of anticholinergics may further aggravate this cortical deficit, which explains the confusional state provoked by them, particularly in patients with mental deterioration (20).

AMANTADINE

Following Schwab et al.'s (2) original observation, several reports confirmed the antiparkinson properties of amantadine HCl. This drug has been shown to benefit 60–70% of patients and to have a synergistic action with levodopa (21,22).

Mechanism of Action

The main effect of amantadine is probably related to its capacity to increase presynaptic synthesis and release of dopamine (23) as well as inhibit dopamine reuptake (24). A nondopaminergic action of amantadine has been postulated on the basis of experimental studies. Thus the effect of amantadine on single neurons following microiontophoretic application was not inhibited by pre- and postsynaptic dopaminergic blockade with reserpine or alpha-flupenthixol nor by the beta-adrenergic blocking action of propranolol (25). An anticholinergic action of amantadine has been suspected on the basis of clinical data alone, because side effects such as dry mouth, urinary retention, and constipation are present in a proportion of patients treated chronically with this drug. However, experimental studies have proved negative regarding a possible anticholinergic action of amantadine (26).

Pharmacokinetics

Peak plasma levels of amantadine are obtained between 2 and 8 hr following a single oral dose (100 mg). Clinical action may become evident 1 hr after ingestion and last for 8 hr, with a mean duration of action of 2–4 hr (27).

Clinical Efficacy

The effect of amantadine compared to placebo in Parkinson's disease has been assessed in several double-blind studies (21,22,28). About two-thirds of patients improved with amantadine alone or in combination with levodopa. Patients not responding initially to amantadine in monotherapy may improve further when this drug is added to levodopa later in the evolution of the disease (21). Amantadine does not appear to have specific actions on the various motor signs seen in Parkinson's disease. However, Butzer et al. (28) noticed that while improvement in tremor and rigidity remained fairly constant over a period of 10–12 months, the effect on movement velocity deteriorated after a few weeks of treatment.

Side Effects

The most frequent side effects of amantadine are ankle edema and livedo reticularis, often occurring together. The exact causes are unknown. Both usually disappear after amantadine is discontinued or improve if the dosage is reduced. Nervousness, dizziness, and insomnia, in addition to the anticholinergic-like side effects mentioned above, are also relatively common complaints.

In patients taking levodopa (Sinemet or Madopar) and/or anticholinergics, dosages of amantadine higher than 300 mg/day usually cause hallucinations, particularly at night. For this reason, we try to avoid giving amantadine in high dosages or in polytherapy. Amantadine is excreted almost completely by the kidneys without metabolization. Therefore this drug should be used with caution in patients with renal disease and avoided altogether in those with a very low glomerular filtration rate.

Anticholinergics and amantadine in combination result in greater improvement of Parkinson's disease than with either used alone. Parkes et al. (29) have suggested that anticholinergics are more effective against rigidity and postural deformity, while amantadine can improve all symptoms. The larger experience now gained with these drugs, in our opinion, does not confirm such differences.

CONCLUSIONS

Anticholinergics and amantadine are, in general, complementary to levodopa in the treatment of the symptoms of Parkinson's disease. Motor disability can effectively be reduced by treatment with amantadine or one anticholinergic drug alone, but it is very seldom that adequate control persists for more than a few months.

The following general considerations represent a summary of the author's view on the value and use of amantadine and anticholinergics in clinical practice.

1.   Amantadine (100 mg two or three times daily) is a very useful initial drug treatment in patients with mild motor disability (stage I or II of Hoehn and Yahr).

2.   Amantadine is added to the drug regimen of patients already taking levodopa when the dosage of levodopa has to be reduced due to side effects or when motor fluctuations in the form of the "wearing off" phenomena develop. The rationale is to delay the initiation of treatment with levodopa and/or other dopamine agonists in mildly affected patients and to reserve other drugs such as bromocriptine, lisuride or pergolide against the possibility that more severe motor complications (the "on-off" phenomena) appear. When amantadine and levodopa fail to improve the "wearing off" phenomena, we turn to deprenyl or start treatment with bromocriptine.

3.   Monotherapy with an anticholinergic drug (Artane, Kemadrin, Akineton) is attempted as initial treatment in patients with hemiparkinsonism with tremor as the main manifestation.

4.   Anticholinergics are not used in patients older than 60, unless they have complete intolerance to levodopa plus dopa-decarboxylase inhibitor as well as to other dopamine agonists.

5.   In our opinion, anticholinergics should be never given to patients with mental impairment.

6.   Biperidin (Akineton) and benztropine (Cogentin) may occasionally be useful for parenteral administration during severe "off" periods in patients with complicated motor fluctuations.

7.   Further improvement of motor disability can be obtained by combining amantadine and one anticholinergic. This is particularly useful in patients with mild symptoms of short duration.

REFERENCES

1.   Ordenstein L. (1867). *Sur la Paralysie Agitante et la Sclérose en Plaque Généralisé*. Paris, Martinet.

2.   Schwab RS, Chafetz ME. (1955). Kemadrin in the treatment of parkinsonism. *Neurology* 5: 273–277.

3.   Fahn S, Calne DB. (1978). Considerations in the management of parkinsonism. *Neurology* 28: 5–7.

4.   Schwab R, Leigh D. (1939). Parpanit in the treatment of Parkinson's disease. *JAMA* 139: 629–634.

5.   Barbeau A. (1962). The pathogenesis of Parkinson's disease. A new hypothesis. *Can Med Assoc J* 87: 802–807.

6.   Stadler H, Lloyd KG, Gadea-Cirea M, Bartholini G. (1973). Enhanced striatal acetylcholine release by chlorpromazine and its reversal by apomorphine. *Brain Res* 55: 476–480.

7. Bartholini G. (1986). Functional neuronal relations in the basal ganglia and their clinical relevance. In: Sandler M, Fenerstein C, Scatton B. (Eds.), *Neurotransmitter Interactions*. New York, Raven Press.

8. Marsden CD. (1982). Neurotransmitter and CNS disease: basal ganglia diseases. *Lancet* 2: 1141–1147.

9. Coyle JT, Snyder SH. (1969). Antiparkinsonian drugs: inhibition of dopamine uptake in the corpus striatum as a possible mechanism of action. *Science* 166: 899–901.

10. Farnebo L, Fuxe K, Hamberger B, Ljungdahl H. (1970). Effect of some antiparkinsonian drugs on catecholamine neurons. *J Pharm Pharmacol* 22: 733–737.

11. Quinn N. (1984). Antiparkinsonian drugs today. *Drugs* 28: 236–262.

12. Burke R, Fahn S. (1982). Pharmacokinetics of trihexyphenidyl after acute and chronic administration. *Ann Neurol* 12: 94.

13. Lang AM. (1984). Treatment of Parkinson's disease with agents other than levodopa and dopamine agonists: controversies and new approaches. *Can J Neurol Sci* 2: 210–220.

14. Doshay LJ, Constable K. (1949). Artane therapy for parkinsonism: preliminary study of results of 117 cases. *JAMA* 140: 1317–1322.

15. Coerlin KB. (1949). Trihexyphenidyl: evaluation of a new agent in treatment of parkinsonism. *JAMA* 141: 377–382.

16. Strang RR. (1965). Kemadrin in the treatment of parkinsonism: a double blind and one year follow-up study. *Curr Med Drugs* 5: 27–32.

17. Fermaglich J, O'Doherty DS. (1972). Effect of gastric motility on levodopa. *Dis Nerv Syst* 33: 624–625.

18. Ruberg M, Ploska A, Javoy-Agid F, Agid Y. (1982). Muscarinic binding and choline acetyltransference activity in parkinsonian subjects with reference to dementia. *Brain Res* 232: 129–139.

19. Dubois A, Ruberg M, Javoy-Agid F, Plasica A, Agid Y. (1983). A subcortico-cortical cholinergic system is affected in Parkinson's disease. *Brain Res* 288: 213–218.

20. Agid Y, Ruberg M, Dubois B, Javoy-Agid F. (1983). Biochemical substrates of mental disturbances in Parkinson's disease. *Adv Neurol* 40: 211–218.

21. Fahn S, Isgreen W. (1985). Long-term evaluation of amantadine and levodopa combination in parkinsonism by double-blind crossover analyses. *Neurology* 25: 695–700.

22. Parkes JD, Curzon G, Knott PJ, et al. (1971). Treatment of Parkinson's disease with amantadine and levodopa. A one year study. *Lancet* 1: 1083–1089.

23. Stromberg V, Svensson TH. (1971). Further studies on the mode of action of amantadine. *Acta Pharmacol Toxicol* 30: 161–171.

24. Von Voigtlander PF, Moore KE. (1971). Dopamine: release from the brain "in vivo" by amantadine. *Science* 174: 408–410.

25. Stone TW. (1977). Evidence for a non-dopaminergic action of amantadine. *Neurosci Letts* 4: 343–346.

26. Gerlak RP, Clark R, Stump JM, Vernier VG. (1970). Amantadine-dopamine interaction. *Science* 169: 203–204.
27. Pacifici GM, Nardini M, Ferrari P. et al. (1976). Effect of amantadine on drug-induced parkinsonism: relationship between plasma levels and effects. *Br J Clin Pharmacol* 3: 883–889.
28. Butzer JF, Silver DE, Sahs AL. (1975). Amantadine in Parkinson's disease. *Neurology* 25: 603–606.
29. Parkes JD, Baxter RC, Marsden CD, Rees JE. (1974). Comparative trial of benzhexol, amantadine and levodopa in the treatment of Parkinson's disease. *J Neurol Neurosurg Psychiatry* 37: 422–425.

17
Levodopa

NIALL P. QUINN
King's College School of Medicine and Dentistry, London, England

EARLY HISTORY

In 1913 Guggenheim isolated and determined the structure of levodopa. Although he himself was extremely nauseated and vomited twice within 10 min of ingesting 2.5 g, nothing seemed to happen to a rabbit to which he fed 1 g, and he therefore concluded that the substance was "not very active from a pharmacological point of view" (1).

Forty-seven years later the discovery by Ehringer and Hornykiewicz (2) that there was a striking deficit of dopamine in the striatum of parkinsonian brains, together with the experience of Carlsson (3) and Degkwitz (4) in reversing reserpine-induced akinesia in mice and man, respectively, with D L-dopa set the stage for the first studies of levodopa in the treatment of the symptoms of human Parkinson's disease. In 1961, two separate groups, one (5) working with oral levodopa 100–200 mg, and the other (6) with intravenous levodopa 50–150 mg, reported temporary striking benefits in parkinsonian subjects. Other workers, however, were often unable to confirm any major effect until Cotzias et al. (7) decided to give much larger oral doses of 1.6–12.6 g D L-dopa/day. The results were so dramatic that the efficacy of levodopa treatment was established beyond any doubt, and a new era in the management of Parkinson's disease began.

From the outset, it was clear that side effects constituted a major problem. Nausea and vomiting caused by peripherally formed dopamine acting on the gut and on receptors of the chemoreceptor trigger zone in the area postrema either caused many patients to abandon the drug completely or so limited the dosage that little useful antiparkinson effect could be obtained. Postural hypotension, confusion, and other mental side effects were recognized early on. Even in the first report of Cotzias et al. drug-induced dyskinesias were mentioned, but these "athetoid movements were observed . . . only when the therapeutic effect was impressive" (7).

PERIPHERAL DECARBOXYLASE INHIBITORS

In order to reduce the peripheral dopaminergic side effects, levodopa was given in association with inhibitors of dopa decarboxylase, the enzyme that converts levodopa to dopamine, which themselves did not cross the blood–brain barrier at clinical dosages. Benserazide (8) caused bone defects in experimental animals, and so has never been approved for use in the United States. However, the association of levodopa with benserazide (9) is widely used in other countries in a 4:1 ratio in the form of Madopar 250 (250 mg levodopa (L-dopa) and 50 mg benserazide), Madopar 125 (100 + 25), and Madopar 62.5 (50 + 12.5) capsules. Carbidopa (Merck, Sharp & Dohme) (10) is the peripheral decarboxylase inhibitor (PDI) associated with levodopa (11) in Sinemet 275 (250 mg L-dopa + 25 mg carbidopa), Sinemet 110 (100 + 10), and Sinemet 125 or Plus (100 + 25) tablets (12). There is no difference in efficacy between Sinemet and Madopar. Some workers have claimed a lower incidence of nausea and vomiting with Madopar (13), but other double-blind studies have found no difference (14). In countries where both drugs are available, the relative frequency of prescription of each compound relates mainly to which preparation came on the market first: Madopar in continental Europe, Sinemet in the United Kingdom and United States. Sinemet is slightly more flexible in application, since by combining half tablets one can give individual doses of 125, 175, and 225 mg levodopa, which is not possible using Madopar capsules. This difference is only of importance in "brittle" parkinsonian patients (see below). Although at standard dosages there is little to choose between Sinemet and Madopar, at very low dosages (for example, on introducing treatment) Sinemet 110 does seem to cause more nausea. This is because a minimum quantity of PDI is needed to inhibit maximally (but not necessarily completely) the peripheral conversion of levodopa to dopamine. Thus some patients taking, for example, two to four tablets of Sinemet 110 per day (and thus receiving 20–40 mg carbidopa) may still have appreciable peripheral formation of dopamine, most of which would be blocked by the same number of tablets of Sinemet Plus (50–100 mg carbidopa). In patients on established therapeutic dosages of Sinemet, however, there is little advantage in prescribing Sinemet Plus.

Since the peripheral decarboxylation of levodopa in gut wall, liver, and brain capillary endothelium is blocked when a PDI is also given, much more of a given dose of levodopa reaches the brain where it is needed. This association thus allows the dosage of levodopa to be reduced by four to five times.

CARDIOVASCULAR SIDE EFFECTS

Although some studies have shown a difference between the drop in blood pressure during usage of plain levodopa vs levodopa plus PDI (15), others have not (16). While peripheral factors are undoubtedly involved in the hypotensive reaction to dopaminergic drugs, central effects seem to predominate, so that postural hypotension remains a clinically important side effect in some patients when a PDI, or even domperidone (a peripherally acting dopamine receptor blocker) is associated with levodopa. Similarly, addition of a PDI does not significantly alter the frequency of cardiac arrhythmias in levodopa-treated patients (16), but domperidone may do so (17). Cardiac arrhythmias hardly ever assume clinical importance when patients are treated with levodopa. On rare occasions, levodopa may cause hypertension when given intravenously, or even orally (18), as a large bolus. Levodopa may also give rise to hypertensive crises when inhibitors of monoamine oxidase (MAO) A are used (19). Their association with levodopa is contraindicated, and there should be an interval of at least 2 weeks between stopping one drug and starting the other. MAO B inhibitors, however, such as selegiline, may safely be associated with levodopa preparations (see Chap. 21). Although there are theoretical risks associated with possible interactions between dopamine and norepinephrine derived from levodopa, and cyclopropane and halothane anesthesia, and both hypo- and hypertensive postoperative reactions have been reported (20), many hundreds of parkinsonian patients have been anesthetized with halothane without any problem. As long as the anesthetist is alerted beforehand, levodopa preparations should be continued up to 4 hr preoperatively, and restarted as soon as practicable afterward. The parkinsonian patient has most to fear from postoperative immobility, the duration of which should be as short as possible. Occasionally, in patients unable to swallow postoperatively, there may be an indication for parenteral levodopa infusion.

PSYCHIATRIC SIDE EFFECTS

Virtually any psychiatric state may be seen during the course of treatment with levodopa, and indeed with any effective antiparkinsonian agent. Particular risk factors are increasing age, underlying dementia, electroencephalographic (EEG) abnormalities, polytherapy, and a prior history of psychiatric disease. The appearance of psychiatric side effects may correspond to a recent change in levodopa dosage, the addition of another drug, or to an intercurrent illness such as urinary or respiratory tract infection, myocardial infarction, or surgery under general anesthesia. Not uncommonly, however, psychiatric events may occur spontaneously on a stable treatment regimen with no apparent precipitating factor. Vivid dreams, nightmares, disturbed sleep pattern, visual illusions, and pseudohallucinations (in which insight is retained) are relatively common. The latter are often nonmenacing, and patients may even refer to groups of small animals or people as "my friends" or "my guests." However, although they may be surprisingly well tolerated by many patients, they may be the precursors of more sinister developments. True visual hallucinations may also occur, and are more serious because insight is lost. Auditory illusions and hallucinations are less common, but undoubtedly occur, and may even take the form of two or more people talking about the patient in the third person. Olfactory illusions and hallucinations, hypersexuality, and sexual deviations may all be related to levodopa treatment. Any of the above may occur in the context of a normal state of alertness, but organic confusional states, which are also common, occur in a delirious setting of altered consciousness. Depression, although common in Parkinson's disease (see Chap. 3), often fails to lift despite the motor improvement attained with levodopa. Although levodopa-induced euphoria, hypomania, and even mania are well recognized, there are also rare patients who respond acutely to levodopa treatment with severe depressive symptoms. Finally, mood swings may occur in parallel with motor fluctuations in "on–off" subjects, with panic, anxiety, depressive affect, and sometimes even depressive psychosis occurring in "off" periods, to be instantly replaced by normal mood or even euphoria in "on" periods. Hence, when psychiatric status needs to be assessed in a fluctuating patient examination in both "off" and "on" periods should be mandatory.

The management of delusions, hallucinations, and organic confusional states in drug-treated parkinsonians is fraught with difficulty. Concurrent treatment with ergots, anticholinergics, selegiline, or amantadine should be stopped, and then the dosage of levodopa reduced. Benzodiazepines or chlormethiazole can be used for sedation if necessary. The problems may settle over a day or 2. If symptoms persist, however, one may be forced to give dopamine-blocking drugs, either by using "mild" neuroleptics such as thioridazine in slowly increasing dosages, or by giving a higher dosage of a more incisive antipsychotic agent from the outset. Alternatively, levodopa may be stopped completely, or, rarely, both measures may be necessary. When one is forced to take these extreme measures, the patient's parkinsonism inevitably returns with a vengeance, and all of the dangers of a "drug holiday" (see below) are introduced. Although psychoses or organic confusional states induced by dopamine agonists may clear gratifyingly early after the offending drug is stopped, they unfortunately can also persist for up to 6 weeks. There is really no "correct" way of managing this problem, since each alternative is equally unsatisfactory for the patient. Favorable results have been reported using L-tryptophan (21,22) but this drug has not been widely used for this indication. The most promising antipsychotic for use in parkinsonian subjects is clozapine, a drug with relatively weak D-1 and D-2 antagonist actions. In some European countries, clozapine (22) is the first-choice drug in this situation, but in others its use is banned because of the occurrence of a cluster of cases of clozapine-associated agranulocytosis in Finland.

OTHER SIDE EFFECTS

Among other reported side effects of levodopa are the rare positive Coombs' test (though hemolytic anemia has never been reported), pupillary dilatation (24) (blindness, though reported after anticholinergic-induced mydriasis in narrow-angle glaucoma, has never been attributed to levodopa), dark discoloration of urine, sweat, and saliva, and profuse sweating (25). Levodopa elevates circulating growth hormone and depresses already low prolactin levels in normal and parkinsonian subjects (26), an effect shared with other dopamine agonists. Paradoxically, all of these drugs will lower pathologically raised growth hormone levels in patients with acromegaly. There is no good evidence to incriminate levodopa as a cause of melanoma (27). However, since levodopa is a precursor of melanin, many physicians would avoid its use in subjects already known to have a melanoma. The yellow dye in Sinemet Plus may rarely cause a skin rash (28). Three successful deliveries to two parkinsonian women treated with levodopa during pregnancy have recently been reported (29).

MOTOR EFFECTS

Although stereotactic surgery, anticholinergics, and amantadine certainly improve tremor and rigidity in many parkinsonian subjects, none of these measures has any major effect on akinesia, the central and most disabling feature of the disease. However, with the advent of levodopa, a powerful antiakinetic treatment was available, which led to the dramatic "awakenings" described by Oliver Sacks (30).

When first treated with plain levodopa, many patients took weeks or even months to attain optimal benefit from a fixed dosage. With the addition of a PDI, this period of progressive improvement is shorter, but may still last days to weeks. The reason for this delay, and for the "lag" of several days that may occur before a final return to baseline disability in a patient whose levodopa is stopped for any reason (long-duration benefit), is unknown.

The improvement in patients with idiopathic Parkinson's disease when they are first treated with adequate and sustained amounts of levodopa with PDI is so dramatic as to be almost without parallel in clinical medicine. Moreover, it is so constant a feature that failure of a patient to improve subjectively or objectively by about 50% should raise doubts concerning the diagnosis. Even in the earliest studies using plain levodopa (and therefore comprising fewer patients tolerating adequate dosages because of sickness), the proportion of patients improving by 50% or more was between 68% (31) (116 patients treated for 6–18 months) and 79% (32) (80 patients treated for 2 months). Improvement of at least 20% was seen in 94% and 90%, respectively, of patients in these series. Not only do a high proportion of patients improve initially, but also most continue to be able to take levodopa with continuing benefit for years. Of Barbeau's initial group (32) of 80 patients with advanced disease, 70% were still taking plain levodopa 6 years later, with 53% still showing more than 50% improvement over pretreatment baseline. Of the 18 withdrawals, 4 were lost to follow-up, and 6 subsequently improved with the addition of a PDI. The remaining 8 (10%) of the original group of 80 patients turned out to have neither idiopathic nor post-encephalitic parkinsonism.

The beneficial motor effects of levodopa do not differ based on patients' sex, age, age at onset, or disease duration or severity (31). All of these categories should show roughly the same proportionate benefit from the drug. Most patients should experience a "levodopa honeymoon" lasting a variable interval, during which they attain smooth, long-duration benefit, usually from three separate daily doses of the drug (but sometimes even on an alternate-day regimen) (33). During this time, they show neither response fluctuations nor unwanted abnormal involuntary movements, and the degree of clinical benefit is usually proportional to the dosage of levodopa taken.

RESPONSE FLUCTUATIONS

With progression of underlying disease and increasing duration of treatment, more and more subjects begin to experience clinical response fluctuations. Their appearance takes the form of a spectrum or continuum from stable response with mild early morning akinesia at one extreme to a chaotic and unpredictable response at the other (34). There is no universal agreement on the staging of fluctuations, and this probably can never be satisfactorily achieved because it is impossible to establish for certain where to draw the line. However, Hoehn (1985) has put forward a clinically useful scheme for grading wearing off (35). Stage 1 is mild, detectable; stage 2 is moderate, activities needing rescheduling, but with the patient still independent when "off"; stage 3 is severe, predictable, with some doses failing to work, and the patient unable to function independently when "off"; stage 4 is severe, unpredictable "on-off". From an extreme standpoint, it could be said that all patients who respond to levodopa experience grade 1 wearing off, since benefit is clearly due to the drug, and not seen in the absence of treatment.

Of itself, grade 1 wearing off is not of functional importance to the patient. Since most subjects initially take levodopa three times a day, the onset of wearing-off is usually related to this regimen. The earliest sign may be increasing early morning akinesia, corresponding to the longest interdose interval. In addition, besides recognizing that he is not as mobile first thing in the morning, the patient is able for the first time to describe a clear change in motor disability occurring at an interval after the first dose of the day. (However, some subjects may experience "early morning benefit," during which they are surprisingly mobile for 15 min to 1 hr on arising, and then deteriorate, only to improve again when the first dose of levodopa takes effect.) Wearing off during the course of the day is usually first noted by the patient as a gradual return of parkinsonian symptoms and signs before the subsequent dose takes effect. When this "end-of-dose deterioration" occurs before the next dose is ingested, the patient will usually appreciate that this is due to the previous dose not lasting long enough. However, this deterioration may sometimes occur after the subsequent dose has been swallowed and before it has taken effect. Many patients may fail to appreciate what is happening, and erroneously blame their deterioration on the dosage of levodopa they have just taken. Sometimes, however, their interpretation is correct because, just as a low dosage of levodopa may initially worsen tremor when patients begin treatment, transient worsening of tremor can indeed be the first sign of the action of a dose of levodopa in a fluctuating patient.

As the clinical duration of action of each dose shortens, patients may need to fractionate their treatment into more frequent and smaller doses. (In this context, it should be stressed that when such patients are admitted to hospital their levodopa *must* be given at appropriate intervals, rather than just at the times of the nurses' routine drug rounds.) Other maneuvers at this stage include the addition of bromocriptine or selegiline (see Chaps. 21 and 22). With the passage of time, the degree and the rapidity of clinical fluctuations alter so that, at their most extreme, patients may be completely mobile and independent, usually with dyskinesias ("on") and deteriorate in seconds into a helpless, chairbound, severe parkinsonian ("off") unable to feed, wash, or even take the next dose of medication to escape this petrified state. The "light-switch" analogy led to the application of the term "on–off" to such fluctuations. Together with the above changes, there may also develop a variably increased latency until each dose "takes." Certain of the smaller individual doses, often in the afternoon, may completely fail to "take" at all. Sometimes this may be the result of a clinical "threshold effect," in which smaller, fractionated doses may fail to "throw the switch." However, sometimes even large single oral doses of levodopa may entirely fail to work at certain times ("dose-resistant off periods").

As a result of the variable latency to central action of individual doses of levodopa, and of certain doses failing to turn a patient "on," response fluctuations may become unpredictable. The term "yo-yoing" (34) was coined for subjects with a totally unpredictable response to treatment. However, since fluctuations (excluding the short-lived paradoxic kinesis and akinesia paradoxica that also occur in untreated subjects) are only seen in patients taking levodopa, all fluctuations must be ultimately dose related. In most, if not all, apparent "yo-yoers," cumulative charting of "off" and "on" periods over a number of days will reveal some relationship between timing of dose and clinical response ("complicated end-of-dose fluctuations") (36). The impact on the patient's lifestyle stems from the prospective unpredictability of the fluctuations. Subjects can no longer plan their daily life around their drug administrations, and dare not venture out in case they are suddenly rendered immobile and helpless. This progression, however, is not necessarily a one-way journey. Many patients experiencing unpredictable and chaotic response fluctuations on frequent small doses of levodopa may regain a predictable response pattern if administration three or four times daily with larger individual amounts of levodopa is recommenced. The almost inevitable price the patient has to pay is increased time "off." Most patients with severe "off" period immobility will not tolerate such a regimen, but those who are still fairly independent in their "off" periods may find this a satisfactory state of affairs. Indeed, the goal of maximizing time "on" may be highly unsuitable for certain patients. Many parkinsonian patients, often because of "on"-period dyskinesias, can best undertake certain activities (for example, cooking and even, surprisingly, playing badminton) only when "off," and depend heavily on their days being predictably apportioned between "on" and "off" conditions.

Although it is natural to be most struck by the dramatic motor changes between the "on" and "off" states, one should not forget that other aspects change as well. Examples are mood (37), bladder function (38), pain (39), blood pressure (40), respiration (41), visual function (at retinal level) (42), and, possibly, eye movements (43). Intellectual function seems to alter little, if at all (44). However, because of their blank expression and slow, poor speech, many patients complain that their "off" periods induce a "does he take sugar?"* attitude in their attendants.

DYSKINESIAS

The development of dyskinesias accompanies that of the "on–off" phenomenon. Although not necessarily present when wearing off is first noticed, dyskinesias almost invariably precede the development of more abrupt motor fluctuations. In most subjects there is a definite relationship between dose of levodopa, degree of clinical benefit, and the presence of dyskinesias.

Peak-dose dyskinesias may initially disappear or markedly decrease with a reduction in levodopa dosage, but later they may be an inevitable accompaniment of "on" periods ("square wave dyskinesias") which the patient must accept as the price of mobility. Most patients will tolerate even the most bizarre and

---

*This phrase is commonly used in England to describe the way "normal" people talk over the heads of the physically disabled, assuming they are incapable of expressing their wants and needs.

dramatic involuntary movements over a state of parkinsonism. Any variety of dyskinesia may occur with levodopa treatment. In subjects with later onset of disease, they focus more on the neck and face (orofacial dyskinesia or chorea), whereas younger-onset patients are more prone to display a variable mixture of chorea and mobile dystonia in the limbs and trunk. This difference interestingly parallels the relationship between age and distribution of signs in idiopathic dystonia, and in tardive dystonia as opposed to tardive dyskinesia.

Peak-dose myoclonus on levodopa is uncommon (as opposed to night-time myoclonic jerks, which are relatively frequent). Methysergide may ameliorate this symptom in some patients (45).

Not all levodopa-associated dyskinesias are peak-dose, however. The most extreme involuntary movements seen in parkinsonian patients occur with a beginning and/or end-of-dose (diphasic "DID") pattern (46–48). They are usually violent, dramatic and disabling, occurring 15–20 min after the patient takes a dose in the "off" condition, lasting 15–20 min, and then settling to be replaced usually by mild axial dyskinesias and sometimes by peak-dose dysphonia and a lurching, staggering, "drunken" gait. They may return for a similar period prior to the patient turning "off." In such subjects, overlapping effective doses of levodopa may be very successful in the short term, but in my experience these patients ultimately always worsen with this maneuver, with the progressive takeover of all their mobile periods by increasingly severe involuntary movements. It becomes impossible to distinguish beginning-from-peak from end-of-dose dyskinesias, and these subjects almost always opt for a return to a sequence of predictable "on–off" cycles. An exception to this rule is the uncommon beginning-of-dose fixed dystonia, which can indeed be avoided by overlapping doses of levodopa, provided that peak-dose mobile dyskinesias are not too severe.

Another type of levodopa-related dyskinesia is "off period" fixed dystonia, which is often painful. This is most frequently seen in the setting of early morning dystonia (49). The patient is usually immobile but dystonia free in bed, but on arising and weight bearing, one (usually on the earliest and more severely affected side) or both legs adopt fixed and often painful dystonic postures. A patient described it as follows:

A peculiarly difficult feature is that since it occurs only in the early morning, doctors don't see it in action, and indeed few of them seem to have heard of it. It happens to me soon after I get up in the mornings (not immediately). I suddenly find that I am standing or walking on the sides of my feet something like a chimpanzee. I generally feel totally incapable of solving the problems of balance involved. I somehow manage to reach the breakfast table and balance myself on a chair. In this state it is difficult for anybody to help because I can't work out what I need to do. Then, in just a few minutes my breakfast coffee dissolves the levodopa, I feel myself sitting up straight, getting my balance, feet straightening out. The relief is very pleasant indeed.

Similar leg dystonias may occur at periods of "wearing off," but much more dramatic episodes may also occur either in the early morning or during "off" periods, and can last up to 4 hr. The most severe examples are terrifying. The entire body may be racked by painful dystonic spasms with forced jaw opening, retrocollis, flexed or extended arms and legs, profuse sweating, mydriasis, severe hypertension and tachycardia, and overwhelming "angst." Although dystonia on action or at rest may sometimes be associated with untreated parkinsonism (50), the painful fixed dystonias described here occur exclusively in levodopa-treated patients. They are relieved when the subject turns "on" with levodopa or another dopamine agonist, and disappear when levodopa is completely stopped (although early morning dystonia may persist for the first few days of a drug holiday). They may also be helped by taking a long-acting dopamine agonist such as bromocriptine or pergolide at night, or by taking the first dose of levodopa immediately on waking, and staying in bed until it begins to work, or by adding baclofen (51). Off period dystonias are often helped by overlapping levodopa doses or by adding day-time bromocriptine or pergolide. If these measures are not successful, the addition of lithium treatment at therapeutic plasma levels often dramatically reduces or abolishes dystonic spasms without necessarily altering duration of time "on" (51a).

Numerous other drugs have been tried in an attempt to reduce "on" period dyskinesias. Although anticholinergics are known to increase levodopa-induced involuntary movements, deanol, a putative cholinergic precursor, does not seem to ameliorate dyskinesias. Titration of a small dosage of a dopamine-blocking drug such as tiapride, oxiperomide, or haloperidol may improve peak-dose dyskinesias, but often at the expense of increasing parkinsonism. Antidyskinetic effects have also been claimed for sodium valproate, naloxone, and apomorphine, but so far none of these drugs has consistently been found useful.

WHAT FACTORS DETERMINE THE ONSET OF DYSKINESIAS AND FLUCTUATIONS?

There is much debate and controversy to whether the development of the "long-term levodopa syndrome" is related more to duration of disease than duration of treatment. The UCLA researchers (52) among others (35) argue that the former is more important, whereas Columbia researchers (53) and others (54) maintain that duration of treatment is the crucial factor. Unfortunately, the two factors are almost inextricably interwoven, and the available data do not allow a conclusive answer to the question. There are also many suggestions that patients treated from the outset with low dosages of levodopa develop a lower incidence of involuntary movements and fluctuations than when higher dosages are used.

The evidence is not conclusive (54), but agrees generally with clinical opinion and experience. A more important factor, however, is "benignity" of the disease in the individual patient. As Barbeau (55) has stated:

> We now recognise . . . a sub-group of patients . . . who essentially do not progress over more than 20 years. Undoubtedly many of our excellent results [with levodopa] belong to this group. They require only moderate doses of L-dopa . . . and almost never have abnormal involuntary movements or oscillations in performance, and represent about 10% of all Parkinsonian patients.

The most important factor determining the subsequent course of events on levodopa treatment is the age of onset of disease. In young-onset parkinsonian patients significant fluctuations frequently begin within weeks or months of the patient starting levodopa, and sometimes from the very first dose. Youth also determines the latency to development of dyskinesias, their severity, distribution, and nature (the vast majority of "diphasic" dyskinesias and of severe off period dystonias occur in subjects with young age at onset). Hoehn (35) has recently drawn attention to the importance of age at disease onset. Of 163 subjects treated with levodopa the percentage of "fluctuators" whose Parkinson's disease was diagnosed before 50 years of age was 65.9%, falling to 29.6% in those aged 50–59, and only 5.9% in those aged 60 or over. Thus geriatricians, who inevitably care for a large proportion of parkinsonians, almost never see the dramatically fluctuating patients that come the way of neurologists and are to be found in specialized Parkinson's disease clinics.

All of these factors conspire to complicate any comparative assessment of new and perhaps better treatments for the symptoms of Parkinson's disease (see, for example, Chap. 21). Take the example of a group of parkinsonian subjects with disease onset in their 60s, and a benign initial course; treat them with a low dosage of a new drug with modest (but useful) clinical benefit, and significant side effects, and one ends up with a "core" of survivors after several years' treatment. Let us say that the incidence of dyskinesias and significant fluctuations is very low among this surviving group. It would be very difficult to know what conclusions to draw about any advantage of the new medication in long-term treatment, since most of the subjects at risk for the long-term complications of levodopa treatment have been selected out. Also, if this new drug is prospectively compared with levodopa treatment, ideally the two groups should be matched for degree of clinical benefit, in which case the dosage of the new drug will have to be high or the dosage of levodopa low. The alternative approach of comparing the incidence of dyskinesias and fluctuations in one patient group taking a new, less potent drug (and hence experiencing a smaller degree of clinical benefit) with a matched patient group taking normal dosages of levodopa with a higher degree of clinical benefit will almost certainly favor the new drug.

WHAT MECHANISM UNDERLIES PROGRESSION
OF THE "ON–OFF" PHENOMENON?

The underlying cause of the observed shortening of clinical duration of action of levodopa over time is unknown. No change in peripheral pharmacokinetics of levodopa in the same patients followed over time from a period of stable response to one of "on–off" occurrence has been shown, and indeed such a study has never been done. Measurement of plasma levodopa levels has, however, in most patients permitted useful correlation between "on" periods and high or rising plasma levodopa levels, and between "off" periods and low or falling levels. If one allows for a variable "lag" corresponding to the latency from the arrival of levodopa in the blood to the action of derived dopamine in the striatum, many "off" periods seem to be related to troughs of plasma levodopa concentration. Although it was suggested (56) that other "off" periods could be caused by "desensitization block" due to the presence of excessive amounts of dopamine in the striatum, the successful reversal or prevention of "off" periods by injections of subcutaneous apomorphine (57), intravenous lisuride (58), or intravenous levodopa infusions added to usual oral levodopa treatment in patients experiencing frequent "off" periods (59) all suggest that central receptors remain available for stimulation. The main problem is of sustained delivery to these receptors of an appropriate agonist at suitable concentrations.

Recent positron emission tomographic (PET) studies (60) examining striatal to surrounding brain ratios of $[^{18}F]$-fluorodopa-derived activity have shown that as well as parkinsonians attaining a lower absolute striatal uptake of isotope in parkinsonians than do controls, patients also lose this activity from striatum faster. Moreover, this decline is more rapid in "on–off" patients than in those showing a stable response, indicating the importance of alterations in central handling of levodopa in the development of response fluctuations.

DRUG HOLIDAYS

In recent years there has been a vogue for levodopa "drug holidays," with claims that after a variable drug-free interval patients experienced greater clinical benefit when treatment with lower dosages of levodopa was reintroduced. It has been suggested (61) that this improvement may be due to up-regulation of dopamine receptors previously chronically down-regulated by bombardment with dopamine (see below). Another equally plausible hypothesis is that drug holidays quite simply permit a "washout" of a chronic accumulation of levodopa and its metabolites, and an opportunity for intensive inpatient physiotherapy and reeducation (61). Various drug holiday regimens have been proposed, from "week-end" holidays (62) to drug-free periods of up to 21 days

(61). In many of these subjects the holiday has not been "elective" but forced because the patient was clearly toxic. No study has compared drug holiday followed by lowered levodopa dosage with simply reducing levodopa dosage without going through "cold turkey" withdrawal. It is quite possible that the results would be comparable. It is interesting to note that the patient reported by Direnfeld et al. in 1978 (63), and widely cited as one of the early examples of a successful drug holiday, only lowered his levodopa dosage but did not stop it. In addition, the later results 1 year after recommencing levodopa therapy are generally disappointing (64). The risks of a drug holiday have to be weighed against any suggested benefit. The patients may need surgical stockings, prophylactic subcutaneous heparin, nasogastric feeding, intensive physiotherapy, and nursing care, and are at risk of all the attendant problems of immobility. In addition, at least one death from possible "neuroleptic malignant syndrome" has been reported due solely to the abrupt cessation of levodopa treatment (65). Finally, the psychologic damage produced by a long period of immobility in which the true stage of progression of underlying disease is revealed to the patient should not be underestimated. Consequently, in practice most neurologists stop levodopa therapy completely only as a last resort, in the context of a clearly toxic patient whom they cannot manage solely by reducing their dosage.

IS LEVODOPA HARMFUL?

Effect on Disease Progression

This has been discussed previously.

Effect on Life Expectancy

In two large studies in the prelevodopa era, subjects with Parkinson's disease were found to have an excess mortality ratio of around 3:1. In the 601 patients evaluated by Hoehn and Yahr (66), mean duration of disease from diagnosis to death was 9 years. If we disregard one of the first postlevodopa studies, which gave a mortality ratio of 0.96:1 (67), the average mortality ratio of 8 similar studies after a mean of 7 years levodopa therapy was 1.56:1. Follow-up to 12 years on the subjects in one of these studies who had a 6-year mortality ratio of 1.45 (68) showed a precipitate rise in later years to 2.59 (69) suggesting a markedly increased late mortality. However, it should be remembered that the proportion of patients with severe pretreatment disability scores in such long-term studies (in which initial commencement of levodopa therapy was determined more by its recent availability than by today's "need to treat" basis) would not be comparable to that in studies starting, for example, after the mid-1970s.

Possible Cytotoxicity

There are a number of theoretical reasons why levodopa treatment could be cytotoxic to dopaminergic neurons. Under certain circumstances, levodopa might be metabolized to 6-hydroxydopamine or 2,4,5-trihydroxyphenylalanine. Both can exert powerful cytotoxic actions on neuroblastoma cells in vitro through the production of superoxide radicals (70). The former is widely used as a specific toxin with which to lesion catecholamine-containing neurons in the nigrostriatal tract of animals (71). The reaction of quinone oxidation products of levodopa with sulfhydryl or other nucleophilic groups might also cause cell damage (72). High dosages of levodopa may also disrupt intracellular trans-methylation reactions. In animals clinically treated with levodopa, S-adenosyl methionine levels are initially lowered, but then overshoot to higher than normal levels (73). However, there is no evidence that any of these reactions assume importance in levodopa-treated parkinsonian patients. Indeed, postmortem examination of one of our patients with parkinsonism who had received more than 2 kg levodopa plus PDI over 4 years showed only cerebral amyloid angiopathy, with lacunae in basal ganglia and no Lewy bodies: there was a normal population and pigmentation of cells in the substantia nigra and locus ceruleus (74).

Receptor Changes

The data on dopamine receptor binding in parkinsonian brains are confusing and conflicting. Although Reisine et al., examining the brains of 10 treated patients, found reduced [3H] spiperone binding in caudate nucleus (75), other workers have found increased dopamine receptor binding in basal ganglia structures in brains of non-levodopa-treated subjects. Thus Lee et al. (76) found increased [3H] haloperidol binding in the putamen of untreated persons but normal levels in levodopa-treated subjects. Similarly, Rinne et al. (77) found increased [3H] spiperone binding in the caudate and putamen of 10 of 15 untreated parkinsonians (but reduced binding in the other 5), and decreased binding in 5 of 10 treated subjects (but normal in the other 5). Bokobsa et al. (78) found [3H] spiperone binding to be normal in both the caudate and putamen once neuroleptic-treated parkinsonian patients were excluded from their study. Although some of these results hint at a possible dopamine receptor supersensitivity in untreated patients, with possible subsensitivity developing when chronic levodopa treatment is given, there is certainly not enough consistent data at present to prove or disprove this hypothesis. Further studies with good clinicopathologic correlation are clearly needed before any conclusions can be drawn.

WHEN SHOULD LEVODOPA BE INTRODUCED?

Many patients with very early Parkinson's disease may not need any drug treatment. When symptoms progress, most neurologists start treatment with an anticholinergic and/or amantadine. In elderly subjects, because of their reduced life expectancy, the likely low incidence of troublesome dyskinesias and "on-off" fluctuations, and the increased risk of organic confusional states with anticholinergics, there is little cause to delay levodopa treatment. However, young patients have many years of life ahead of them, and are likely to develop the "long-term levodopa syndrome" earlier and more severely. Yet these are precisely the subjects likely to be still holding down a job, paying off a mortgage, and raising young children, all of which are arguments for not delaying the dramatic benefits that levodopa can give. In the final analysis, all of these factors have to be considered separately in each individual. The decision to move from initial treatment to "stronger" levodopa-based therapy should ultimately be the patient's decision, made in conjunction with an impartial discussion of the available evidence with a neurologist.

HOW SHOULD LEVODOPA BE INTRODUCED?

Most neurologists usually introduce levodopa in the form of Madopar 62.5 three times daily or Sinemet Plus, half a tablet three times daily taken with meals, increasing to Madopar 125 or Sinemet Plus, 1 tablet three times daily. After some days or weeks, but occasionally after a month or 2, the degree of clinical benefit achieved will be apparent, and some subjects will need a further increase in dosage. Since tolerance to any possible gastrointestinal side effects will have developed in most patients by this stage, subjects can then be told that they do not necessarily have to take each dose with a meal. If an adequate dosage of Sinemet has been attained, a change to the cheaper Sinemet 110 (or to whole or half tablets of Sinemet 275) can be attempted. The addition of domperidone 20 mg orally three times a day may be helpful in the early stages of treatment of the minority of patients who are initially troubled by nausea and vomiting despite peripheral decarboxylase inhibitors. This can usually be stopped when tolerance develops. However domperidone is not currently available in the United States except in certain investigative clinical settings. Once significant clinical benefit has been obtained, I usually attempt to withdraw anticholinergics and/or amantadine and reassure the patient that any lost ground can be made up by a slight further increase in levodopa. In patients with response fluctuations, attention to protein intake (see Chap. 18) may be necessary. Some subjects find that they achieve rapid and sometimes more reliable benefit from individual doses by crushing their tablets of Sinemet and taking them in liquid.

RESPONSE TO LEVODOPA

Lack of Response

There can be a number of reasons for a patient failing to respond to levodopa. The patient may not be able to tolerate an adequate dosage of levodopa because of side effects. Some other patients, for whatever reasons, may require higher dosages of levodopa to obtain a response. I would not label a patient as a definite response failure until he or she has taken between six and eight doses of Madopar 250 or Sinemet 275 per day for a period approaching 3 months. In a few centers, measurement of plasma levels of levodopa and its metabolites may possibly unearth the rare patient who either fails to absorb levodopa or displays unusually high levels of 3-0-methyldopa (79).

By far the most common cause for a patient not responding to adequate dosages of levodopa is misdiagnosis. Any patient should have been assessed on presentation for evidence of disturbance of sexual function, micturition, sweating, cardiovascular reflexes, eye movements, and intellect. If a patient fails to respond to levodopa, all of these aspects should be scrutinized even more closely. Autonomic function tests should be performed with the patient off treatment, and a computed tomographic (CT) scan is indicated. This may show brain stem or cerebellar atrophy in subjects with multiple system atrophy, or progressive supranuclear palsy, unsuspected deep lacunar infarcts in basal ganglia of elderly hypertensive subjects with arteriosclerotic pseudoparkinsonism, or cerebral atrophy in subjects with the association of dementia and parkinsonism. A dramatic clinical response to levodopa is usually synonymous with idiopathic Lewy body Parkinson's disease, but some patients with other conditions may occasionally show a very favorable response, even with clinical fluctuations and dyskinesias. A larger number may show a partial response to levodopa. The best approach is to remain open to the possibility that one's initial diagnosis of Parkinson's disease may have been incorrect. The more experience one has had with Parkinson's disease, the higher the proportion of patients in whom one has doubts about the diagnosis. Certain features such as definite cerebellar or pyramidal signs or gross selective brain stem atrophy on CT may make it certain that one is not dealing with idiopathic Parkinson's disease. In the remainder only the absence of Lewy bodies in the brain at postmortem may reveal for certain that the diagnosis during life was mistaken. However, the converse is not necessarily true. The prevalence of Lewy bodies in pigmented brain stem nuclei in aged brains is, at about 10%, a factor of 10 greater than the prevalence of clinical Parkinson's disease at that age. Thus the finding of Lewy bodies postmortem is not synonymous with clinical Parkinson's disease during life (80). The impetus to cross the threshold to clinical parkinsonism in some of these subjects harboring Lewy bodies could have been provided by the superimposition of co-existent Alzheimer's change or cerebrovascular disease, rather than by the severity of the Lewy body pathology alone.

Loss of Response

Contrary to accepted wisdom, complete loss of response to levodopa in patients with a previous definite clinical improvement is rare. Many subjects may appear to have lost a previous good response to levodopa because they no longer appear to fluctuate during the day. However, in most of these patients clinical deterioration will be seen if levodopa is stopped for several days. In addition, because of progressive loss of striatal as well as nigral neurons in subjects with multiple system atrophy and progressive supranuclear palsy, the group of "loss of response" patients will certainly include some with these diseases who initially responded to levodopa with a mild to moderate degree of benefit.

NEW DIRECTIONS

Sustained continuous intravenous infusions of levodopa are very successful in abolishing "on–off" fluctuations in the short term (58,59,81), but are not a practicable long-term solution because of problems of access, acidity, and volume. Levodopa is not absorbed through rectal mucosa (82), so this route cannot be used either. Intraduodenal and intragastric infusions of levodopa can certainly improve fluctuations in some patients (83), but current practical approaches for long-term management are focusing on two alternative strategies.

Methods of parenteral infusion work are moving away from levodopa and the intravenous route toward the use of more soluble dopamine agonists such as lisuride (see Chap. 20) given by continuous subcutaneous infusion (84). Given a suitable agonist, it may even be possible to utilize the transdermal route.

In parallel with these developments, much effort is being directed toward developing an effective sustained-release oral formulation of levodopa. In the early 1970s, a number of supposed slow-release preparations of plain levodopa were subjected to trial. Clinical results and the little pharmacokinetic data available were both disappointing. Recent technologic advances in sustained-release formulations for all kinds of drugs, paired with a renewed interest in the pharmacokinetics of levodopa (see Chap. 18), have given impetus to the development of such formulations for the treatment of the symptoms of Parkinson's disease. Trials of sustained-released formulations of both Sinemet (85) and Madopar (86) have recently begun.

Although some patients have achieved more stable clinical benefit with these formulations, others complain of increased unpredictability of response and unacceptable delays before the first morning dose takes effect. It is apparent that the bioavailability of both formulations relative to standard preparations is reduced to a varying degree in different subjects. Thus there is still considerable room for improvement in delivery of oral levodopa to patients with response fluctuations. Other as yet unexplored aspects of any sustained-release oral preparation of levodopa are its potential to improve night-time disability and to reduce early morning akinesia and dystonia. In addition, it will be important to establish whether patients treated de novo with sustained-release preparations (thus avoiding the periodic flooding and starving of the brain with levodopa), develop a lower or later incidence of dyskinesias and motor fluctuations.

CONCLUSIONS

It is clear that dopamine deficiency, although the central deficit in idiopathic Parkinson's disease, is but one of a series of changes in neurotransmitter and neuromodulator function in this condition. Alterations in central noradrenergic, serotonergic, cholinergic, and peptidergic function have also been demonstrated. However, levodopa remains without any doubt the single most effective treatment for Parkinson's disease symptoms, the "gold standard" against which all other treatments must be compared. After more than 15 years of its widespread clinical use, many questions concerning when, how, and in what dosage to use the drug remain unanswered. While the search for alternative dopamine agonists continues, much can be done to improve levodopa treatment. Future developments will see improved methods of drug delivery, together with efforts to develop treatment strategies that will dissociate involuntary movements and unwanted psychiatric side effects from the remarkably beneficial motor effects of the drug.

REFERENCES

1. Guggenheim M. (1913). *J Physiol Chem* 88: 276.
2. Ehringer H, Hornykiewicz O. (1960). *Klin Wochenschr* 38: 1236.
3. Carlsson A, Lindqvist M, Magnusson T. (1957). *Nature* 180: 1200.
4. Degkwitz R, Frowein R, Kulenkampff C, Mohs U. (1960). *Klin Wochenschr* 38: 120.
5. Barbeau A, Sourkes TL, Murphy GF. (1962). In: de Ajuriaguerra J. (Ed.), *Monoamines et Système Nerveux Central.* Paris, Masson.
6. Birkmayer W, Hornykiewicz O. (1961). *Wien Klin Wochenschr* 73: 787.
7. Cotzias GC, van Woert MH, Schiffer LM. (1967). *N Engl J Med* 276: 374.
8. Bartholini G, Burkard WP, Pletscher A, Bates HM. (1967). *Nature* 215: 852.
9. Birkmayer W. (1969). *Wien Klin Wochenschr* 81: 677.
10. Porter CC, Watson LS, Titus DC, Tolaro JA, Byer SS. (1962). *Biochem Pharmacol* 11: 1067.
11. Calne DB, Reid JL, Vakil SD, Rao S, Petrie A, Pallis CA, Gawler J, Thomas PK, Hilson A. (1971). *Br Med J* 3: 729.
12. Tourtellotte W, Syndulko K, Potvin AR, Hirsch SB, Potvin JH. (1980). *Arch Neurol* 37: 723.
13. Rinne UK, Molsa P. (1979). *Neurology* 29: 1584.
14. Diamond SG, Markham CH, Treciokas LJ. (1978). *Ann Neurol* 3: 267.
15. Calne DB, Petrie A, Rao S, Reid JL, Vakil SD. (1972). *Br J Pharmacol* 44: 162.

16. Leibowitz M, Lieberman A. (1975). *Neurology* 25: 917.
17. Quinn N, Parkes J, Jackson G, Upward J. (1985). *Lancet* 2: 724.
18. Cotzias GC, Papavasiliou PS, Gellene R. (1969). *N Engl J Med* 280: 337.
19. Teychenne PF, Calne DB, Lewis PJ, Findley LJ. (1975). *Clin Pharmacol Ther* 18: 273.
20. Bevan DR, Monks PS, Calne DB. (1973). *Anaesthesia* 28: 29.
21. Miller EM, Nieburg HA. (1974). *Dis Nerv Syst* 35: 20.
22. Rabey JM, Vardi J, Askenazi JJ, Streifler M. (1977). *Gerontology* 23: 438.
23. Gerlach J, Koppelhus T, Helwig E, Monrad A. (1974). *Acta Psychiatr Scand* 50: 410.
24. Weintraub MI, Gaasterlan DD, van Woert MH. (1970). *N Engl J Med* 283: 120.
25. Tanner CM, Goetz CG, Klawans HL. (1982). *Neurology* 32(2): A162.
26. Malarkey WB, Cyrus J, Paulson GW. (1974). *J Clin Endocrinol Metab* 39: 229.
27. Rampen FHJ. (1985). *J Neurol Neurosurg Psychiatry* 48: 585.
28. Goetz CG. (1984). *Clin Neuropharmacol* 7: 107.
29. Cook DG, Klawans HL. (1985). *Clin Neuropharmacol* 8: 93.
30. Sacks O. (1982). *Awakenings*. London, Pan Books Ltd.
31. Yahr MD. (1970). In: Barbeau A, McDowell FH. (Eds.), *L-Dopa and Parkinsonism*. Philadelphia, F.A. Davis Co.
32. Barbeau A. (1969). *Can Med Assoc J* 101: 59.
33. Koller WC. (1982). *Neurology* 32: 324.
34. Marsden CD, Parkes JD. (1976). *Lancet* 1: 292.
35. Hoehn MM. (1985). *Acta Neurol Scand* 71: 97.
36. Marsden CD, Parkes JD, Quinn N. (1982). In: Marsden CD, Fahn S. (Eds.), *BIMR Neurology 2: Movement Disorders*. London, Butterworths.
37. Damasio AR, Lobo-Antunes J, Macedo C. (1971). *J Neurol Neurosurg Psychiatry* 34: 502.
38. Fitzmaurice H, Fowler CJ, Rickards D, Kirby RS, Quinn NP, Marsden CD, Milroy EJG, Turner-Warwick RT. (1985). *Br J Urol* 57: 652.
39. Quinn N, Koller WC, Lang AE, Marsden CD. (1986). *Lancet* (in press).
40. Baratti M, Calzetti S. (1984). *J Neurol Neurosurg Psychiatry* 47: 1241.
41. Ilson J, Braun N, Fahn S. (1983). *Neurology* 33 (Suppl 2): 113.
42. Bodis-Wollner I, Yahr MD, Mylin LH. (1984). *Adv Neurol* 40: 289.
43. Gibson JM, Pimlott R, Kennard C. *J Neurol Neurosurg Psychiatry* (in press).
44. Brown RG, Marsden CD, Quinn NP, Wyke MA. (1984). *J Neurol Neurosurg Psychiatry* 47: 454.
45. Klawans HL, Goetz CG, Bergen D. (1975). *Arch Neurol* 32: 331.
46. Tolosa ES, Martin WE, Cohen HP, Jacobson RL. (1975). *Neurology* 25: 177.
47. Muenter MD, Sharpless NS, Tyce GM, Darley FL. (1977). *Mayo Clin Proc* 52: 163.
48. Lhermitte F, Agid Y, Signoret J-L. (1978). *Arch Neurol* 35: 261.
49. Melamed E. (1979). *Arch Neurol* 36: 308.

50. Lees AJ, Hardie RJ, Stern GM. (1984). *J Neurol Neurosurg Psychiatry* 47: 885.
51. Lees AJ, Shaw KM, Stern GM. (1978). *J Neurol Neurosurg Psychiatry* 41: 707.
51a. Quinn N, Marsden CD. (1986). *Lancet* 1: 1377.
52. Markham CH, Diamond SG. (1981). *Neurology* 31: 125.
53. Lesser RP, Fahn S, Snider SR, Cote LJ, Isgreen WP, Barrett RE. (1979). *Neurology* 29: 1253.
54. Rajput AH, Stern W, Laverty WH. (1984). *Neurology* 34: 991.
55. Barbeau A. (1981). *TIPS* 2: 297.
56. Fahn S. (1974). *Neurology* 24: 431.
57. Yahr MD, Clough CG, Bergmann KJ. (1982). *Lancet* 2: 709.
58. Hardie RJ, Lees AJ, Stern GM. (1984). *Brain* 107: 487.
59. Quinn NP, Marsden CD, Parkes JD. (1984). *Neurology* 34: 1131.
60. Leenders KL, Palmer AJ, Quinn N, Clark JC, Firnau G, Garnett ES, Nahmias C, Jones T, Marsden CD. (1986). *J Neurol Neurosurg Psychiatry* 49: 853.
61. Direnfeld LK, Feldman RG, Alexander MP, Kelly-Hayes M. (1980). *Neurology* 30: 785.
62. Goetz CG, Tanner CM, Nausieda PA. (1981). *Neurology* 31: 1460.
63. Direnfeld L, Spero L, Marotta J, Seeman P. (1978). *Ann Neurol* 4: 573.
64. Koller WC, Weiner WJ, Perlik S, Nausieda PA, Goetz CJ, Klawans HL. (1981). *Neurology* 31: 473.
65. Sechi GP, Tanda F, Mutani R. (1984). *Neurology* 34: 249.
66. Hoehn MM, Yahr MD. (1967). *Neurology* 17: 427.
67. Diamond SG, Markham CH, Treciokas LJ. (1976). In: Birkmayer W, Hornykiewicz O. (Eds.), *Advances in Parkinsonism*. Basle, Roche.
68. Shaw KM, Lees AJ, Stern GM. (1980). *Q J Med* 49: 283.
69. Curtis L, Lees AJ, Stern GM, Marmot MG. (1984). *Lancet* 2: 211.
70. Graham DG, Tiffany SM, Bell WR, Gutknecht WF. (1978). *Mol Pharmacol* 14: 644.
71. Ungerstedt U. (1971). *Acta Physiol Scand* 82 (Suppl. 367): 49.
72. Sandler M. (1973). *Adv Neurol* 2: 255.
73. Wurtman RJ, Romero JA. (1972). *Neurology* 22 (Suppl. 511): 72.
74. Quinn N, Parkes D, Janota I, Marsden CD. (1986). *Movement Disorders* 1:65.
75. Reisine TD, Fields JZ, Yamamura HI, Bird ED, Spokes E, Schreiner PS, Enna SJ. (1977). *Life Sci* 21: 335.
76. Lee T, Seeman P, Rajput A, Farley IJ, Hornykiewicz O. (1978). *Nature* 273: 59.
77. Rinne UK, Lonnberg P, Koskinen V. (1981). *J Neural Transm* 51: 97.
78. Bokobsa B, Ruberg M, Scatton B, Javoy-Agid F, Agid Y. (1984). *Eur J Pharmacol* 99: 167.
79. Rivera-Calimlim L, Tandon D, Anderson F, Joynt R. (1977). *Arch Neurol* 34: 228.
80. Quinn N, Rossor MN, Marsden CD. (1986). *Br Med Bull* 42: 86.

81. Nutt JG, Woodward WR, Hammerstad JP, Carter JH, Anderson JL. (1984). *N Engl J Med* 310: 483.
82. Eisler T, Eng N, Plotkin C, Calne DB. (1981). *Neurology* 31: 215.
83. Kurlan R, Rubin AJ, Miller C, Rivera-Calimlim L, Shoulson I. (1985). *Ann Neurol* 18: 139.
84. Obeso JA, Luquin MR, Martinez-Lage JM. (1986). *Lancet* 1: 467.
85. Juncos J, Serrati C, Fabbrini G, Chase TN. (1985). *Lancet* 2: 440.
86. Marion M-H, Stocchi F, Quinn NP, Jenner P, Marsden CD. Eighth International Symposium on Parkinson's Disease, June 1985, New York, Abstract, p. 105.

18

Pharmacokinetics of Levodopa
Clinical Implications

JOHN G. NUTT
Oregon Health Sciences University, Portland, Oregon

Levodopa, the most effective agent for the treatment of the symptoms of Parkinson's disease, differs from most other drugs used in central nervous system disorders in three interesting ways: (a) metabolism in the periphery and brain is very rapid and produces compounds that may have other pharmacologic effects; (b) levodopa crosses cell membranes by a saturable, carrier-mediated transport system rather than by diffusion; and (c) enzymatic barriers to levodopa's absorption and transport into brain are present. These unique features must be understood by the clinician to achieve the optimal clinical response to levodopa. This chapter will first consider levodopa metabolism, transport, and enzymatic barriers in general terms and then review the clinical aspects of absorption, distribution, and elimination of levodopa and conclude with a discussion of the relationship between plasma levodopa concentrations and clinical response.

BIOCHEMISTRY

Metabolism

Levodopa is extremely rapidly metabolized (Fig. 1) in the periphery, a large percentage of the metabolism occurring during absorption. In the absence of decarboxylase inhibitors it is estimated that only about one-half to one-quarter of an orally administered dose reaches the systemic circulation as levodopa (1-3). In patients not receiving decarboxylase inhibitors such as carbidopa, levodopa is predominantly decarboxylated in gut and liver to dopamine (3-7). The dopamine is either conjugated with sulfate (8-10) or converted to dihydroxyphenylacetic acid (DOPAC) and homovanillic acid (HVA) (3-7). When de-

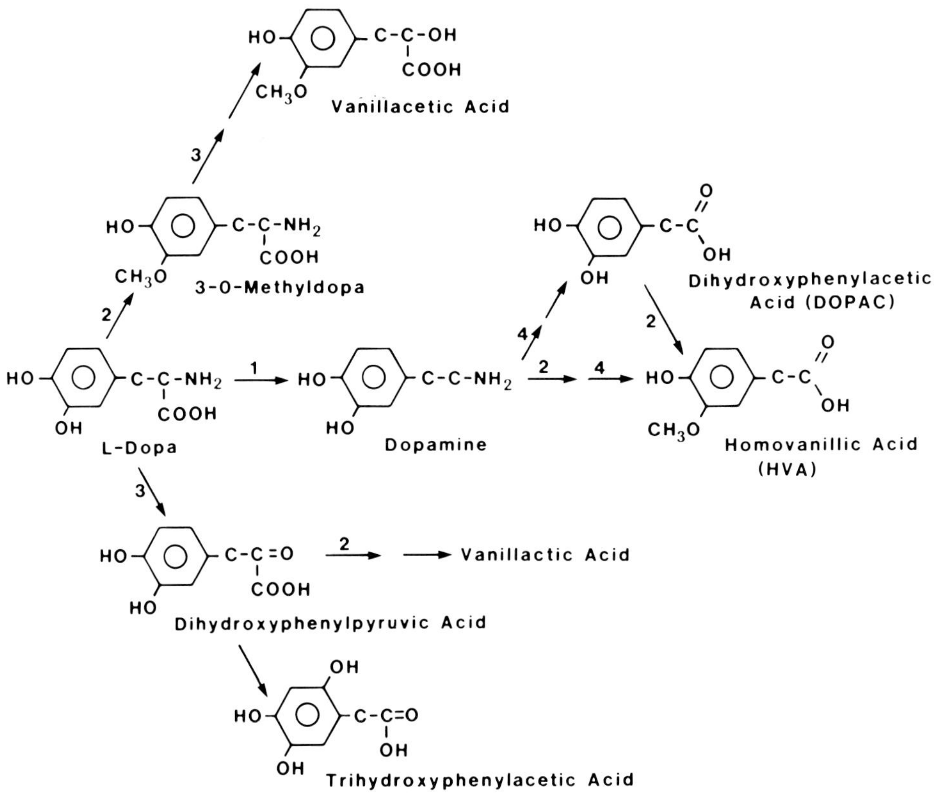

FIGURE 1 Major metabolic routes of levodopa. Enzymes are indicated by the numbers: 1, aromatic amino acid decarboxylase; 2, catechol-O-methyltransferase; 3, tyrosine aminotransferase; 4, monoamine oxidase. Adapted with permission from *Clin Neuropharmacol* 1984; 7(1):35–49.

carboxylase inhibitors are administered concomitantly, approximately one-quarter of the usual oral dose is required to produce the same plasma concentrations (11–13). Conjugated dopamine and dopamine metabolites become minor products and the side effects that may represent peripheral effects of dopamine (nausea and cardiac arrhythmias) are reduced (14). With the reduction of decarboxylation, proportionally more of the levodopa is O-methylated to 3-O-methyldopa (3OMD) (11,15) and is transaminated and excreted as vanillactic acid (16) and trihydroxyphenylacetic acid (17). 3OMD is of interest because high plasma levels have been associated with poor response to levodopa and dyskinesia (18–20). Transamination is reversible so that the immediate product of levodopa transamination, 3,4-dihydroxyphenylpyruvic acid, is of interest because it could serve as a precursor to levodopa (21). There are also a large number of metabolites of levodopa, many unidentified, that could be of pharmacologic or neurotoxic importance (4,6).

The cerebral metabolism of levodopa appears to be primarily to 3OMD in brain areas without significant catecholamine innervation, such as the cerebellum, and to dopamine and its metabolites as well as 3OMD in the striatum and other areas with rich catecholamine innervation (22). Biochemical and positron emission tomographic studies suggest that the half-life of dopamine in the striatum, formed after levodopa administration, ranges from minutes to several hours (22–24) and is reduced by lesions of nigrostriatal dopaminergic projections (22,25, 26).

Transport

Levodopa is a large neutral amino acid (LNAA) which enters cells by a saturable carrier system also utilized by other LNAAs such as phenylalanine, tyrosine, tryptophan, leucine, isoleucine, valine, methionine, and histidine (27,28). In most tissues the equilibrium constant for transport (Kt) of LNAAs is much higher than the normal physiologic concentrations of the amino acids and therefore there is no competition among the various members of the LNAAs for transport (29–31). However, extremely high concentrations of amino acids may be present in the gut after a meal and competition for transport can occur. A second site at which competition can occur is the blood–brain barrier. The Kt for LNAA transport in the brain capillary endothelial cells is approximately tenfold less than in other tissues and approximates the plasma concentrations of the LNAAs. This means that there will always be competition among these amino acids for entry into the brain (29–31). The transport of LNAAs into neurons is believed to be of high capacity and thus competition at the neuronal membrane is unlikely (30,31).

Enzymatic Barriers

Intracellular aromatic amino acid decarboxylase (AAAD) in stomach and intestinal mucosa (32–34) and brain capillary endothelial cells (35–37) form an enzymatic barrier to the absorption of levodopa and to its entry into brain. The gut AAAD decarboxylates between one-half and three-quarters of an orally administered dose of levodopa (1,2). Inhibition of this decarboxylase with carbidopa or benserazide reduces the amount of levodopa required for equivalent plasma concentrations by three-quarters (11). The brain capillary decarboxylase activity is probably not altered by carbidopa in the usual clinical dosages (38), although this is a subject of controversy (37). The enzymatic barrier produces a curvilinear relationship between plasma and brain concentrations of levodopa;

proportionally more levodopa enters at high plasma concentrations (35) when the decarboxylase approaches saturation.

PHARMACOKINETICS

Absorption

Gastric Role

Levodopa is poorly or not at all absorbed from the stomach (32), but may be decarboxylated by AAAD in the gastric mucosa (32,33) (Fig. 2). Thus the stomach may hinder absorption by delaying levodopa's passage into proximal bowel and the vicinity of its absorptive sites as well as by metabolizing the drug so that less

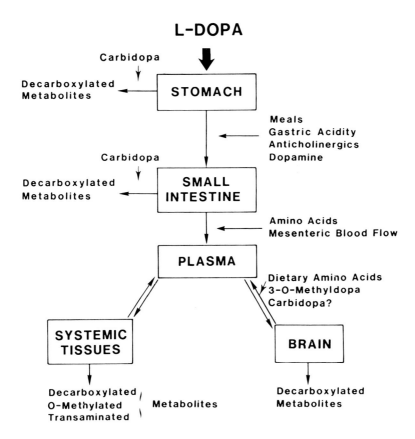

FIGURE 2 Schematic overview of levodopa pharmacokinetics, with permission from *Clin Neuropharmacol* 1984: 7(1):35–49.

is available for absorption (32). What factors influence gastric emptying and thus levodopa absorption? The most obvious is food, particularly high-protein or high-fat meals. The administration of levodopa with meals will frequently delay and reduce absorption (2,5,39) (Fig. 3). The effect of snacks is less clear; a clinical study suggested that snacks had no effect on the response to levodopa (40). However, for a more predictable response to each dose of levodopa, administration of the drug away from the time of meals is preferable. Meals taken 15–30 min after the medicine probably have little effect on absorption of levodopa (unpublished results). For patients who experience nausea when the medicine is taken on an empty stomach, the drug can be given with a small snack. The antinausea effect of taking levodopa with snacks may, in fact, be due

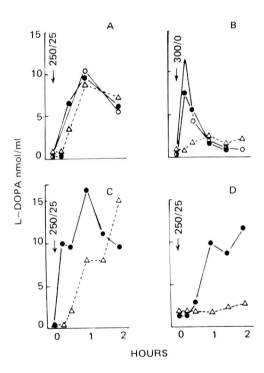

FIGURE 3 Effect of meals on absorption of levodopa in four patients. Open and closed circles represent plasma concentrations of levodopa when the medicine was taken after fasting overnight (patients A and B were tested twice under these conditions). Triangles represent plasma concentrations when the same dosage was taken after a routine breakfast. The meal had no effect on appearance of levodopa in the plasma of patient A, delayed it in patient C, and virtually eliminated absorption in patients B and D. (From ref. 39, with permission.)

to a reduction of absorption and blunting of the peak plasma concentration of levodopa.

Gastric emptying may also be influenced by gastric acidity. Low gastric pH is associated with delayed gastric emptying and consequently delayed and reduced levodopa absorption (32). The administration of antacids to patients with excessive gastric acidity will improve levodopa absorption by hastening gastric emptying (41). Administering antacids routinely to nonselected patients does not improve absorption (42). An antidepressant with anticholinergic properties delayed gastric emptying and reduced levodopa absorption in normal volunteers (43). However, patients using anticholinergics did not have lower plasma levodopa concentrations after a single dose of levodopa than those patients not receiving anticholinergics (44). Other factors known to influence gastric emptying and that could theoretically alter levodopa absorption include exercise, meal temperature, and meal osmolality. The sum of all of these factors modifying gastric emptying may be responsible for the considerable inter- and intrasubject variability in levodopa absorption (45,46).

Enhanced gastric emptying occurs with gastrectomy; patients who have had this procedure do absorb the drug more quickly and completely than do other patients (2,32). Likewise, infusion of levodopa directly into the duodenum by tube (bypassing the stomach) produces very rapid absorption (32). Metoclopramide increases gastric emptying and consequently levodopa absorption (47), but the central dopamine antagonist properties of the drug contraindicate its use in the parkinsonian patient.

Intestinal Role

Levodopa is absorbed preferentially from the proximal bowel. This has been shown by the rapid absorption when levodopa is infused into the proximal bowel (32,48) and by comparing absorption from isolated bowel segments in animals (49). This absorption is by active transport and can be inhibited by other large neutral amino acids (50). In humans the coadministration of levodopa with 3-0-methyldopa or tryptophan results in reduced absorption of levodopa (51,52) most likely due to competition between the compounds for transport. Conversely, levodopa administered with phenylalanine reduced the absorption of phenylalanine (53). Amino acid transport systems are absent from the large bowel (54) and therefore it is not surprising that levodopa is not absorbed when administered rectally (55).

Absorption from the gut is also dependent upon mesenteric blood flow. Exercise reduces mesenteric blood flow and could reduce the absorption of levodopa. This, coupled with delayed gastric emptying, could be the reason that many patients say that they require more medicine when exercising.

The small intestine is a formidable barrier to levodopa absorption; although the majority of each administered dose is absorbed, only 25–50% reaches the systemic circulation as levodopa if decarboxylase inhibitors are not administered concomitantly (1,2). This first-pass metabolism, for the most part, takes place in the gut and not the liver: peripheral and hepatoportal vein injections of levodopa yield similar plasma concentrations of levodopa (34,56,57). Furthermore, hepatectomy does not produce major alterations in the disposition of injected levodopa (58). The gut is important not only in this first-pass capacity but also in the decarboxylation and conjugation of intravenously injected levodopa (59). Since the gut will be exposed to the highest concentrations of the poorly absorbed decarboxylase inhibitor, carbidopa, it is possible that the majority of carbidopa's action on the absorption and plasma clearance of levodopa is by inhibition of gut decarboxylase.

The variability of absorption of levodopa is considerable (2,5,39,45,46). This becomes exceedingly important when the drug has a short plasma half-life and delays or reductions in absorption are immediately translated into large swings in the plasma concentration of the drug. This is probably the largest single factor contributing to the seemingly unpredictable response to levodopa in the "brittle" parkinsonian patient. The variable rate of progression of drug tablets through the gastrointestinal tract, the metabolism of the drug throughout the gut, and the preferential absorption in the small bowel by a saturable transport system has made the development of sustained-release preparations very difficult (60).

Distribution

Levodopa very rapidly disappears from the plasma in a biphasic manner (Fig. 4). The first phase represents redistribution of levodopa from the plasma compartment into other tissues, primarily muscle (61). This distribution phase has a half-life of 5–10 min, thus plasma levels may be halved in 10 min (38). Furthermore, tissue does not appear to become saturated with the drug; the distribution phase is generally evident even after 1 and 2 days of constant L-dopa infusion (38) (Fig. 5). With oral administration of levodopa, the rapid distribution phase is often masked by the concomitant absorption of the drug, but nevertheless may be apparent during oral dosing (see Fig. 3B). Redistribution rather than metabolism of the drug may be largely responsible for terminating the action of levodopa. This could explain why carbidopa does not materially prolong the duration of the clinical effects of levodopa (11,38).

The distribution of levodopa into brain can be a critical step in its clinical action. As described above, levodopa enters the brain by a saturable carrier system that is more than half saturated at normal plasma concentrations of the large neutral amino acids (LNAA) (30,31). Levodopa flux into brain is then proportional to the ratio of levodopa to the other LNAAs (62). Flux can be increased by raising the levodopa concentration or lowering the concentration of the other LNAAs and vice versa. For example, administering a large oral bolus of phenylalanine during a constant-rate levodopa infusion will reverse the clinical

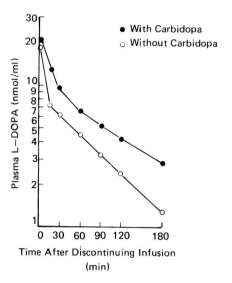

FIGURE 4 Disappearance of levodopa from plasma of a single patient after levodopa infusions were stopped at time zero. On one occasion carbidopa was concomitantly administered (closed circles) and during another infusion it was omitted (open circles).

response to the infused levodopa (39 (Fig. 5). Conversely, administration of a high-carbohydrate snack, which would be expected to cause insulin secretion and consequently promote the branched amino acids' passage into cells and lower the plasma concentration of the LNAAs, has been reported to augment the action of levodopa (63). Similarly, the fluxes of the LNAAs alpha-methyl-dopa and L-tryptophan have been shown to depend upon the concentrations of other plasma LNAAs (64,65). From these results it would be predicted that low-protein diets would reduce the dosage of levodopa required for a therapeutic effect. This is true (66), although it is not possible to differentiate an effect of the diet on absorption of the drug from an effect on blood–brain barrier transport. Low-protein diets do not reduce the fluctuations (66).

The levodopa metabolite 3OMD is also a large neutral amino acid and can compete with levodopa for entry into the brain. The concomitant injection of levodopa and 3OMD into rats will reduce the rise of levels of dopamine and its metabolites in the brain and attenuate the pharmacologic response to levodopa (67–69). Elevated levels of 3OMD have been associated with poor clinical response (18,20) and dyskinesia (19); this could be related to altered levodopa transport. Arguing against this hypothesis is the observation that the levels of 3OMD during chronic levodopa dosing, although several times higher than levodopa concentrations, are still only 5–15% of the concentration of LNAAs competing for entry into the brain.

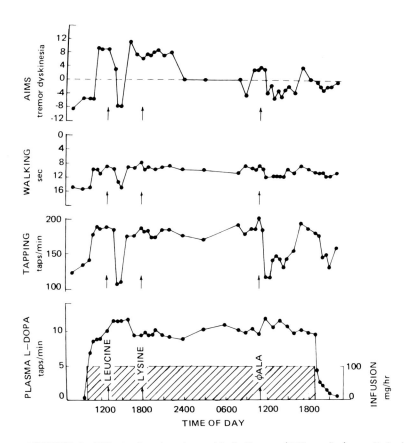

FIGURE 5 Effect of oral amino acid challenges (100 mg/kg) on clinical response to a constant infusion of levodopa. The LNAAs leucine and phenylalanine reduced tapping speed, walking speed, and dyskinesia without decreasing the plasma levodopa. Lysine, a basic amino acid, had no effect on the clinical response. Note also the rapid disappearance of levodopa from the plasma after 33 hr of constant infusion, indicating no saturation of tissue sinks for levodopa. (From ref. 39, with permission.)

Elimination

The elimination half-life of levodopa is estimated to be about 40 min (70) to about 80 min (38) without concomitant carbidopa and about 130 min (38) with carbidopa, but with considerable interpatient variability in the response to carbidopa. The variable prolongation of the elimination half-life by carbidopa has not translated into longer duration of action for each dose of levodopa (11). One possibility, discussed above, is that redistribution rather than elimination determines the duration of action in the fluctuating patient. The extremely rapid distribution phase and moderately rapid elimination phase are responsible for the rapid fluctuations in plasma levodopa, which in turn contribute to the fluctuating clinical response.

PHARMACODYNAMICS

What is the relationship between the plasma concentrations of levodopa and clinical response? Although most investigators have found some association between plasma levels and response, it has not bee consistent. This has raised the suspicion that something other than plasma drug concentration determines clinical response. Part of these seemingly discrepant results may reflect that plasma levodopa concentrations rather than striatal dopamine concentrations are monitored. The time required for the passage of levodopa into the brain and its conversion into dopamine may produce a lag between plasma peaks and clinical response (71) (Fig. 6) although other explanations for this lag need to be explored. Another problem is that levodopa flux into brain is proportional to the ratio of plasma levodopa to other plasma LNAAs, so there may be apparent discrepancies between plasma levodopa levels and clinical response (39). A final observation is that clinical responses are more unpredictable with plasma concentrations maintained in the vicinity of the therapeutic threshold. Concentrations clearly below or above the threshold are associated with "off" or "on" states, respectively (71).

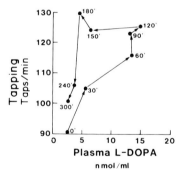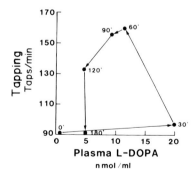

FIGURE 6   Lag between clinical response and plasma levodopa is illustrated by a plot of clinical response against plasma levodopa in temporal sequence. Numbers are minutes after starting a 2-hr levodopa infusion in left panel and after an oral dose of levodopa (25/250) in the right panel. (From ref. 71, with permission.)

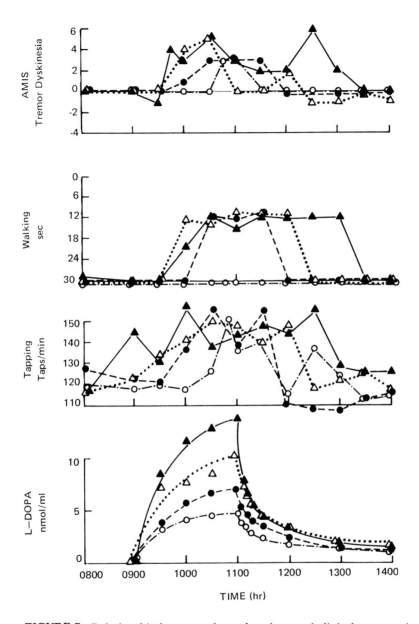

FIGURE 7 Relationship between plasma levodopa and clinical response in a single patient who underwent 2-hr levodopa infusions at different rates, 0.45 mg/kg/hr (open circles), 0.68 mg/kg/hr (solid circles), 0.91 mg/kg/hr (open triangles) administered with carbidopa and 1.82 mg/kg/hr (solid triangles) without carbidopa. The magnitude of the clinical response was similar for all infusions (except that the patient was never able to walk with the lowest infusion rate), but the duration of the response was proportional to the peak plasma levodopa level. (From ref. 71, with permission.)

One other pharmacodynamic relationship is very pertinent to the clinician. The duration of clinical response is proportional to the plasma concentration or, more precisely, to the plasma concentration minus the threshold concentration (71) (Fig. 7). Thus, the strategy of reducing the size of each dose and giving more doses when a patient develops a fluctuating response will predictably lead to shorter duration of response for each dose and less safety factor (i.e., plasma levodopa concentration will not always exceed the threshold concentration). The unpredictable fluctuating condition ("on-off") may be partially a product of this treatment strategy.

Finally, it is important for the clinician to realize that most patients have no therapeutic window at which they are completely mobile without dyskinesia. In fact, a large portion of the patients may have more marked tremor and dyskinesia as they switch between immobility and mobility. The magnitude of the clinical response (including the dyskinesia) is to a great extent all or nothing and is not linearly related to plasma levodopa levels (71,72).

CONCLUSION

Levodopa has unique and interesting pharmacokinetic features that determine the clinical response to the drug. The clinician must appreciate these to use the drug for optimal control of the symptoms of parkinsonism.

REFERENCES

1. Granerus AK, Jagenburg R, Svanborg A. (1973). Intestinal decarboxylation of L-DOPA in relation to dose requirement in Parkinson's disease. *Naunyn Schmiedebergs Arch Pharmacol* 180: 429–439.
2. Andersson I, Granerus AK, Jagenburg R, Svanborg A. (1975). Intestinal decarboxylation of orally administered L-DOPA. *Acta Med Scand* 198: 415–420.
3. Bianchine JR, Messiha FS, Hsu TH. (1973). Peripheral aromatic L-amino acids decarboxylase inhibitor in parkinsonism. II Effect on metabolism of L-2-^{14}C-DOPA. *Clin Pharmacol Ther* 13: 584–594.
4. Calne DB, Karoum F, Ruthven CRJ, Sandler M. (1969). The metabolism of orally administered in L-DOPA in parkinsonism. *Br J Pharmacol* 37: 57–68.
5. Morgan JP, Bianchine JR, Spiegel HE, Rivera-Calimlin L, Hersey RM. (1971). Metabolism of levodopa in patients with Parkinson's disease. *Arch Neurol* 25: 39–44.
6. Goodall McC, Alton H. (1972). Metabolism of 3,4-dihydroxyphenylalanine (L-DOPA) in human subjects. *Biochem Pharmacol* 21-2401-2408.
7. Hinterberger H, Andrews CJ. (1972). Catecholamine metabolism during oral administration of levodopa. *Arch Neurol* 26: 245–252.
8. Rutledge CO, Hoehn MM. (1973). Sulphate conjugation and L-DOPA treatment of parkinsonism patients. *Nature* 244: 447–450.

9. Tyce GM, Sharpless NS, Muenter MD. (1975). Free and conjugated dopamine in plasma during levodopa therapy. *Clin Pharmacol Ther* 16: 782–788.

10. Jenner WN, Rose FA. (1974). Dopamine 3-0-sulphate, an end product of L-DOPA metabolism in parkinsonian patients. *Nature* 252: 237–238.

11. Fahn S. (1974). "On-off" phenomenon with levodopa therapy in parkinsonism. Clinical and pharmacological correlations and the effect of intramuscular pyridoxine. *Neurology* 24: 431–441.

12. Preziosi TJ, Bianchine JR, Hsu TH, Messiha FS. (1972). L-methyldopa hydrazine (MK 486) and L-DOPA: a double-blind study in parkinsonism. *Trans Am Neurol Assoc* 97: 321–322.

13. Mars H. (1973). Modification of levodopa effect by systemic decarboxylase inhibition. *Arch Neurol* 28: 91–95.

14. Pinder RM, Brogden RN, Sawyer PR, Speight TM, Avery GS. (1976). Levodopa and decarboxylase inhibitors: a review of their clinical pharmacology and use in the treatment of parkinsonism. *Drugs* 11: 329–377.

15. Messiha FS, Hsu TH, Bianchine JR. (1972). Peripheral aromatic L-amino acids decarboxylase inhibitor in parkinsonism: I. Effect on O-methylated metabolites of L-DOPA-[14]C. *J Clin Invest* 51: 452–455.

16. Sandler M, Johnson RD, Ruthven CRJ, Reid JL, Calne DB. (1974). Transamination is a major pathway of L-DOPA metabolism following peripheral decarboxylase inhibition. *Nature* 247: 364–366.

17. Fellman JH, Roth ES, Heriza EL, Fujita TS. (1976). Altered pattern of dopa metabolism. *Biochem Pharmacol* 25: 222–223.

18. Rivera-Calimlin L, Tandon D, Anderson F, Joynt R. (1977). The clinical picture and plasma levodopa metabolite profile of parkinsonian nonresponders. *Arch Neurol* 34: 228–232.

19. Feuerstein C, Tanche M, Serre F, Gavend M, Pellat J, Perret J. (1977). Does O-methyldopa play a role in levodopa-induced dyskinesias? *Acta Neurol Scand* 56: 79–82.

20. Reilly DK, Rivera-Calimlun L, Van Dyke D. (1980). Catechol-O-methyltransferase activity: a determinant of levodopa response. *Clin Pharmacol Ther* 28: 278–286.

21. Linden I-B. (1980). Effects of 3,4-dihydroxyphenylpyruvic acid and L-glutamic acid on some pharmacokinetic parameters of L-DOPA in the rat. *J Pharm Pharmacol* 32: 344–348.

22. Horne MK, Cheng CH, Wooten GF. (1984). The cerebral metabolism of L-dihydroxyphenylalanine: an autoradiographic and biochemical study. *Pharmacology* 28: 12–26.

23. Doller HJ, Connor JD. (1980). Changes in neostriatal dopamine concentrations in response to levodopa infusions. *J Neurochem Res* 34: 1264–1269.

23a. Lloyd KG, Davidson L, Hornykiewicz O. (1975). The neurochemistry of Parkinson's disease: effect of L-DOPA therapy. *J Pharmacol Exp Ther* 195: 453–464.

24. Millar J, Stanford JA, Kruk ZL, Wightman RM. (1985). Electrochemical, pharmacological and electrophysiological evidence of rapid dopamine re-

lease and removal in the rat caudate nucleus following electrical stimulation of the median forebrain bundle. *Eur J Pharmacol* 109: 341–348.

25. Spencer SE, Wooten GF. (1984). Altered pharmacokinetics of L-DOPA metabolism in rat striatum deprived of dopaminergic innervation. *Neurology* 34: 1105–1108.

26. Calne DB, Langston JW, Martin WR, Stoessl AJ, Ruth TJ, Adam MJ, Pate BD, Schulzer M. (1985). Positron emission tomography after MPTP: observations relating to the cause of Parkinson's disease. *Nature* 317: 246–248.

27. Oldendorf WH. (1971). Brain uptake of radiolabeled amino acids, amines, and hexoses after arterial injection. *Am J Physiol* 221: 1629–1639.

28. Wade LA, Katzman R. (1975). Synthetic amino acids and the nature of L-DOPA transport at the blood-brain barrier. *J Neurochem* 25: 837–842.

29. Guroff G, Udenfriend S. (1962). Studies on aromatic amino acid uptake by rat brain in vivo. *J Biol Chem* 237: 803–806.

30. Pardridge WM, Oldendorf WH. (1977). Transport of metabolic substrates through the blood-brain barrier. *J Neurochem* 28: 5–12.

31. Pardridge WM. (1977). Kinetics of competitive inhibition of neutral amino acid transport across the blood–brain barrier. *J Neurochem* 28: 103–108.

32. Rivera-Calimlin L, Dujovne CA, Morgan JP, Lasagna L, Bianchine JR. (1971). Absorption and metabolism of L-DOPA by the human stomach. *Eur J Clin Invest* 1: 313–320.

33. Rivera-Calimlin L, Morgan JP, Dujovne CA, Bianchine JR, Lasagna L. (1971). L-3,4-dihydroxyphenylalanine metabolism by the gut in vitro. *Biochem Pharmacol* 20: 3051–3057.

34. Sasahara K, Nitanai T, Habara T, Kojima T, Kawahara Y, Morioka T, Nakajima E. (1981). Dosage form design for improvement of bioavailability of levodopa IV: possible causes for low bioavailability of oral levodopa in dogs. *J Pharm Sci* 70: 730–733.

35. Wade LA, Katzman R. (1975). Rat brain regional uptake and decarboxylation of L-DOPA following carotid injection. *Am J Physiol* 228: 352–359.

36. Hardebo JE, Emson PC, Falck B, Owman C, Rosengren E. (1980). Enzymes related to monoamine transmitter metabolism in brain microvessels. *J Neurochem* 35: 1388–1393.

37. Hardebo JE, Owman C. (1980). Barrier mechanisms for neurotransmitter monoamines and their precursors at the blood–brain interface. *Ann Neurol* 8: 1–11.

38. Nutt JG, Woodward WR, Anderson JL. (1985). Effect of carbidopa on pharmacokinetics of intravenously administered levodopa: implications for mechanism of action of carbidopa in the treatment of parkinsonism. *Ann Neurol* 18: 537–543.

39. Nutt JG, Woodward WR, Hammerstad JP, Carter JH, Anderson JL. (1984). The "on–off" phenomenon in Parkinson's disease: relation to levodopa absorption and transport. *N Engl J Med* 310: 483–488.

40. Bozek CB, Calne DB, Purves S, Calne S. (1984). A blind evaluation of Sinemet efficacy on different diets in Parkinson's disease. *Neurology* 34 (Suppl 1): 208.

41. Rivera-Calimlin L, Dujovne CA, Morgan JP, Lasagna L, Bianchine JR. (1970). L-DOPA treatment failure: Explanation and correction. *Br Med J* 4: 93-94.

42. Leon AS, Spiegel HE. (1972). The effect of antacid administration on the absorption and metabolism of levodopa. *J Clin Pharmacol* 12: 263-267.

43. Morgan JP, Rivera-Calimlin L, Messiha FS, Sundaresan PR, Trabert N. (1975). Imipramine-mediated interference with levodopa absorption from the gastrointestinal tract in man. *Neurology* 25: 1029-1034.

44. Bergman S, Curzon G, Friedel J, Godwin-Austen RB, Marsden CD, Parkes JD. (1974). The absorption and metabolism of a standard oral dose of levodopa in patients with parkinsonism. *Br J Clin Pharmacol* 1: 417-424.

45. Wade DN, Mearrick PT, Birkett DJ, Morris J. (1974). Variability of L-DOPA absorption in man. *Aust NZ J Med* 4: 138-143.

46. Evans MA, Triggs EJ, Broe GA, Saines N. (1980). Systemic availability of orally administered L-DOPA in the elderly parkinsonian patient. *Eur J Clin Pharmacol* 17: 215-221.

47. Mearrick PT, Wade DN, Birkett DJ, Morris J. (1974). Metoclopramide, gastric emptying and L-DOPA absorption. *Aust NZ J Med* 4: 144-148.

48. Gundert-Remy V, Hildenbrandt R, Stiehl A, Weber E, Zurcher G, DaPrada M. (1983). Intestinal absorption of levodopa in man. *Eur J Clin Pharmacol* 25: 69-72.

49. Sasahara K, Nitanai T, Habara T, Moroika T, Nakajima E. (1981). Dosage form design for improvement of bioavailability of levodopa V: absorption and metabolism of levodopa in intestinal segments of dogs. *J Pharm Sci* 70: 1157-1160.

50. Wade DN, Mearrick PT, Morris JL. (1973). Active transport of L-DOPA in the intestine. *Nature* 242: 463-465.

51. Muenter MD, Dinapoli RP, Sharpless NS, Tyce GM. (1973). 3-O-methyl-dopa, L-DOPA, and trihexyphenidyl in the treatment of Parkinson's disease. *Mayo Clin Proc* 48: 173-183.

52. Weitbrecht WU, Weigel K. (1976). Der einflus von L-tryptophan auf die L-DOPA resorption. *Dtsch Med Wochenschr* 101: 20-22.

53. Granerus AK, Jagenburg R, Rodjer S, Svanborg A. (1971). Inhibition of L-phenylalanine absorption by L-DOPA in patients with parkinsonism. *Proc Soc Exp Biol Med* 137: 942-944.

54. Binder HJ. (1970). Amino acid absorption in the mammalian colon. *Biochem Biophys Acta* 219: 503-506.

55. Eisler T, Eng N, Plotkin C, Calne DB. (1981). Absorption of levodopa after rectal administration. *Neurology* 31: 215-217.

56. Mearrick PT, Graham GG, Wade DN. (1975). The role of the liver in the clearance of L-DOPA from plasma. *J Pharmacokin Pharm* 3: 13-23.

57. Cotler S, Holazo A, Borenbaum HG, Kaplan SA. (1976). Influence of route of administration on physiological availability of levodopa in dogs. *J Pharm Sci* 65: 822-827.

58. Tyce GM, Owen CA. (1979). Administration of L-3, 4-dihydroxy-phenylalanine to rats after complete hepatectomy-II. Excretion of metabolites. *Biochem Pharmacol* 28: 3279-3284.

59. Landsberg L, Berardino MB, Stoff J, Young JB. (1978). Further studies on catechol uptake and metabolism in rat small bowel in vivo: (1) A quantitatively significant process with distinctive structural specifications; and (2) The formation of dopamine glucuronide reservoir after chronic L-DOPA feeding. *Biochem Pharmacol* 27: 1365–1371.

60. Nutt JG, Woodward WR, Carter JH. (1986). Clinical and biochemical studies with controlled-release Sinemet. *Neurology* 36: 1206–1211.

61. Romero JA, Lytle LD, Ordonez LA, Wurtman RJ. (1973). Effects of L-DOPA administration on the concentrations of DOPA, dopamine and norepinephrine in various rat tissues. *J Pharmacol Exp Ther* 184: 67–72.

62. Daniel PM, Moorhouse SR, Pratt OE. (1976). Do changes in blood levels of other aromatic amino acids influence levodopa therapy? *Lancet* 1: 95.

63. Muenter MD, Sharpless NS, Tyce GM, Darley FL. (1977). Patterns of dystonia ("I-D-I" and "D-I-D") in response to L-DOPA therapy for Parkinson's disease. *Mayo Clin Proc* 52: 163–174.

64. Markovitz DC, Fernstrom JD. (1977). Diet and uptake of aldomet by the brain: competition with natural large neutral amino acids. *Science* 197: 1014–1015.

65. Fernstrom JD, Wurtman RJ. (1972). Brain serotonin content: physiological regulation by plasma neutral amino acids. *Science* 178: 414–416.

66. Mena I, Cotzias GC. (1975). Protein intake and treatment of Parkinson's disease with levodopa. *N Engl J Med* 292: 181–184.

67. Gervas JJ, Murádas V, Bazán E, Aguado EG, deYebenes JG. (1983). Effects of 3-OM-dopa on monoamine metabolism in rat brain. *Neurology* 33: 278–282.

68. McLean JR, Ensor CR, McCarthy DA, Bohner B, Potoczak D. (1973). Effects of L-DOPA and L-3-methoxytyrosine on D-methamphetamine-induced motor activity and seizures induced by electroshock. *Proc Soc Exp Biol Med* 143: 1083–1087.

69. Reches A, Fahn S. (1982). 3-O-methyldopa blocks dopa metabolism in rat corpus striatum. *Ann Neurol* 12: 267–271.

70. Sasahara K, Nitanai T, Habara T, Morioka T, Nakajima E. (1980). Dosage form design for improvement of bioavailability of levodopa II: bioavailability of marketed levodopa preparations in dogs and parkinsonian patients. *J Pharm Sci* 69: 261–265.

71. Nutt JG, Woodward WR. (1986). Levodopa pharmacokinetics and pharmacodynamics in fluctuating parkinsonian patients. *Neurology* 36:739–744.

72. Hardie RJ, Lees AJ, Stern GM. (1984). On–off fluctuations in Parkinson's disease: a clinical and neuropharmacological study. *Brain* 107: 487–506.

19
Mechanism of Action of Levodopa

ELDAD MELAMED
Hadassah University Hospital, Jerusalem, Israel

In the central nervous system, dopamine has an essential role in the control and regulation of voluntary movement. The major pathogenic substrate in Parkinson's disease is death of the neuromelanin-containing dopaminergic cell bodies in the pars compacta of the substantia nigra, leading to degeneration of the nigrostriatal axonal projections and their nerve terminals, depletion of dopamine content in the corpus striatum (caudate and putamen nuclei), and suppression of the nigrostriatal dopaminergic neurotransmission. Parkinson's disease can therefore be regarded as a dopamine deficiency state within the striatum. However, systemic administration of even high dosages of dopamine is without benefit because it cannot cross the blood–brain barrier. Inability of exogenous dopamine to penetrate into brain parenchyma is due to the polarity of the neurotransmitter molecule and also to the presence of the monoamine degrading enzymes monoamine oxidase and catechol-O-methyltransferase in the endothelial cells of cerebral microvessels, which act as an enzymatic trapping mechanism and readily metabolize dopamine before it can gain access into the brain. Under normal circumstances, the biosynthesis of dopamine within dopaminergic neurons involves the hydroxylation of tyrosine catalyzed by tyrosine hydroxylase and the decarboxylation of the formed levodopa (L-dopa) (L-3,4-dihydroxyphenylalanine) catalyzed by the enzyme dopa decarboxylase. Systemic administration of tyrosine is of little or no benefit in Parkinson's disease because tyrosine hydroxylase is a rate-limiting enzyme in the synthesis of dopamine, has a high affinity for its substrate, and is contained almost exclusively within dopaminergic neurons in the striatum.

Systemic oral administration of levodopa, the immediate biosynthetic precursor of dopamine, was undoubtedly the major breakthrough in the treatment of the symptoms of Parkinson's disease (1). Levodopa corrects the motor symptoms of parkinsonism, particularly the akinesia and rigidity, and improves not only the quality of life but also the survival of afflicted patients. It remains the most important therapeutic approach to the disease. It is generally assumed that levodopa is beneficial in Parkinson's disease because, unlike dopamine, it is capable of penetrating the blood–brain barrier into the striatum where it is converted to dopamine. It thus increases neurotransmitter concentrations, corrects the depletion of striatal dopamine content, and restores the arrested nigrostriatal dopaminergic neurotransmission (2). However, the mechanisms of action of short- and long-term levodopa therapy in Parkinson's disease are far from simple. They are highly complex and pose many puzzling and intriguing questions, only some of which can be answered.

PERIPHERAL MECHANISMS

After levodopa is ingested, it is absorbed through the gut and increases its concentrations in the plasma. The biological half-life of plasma levodopa is 3–4 hr. Part of the systemically administered levodopa is transaminated in the liver. A major fraction of the drug is decarboxylated to dopamine outside the brain by dopa decarboxylase present in many peripheral tissues including gut, kidney, spleen, and liver. Exogenous levodopa does not freely enter the brain. It is neutral aromatic amino acid and shares mechanism of transport into the brain with the other circulating neutral amino acids such as tyrosine, tryptophan, valine, leucine, and isoleucine. Therefore, its entry into brain is partly controlled by blood levels of the other amino acids. For instance, relative increases in plasma tyrosine and tryptophan following a protein meal can suppress transport of levodopa from blood into brain. More importantly, the enzyme dopa decarboxylase is also present in endothelial cells of cerebral microvessels, where it acts as an enzymatic trapping mechanism for circulating levodopa. It converts levodopa to dopamine in the capillary wall outside the brain parenchyma. The formed dopamine is then avidly metabolized by monoamine oxidase and catechol-O-methyltransferase also present in the endothelium. Thus only a small portion of the systemically administered levodopa, 2–3%, gains access to the brain. This is the reason why beneficial effects in Parkinson's disease are achieved only with high oral dosages (4–6 g daily) of levodopa.

It also explains, in part, why the dopa-induced amelioration in parkinsonian patients does not occur soon after initiation of treatment and arrival at optimal daily maintenance dosages, but takes a relatively long time. Also, the high dosages of levodopa and the peripheral decarboxylation of the drug to dopamine can give rise to some of the early side effects associated with L-dopa therapy, such as gastrointestinal symptoms and orthostatic hypotension. For instance, conversion of exogenous levodopa to dopamine in the "vomiting center" at the area postrema located outside the blood–brain barrier can cause nausea and vomiting, which are quite common in the initial stages of levodopa treatment.

An important milestone in the evolution of levodopa therapy was the addition of peripheral dopa decarboxylase inhibitors to the treatment regimen (3). These drugs block dopa decarboxylase in peripheral tissues and endothelial cells of cerebral microvessels and are, themselves, incapable of penetrating the blood-brain barrier and inhibiting the enzyme centrally. Consequently, these agents prevent the extracerebral conversion of levodopa to dopamine and weaken the blood–brain barrier to circulating levodopa, permitting better penetration of exogenous levodopa into brain. Therefore, their use allows the administration of far smaller daily doses of levodopa, achievement of better and earlier drug efficacy, and prevention of the adverse reactions due to peripheral utilization of levodopa. Unfortunately, the "central" side effects of levodopa treatment seem to occur earlier and in greater frequency with such therapy. To date, most patients are given combined treatment with pills that contain levodopa and a peripheral dopa decarboxylase inhibitor such as carbidopa (Sinemet) or benserazide (Madopar), usually at a ratio of 10:1.

CENTRAL MECHANISMS OF LEVODOPA

Does Levodopa Work Through Conversion to Dopamine?

In Parkinson's disease there is depletion of dopamine in the striatum. Administration of exogenous levodopa increases dopamine concentrations in the normal as well as in the parkinsonian striatum and improves the motor symptoms and signs of Parkinson's disease (4). These considerations led to the universal hypothesis that levodopa is beneficial through its conversion to dopamine molecules, which become accessible to and activate postsynaptic dopaminergic receptors in the striatum and thus correct the deficient nigrostriatal transmission. However, levodopa itself is an agonist for dopaminergic receptors and it might, after its entry into the striatum, directly stimulate the receptors independently of dopamine formation. Studies in experimental animals, however, indicate that a decarboxylation step of levodopa to dopamine is indeed mandatory for the beneficial effect of levodopa in parkinsonism.

Does Levodopa Work Through Conversion to Dopamine Only in the Striatum or Also in Other Brain Regions?

In MPTP-induced parkinsonism there is a highly selective degeneration of the nigrostriatal dopaminergic projections. The signs and symptoms are closely similar to those of idiopathic Parkinson's disease and respond to levodopa therapy. This suggests that the major site of action of levodopa is within the corpus striatum. However, in Parkinson's disease there is a degeneration not only of the nigrostriatal pathways but also of the nigromesolimbic and nigromeso-cortical dopaminergic projections, which originate from the A_9 and A_{10} nuclear populations in the midbrain. It is possible that part of the parkinsonian signs and symptoms are due to dopamine depletions in limbic and cortical structures. Exogenous levodopa increases dopamine concentrations not only in the striatum but also in other brain regions dopaminergically innervated by the mesolimbic and mesocortical neuronal systems. Therefore, some of the beneficial effects of (as well as the adverse reactions to) L-dopa may be due to repletion of dopamine at extrastriatal sites within the central nervous system.

Does Levodopa Completely Correct Dopamine Depletions in the Parkinsonian Striatum?

Under normal circumstances and when the nigrostriatal projections are intact, most of the systemically administered levodopa is converted to dopamine in dopaminergic nerve terminals within the striatum. There seems to be a close correlation between the number of dopaminergic nerve endings and the increases in striatal dopamine concentrations produced by levodopa. Postmortem studies in levodopa-treated parkinsonian patients and in experimental animals with lesions of the nigrostriatal projections indicate that the dopa-induced elevations in striatal dopamine levels are far smaller than those that occur in tissues not deprived of dopaminergic innervation. When the nigrostriatal dopaminergic nerve terminals are lost, the capacity of the striatum to synthesize dopamine from exogenous levodopa greatly diminishes. Therefore, although levodopa is capable of increasing dopamine concentrations in the parkinsonian striatum, this treatment does not restore the deficient neurotransmitter to normal preillness levels. Nevertheless, even the small and subnormal dopamine elevations induced by exogenous levodopa are apparently sufficient to "turn on" the suppressed nigrostriatal function and generate the beneficial response in patients with Parkinson's disease. The cause of this apparent paradox may be linked to changes in the postsynaptic dopaminergic receptors within the striatum. In Parkinson's disease as well as in experimental animals with lesions of the dopaminergic pathways, degeneration of the nigrostriatal projections and the resultant reduction of dopamine molecules available at receptor sites may lead to postsynaptic dopaminergic receptor denervation supersensitivity. The number of receptor sites increases and their affinity for the neurotransmitter may also be enhanced. Studies in experimental animals suggest that such denervation supersensitivity occurs when more than 90% of the nigrostriatal tract has been destroyed. It is interesting that parkinsonian signs and symptoms first emerge when approximately the same percentage of dopaminergic nerve terminals in the striatum have been lost. Exogenous levodopa increases not only the concentrations of dopamine molecules but also their release and availability at receptor sites in the striatum.

Therefore, although levodopa causes only small elevations in striatal dopamine, such supersensitive dopaminergic receptors can amplify the postsynaptic response and thus accelerate the suppressed nigrostriatal transmission. It is possible that the unusual sensitivity of some patients with postencephalitic parkinsonism to even low dosages of levodopa may be due to more enhanced supersensitivity of the dopaminergic receptors in their striata.

How Does the Dopaminergic Neuron Handle Exogenous Levodopa?

Under normal physiological conditions most of the dopamine synthesized from endogenous tyrosine and the levodopa derived from tyrosine hydroxylation is stored within vesicles in nigrostriatal nerve endings. It is tonically released into the synaptic cleft, where it activates postsynaptic as well as presynaptic dopaminergic receptors. Tyrosine hydroxylase activity and synthesis, and release of the dopamine stored within the vesicles, are coupled to and are controlled and regulated by the state of activity and firing rates of the dopaminergic neurons. Thus, acceleration or suppression of dopaminergic neuronal impulse flow enhances or decreases, respectively, formation, storage, and release of the dopamine derived from endogenous levodopa. Within the dopaminergic nerve terminal, the enzyme dopa decarboxylase is not rate-limiting in the neurotransmitter biosynthesis, its activity is not coupled to changes in neuronal firing rates, and it will convert to dopamine any amounts of levodopa synthesized from tyrosine hydroxylation. These events are highly important for the control and regulation of voluntary movement. At least part of the exogenous levodopa is converted to dopamine in dopaminergic neurons in the parkinsonian striatum. It is unknown whether endogenous levodopa (formed from tyrosine) and exogenous levodopa (derived from systemic administration) and the dopamine synthesized from each are handled in similar or different ways within the nigrostriatal terminals. It is possible that the dopamine formed from exogenous levodopa is also stored within the vesicles and that its release is also regulated by dopaminergic neuronal firing. In that case, levodopa treatment may truly mimic the natural physiologic state of dopaminergic neuronal activity, in that the release of the formed dopamine would be subject to synaptic demand. An alternative and totally contrasting possibility is that the dopamine synthesized from exogenous levodopa within nigrostriatal nerve endings is not packaged into vesicles and its release is not coupled to state of activity and firing of the dopaminergic neurons.

Recent studies seem to favor the latter theory. In experimental animals, acceleration (by direct electrical stimulation of the substantia nigra with implanted electrodes and by treatment with dopamine-receptor-blocking agents such as haloperidol) and suppression (by treatment with direct dopaminergic receptor agonists such as apomorphine and bromocriptine) of dopamine neuronal firing rates had no effect on the synthesis and release of dopamine formed from exogenously administered levodopa. In rats given reserpine to destroy vesicular storage mechanisms in nigrostriatal terminals, the incremental increases in striatal dopamine accumulation induced by systemic administration of levodopa were similar to those in control animals with intact dopaminergic vesicles.

These data suggest that the dopamine formed from exogenous levodopa is not stored within vesicles in dopaminergic terminals and that its release is not governed by rates of neuronal firing. It probably accumulates in the cytosol in a free form or bound in part to macromolecules (perhaps glycoproteins) and leaks out of the neuron when a critical level is reached. Therefore, part of the efficacy of levodopa in Parkinson's disease may be due to unregulated spillage of non-stored cytoplasmic dopamine into the synaptic cleft. In that case, treatment with levodopa does not restore the normal physiologic state within the striatum but instead completely bypasses the natural demand-controlled synthesis and release of dopamine. it is also likely that the dopa decarboxylase that decarboxylates tyrosine-derived endogenous L-dopa and the decarboxylase that converts exogenous L-dopa to dopamine exist in different subcellular compartments within nigrostriatal terminals.

WHERE IS EXOGENOUS LEVODOPA CONVERTED TO FUNCTIONAL DOPAMINE IN THE PARKINSONIAN STRIATUM AFTER DEGENERATION OF THE NIGROSTRIATAL DOPAMINERGIC NEURONS?

In the mammalian striatum, the enzyme dopa decarboxylase, which catalyzes the conversion of levodopa to dopamine, is predominantly localized within dopaminergic nerve terminals. In Parkinson's disease, degeneration of the nigrostriatal projections causes marked reduction not only of dopamine concentrations but also of dopa decarboxylase activity in the striatum. Nevertheless, systemic administration of levodopa increases striatal dopamine concentrations in parkinsonian patients and in animals with almost total lesions of the nigrostriatal projections. Levodopa is also capable of functionally restoring dopaminergic transmission despite the massive loss of dopaminergic terminals and their content of dopa decarboxylase activity.

These considerations unavoidably lead to an obvious paradox: how can exogenous levodopa be effective at all in Parkinson's disease and since it is, where is it converted to receptor-accessible dopamine molecules in a striatum deprived of its dopaminergic innervation? Levodopa must therefore be converted to dopamine by the dopa decarboxylase that persists in the striatum despite remarkable loss of dopaminergic neurons. Postmortem studies in parkinsonian striata indeed showed that the enzyme never disappears completely; there is always some residual activity left even when dopamine is undetectable. In experimental animals with near total lesions of the nigrostriatal projections, striatal dopa decarboxylase activity is relatively less reduced than tyrosine hydroxylase activity and dopamine concentrations. In the rat, when all dopaminergic terminals are destroyed, about 15–20% of the original dopa decarboxylase activity remains in the striatum. All these data indicate that a fraction of striatal dopa decarboxylase activity also exists at extradopaminergic sites. Therefore, in the parkinsonian striatum, exogenous levodopa may be converted to dopamine in the surviving dopaminergic nerve terminals and/or in other nondopaminergic decarboxylase-containing compartments.

Surviving Dopaminergic Neurons

When the first symptoms of Parkinson's disease emerge and when levodopa therapy is usually initiated, there has already been an enormous (more than 90%) depletion of the nigrostriatal dopaminergic neurons. It was argued that the remaining dopaminergic nerve terminals constitute the main locus for the decarboxylation of exogenous levodopa to dopamine in the parkinsonian striatum because they contain the necessary enzyme, dopa decarboxylase. In addition, it is known from postmortem and experimental animal studies that when the nigrostriatal projection is partially destroyed, the residual neurons become hyperactive and accelerate synthesis and release of dopamine from endogenous tyrosine and levodopa to compensate for the loss of the other neurons. It was postulated that they can also utilize exogenous levodopa more rapidly and thus correct the dopamine depletions despite their exceedingly small numbers. However, levodopa treatment can raise striatal dopamine levels even after complete elimination of nigrostriatal terminals. It also increases dopamine concentrations in brain regions that do not receive dopaminergic inputs, such as the cerebellum.

Recent evidence suggests that hyperactive striatal dopaminergic neurons do not accelerate synthesis and release of dopamine from exogenously administered levodopa (see above). Furthermore, initiation of levodopa therapy is effective even in patients with "end-stage" MPTP-induced, and postencephalitic parkinsonism in whom there is a near-total loss of dopaminergic nerve terminals. All these considerations indicate that the surviving nigrostriatal dopaminergic neurons cannot be the only sites for the formation of dopamine from exogenous levodopa in the parkinsonian striatum.

Nondopaminergic Sites

Except for the dopaminergic nerve endings, dopa decarboxylase was known to exist in the striatum and also in the capillaries and noradrenergic and serotonergic neurons (5). Although the enzyme located in endothelial cells of striatal microvessels can and does decarboxylate exogenous levodopa, the formed dopamine cannot be of functional significance in Parkinson's disease since it cannot penetrate the blood–brain barrier and reach the postsynaptic dopaminergic receptors in the parenchyma. Also, this fraction of dopamine formation is greatly diminished or even eliminated by the combined use of levodopa with peripheral decarboxylase inhibitors. The number of noradrenergic neurons in the mammalian striatum is very small and their destruction does not affect the utilization of exogenous levodopa. It seems that the dopa decarboxylase they contain does not contribute meaningfully to the decarboxylating capacity of the striatum.

Serotonergic neurons originating from the midbrain raphe nuclei innervate the striatum. They contain dopa decarboxylase that is not specific only for levodopa as a substrate but also converts 5-hydroxytryptophan to serotonin. It was theorized that exogenous levodopa can be taken up by striatal serotonergic nerve terminals and converted to dopamine which can, in turn, be released as a false neurotransmitter and restore the suppressed nigrostriatal transmission in parkinsonism. Indeed, administration of high dosages of levodopa causes reductions in striatal serotonin concentrations since serotonin is displaced from serotonergic nerve endings by the formed dopamine. However, it seems unlikely that these neurons represent a major decarboxylation site in parkinsonism since, in animals with total nigrostriatal lesions, additional destruction of the afferent striatal serotonergic projection did not further reduce the residual dopa decarboxylase and the conversion of exogenous levodopa to dopamine in the striatum and did not affect the dopa-induced behavior patterns in such animals. Elimination of the massive corticostriatal afferent projections by decortication did not affect striatal dopa decarboxylase activity and utilization of systemically administered levodopa. This suggests that the glutamatergic corticostriatal nerve terminals do not contain dopa decarboxylase. It was even proposed that the decarboxylation of exogenous levodopa in the parkinsonian striatum is nonenzymatic and does not depend on dopa decarboxylase. However, such possibility is ruled out because when levodopa is administered with drugs that can block dopa decarboxylase centrally, the elevations in striatal dopamine concentrations produced by levodopa are totally prevented.

Recent findings in experimental animals raise an additional interesting possible location for the decarboxylation of levodopa in the striatum after degeneration of its dopaminergic innervation (6). Intrastriatal injections of the neurotoxin kainic acid selectively destroy neurons that originate in the striatum, including interneurons and afferent neurons, but spare axons of passage and afferent projections, such as the dopaminergic and serotonergic nerve-endings. In rats, kainic acid lesions markedly reduce (by 15–20%) striatal dopa decarboxylase activity without damaging the dopaminergic terminals. In animals with lesions of the nigrostriatal dopaminergic projections, the addition of striatal kainic acid lesions further decreases the residual dopa decarboxylase activity in the striatum. In addition, kainic acid markedly diminished (by about 30%) the increases in striatal dopamine concentrations induced by exogenous levodopa. These data suggest that a substantial amount of striatal dopa decarboxylase activity is located in an intrinsic and efferent nonaminergic neuronal compartment, which is susceptible to kainic acid lesions. Such neurons utilize, among others, acetylcholine, GABA, substance P, and enkephalins as neurotransmitters. Lack of more selective neurotoxins makes it impossible at present to determine either which of these neuronal systems contains the extradopaminergic dopa decarboxylase in the striatum or the functional significance of the presence of this enzyme within neurons that do not normally synthesize monoamines. Peptidergic (e.g., substance-P- and enkephalin-containing) neurons may be more likely candidates since monoamines and peptides are known to coexist in such neurons in the nervous system. Therefore, even though these striatal peptidergic neurons do not synthesize monoamines, they may contain dopa decarboxylase activity for evolutional if not functional reasons. Presence of the enzyme in these striatal neuronal elements may be very fortuitous in parkinsonian patients. In the normal striatum, the fraction of dopa decarboxylase located in the nonaminergic neurons is small compared with that contained in dopaminergic nerve terminals. However, when the striatal dopaminergic neurons degenerate in Parkinson's disease, the relative contribution of each compartment is changed drastically and the interneurons may now contain a major portion of the residual dopa decarboxylase in the striatum.

It is therefore possible that the decarboxylation of exogenous levodopa in Parkinson's disease takes place, at least in part, in such decarboxylase-containing nonaminergic striatal neurons. These neurons, in all likelihood, lack vesicular storage mechanisms for dopamine and are unable to store the dopamine formed from exogenous levodopa. Such molecules would therefore leak out of the neurons and by diffusion, reach and activate postsynaptic dopaminergic receptors and thus participate in restoring deficient nigrostriatal function. Some of the administered levodopa is probably converted to dopamine in the surviving nigrostriatal neurons. Dopaminergic nerve terminals are also incapable of storing the dopamine formed from exogenous levodopa in their dopamine-containing vesicles (see above). Therefore, regardless of the precise relative contribution of each of the two compartments to the decarboxylation process in the parkinsonian striatum, the beneficial effects of exogenous levodopa are dependent on nonregulated leakage of the formed dopamine into the dopaminergic synapse.

All of the above and perhaps other unknown and even yet unconsidered highly complex mechanisms might be involved in mediating the therapeutic efficacy of levodopa in Parkinson's disease (6). When levodopa was introduced and rapidly gained widespread use as a successful antiparkinson drug, it was enthusiastically, rather naively, and prematurely believed that such precursor replacement treatment was the definitive solution because it can correct the basic biochemical deficiency of Parkinson's disease. However, after an initial "honeymoon," problem-free, period averaging 2–5 years, many patients who responded favorably and sometimes even dramatically to levodopa develop a variety of limiting and disturbing adverse reactions. These include dyskinesias, "off" period and early morning dystonia, psychiatric reactions and hallucinosis and particularly a global decline in efficacy and fluctuations in responsiveness to levodopa. The biochemical substrates of the complications associated with long-term levodopa administration are even more complex and enigmatic than those responsible for the beneficial response to the drug.

DOES CHRONIC LEVODOPA THERAPY CHANGE THE NATURAL HISTORY OF PARKINSON'S DISEASE?

Parkinson's disease is a chronic progressive disorder. Rates of progression may be predetermined and vary among different patients, ranging from very slow to very rapid deterioration with time. It is generally accepted that since levodopa only corrects the deficient dopamine content in the striatum and the suppressed nigrostriatal transmission, it does not interfere with the basic and yet unidentified cause of idiopathic Parkinson's disease and therefore does not arrest or slow the progression of illness. Death of substantia nigra/pars compacta dopaminergic neurons in parkinsonism may be linked to excess intraneuronal formation of cytotoxic free radicals, perhaps mediated by exogenous or endogenous neurotoxins or by premature aging. Auto-oxidation of levodopa may generate similar toxic substances.

It is theoretically possible that continuous loading of the surviving dopaminergic neurons with high dosages of exogenous levodopa may, through chronic production of noxious agents, accelerate the predetermined rate of nigrostriatal degeneration and thus the disease progression. However, chronic administration (for about 18 months) of levodopa to mice did not damage dopaminergic neurons in their striata. Likewise, long-term treatment with levodopa did not augment the toxic effects of MPTP on nigrostriatal neurons in mice. These data suggest that chronic levodopa treatment is probably not toxic to and does not increase degeneration of nigrostriatal neurons even when they are rendered vulnerable by the basic causes of Parkinson's disease (8,9).

SIDE EFFECTS

Mechanism of Levodopa-Induced Dyskinesias

Paradoxically, while correcting the basic akinesia of Parkinson's disease, treatment with levodopa overshoots and causes hyperkinetic abnormal involuntary movements in the majority of patients. The dyskinesias are dosage- and time-dependent on levodopa administration, decline with dosage reduction, and totally disappear when levodopa is discontinued or given with neuroleptics that block postsynaptic dopaminergic receptors. These involuntary movements are similar in form to the tardive dyskinesia that occurs as a complication of chronic neuroleptic therapy. Dyskinesias do not happen in normal subjects given even high dosages of levodopa for long durations, which suggests that the combination of Parkinson's disease and levodopa treatment is mandatory for their development. These considerations and studies in experimental animals suggest that the levodopa-induced dyskinesias may be due to excess formation of dopamine from exogenous levodopa, its uncontrolled and unregulated spillage into striatal synapses, and overstimulation of postsynaptic dopaminergic receptors rendered supersensitive by denervation of the nigrostriatal projections.

Early Morning and "Off" Period Dystonia

Certain patients on long-term levodopa therapy may develop a peculiar and disabling dystonia affecting one or both feet immediately upon awakening in the morning, while still in bed, or, more commonly, when attempting to take their first steps. This dystonia occurs before the first morning dose of levodopa, when the patient is akinetic, rigid and without dyskinesias, persists for periods ranging from several minutes to about an hour and subsides spontaneously. In some patients, it may recur once or more often, later in the day, often when a dose-induced benefit of levodopa wears off. The causes of this puzzling phenomenon are unknown. This dystonia is definitely due to levodopa because it disappears after discontinuation of treatment and reemerges upon its renewal. It occurs when plasma levodopa levels are low. Therefore, it may paradoxically be linked to reduction of dopamine available at receptor sites, perhaps in the putamen.

Psychiatric Reactions and Hallucinosis

These may occur both early and late during the course of levodopa therapy and are more frequent in demented and older parkinsonian patients. Similar to dyskinesias, they may be dosage- and time-linked to levodopa administration, decline or disappear upon dosage reduction, and are abolished by cotreatment with neuroleptics. The causes for these phenomena are not entirely clear. They may be due to excess formation of dopamine from exogenous levodopa and its action on supersensitive postsynaptic receptors outside the striatum, perhaps in cortex and limbic structures innervated by the nigromesocortical and nigromesolimbic dopaminergic pathways which also degenerate in Parkinson's disease. Alternatively, they may be caused by interference with serotonergic mechanisms in the central nervous system, for example, by forced displacement of serotonin from its nerve terminals by levodopa and/or the formed dopamine.

Does Chronic Levodopa Therapy Cause Dementia?

The causes of the high prevalence of cognitive impairment in patients with Parkinson's disease are not well-understood. As in Alzheimer's disease, the ascending cortical cholinergic projections that originate in the nucleus basalis of Meynert may also undergo degeneration in Parkinson's disease. The dementia may be due to superimposed Alzheimer's disease or to participation of the innominatocortical cholinergic neurons in the basic pathogenesis of Parkinson's disease. It was proposed that chronic levodopa treatment may cause or contribute to the development of dementia in parkinsonian patients. However, we found that the presence and severity of cognitive dysfunction in patients with Parkinson's disease were unrelated to duration and total daily dosage of levodopa therapy. Furthermore, in normal as well as in MPTP-treated mice, long-term administration of levodopa did not damage cholinergic neurons in the central nervous system.

Mechanisms Responsible for Tolerance Phenomenon

After several years of sustained levodopa treatment, there is a global decline in its efficacy. In addition, the response pattern to levodopa may change entirely. Initially, response to levodopa doses is stable, smooth, and long-lasting (10). Patients do not notice the effect of each single dose and may even miss occasional doses without feeling any discomfort. Later, they become aware of the onset and termination of benefit produced by individual doses and the need to take a dose when the effect of the previous one deteriorated. Patients' daily performance fluctuates and becomes dependent on the schedule of levodopa intake. The duration of each dose-produced benefit shrinks progressively, giving rise to the "wearing-off" phenomenon or "end-of-dose" akinesia and necessitates increases in the number of daily doses of levodopa. There is also a progressive delay in the onset of clinical response produced by single doses of levodopa. Patients complain that doses ingested in the afternoons and evening are less effective than those taken in the mornings. There are occasional episodes of total unresponsiveness to certain doses of levodopa. Some patients develop the "on-off" phenomenon, manifested by sudden and unpredictable onset of severe akinesia at the peak of a dose-produced successful response. Combinations of these complications make the patient severely incapacitated and greatly decrease the daily duration of functional "on" periods of relief induced by levodopa. Various theories were proposed to explain these unique and puzzling tolerance phenomena but there are many arguments for and against each. No one mechanism can be singled out as the only cause for such complex side effects. They may be due to several of the following possibilities.

Disease Progression

It was suggested that loss of levodopa efficacy is due to progression of Parkinson's disease, with continuous loss of nigrostriatal neurons that proceeds under the cover of levodopa therapy. This hypothesis was based mainly on the assumption that the surviving striatal dopaminergic neurons represent the only or major site of decarboxylation of exogenous levodopa to dopamine and its storage. Therefore, when degeneration of the remaining neurons reaches a critical point, the capacity of the striatum to form and store dopamine from exogenous levodopa is lost and drug efficacy declines. However, dopaminergic neurons do not represent the only locus of dopa decarboxylation in the parkinsonian striatum. Furthermore, the formed dopamine is probably not stored within vesicles in the nigrostriatal terminals. Also (see above), there is no negative correlation between initial benefit from levodopa and the number of remaining neurons. In addition, several studies, although not all, indicate that declining responsiveness to levodopa is not linked to duration of disease. Nevertheless, diminution in number of residual dopaminergic nerve terminals may play a role.

Experimental studies in animals with near-total lesions of the nigrostriatal projections show that dopamine elevations induced by exogenous levodopa are smaller and of shorter duration in dopaminergically lesioned animals than in intact striata. It is possible that although the dopamine formed from levodopa is not packaged into vesicles, it is nevertheless bound, in part, to macromolecules in the cytosol. This may represent some storage within the surviving dopaminergic terminals that eventually declines when their numbers diminish. In addition, it is possible that a fraction of the dopamine formed from exogenous levodopa is retaken up by the dopaminergic terminals after its leakage into the synapse and can be recycled. When the number of these terminals decline with disease progression, the chances for reuptake of levodopa-derived dopamine can be greatly reduced. Most of such molecules may be subject to rapid degradation by extraneuronal monoamine oxidase and catechol-O-methyltransferase. Such mechanisms could explain not only the global decline in efficacy but perhaps also the "wearing-off" phenomenon. It cannot be ruled out that other decarboxylase-containing elements in the striatum, such as nonaminergic and serotonergic neurons, also degenerate during the course of Parkinson's disease and thus contribute to reduction in the striatal decarboxylating capacity.

Receptor Dysfunction

It was suggested that although the striatal postsynaptic dopaminergic receptors are initially supersensitive due to denervation of the nigrostriatal projections, they are down-regulated and become desensitized due to their chronic "bombardment" by large amounts of dopamine formed under chronic levodopa therapy and that their responsiveness to the neurotransmitter molecules declines.

However, postmortem studies of parkinsonian patients and in vivo experimental animals yield conflicting results concerning this theory. Decreases, no change, and even increases in receptor sensitivity were reported after long-term levodopa administration. Postsynaptic dopaminergic receptors are located on interneurons and perhaps also on efferent neurons in the striatum. If these neuronal targets for the presynaptic nigrostriatal nerve terminals are also involved in the degenerative process of Parkinson's disease, there may be actual depopulation of the dopaminergic receptors. It is also possible that episodic overstimulation of such receptors by dopamine formed from exogenous levodopa may cause depolarization block of the postsynaptic membrane and arrest information transport downs the chain of striatal interneurons and efferents. Another possibility is that aberrant metabolites may be formed from exogenous levodopa and its dopamine, act as false neurotransmitters, and block the striatal postsynaptic receptors and their ability to respond to dopamine stimulation. The latter mechanisms could be responsible for the "on–off" phenomenon.

Effect of Chronic Levodopa Therapy on Its Own Utilization

There is a continuing debate about the relative role of disease progression and long-term levodopa treatment on the development of declining efficacy. Clinical evidence (although not universally accepted) indicates that emergence of tolerance phenomena is linked to duration of therapy rather than to duration of disease. Studies in rats with intact nigrostriatal projections show that after chronic oral or intraperitoneal pretreatment with levodopa, the increases in striatal dopamine concentrations induced by a challenge with levodopa are smaller and persist for less time than in controls. This suggests that long-term levodopa administration may suppress its own utilization and conversion to dopamine in the striatum independently of degeneration of nigrostriatal dopaminergic neurons. It was long known that chronic levodopa treatment suppresses dopa decarboxylase activity in peripheral tissues such as the liver. Recent studies show that it also suppresses dopa decarboxylase activity in the striatum of experimental animals. The causes for this enzymatic suppression by its own substrate are unknown, but may be related to chronic depletion of essential cofactors induced by the chronic overloading of the decarboxylating process by exogenous levodopa or to blockade of the enzyme by aberrant metabolites of levodopa or dopamine. Regardless of the precise underlying mechanism, the parkinsonian striatum may be particularly susceptible to the enzyme suppression induced by long-term levodopa administration because, at the start of levodopa therapy, its dopa decarboxylase activity is already diminished due to degeneration of the decarboxylase-containing nigrostriatal nerve endings.

Peripheral Mechanisms

Accumulating evidence suggests that peripheral mechanisms and particularly faulty absorption may be important in mediating at least part of the tolerance to long-term levodopa treatment. There is a delay (sometimes up to 2 hr) in "start up" of a response after ingestion of levodopa in many parkinsonian fluctuators, suggesting slow and tardy absorption of levodopa from the gut. In some patients there are episodes of complete lack of benefit after intake that coincide with total failure of the same dose to produce elevations in plasma levodopa levels.

Bypassing the oral route by administration of levodopa and dopamine agonists intravenously for short periods, and lisuride subcutaneously via an automatic pump for longer durations, may sometimes overcome and prevent the response fluctuations. Presence of food in the gastrointestinal tract may interfere with dissolution of the levodopa-containing pills. Excess neutral amino acids in the gut and in the circulation induced by a heavy protein meal may compete with and prevent absorption of levodopa and its penetration through the blood–brain barrier, respectively.

A major fraction of levodopa is metabolized in peripheral tissues to 3-O-methyldopa, which may also interfere with levodopa absorption from the gut and entry into brain. Dopaminergic receptors are present in the stomach wall and chronic levodopa ingestion might reduce gastric motility and delay or prevent its dissolution and absorption. It is not unlikely that long-term overloading with oral levodopa might affect and suppress its own absorption mechanisms in the gut. There may also be a role for chronic ingestion of peripheral dopa decarboxylase inhibitors. Prolonged levodopa therapy may cause induction of enhanced transamination processes and accelerated inactivation of absorbed levodopa by the liver.

Almost no information is available on the possible effect of levodopa and peripheral dopa decarboxylase inhibitors on the physiological blood–brain barrier to circulating levodopa. The regional cerebral blood flow (rCBF) is reduced in patients with Parkinson's disease compared with their age-matched controls. Theoretically, chronic levodopa administration might further decrease the rCBF in parkinsonian patients and interfere with its own delivery to the striatum. However, recent studies show that long-term levodopa therapy does not affect the rCBF in patients with Parkinson's disease.

Apparently the mechanisms of action of short- and long-term levodopa therapy are far from simple. Only some are scientifically elucidated and proved while others remain theoretical and speculative. There is not doubt that further intensive studies are needed to clarify the action of exogenous levodopa in Parkinson's disease and to understand better not only the causes of its beneficial effects but also those mechanisms responsible for failing responsiveness to the drug. Only through this approach is there hope for new pharmacologic strategies to manage parkinsonian patients better, decrease their disability, and improve their quality of life.

ACKNOWLEDGMENT

This work was supported by the Jacob and Hilda Blaustein Foundation.

REFERENCES

1. Cotzias GC, Papvasiliou PS, Gellene R. (1969). Modification of parkinsonism. Chronic treatment with L-dopa. *N Engl J Med* 280: 337–345.
2. Hornykiewicz O. (1974). The mechanisms of action of L-dopa in Parkinson's disease. *Life Sci* 15: 1249–1259.
3. Calne DB. (1977). Developments in pharmacology and therapeutics of parkinsonism. *Ann Neurol* 1: 111–119.
4. Rinne UK. (1978). Recent advances in research in parkinsonism. *Acta Neurol Scand* 57 (suppl 67): 77–113.
5. Melamed E, Hefti F, Wurtman RJ. (1980). Nonaminergic striatal neurons convert exogenous L-dopa to dopamine in parkinsonism. *Ann Neurol* 8: 558–563.
6. Hefti F, Melamed E. (1980). L-dopa's mechanisms of action in Parkinson's disease. *Trends Neurosci* 3: 229–231.
7. Melamed E, Hefti F. (1983). Mechanism of action of short- and long-term L-dopa treatment in parkinsonism: role of the surviving nigrostriatal dopaminergic neurons. *Adv Neurol* 40: 149–157.
8. Melamed E, Globus M, Friedlender E, Rosenthal J. (1983). Chronic L-dopa administration decreases striatal accumulation of dopamine from exogenous L-dopa in rats with intact nigrostriatal projections. *Neurology* 33: 950–953.
9. Spencer SE, Wooten GF. (1984). Altered pharmacokinetics of L-dopa metabolism in rat striatum deprived of dopaminergic innervation. *Neurology* 34: 1105–1108.
10. Marsden CD, Parkes JD, Quinn NP. (1981). Fluctuations of disability in Parkinson's disease—clinical aspects. In: Marsden CD, Fahn S (Eds.), *Movement Disorders*. London, Butterworth Scientific.

20
Sleep Disorders

PAUL A. NAUSIEDA
St. Mary's Hospital, Milwaukee, Wisconsin

Disorders of sleep are not uncommon in the general population and tend to be more frequently encountered with advancing age. Sleep disorders can be grouped into three major categories: disorders of sleep initiation and maintenance (insomnia), disorders of excessive daytime somnolence, and parasomnias (behavioral events during sleep such as nightmares, sleep walking, or sleep talking). In parkinsonian patients multiple sleep problems in all three categories are frequently encountered. In some instances the complaint is unrelated to the disease or its treatment while in other situations specific sleep disorders appear that seem to be unique to this group of patients. This chapter discusses the various sleep complaints likely to be encountered, the various theories for their occurrence, and clinical strategies that may be employed in treatment.

PHYSIOLOGY OF SLEEP

Sleep is recognized as a complex behavioral state with its own neural substrate. In the study of sleep it is important to recognize that wakefulness and sleep are intimately related and that alterations in one are likely to be reflected in the other. It is impossible rationally to approach a complaint of daytime fatigue without considering the nature of nocturnal sleep, and insomnia must always be evaluated relative to its impact on daytime performance. While this seems to be too obvious a point to mention, it is the critical element in this area most often overlooked by the physician.

The sleep cycle appears to be modulated by a number of neurochemical systems, each of which appears to influence a specific stage of sleep. Slow-wave sleep appears to depend, in part, on central serotonergic activity arising in cell bodies of the midline raphe nucleus of the pons (1,2). Rapid eye movement sleep (REM) appears to depend to some degree on the integrity of the noradrenergic projections arising in the cell bodies of the locus ceruleus (3,4). The timing of the initial REM cycle appears to be partially dependent on cholinergic activity within the central nervous system (5,6). In addition, evidence suggests that various peptidergic systems influence sleep behavior (7,8).

The complex interactions of these neurochemical systems appear to be under the control of a circadian "clock" that synchronizes the various systems involved in sleep and allows sleep to occur in a consolidated, internally organized fashion with a relatively predictable time of onset, sequence of architectural development, and termination. Normal sleep can be characterized polygraphically and defined with respect to sleep latency (the amount of time needed to fall asleep), sleep staging, REM latency, REM periodicity, and the various times spent in each stage of sleep. Sleep efficiency can be defined (percentage of time asleep relative to total sleep time) and the efficacy of sleep determined by evaluating sleep latency in a sequence of five daytime nap sessions (multiple sleep latency test).

Sleep disorders are frequently psychogenic. Defining whether a complaint is organic or psychogenic is frequently difficult. The problems are compounded in Parkinson's disease, in which the neuropathology of the disorder is known to involve structures such as the locus ceruleus and neurochemical determinations have identified abnormalities in brain serotonin levels. The treatment of Parkinson's disease symptoms involves agents that induce acute and chronic alterations in central neurotransmitter levels. Given all the variables, it is surprising that all parkinsonian patients do not complain of significant sleep abnormalities. While there appear to be a number of sleep-related complaints directly related to the presence of Parkinson's disease or the pharmacologic agents employed in its symptomatic treatment, it is important to recognize that patients with this disorder may also have one of the many sleep disorders common to the general population. To provide the reader with an organized approach to sleep complaints in the parkinsonian patient, we have organized the topic according to specific categories of sleep disruption rather than disease-specific complaints. Those instances in which a particular relationship to the disease or treatment exists are discussed at the end of each section.

SLEEP IN THE PARKINSONIAN PATIENT WITHOUT SLEEP COMPLAINTS

Few studies have investigated the sleep of untreated parkinsonian patients, but the lack of sleep-related complaints noted in early descriptions of the disease suggests that they are uncommon (9). In general, the motor manifestations of Parkinson's disease are abolished during sleep. Electromyographic evidence of tremor and rigidity disappear as the subject enters stage 1 sleep. Sleep architecture in parkinsonian patients has been reported to be similar to that observed in nonparkinsonian patients of the same age (10). No specific abnormalities of ocular motility, respiratory control, or sleep-related autonomic function have been reported. Although the amount is very limited, currently available data suggest that sleep physiology is not appreciably affected by the pathologic changes of Parkinson's disease.

INSOMNIA

Insomnia can be differentiated into three separate symptom complexes that may coexist or be present in isolation: sleep initiation insomnia, sleep fragmentation, or early morning awakening. Sleep initiation insomnia describes the patient who "can't get to sleep" but is likely to remain asleep for the night once sleep begins. Although a common problem in the general population, this complaint is unusual in parkinsonian patients (11). In most instances, sleep initiation problems can be related to anxiety or agitated depression, which constitute the appropriate focus of treatment. In some cases, late evening administration of phenylethylamine-containing decongestants may be at fault, and theophylline-based bronchodilators may cause similar problems. Eliminating the medication or administering it earlier may clear the problem without the need for additional treatment.

Patients in the initial phases of levodopa therapy may experience insomnia, a side effect of treatment also observed in normal patients (11-17). This has been related to the fact that levodopa is a phenylethylamine with potential amphetamine-like effects. As with other drugs of this class, sleep suppression and REM suppression appear to be dosage-dependent. Studies have suggested that the sleep-suppressing effect of levodopa undergoes rapid tachyphylaxis (18) in a manner similar to that observed with the amphetamines (19). For this reason, sleep initiation insomnia at the outset of levodopa therapy is probably best treated with early administration of the agent and patience. In the event that the symptoms are of major concern, the use of short-acting benzodiazepines is justifiable. In our clinical experience the most useful agents have been temazepam (15--30 mg), alprazolam (0.125-0.25 mg), and triazolam (0.125 mg). Benzodiazepines with a longer biologic half-life may have applicability in patients with generalized anxiety but should be used with caution in elderly patients. In situations where a generalized anxiolytic effect is desired, it seems more prudent to use agents with a shorter half-life (alprazolam) that can be titrated with multiple administration times during the course of the day.

Early morning awakening in the parkinsonian patient usually signals the appearance of depression. In the parkinsonian patient the usual vegetative symptoms (i.e., weight loss, psychomotor retardation, limitation in social activity, constipation) may be related to the disease or are drug-related side effects. While depression is probably not more common in parkinsonian patients than in patients with other chronic diseases (20), its occurrence in this patient group is not surprising. Appropriate treatment is aimed at the primary cause rather than the sleep complaint per se. Antidepressant medications may be utilized (keeping in mind that their anticholinergic effects may be synergistic with the effects of many of the antiparkinson medications used in the symptomatic treatment of the disease). In our experience depressive symptoms tend to abate with supportive care; the presence of an active support program seems more effective in most patients than any specific drug therapy.

Two major pitfalls in diagnosis remain to be discussed regarding the patient with early morning awakening. The use of ethanol as a sedative needs to be carefully scrutinized. Patients using ethanol as a sedative frequently experience early morning awakening that clears following a period of abstinence. Another problem in the elderly population reflects a disorder of circadian rhythmicity, that of phase advance of sleep onset time. When a patient complains of early morning awakening, it is useful to ask the time of sleep initiation. In many patients, sleep onset is extremely early and the fact that the patient awakens early in the morning is not surprising (after all, if you go to bed at 6 P.M., waking up at 3 A.M. is not a cause for concern). Progressive delay in the sleep onset time may prove useful in some cases; in most instances reassurance that the problem is not of major concern is sufficient.

Sleep fragmentation is the most common complaint in parkinsonian patients (12). Routinely, patients find they have no difficulty in falling asleep, but awaken 2–3 hr later feeling relatively refreshed. Upon returning to sleep patients may find that spontaneous arousals continue throughout the night. Initially, these arousals may have no effect on daytime alertness, but many patients develop progressive daytime somnolence and begin napping intermittently throughout the day (12). Analysis of patients with these complaints suggests that a progressive loss of consolidated nocturnal sleep occurs, with total 24-hr sleep times remaining in the normal range. Patients with this complaint often identify a number of somatic reasons: joint pains, tremor, rigidity, or a need to urinate. Polysomnographic studies of these patients reveal spontaneous awakening, usually from stage 1 to 2 sleep, in the absence of any clear precipitating factors (21). Within minutes of patients awakening, electromyographic recordings demonstrate tremor or increased muscle activity that suggests rigidity. While the patient may identify parkinsonian symptoms as the "cause" of the awakening, data suggests that spontaneous arousal is the initial event and that symptoms of the disease follow. In general, sleep fragmentation appears to be more likely in patients taking dopaminergic agents immediately before sleep onset, and often responds to alterations in drug administration that restrict administration after 6–7 P.M. (12).

Other causes of sleep fragmentation appear to be unusual in the parkinsonian population. Sleep apnea and periodic movements of sleep may also cause spontaneous awakening. In our experience, the prevalence of sleep apnea is no greater in Parkinson's patients than in the general population. Periodic movements of sleep are frequently seen in patients with Parkinson's disease, but are rarely associated with spontaneous awakening. In the event that a bedpartner reports loud snoring, respiratory arrest, or intermittent withdrawal movements of the legs during sleep, full polysomnographic studies would appear to be justified. In our own clinical population the yield of such studies has been very low and routine polysomnographic recordings would appear to be of little value.

Treatment of sleep fragmentation in Parkinson's disease patients has limited success. Initially, short-acting benzodiazepines are of value (see above), but prolonged treatment usually results in tolerance. Amitriptyline (10–50 mg at bedtime) is often of value, but tends to precipitate confusion and overt hallucinosis in patients with associated parasomnias (see section on parasomnias below) (22). Many clinicians tend to use evening doses of sedative antihistaminic–anticholinergics (diphenhydramine 25-50 mg), though these agents are of limited value in this setting.

EXCESSIVE DAYTIME SOMNOLENCE

Excessive daytime somnolence is characterized by a tendency to fall asleep readily during the day. Many patients complain of feeling fatigued during the day; others identify a host of complaints which they relate to the fact that they have not slept soundly the previous night. In many cases these complaints are generalized into a complaint of "sleepiness." While there is a commonality to the term "sleepy" that everyone recognizes, it is important for the clinician to question patients and their families specifically on the presence of daytime napping before assuming that excessive somnolence is present. The patient who complains of being "sleepy all day" and yet never falls asleep inappropriately is probably suffering from an unrelated systemic disorder (electrolyte imbalance, endocrine disease, megaloblastic anemia, iron deficiency anemia) or is depressed. Before assuming the symptom is psychogenic in origin, it is important to exclude treatable causes. Vitamin B12 deficiency is occasionally present in parkinsonian patients as a result of physiological blind loop syndrome secondary to slowed bowel motility (unpublished observation), and commonly presents as daytime fatigue. Patients with Parkinson's disease are not immune to other diseases and a careful search for treatable causes of fatigue should be undertaken.

A significant percentage of patients have true daytime somnolence. Two patterns appear to exist. In some patients the symptom seems related to a breakdown in the circadian control of sleep. These patients are insomniac at night and tend to disperse sleep into multiple brief naps throughout the day. In other patients, daytime somnolence is directly related to the time dopaminergic drugs are administered. While levodopa is a phenylethylamine with amphetamine-like effects in normals, a number of patients experience uncontrollable somnolence within 30-60 min of taking the drug.

We have studied a number of these patients in the sleep laboratory and have identified two groups of patients. In one group the baseline electroencephalogram is normal and transition into stage 1–2 sleep routinely follows the administration of levodopa, with a latency of 30–60 min. Sleep architecture is unremarkable, and multiple sleep latency testing is normal on days when the drug is withheld. In other patients the resting electroencephalogram is slowed; the usual resting 9–11 Hz occipital frequency is slowed in the range of 4–8 Hz. These patients usually show signs of cognitive impairment on clinical examination. In this group of patients, behavioral transition into sleep (i.e., lack of communication with an observer, loss of tremor artifact from electromyographic recordings, roving eye movements on electro-oculogram recordings) is unassociated with alterations in the electroencephalographic characteristics. In this setting one is hard pressed to define whether the patient is awake or asleep the majority of the time. No convincing explanation for this phenomenon has been advanced.

Treatment of this complication of therapy is difficult. When daytime somnolence is unrelated temporally to the times of levodopa administration, consolidation of nocturnal sleep appears to be effective (see section on insomnia). In patients showing a direct relationship between drug administration and somnolence, two approaches have been utilized. The use of amphetamines has been explored (unpublished observations) and they appear to be of marginal value. Pemoline (18.75–75 mg/day) is occasionally useful, as is dextroamphetamine (5–20 mg/day) or methylphenidate (10–30 mg/day). In our experience the effects of these agents are transitory and rapidly lost.

A more effective, though less than satisfactory, solution has been identified: alternate-day levodopa administration. We have found that discontinuing levodopa-containing medications on alternate days results in the patient being quite awake on the days "off" levodopa with no loss in motor control, but somnolent on the days levodopa is taken. In most patients the total daily dose on the "on" days needs to be increased (average range, 25–50%) to maintain adequate symptomatic control on the days the drug is withheld. Longer periods of withdrawal do not appear to be useful, since severe motor manifestations of the disease appear after 48–72 hr. Although the solution allows relatively normal function only 50% of the time, patients and families have found this compromise preferable to a situation in which the patient is constantly in a state of sedation. The institution of a "drug holiday" has been of minimal success in the treatment of this side effect of chronic levodopa therapy. The use of direct dopamine agonists (bromocriptine) has not proven effective in alleviating this complication and commonly worsens the daytime somnolence.

PARASOMNIAS

Parasomnia describes a variety of sleep-related behavioral phenomena. In parkinsonian patients the major disorders are sleep talking, sleep walking (somnambulism), altered dream content, nocturnal terrors (pavor nocturnus), and nocturnal myoclonus. Studies have suggested that parasomnias in this patient group reflect a side effect of treatment with levodopa (12,22). Alterations in dream content are frequently reported by patients in the initial phases of treatment with levodopa (12,23,24). Patients report that their dreams are more "vivid" and "lifelike" with little alteration in content. As treatment continues many patients report an alteration in the qualitative nature of dream content and a peculiar tendency of dreams to incorporate deceased relatives or particularly significant household pets. Bedpartners may report an increase in nocturnal vocalizations— sleep talking initially, with later development of loud nocturnal vocalizations reflecting a state of panic or sense of imminent danger.

Polysomnographic studies of patients with these complaints do not demonstrate any distinct alterations in sleep architecture, although phasic elements of stage 2 slow-wave sleep appear to decrease (sleep spindles and K complexes) (10, 12). Episodes of what appear to be "nocturnal terrors" are noted in some patients (12). Nocturnal terrors are slow-wave sleep phenomena (25) common in children. In classic form the dream content is monothematic, lacking the plot development of REM-related dreams. Patients imagine themselves in a dangerous situation with a threat of immediate harm or death that requires an immediate response. In some instances the patient may cry out during sleep, while in others the patient may exhibit motor responses appropriate to the situation. Patients usually do not remember the episode, but bedpartners may relate a violent motor behavior in association with diffuse autonomic symptoms such as flushing or diaphoresis. Polysomnographic recordings identify these episodes arising from slow-wave sleep (12).

Treatment of these complications is only partially successful. While nocturnal terrors in nonparkinsonian patients may respond to benzodiazepines that suppress stage 3–4 slow-wave sleep, these agents have not been found to be of use in parkinsonian patients (12). Restriction of levodopa to daytime hours may offset the problem for a time but symptoms tend to recur. Data suggest that these nocturnal symptoms are an initial feature of the hallucinatory syndrome that may occur in some patients receiving chronic levodopa (12). The development of sleep-related complaints should alert the physician to the possibility that psychiatric decompensation is likely if a further escalation in dosage is attempted.

Occasionally patients with nocturnal terrors may exhibit episodes of somnambulism. These episodes probably reflect an alteration in sleep behavior similar to that underlying the nocturnal terrors. For unknown reasons somnambulism is less frequent than nocturnal terrors; treatment is identical to that for the latter disorder (12).

Nocturnal myoclonus may present a distinct problem to the bedpartners of patients with Parkinson's disease (12). Most individuals experience occasional axial myoclonus immediately after sleep onset. The motor movements are frequently associated with an acute sensation of falling and may precipitate an abrupt arousal from sleep. In the parkinsonian patient, similar phenomena may occur, but the appearance of frequent axial myoclonic movements appears to be related to the chronic administration of levodopa and the prevalence of this complaint increases with chronic levodopa administration (12,26). In most instances these myoclonic movements are unassociated with significant sleep disruption. Similar movements are often observed in patients receiving tricyclic antidepressants (whether they are parkinsonian or not); in patients concomitantly receiving antidepressants withdrawal of these drugs may cause the movements to stop. Some studies have suggested that central serotonin-blocking agents such as methysergide may block the appearance of myoclonic movements (22). While this suggests that myoclonic movements induced by chronic levodopa arise from altered central serotonergic activity, clinical use of serotonin-blocking agents to treat this sleep-related phenomenon does not seem warranted.

Myoclonic movements may be confused with a similar sleep-related disorder: periodic movements of sleep (27). Periodic movements of sleep tend to be more prolonged, are often unilateral, and are characterized by a flexor withdrawal movement of the lower extremities. The movement resembles the triple flexor withdrawal response and is frequently seen in the context of peripheral neuropathic disorders or segmental radiculopathy. Periodic movements of sleep are sometimes associated with brief arousals from sleep and may result in sleep fragmentation, lowered sleep efficiency, and excessive daytime somnolence. While periodic movements of sleep do not appear to be more common in the parkinsonian population and have no recognized relationship to the administration of antiparkinson medications, their presence may cause a sleep derangement that superficially mimics drug-induced sleep alteration. While a careful history from a spouse or bedpartner may clarify the nature of the problem, all-night polysomnographic studies may be required to identify the problem properly. Periodic movements of sleep are often suppressed by clonazepam (1-2 mg at bedtime) or by oxycodone (5-15 mg at bedtime) with resultant improvement in nocturnal sleep and daytime alertness.

Leg cramps may constitute an independent problem in parkinsonian patients. While nocturnal leg cramps may reflect electrolyte imbalance, hypothyroidism, or the presence of focal disorders of perfusion, their usual cause is focal dystonia. This appears to increase in prevalence as the duration of treatment with levodopa lengthens but may be seen as an initial feature of the disease in a small percentage of patients (28). The complaint is most often reported in the early morning hours, but may occur sporadically during the day. Foot dystonias are usually recognizable by the flexion movements of the toes, internal rotation and plantar flexion of the foot, and occasional tonic extension of the great toe readily observable when the movements occur. Screening for electrolytes usually gives normal results; the movements appear to be a component of the disease or of chronic dopaminergic treatment. Treatment with nocturnal anticholinergics may be of benefit, as will treatment with evening doses of quinine (300 mg). The administration of 10-40 mg lioresal at bedtime may be of benefit in such cases. In some cases the administration of levodopa (Sinemet) at night may be the only means of alleviating symptoms. It is important to eliminate metabolic causes of this symptom before concluding that the complaint is an inevitable component of the disease or its treatment.

Many patients will insist that they are awakened from sleep by tremor, rigidity, or some combination of symptoms immediately referable to their disease. Initially these reports may suggest that nocturnal treatment with anti-parkinson agents is required. We have monitored a number of patients with this complaint and have universally found that spontaneous awakening in the absence of a clear precipitant is the primary event. Electromyographic evidence of tremor or increasing muscle tone appears within a minute or 2. It has been our conclusion that sleep fragmentation induced by dopaminergic agents is the primary disorder in these patients and nocturnal symptoms improve with any technique aimed at consolidating nocturnal sleep (see above). Treatment of emergent parkinsonian symptoms following arousal may be necessary when sleep consolidation is impossible but should be regarded as a less than satisfactory approach, to be reserved for difficult management situations.

SUMMARY

Sleep-related complaints are extremely common in patients with Parkinson's disease. In some instances the sleep complaints reflect disorders common to the general population, while in other situations the complaints seem related to the agents employed in treatment. A detailed history with parallel reporting by the bedpartner is the best way of substantiating the validity of the sleep complaints and should be routinely employed. Sleep disorders in the parkinsonian population are amenable to logical forms of therapy once their nature is identified.

REFERENCES

1. Mouret J, Bobillier P, Jouvet M. (1968). *Eur J Pharmacol* 5: 17–22.
2. Jouvet M. (1969). *Science* 163: 32–41.
3. Rousell B, Bouguet A, Bobillier P, Jouvet M. (1967). *C R Soc Biol* 161: 2537–2541.

4. Laguzzi R, Petitjean F, Pujol J, Jouvet M. (1972). *Brain Res* 48: 295–310.
5. Cordeau J, Moreau A, Beaulnes A, Lawrin C. (1963). *Arch Ital Biol* 101: 30–47.
6. Gillin J, Mendelson B, Sitaram N, Wyatt R. (1978). *Annu Rev Pharmacol Toxicol* 18: 563–579.
7. Pappenheimer J, Miller T, Goodrich C. (1967). *Proc Natl Acad Sci (USA)* 58: 513–517.
8. Drucker-Colin R, Rojas-Ramirez J, Vera-Treuba J, Monroy-Ayala G, Hernandez-Peon R. (1970). *Brain Res* 23: 269–273.
9. Wilson SAK. (1970). *Neurology* 787–804.
10. Mouret J. (1975). *Electroencephalogr Clin Neurophysiol* 38: 653–657.
11. Kales A, Ansel R, Markham C, Schart M, Tan T. *Clin Pharmacol Ther* 12: 397–401.
12. Nausieda P, Weiner WJ, Kaplan L, Weber S, Klawans H. (1982). *Clin Neuropharmacol* 5: 183–194.
13. Wyatt R, Chase TN, Scott J, Synder F, Engelman K. (1970). *Nature* 228: 999–1001.
14. Gillin J, Post R, Wyatt R, Goodwin F, Synder F, Bunney W. (1973). *Electroencephalogr Clin Neurophysiol* 35: 181–186.
15. Azumi K, Jinnai S, Takahashi S. (1972). *Sleep Res* 1: 40 (abstract).
16. Greenberg R, Perlman C. (1970). *Psychophysiology* 7: 314.
17. Fram D, Murphy D, Goodwin F, Brodie H, Bunney W, Snyder F. (1970). *Psychophysiology* 7: 316–317.
18. Kendel K, Beck U, Wita C, Hohneck E, Zimmerman H. (1972). *Arch Psychiatr Nervenkr* 216: 82–100.
19. Nausieda PA. (1979). In: Vinken, Bruyn (Eds.), *Handbook of Clinical Neurology*. Amsterdam, Elsevier, North Holland.
20. Nausieda PA, Carter R.
21. Nausieda PA, unpublished observations.
22. Nausieda PA, Tanner CM, Klawans H. (1983). In: Fahn, Calne, Shoulson (Eds.), *Advances in Neurology*. New York, Raven Press.
23. Scharf B, Moskovitz C, Lupton M, Klawans H. (1978). *J Neural Transm* 43: 143–151.
24. Moskovitz C, Moses H, Klawans HL. (1978). *Am J Psychiatry* 136: 6–10.
25. Broughton R. (1968). *Science* 159: 1070–1078.
26. Klawans HL, Goetz CG, Bergen D. (1975). *Arch Neurol* 32: 331–334.
27. Coleman R, Pollak C, Weitzman E. (1980). *Ann Neurol* 8: 416–421.
28. Nausieda PA, Weiner WJ, Klawans HL. (1980). *Arch Neurol* 37: 132–136.

21

Therapy with Dopaminergic Drugs in Parkinson's Disease

PETER A. LE WITT
Lafayette Clinic and Wayne State University School of Medicine, Detroit, Michigan

Options for the treatment of parkinsonian symptoms have expanded over the past decade to include drugs which duplicate or enhance the effects of levodopa. Levodopa is capable of producing sustained benefit for most Parkinson's disease patients, but sometimes at a great price in long-term adverse effects, particularly dyskinesias and motor fluctuations. Furthermore, the decline of levodopa efficacy in advanced parkinsonism may result from continuing loss of presynaptic neurons in nigrostriatal pathways. Even though postsynaptic neurotransmission may remain responsive to dopamine and dopamine-like compounds, the failure of metabolism, storage, and release of dopamine by presynaptic neurons may be one basis for the progression of parkinsonian symptomatology in the face of previously adequate therapy. A major goal of antiparkinson drug development has been the discovery of alternative medications which, unlike levodopa, would not require intraneuronal activation within the impaired nigrostriatal dopamine pathways, and which possess increased potency and selectivity of action as compared to dopamine.

Though a number of neurochemical alterations do occur in the brain of Parkinson's disease patients, most of the primary clinical features of the disease and related syndromes can be linked solely to deficiency of striatal dopamine. This understanding has been highlighted by recent human and animal studies of the motor deficits caused by MPTP, a neurotoxin highly selective for the substantia nigra dopaminergic neurons projecting to striatum. Remedies for alleviating tremor, rigidity, bradykinesia, and decreased dexterity have been sought among drugs that can selectively stimulate dopamine receptors. Although drugs with such properties have been generally regarded as "dopamine agonists," the term is somewhat misleading in that their pharmacological actions can differ in several ways from those of dopamine. This point is well illustrated by the multiplicity in pharmacological effects of the antiparkinson ergot derivatives, which so far have been the most successful of the "dopaminergic" alternatives or adjuncts to levodopa therapy. In addition to their actions in other neurochemical systems (e.g., serotonergic, adrenergic) (1), the effects of dopaminergic ergot derivatives may differ greatly among the various dopaminergic systems and receptor populations as a function of concentration or chronicity of use, and depending on the endogenous monoamine content of neurons upon which they act. Animal behavior, receptor binding, and hormonal effects have been used to define the dopaminergic properties and antiparkinson potential of these drugs. To some extent, these methods have been useful for predicting potency or selectivity of effect. However, clinical trials with the drugs depicted in Figure 1 have disclosed similarities and differences among dopaminergic drugs which, in some instances, were not anticipated by preclinical testing in animals. It may be that the model of parkinsonian motor and neurochemical deficits brought about by MPTP will provide in future a better replica of human parkinsonism for evaluating the acute and chronic pharmacology of dopaminergic therapy.

The understanding that dopamine serves as a neurotransmitter mediating movement via the striatum emerged several years after the finding of striatal dopamine deficiency in Parkinson's disease by Ehringer and Hornykiewicz in 1960 (2). However, the first clinical experience with dopaminergic therapy preceded these pathophysiological insights by a decade. In 1951, Schwab and colleagues described transient improvement of rigidity and tremor from injections of apomorphine (3), long before its recognition as a "classical" dopaminergic agonist (4). Following the development of levodopa therapy for Parkinson's disease patients, Cotzias and colleagues re-evaluated apomorphine and a congener, N-propyl-noraporphine, for the treatment of parkinsonian symptoms (5). With the latter compound, they found considerable antiparkinson effect with fewer adverse reactions than with apomorphine, although efficacy was generally lost within several weeks. Another drug with dopaminergic properties that underwent trials in the early 1970s was piribedil, a piperazine derivative. Its antiparkinson benefits were relatively mild compared to levodopa, and psychiatric side effects frequently resulted (6). It was against the background of relatively unsatisfactory clinical experience with direct-acting dopamine-like compounds that ergot derivatives entered into the therapeutic arena, and until recently have dominated the search for such therapy.

In the past decade, the roles for dopamine as a neurotransmitter in several systems of the brain have been expanded with the recognition of alternative functional patterns and subcategories of receptors (7). The pharmacological principles for treating the pathophysiology of Parkinson's disease have become far more complicated than the notion that dopamine, like apomorphine (and

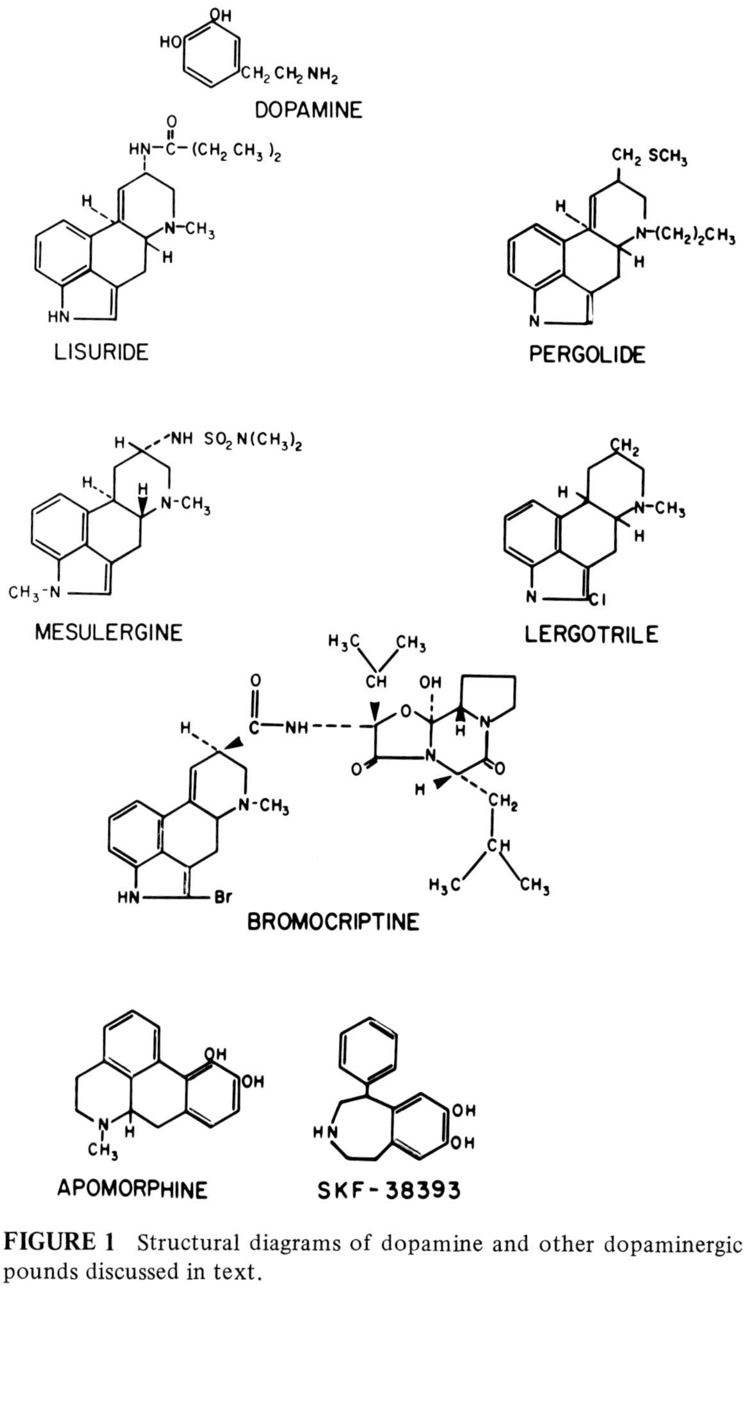

FIGURE 1 Structural diagrams of dopamine and other dopaminergic compounds discussed in text.

other artificial substances sharing similar receptor effects), simply reverses the motor and behavioral deficits of dopamine depletion. In the nigrostriatal system, nigral efferents also have sites, termed "autoreceptors," at which dopamine can exert a presynaptic feedback control on its turnover and release. These mechanisms, part of a physiological self-regulatory system, may explain why administration of dopaminergic agonists at low-dosage (which preferentially activates "autoreceptors") can lessen dyskinesia and worsen control of parkinsonian symptoms. Animal studies, confirmed by human experience, revealed that receptors not linked to adenylate cyclase (D-2 type) mediate prolactin suppression as well as the motor effects desired in relieving parkinsonian symptoms. In contrast, the roles for D-1 (cyclase-linked) dopaminergic receptor systems in movement and behavior are less well understood. Some sets of D-1 receptors may be important in regulating dopamine turnover and release in striatal nerve terminals (8), while other properties of D-1 activation include a diminution of D-2 receptor binding (9). Acetylcholine has an antagonistic role of the function of dopamine in the striatum; D-2 agonist-mediated suppression of acetylcholine release is antagonized in turn by D-1 activation (10).

Other findings pertinent to parkinsonian neuropharmacology are the results of animal studies involving the lesioning of presynaptic dopaminergic neurons: for maximal return of motor functioning, postsynaptic activation of both D-1 and D-2 receptor systems is necessary (11). All of the highly effective dopaminergic ergots—bromocriptine (BCP), lergotrile, lisuride, pergolide, and mesulergine (Fig. 1)—have effects as D-2 agonists roughly proportional to their intrinsic potency as antiparkinson agents in clinical use. Both BCP and lisuride are weak antagonists of the cyclase-linked D-1 systems, while lergotrile, pergolide, and mesulergine share with dopamine the additional property of D-1 agonism. Trials comparing optimized regimens each of these ergot derivatives have revealed no major differences in their clinical efficacy or side-effect profile (12–15). It would seem from this evidence that either D-1 agonism or antagonism in the presence of potent D-2 agonism confers no alteration of antiparkinson effect. In studies with animal models of parkinsonism, maximal activation of locomotor behaviors from BCP is not achieved until presynaptic dopamine content is restored (16) (even though the actions of the ergot compound are thought to be entirely postsynaptic). Lisuride, pergolide, and mesulergine do not share this requirement for the presence of dopamine in the nerve terminal. In clinical practice, however, all of these compounds attain their best outcome when combined with levodopa therapy. One speculation has been that the antiparkinson actions of BCP and other dopaminergic agonists are enhanced by an effect of synaptic dopamine (or, possibly, other sources of D-1 agonism) in producing a conformational change of the D-2 receptor, resulting in greater affinity or increased potency of effect (17). Despite the loss of serotonergic neurotransmission in Parkinson's disease, the potent serotonergic agonism of lisuride apparently adds nothing to its clinical effects except possibly an increased incidence of sedation, hallucination, and vivid dreams (13). The basis for both hallucination and dyskinesia appears to be through activation of D-2 mechanisms, since highly selective antagonists of this system can readily abolish these features (though at the expense of antiparkinson control).

One concern raised by the use of potent dopaminergic agonists is that progressive loss of efficacy might result from chronic therapy. Sustained treatment with pergolide and levodopa treatment in animals with intact and dopaminergically denervated striatums leads to functional "down-regulation," attributable to change at the dopamine receptor (18). The deterioration of clinical response sometimes evolving with long-term dopaminergic therapy (19) might, in part, result from treatment. On the other hand, other studies have indicated that sustained BCP therapy produces a persistent up-regulation of behavioral and motor responsiveness to dopaminergic challenges (20). It is not known if the other dopaminergic agonists have comparable propensities for altering the responsiveness of receptor-mediated functions, or whether these receptor changes offer any advantages for the long-term management of symptoms of Parkinson's disease.

Several recent symposia and publications have collected the clinical experience and neuropharmacology reported with BCP and other dopaminergic agonists (21–26). Though necessarily selective in reviewing the extensive literature, this chapter will evaluate some practical issues from studies performed over the past decade with these drugs. Most of the benefits, adverse effects, and principles of treatment with BCP are common to the other ergot derivatives; experience with other classes of dopaminergic compounds has been extremely limited.

BROMOCRIPTINE AND OTHER ERGOT DERIVATIVES: CLINICAL AND PHARMACOKINETIC CONSIDERATIONS

BCP was introduced slightly over a decade ago as a the first direct-acting dopaminergic drug for treatment of Parkinson's disease. Though it followed the introduction of Sinemet (levodopa plus carbidopa) in the United States by only a few years, its mode of action and therapeutic applications have characterized a new generation of pharmacological strategies for treating Parkinson's disease and related disorders. BCP has been promoted widely as a treatment for managing problems of Parkinson's disease with declining efficacy or levodopa-related complications. Despite the obvious need for drugs with such capabilities, some surveys have indicated that relatively few clinicians make regular use of BCP. The reasons likely are related to the complex, frustrating challenges that advanced or fluctuating parkinsonian symptoms present. Although many difficulties may accompany attempts to optimize therapy with the addition of BCP, some fortunate patients experience a major rejuvenation or enhancement of levodopa effects. Since this outcome may be difficult to achieve with an unfamiliar drug, this review will emphasize the practical aspects of BCP therapy and highlights of its clinical pharmacology.

Certain ergot derivatives were found to cause prolactin inhibition and other endocrine effects which can be linked to dopaminergic properties (27). Based on the studies of Corrodi and colleagues (16), ergot drugs were recognized to be direct stimulants of central nervous system (CNS) dopaminergic receptors and trials with them were proposed for parkinsonism. Within a year, studies by Calne and colleagues confirmed that BCP alone could be as efficacious as levodopa in some patients. Later observations confirmed that, when added to or partially substituted for levodopa, BCP could greatly improve control of most features of Parkinson's disease. Like levodopa, it is least effective against postural instability, and BCP does not appear to improve cognitive deficits of parkinsonism. While comparisons to amantadine and trihexyphenidyl have shown BCP to offer greater benefit for parkinsonian control as monotherapy, there has been some evidence that symptom control can deteriorate with substitution of BCP for levodopa. Although like levodopa it can exacerbate dyskinesias or hallucinations, BCP can improve on the therapeutic index achieved with levodopa. Adjunctive use of BCP can result in lessening of "wearing-off" fluctuations, dyskinesias, and overall enhancement of antiparkinson effect, even when additional levodopa fails to help. Such observations were made in studies using a variety of methodologies, dose ranges, observation intervals, and patient groups. Not surprisingly, the conclusions reached have varied greatly. For example, several involved using a fixed or an arbitrary upper limit of BCP dosage below what might be an optimal quantity (which for some patients can exceed 80 mg/day) (28,29).

BCP has a number of specific indications in treating parkinsonism and related problems. Among its most dramatic effects are the relief of early morning dystonia (when taken the night before) (30), end-of-dose dystonic reactions, leg pains (31), and dystonia present before the onset of antiparkinson therapy (32). The occurrence of unpredictable episodes of start hesitation or "freezing" can be substantially lessened, and total daily "on" time can be increased. Though similar outcomes are sometimes achieved by adding to or rearranging the levodopa schedule, the nature of improvements achieved with BCP for many patients suggests a synergistic effect with levodopa. Although BCP is generally not as effective when substituted completely for levodopa, used in combined therapy it permits reduction from one-quarter to one-half of the previous levodopa dosage. In patients with a "delicate balance" between too little and too much dopaminergic effect (e.g., "freezing," dyskinesias, dystonia, hallucinations), the partial substitution with the longer-acting ergot compound can improve on what can be optimally achieved by levodopa alone. For pharmacological or pharmaco-kinetic reasons (or both), the addition of BCP can result in a smoothing out of fluctuations that so commonly disable patients with advanced Parkinson's disease. Rarely, patients who fail to respond to levodopa (33) or who have intolerable side effects, achieve highly satisfactory benefits from BCP mono-therapy.

The practical role that BCP can play in improving symptom control is il-lustrated in Figure 2. This data was obtained by a parkinsonian patient with prominent wearing-off responses and dyskinesia after several years of levodopa therapy, whose problems were not improved by changes in his dosage or schedule of levodopa/carbidopa (Sinemet). The speed of thumb movements roughly paralleled the patient's bradykinetic state and so followed the 3-4 hour pattern of effectiveness from each Sinemet tablet (Fig. 2a). Moderately severe dyskinesia on the right side would develop at 1 to 2 hours after each dose, in association with maximal improvement of mobility. Figure 2b portrays the limited improvement from a stable regimen of amantadine added to Sinemet: while the starting point and drop-off of the levodopa therapy-related "troughs" are not as low, there was no change in wearing-off phenomena, dyskinesia, or mobility. With bromocriptine 5 mg three times a day added to Sinemet (Fig. 2c), however, a more substantial proportion of "on" time and less wearing-off im-mobility resulted, and there was no increase of dyskinesia. There is also a cumu-lative effect from the added BCP as the day progresses, suggesting that this regimen resulted in a longer duration of clinical effect than that produced by Sinemet alone. These observations exemplify the improvement possible from adjunctive use of a dose of BCP, using a dose as low as 15 mg/day.

Other examples of benefits from BCP therapy include the patient experiencing severe dyskinesia from an amount of levodopa insufficient to improve mobility; only minimal dyskinesia may result from BCP in the context of satisfactory anti-bradykinetic effect (28). Substituting BCP for levodopa in patients with severe peak-dose or wearing-off dyskinesia may also result in relatively less adverse symptomatology than comparably effective doses of levodopa.

Not all patients are as fortunate to achieve benefit or acceptable freedom from side effects with BCP. Some patients receiving as much as 30 mg/day fail to respond or may even worsen, despite marked responses to levodopa. Patients with severe bradykinesia or rigidity are more likely not to respond to BCP or to lose effectiveness within months of starting the drug. Although symptoms may worsen in apparent nonresponders to BCP when the drug is stopped acutely (34), some patients have shown a paradoxical worsening of symptoms as they progress from the introduction of the drug to 20 mg/day or more (12,35). Nevertheless, the rejuvenation of clinical benefit can be especially gratifying for the patient who does not benefit from advance of levodopa dosage. In this regard, BCP and

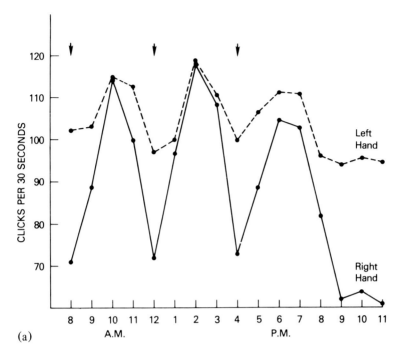

FIGURE 2 Data averaged from tally counter clicks operated by a patient's left and right thumb (as many movements as possible in 30 seconds tested hourly; points represent mean values hourly for each day of 2 weeks of continuous data collection in each instance). Each arrow represents the time of oral intake of Sinemet (carbidopa/levodopa) 25/100, Sinemet plus amantadine 100 mg, or Sinemet plus bromocriptine 5 mg after 2 weeks of medication build-up. The patient's left side, clinically unaffected by parkinsonian deficit, nonetheless shows the pattern of levodopa responsiveness similar to the more affected side.

related ergots can offer some symptomatic improvement for patients with Parkinson's disease associated with Shy-Drager syndrome, olivopontocerebellar degeneration, and progressive supranuclear palsy (36,37).

   Though most evaluation of BCP has been as adjunctive therapy with levodopa, there have been several studies of BCP as an initial alternative to levodopa (38–41). While it is clear that parkinsonian symptoms progress under BCP therapy, there has been speculation that the risk of dyskinesias and motor fluctuations commonly developing with chronic levodopa therapy could be lessened. As a low-dosage monotherapy, BCP can give at least several months of sustained benefit using 15 mg or less for some patients with mild symptoms, but more affected patients required larger doses or levodopa supplementation in one

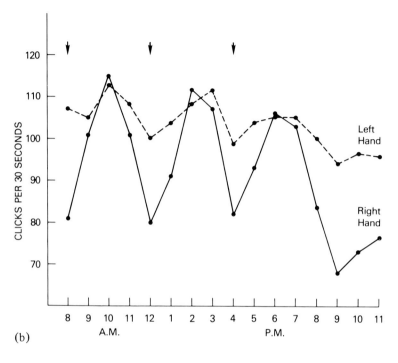

(b)

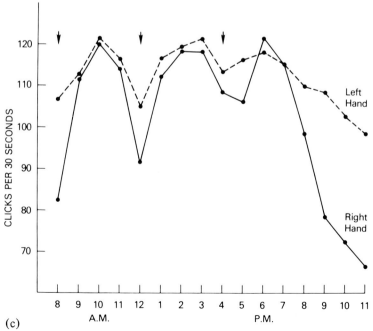

(c)

double-blind study (41). In another evaluation, the BCP dosage ranging between 17.5 and 120 mg/day (mean: 56.5) gave satisfactory symptom control for half of the patient group. However, side effects were frequent, and insufficient response to this monotherapy regimen required the addition of levodopa for the others, sometimes within months (39). In those patients with benefit, follow-up for 4 to 8 years after initiation of BCP showed no peak-dose dyskinesia, dystonia, "freezing," or other motor fluctuations, in contrast to the usual frequent incidence from a comparable period of levodopa therapy. In another BCP monotherapy study with a similar format, there were similar results (though one case of dyskinesia occurred), including a high incidence of adverse effects and treatment failure necessitating addition of levodopa (38). Fewer than one third of 76 patients initiated on a dose of BCP (averaging 28 mg/day) were able to continue with this treatment in a third study, the reason in more than half being insufficient response or significant side effects (40). Response to BCP therapy tended to decline more prominently than is the usual outcome with comparable levodopa therapy, although increased BCP dosage may give further improvement (39). Combination of an initial regimen of BCP (averaging 16.6 mg/day) with a standard levodopa regimen gave a much lower incidence of dyskinesia and fluctuations after 3 years as well as antiparkinson control comparable to results from levodopa therapy alone (40). Whether the latter therapeutic strategy will prove to combine optimal symptomatic control with avoidance of long-term levodopa-related problems awaits confirmation by prospective studies now underway.

Perhaps no other drugs in current use have as wide a range of optimal dosage as has been found with BCP and related antiparkinson ergots. Any consideration of what constitutes ideal regimens with these drugs must consider the wide interpatient variability as to blood levels following standard oral doses (42). In the author's studies for which patients with advanced Parkinson's disease ("on-off", loss of efficacy, and dyskinesia problems) received supplemental BCP, dose ranges leading to improvement without significant side effects have ranged from 5.8 to 87.5 mg/day (mean: 42.7) (13) and 12.5 to 150.0 mg/day (mean: 56.5) (14). In the same studies, optimal doses of lisuride ranged from 0.6 to 10.0 mg/day (mean: 4.5) and for pergolide, 0.7-7.2 mg/day (mean: 3.3). Other studies with pergolide and lisuride have used similar doses for good effect. Optimal lisuride dosage in one patient has been as high as 17 mg/day (37), and in one study in which BCP was substituted for levodopa, doses in excess of 200 mg/day (mean: 148) were used (29).

As BCP is an expensive drug and side effects are in part dose related, the effectiveness of low-dose regimens has undergone a great deal of review and controversy (26). Teychenne (43) has reviewed the efficacy of BCP as an adjunct to levodopa using an arbitrary maximum of 30 mg/day. Using a dose build-up of no more than 1 mg/week for the first 6 weeks, patients were slowly brought to a dose range of 8-18 mg/day over several months. With this approach, maximal improvement is delayed longer than in regimens using BCP advances as rapidly as 2.5 (44) to 70 (45) mg increments/week to the maximal daily ranges of 75–150 mg/day attained within a month. Although such large doses may be necessary for some patients, rapid escalation of dosage may overlook potential benefit that could come weeks or months lafter from a stable dose (46). Furthermore, there has been some evidence that a therapeutic "ceiling" may exist (estimated at 100 mg/day for some patients (35), but likely to be lower for others), and so a too-rapid advance in dosage may bring patients into a range in which further increases bring deterioration rather than progressive improvement. With no more than 20 mg/day, there has been good toleration of BCP (only 15% of patients having adverse effects necessitating discontinuation of BCP in one study, which also found marked improvement of disabilities) (31).

In a large clinic of patients with advanced parkinsonism and levodopa-related problems, optimal regimens with BCP used an average of 49 mg/day (28). Other researchers have concluded that the greatest benefit from BCP came from dosage in excess of 30 mg/day (47–49) over long periods of follow-up. The effectiveness of lower-dosage BCP in controlling the primary symptoms of Parkinson's disease, as well as fluctuations and dyskinesias, may be in part a function of the disease severity and duration, and age of patients (50). With the controversial status that has attached itself to the issue of what is optimal dosage with BCP, the question in any one patient is best dealt operationally with the strategy to advance medication slowly to maximize tolerance and minimize the amount of drug needed.

The decision to use BCP or other ergot derivatives as adjuncts to levodopa should consider a reduction in levodopa dosage, particularly if dose-limiting effects of levodopa (such as dyskinesia) contribute to the disability. Even with toleration of large levodopa dosage, adverse effects with the introduction of dopaminergic ergots are common and potentially severe (especially nausea, hypotension, and hallucination). An ideal starting dosage of BCP is 1.25 mg (half a tablet) daily for the first few days. Taking the drug after a meal slows absorption and so may lessen any potential side effects, though if tolerated, the drug is best administered between meal times for achieving uniform absorption. With end-of-dose failure, it may be necessary to use BCP or other dopaminergic ergots as frequently as every 2–3 hours (13,14), though for many patients the drug is effective at 2–3 times per day dosing (48). A sustained-release preparation of BCP currently under development may add to its usefulness. The control of early morning dystonia of the feet can be relieved by as little as 2.5–5 mg taken at bedtime.

It is common for patients started on BCP to experience a transient worsening of parkinsonian symptoms with the introduction of 1.25 to 2.5 mg/day. This low-dose effect probably caused by preferential activation of presynaptic mechanisms (which can also initiate a marked reduction of dyskinetic movements). Gradual increase of BCP dose by no more than 5 mg every week may be rewarded by avoidance or early warning of side effects resulting from larger dosage. While the slow build-up of drug may be one way to avoid hypotension or nausea, a similar tolerance to other side effects may not develop.

The success of BCP prompted searches for related compounds with less costly synthesis and improved therapeutic indices. Lergotrile, an ergoline (lacking the synthetic peptide adduct of BCP) was the next analogue to undergo clinical study. Though equipotent and highly comparable to BCP as an antiparkinson agent (12), lergotrile frequently caused hepatotoxicity, which necessitated its withdrawal. Two other ergolines, lisuride (13,37,51–53) and pergolide (14,54), were next to be evaluated. Each has a 10- to 15-fold increase over BCP's intrinsic potency in antiparkinson effect. Although the duration of effect after oral dosage of lisuride has been regarded as shorter (53) and pergolide as longer (54) than that of BCP, studies evaluating the clinical efficacy of each in the same patients revealed no such differences (12,13). Lisuride is water soluble, permitting intravenous delivery. Subcutaneous administration by portable pump for maintaining constant blood levels has resulted in marked improvement of predictable and random fluctuations associated with oral levodopa therapy (55). Pharmacokinetic studies with lisuride have demonstrated marked dose-to-dose variability of plasma drug levels even in the same patient (51). These findings may have important implications for interpreting the relationship between stable oral regimens of antiparkinson ergots and their clinical effects.

Pergolide has been evaluated in a number of short- and long-term trials in which it has achieved clinical outcomes similar to those with BCP. Like lisuride and BCP, pergolide generally needs concomitant levodopa to achieve an optimal antiparkinson effect, as shown by attempts to substitute the drug for levodopa therapy (56). Studies with pergolide (14,26,54,57) have used a dose range of 0.1–7.2 mg/day, and have concluded that three times daily regimens are adequate for some patients, while others require the drug as frequently as every 2–3 hours for optimal effect (56). Most patients in one study experienced their peak benefit during the first 3 months of therapy, with some decline thereafter in scores of antiparkinson efficacy. However, at 28 months the mean total disability score was still significantly improved over earlier scores from levodopa therapy alone (58). Studies of patients for up to 50 months follow-up with pergolide therapy have shown maintenance of its effectiveness (59).

The latest ergot derivative to be studied has been mesulergine (CU 32-085), an 8-alpha-ergoline (like lisuride) with D-1 and D-2 agonism (like pergolide). Mesulergine differs from the other analogues in that a demethylation metabolite, rather than the parent drug, appears to be responsible for its antiparkinson effect (60). In studies similar to those discussed above, its clinical profile was extremely promising: it was as effective as BCP for antiparkinson actions (15) and had other desirable properties as well. In some patients, antidepressant effect was found, postural instability improved in some instances, orthostatic blood pressure drop was less common than with other dopaminergic drugs, and other adverse effects seemed milder (61). Using a daily dose ranging between 2 to 60 mg/day, various studies showed effectiveness sustained for as long as 18 months. Unfortunately, this drug had to be discontinued from further clinical trials because of carcinogenic potential found in rodent studies.

The pharmacokinetic profile of BCP and the other ergot compounds are related to their clinical pattern of action. With BCP (62,63) and with lisuride (51,53), antiparkinson effect correlates well with oral dose and with plasma levels. Using radiolabelled BCP, the T 1/2 of oral absorption has been shown to be 0.12 hour (65). A biphasic decay curve was found, with the first phase of decline in blood level having a half-life of 6 hours and a second-phase half-life of 50 hours. BCP has a high extraction ratio by the liver (first-pass metabolism); this pattern of drug metabolism probably contributes to the considerable inter-subject variability of BCP levels from the same oral dose (42). Similar conclusions have been reached with lisuride pharmacokinetics (51). Bioavailability studies with BCP, repeated at 3 and 6 months, have confirmed a stable effect in the same individual (62). With a single oral dose of BCP ranging from 12.5 to 100 mg, a peak blood dose is achieved at approximately 100 minutes, preceding the maximal antiparkinson effect at approximately 130 ± 12 minutes. However, abnormal involuntary movements (thought to be derived from dopaminergic effect) do not always follow this timing (62,63). Optimal antiparkinson effect occurred with plasma BCP levels between 2 and 5 ng/ml (62). Curiously, for some patients, peak plasma levels were lower as oral BCP dosage was increased. Pretreatment with metoclopramide elevated peak BCP levels. Erythromycin also interacts with BCP to cause increased blood levels and effect, through an as-yet undefined mechanism (64).

ADVERSE EFFECTS FROM BROMOCRIPTINE AND OTHER DOPAMINERGIC ERGOTS

The occurrence of dose-related or idiosyncratic side effects often decide the dosage or ability to use BCP or other dopaminergic drugs. As many of these side effects are dose and tolerance related, slow, gradual escalation of dose can lessen their occurrence. The author has followed several patients who, though initially intolerant (having gastrointestinal or psychiatric side effects) of 5–20 mg of BCP daily, ultimately could use as much as three times that amount. The cross-tolerance that develops in switching from BCP to other ergot derivatives such as pergolide, lisuride, and lergotrile (37,66) indicates that the D-2 dopamine receptor agonism common to these drugs is likely the basis for the adverse effects as well as the antiparkinson benefits.

The most common adverse effects with BCP and the other ergots are qualitatively similar to those of levodopa and amantadine. In the order of usual frequency, these include constipation, fatigue, sedation, nausea, vomiting, postural hypotension, vivid dreaming, hallucination, and confusion. Other common effects have included dryness of mouth, lightheadedness, diplopia, irritability, hiccups, insomnia, headache, nasal stuffiness, palpitations, exacerbation of myopia, and abdominal cramping. Movement disorders comparable to those caused by levodopa include dyskinesia, painful dystonic spasms (peak-dose and wearing-off), and blepharospasm. Increased loss of hair (67), diarrhea (68), chest pain resembling angina (31), and exacerbation of myoclonus during sleep (69) have been described. The use of alcohol concomitantly with BCP has been associated with development of nausea and vomiting at a BCP dose previously tolerated (70). More uncommon reactions with BCP have been urinary urgency or incontinence (71), and facial puffiness. Digital vasospasm (lacking the full picture of Raynaud syndrome) (72) and gastrointestinal bleeding (73) have also been described.

Several of the dose-related side effects merit further consideration. Both nausea and vomiting and postural hypotension (74) are common at initiation of therapy, even with a starting dose as low as 1 mg of BCP. Both systolic and diastolic blood pressure are decreased by BCP in relation to dose (75), though the occurrence of symptomatic postural faintness is less predictable (29,76) than blood pressure readings might suggest. Orthostatic hypotension can resolve for some patients within days to weeks of starting medication. With the use of metoclopramide or domperidone pretreatment with antiparkinson ergots (29,62), nausea and vomiting induced by BCP (in excess of 200 mg/day) can be abolished. Though highly effective, metoclopramide has the potential drawback of exacerbating parkinsonian symptoms. Domperidone, which may soon become available in the United States, can protect against nausea and vomiting from the initial, rapidly increasing, or sustained high dosage of BCP. Although a potent dopamine receptor blocker, domperidone is excluded from access to the striatum and so does not interfere with antiparkinson effect. Orthostatic hypotension and other central adverse effects of the dopaminergic ergots, however, are not avoided with these drugs.

Among the spectrum of psychiatric side effects that can occur from dopaminergic therapy are apathy, irritability, anxiety, restlessness, emotional lability, obsessive thoughts, paranoid ideation, manic states, confusion, and delirium (77-80). Though cognitive impairment is common in Parkinson's disease, no significant changes in intellect or cognitive operations were found in a careful study of patients treated with pergolide (80). Hallucinations and similar psychotic phenomena are experienced by up to one-quarter of patients treated with dopaminergic ergots (81). While they may occur in similar fashion from levodopa and amantadine, the increased potency of these drugs as D-2 agonists adds to their likelihood. In several studies, psychiatric side effects have been the most common reason for the need to discontinue BCP or other dopaminergic ergots. The prior occurrence of hallucinations with other therapy, advanced age, and stage of parkinsonism, and significant dementia seem to be the major risk factors for dose-related hallucinations, though such patients have been excluded from most studies in which the incidence of these events might have been evaluated. Concomitant use of anticholinergics does not seem to increase the incidence of hallucination.

Hallucinations can be brief and benign, often with recurrent themes of a non-frightening or pleasurable nature and without distortion of reality. With full insight into their identity, many patients have described them as single or multiple human or animal faces (often in the periphery of vision), or else as small figures crowding a room. Hallucination can regularly follow each dose of medication, though it may be more common at the end of day with the onset of darkness. Vivid dreaming, with talking out in sleep, or daytime hallucination can also occur. Although hallucinations can occur for years on a stable dosage regimen without worsening, disorientation, delusions, or paranoid states may evolve insidiously in some patients. These psychotic features are generally dose related, but even with discontinuation of medication can persist for several days or longer before resolution. As with psychiatric effects from levodopa therapy (82), continuing use of dopaminergic ergots may ultimately permit oral dosage to be used much in excess of that initially causing intolerable hallucinations. The isolated occurrence of hallucinations in patients free of other psychiatric adverse effects and experiencing good motor control can be particularly distressing and disabling. Although reduction in medication is generally necessary, use of small doses of low-potency neuroleptics (like molindone), or methysergide (83) can block hallucinations in some patients.

Dopaminergic compounds could theoretically induce cardiac arrhythmias, as have been reported as a consequence of pergolide therapy (84). However, more controlled investigations, which have studied patients with pre-existing heart disease (85), have shown no occurrence of arrhythmia or other cardiotoxicity (though an additional evaluation has reported a mild but clinically insignificant bradycardic effect with pergolide) (86).

A number of other rare but potentially serious adverse symptoms have been linked to BCP and other ergots on an apparently idiosyncratic basis. Prominent capillary networks can develop on the feet (Fig. 3). A tender, swollen, erythromelalgia-like rash has been described that can develop uni- or bilaterally in the ankle-foot region, generally following a period of edema (87) (Fig. 4). This generally has occurred after prolonged high-dose therapy, and can remit with reduction in dosage. The author has observed prompt resolution of this disorder with administration of cyproheptadine, 4 mg/day. Erythromelalgia-like reactions have been reported with pergolide (88) and mesulergine (61), but the reaction does not result from levodopa, nor does it resemble the livedo reticularis commonly associated with amantadine therapy. One patient receiving pergolide de-

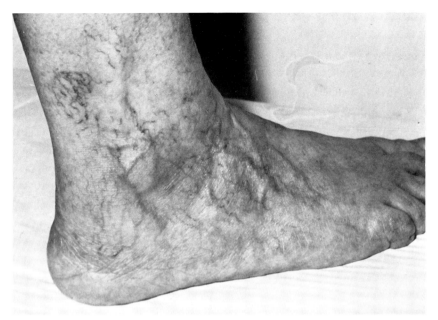

FIGURE 3 Prominent violaceous capillary networks developing asymptomatically over the surfaces of both feet several weeks after initiation of bromocriptine therapy.

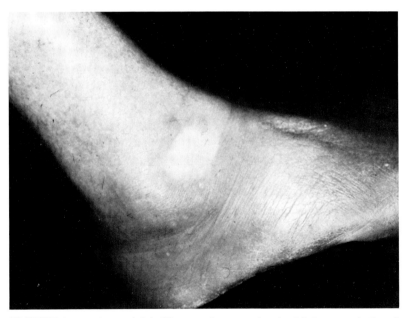

FIGURE 4 Erythromelalgia-like reaction associated with bromocriptine therapy typically occurs in the ankle or shin region. The reddened edematous skin is warm, extremely tender, and can simulate cellulitis or thrombophlebitis. This idiopathic reaction, which can be unilateral, may suddenly develop after months to years of therapy at stable bromocriptine dosage.

veloped migratory arthralgias, rash, and antibody studies suggestive of lupus ery-thematosus, a condition which resolved upon discontinuation of the drug (58). Rarely, pleural thickening and pulmonary infiltrates and effusions have developed in patients maintained on chronic, high-dose BCP regimens (14,28), in some in-stances developing asymptomatically (Fig. 5a and b). Screening on a regular basis for these changes in BCP-treated patients with chest x-rays is advised. A recent case report concerned retroperitoneal fibrosis evolving after a period of high-dose BCP therapy and previous development of an erythromelalgia-like reaction (89). Retroperitoneal fibrosis and pleural thickening has frequently been de-scribed with another ergot compound, methysergide, but the relationship be-tween these idiosyncratic events and BCP therapy is unclear. One adverse effect of theoretical concern is potentially fatal hyperpyrexia similar to "neuroleptic malignant syndrome" were BCP to be abruptly discontinued; this situation has followed the stopping of levodopa (90).

NEW DIRECTIONS IN DOPAMINERGIC DRUGS

Currently, BCP is the only dopaminergic ergot commercially available in the United States; pergolide is awaiting approval by the Food and Drug Administra-tion for marketing (as of October, 1986), and lisuride is not planned for marketing in the United States, but will be available elsewhere. The development of other antiparkinson drugs of this class may involve analogues with modifica-tions to the tetracyclic structure for an improved therapeutic index. 6-N-propyl lisuride has more sustained dopaminergic properties than its parent compound, and so may have improved clinical utility (52). Clinical trials with the partial dopaminergic agonist *trans*-9,10-dihydrolisuride (terguride) showed, as compared to lisuride, the same profile of activity in controlling "off" periods and lessening dyskinesia, but fewer side effects in comparable dosage (91). LY 141865, a tri-cyclic compound with some structural similarities to the tetracyclic ergoline pergolide, has dopaminergic effects limited to the D-2 system, in contrast to ad-ditional interactions with D-1 mechanisms of the other ergot-related compounds. Although not used in clinical trials to date, LY 141865 might be a useful probe of the role that a "pure" D-2 agonist might play in treating Parkinson's disease.

Several non-ergot compounds have been investigated for their antiparkinson potential. Ciladopa (AY 27,110) has been described as a partial dopaminergic agonist equipotent to BCP, with increased affinity for supersensitive dopamine receptors (as can develop in parkinsonism). In pilot studies with ciladopa (92,93), clinical signs and disability improved for most patients and adverse ef-fects were minimal, although the drug had to be withdrawn because of animal toxicity. (+)4-Propyl-9-hydroxynaphthoxazine, a potent dopaminergic com-pound with the potential for transdermal administration, has shown some effectiveness against tremor and overall features of Parkinson's disease, though adverse effects may be prominent (94). The antiparkinson potential of a novel

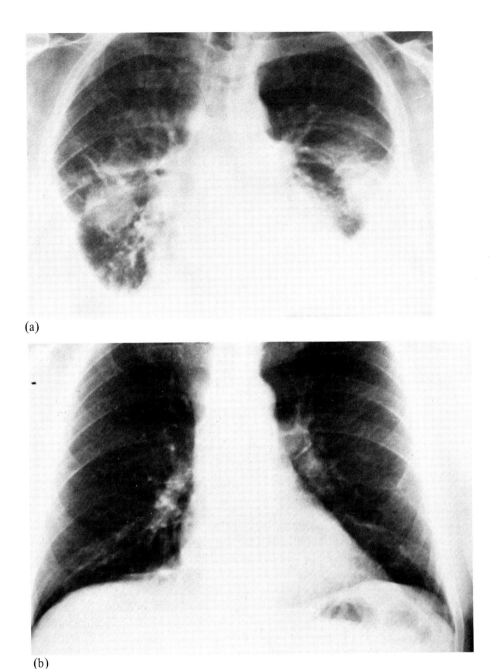

(a)

(b)

FIGURES 5a and b Chest x-rays before (Figure 5a) and during (Figure 5b) bromocriptine therapy, 80-100 mg/day for 3 years, in a 61-year-old man with no prior pulmonary disease. The patient presented with exertional dyspnea that progressed in severity over several weeks (28). The pleural thickening and effusion was associated with an inflammatory exudate. These abnormalities resolved by 2 months after discontinuation of bromocriptine.

abeorphine compound with D-1 and D-2 dopaminergic effects as well as alpha-$_2$-adrenergic effects, is currently under study (95). SK&F 38393 is a benazepine compound with dopaminergic agonism limited to the D-1 system. In rodent studies, it has shown some effects similar to other antiparkinson agents when given in combination with D-2 agonists (11); given to MPTP-parkinsonian monkey, however, it has no effect alone (96). Trials in parkinsonian patients have suggested slight therapeutic effect in 2 patients in the author's pilot studies but not in another evaluation (97).

REFERENCES

1. Berde B, Schild HO. (Eds.). (1978). *Ergot Aklaloids and Related Compounds*. Berlin, Springer Verlag.
2. Ehringer H, Hornykiewicz O. (1960). *Klin Wnschr* 38: 1236.
3. Schwab RS, Amador LV, Lettvin LY. (1951). *Trans Am Neurol Assoc* 76: 251.
4. Anden NE, Rubenson A, Fuxe K. (1967). *J Pharm Pharmacol* 19: 627.
5. Cotzias GC, Papavasiliou PS, Ginos JZ. (1976). In: Yahr MD (Ed.), *The Basal Ganglia*. New York, Raven Press.
6. Rinne UK, Sonninen V, Marttila R. (1975). *Adv Neurol* 9: 383.
7. Kebabian JW, Kebabian PR, Munemura M, Calne DB. (1979). In: Fuxe K, Calne DB (Eds.), *Dopaminergic Ergot Derivatives and Motor Function*. New York, Pergamon Press.
8. Fuxe K, Agnati LF, Ogren SO, Kohler C, Calza L, Benfenati F, Goldstein M, Andersson K, Eneroth P. (1983). In: Carlsson A, Nilsson JLG (Eds.), *Dopamine Receptor Agonists*. Stockholm, Swedish Pharmaceutical Press.
9. Stoof JC, Kebabian JW. (1981). *Nature* 294: 366.
10. Gorell JM, Czarnecki B, Hubbell S. (1985). *Neurology* (Suppl 1) 35: 158.
11. Gershanik O, Heikkila RE, Duvoisin RC. (1983). *Neurology* 33: 1489.
12. Teychenne PF, Pfeiffer R, Bern SM, McInturff D, Calne DB. (1978). *Ann Neurol* 3: 319.
13. LeWitt PA, Gopinathan G, Ward CD, Sanes JN, Dambrosia JM, Durso R, Calne DB. (1982). *Neurology* 32: 69.
14. LeWitt PA, Ward CD, Larsen TA, Raphaelson MI, Newman RP, Foster N, Dambrosia JM, Calne DB. (1983). *Neurology* 33: 1009.
15. Burton K, Larsen TA, Robinson RG, Bratty PJ, Martin WRW, Schulzer M, Calne DB. (1985). *Neurology* 35: 1205.
16. Corrodi H, Fuxe K, Hokfelt T, Lidbrink P, Ungerstedt U, (1973). *J Pharm Pharmacol* 25: 409.
17. Goldstein M, Lieberman AN, Meller A. (1985). *Trends Pharmacol Sci* 7: 436.
18. Reches A, Wagner HR, Jackson-Lewis V, Yablonskaya E, Fahn S. (1984). *Neurology* 34: 1208.
19. Lieberman AM, Goldstein M, Leibowitz M, Gopinathan G, Neophytides A, Hiesiger E, Nelson J, Walker R. (1984). *Neurology* 34: 223.

20. Nausieda PA, Weiner WA, Kanapa DJ, Klawans HL. (1978). *Neurology* 28: 1183.

21. Fuxe K, Calne DB. (Eds.). (1979). *Dopaminergic Ergot Derivatives and Motor Function.* New York, Pergamon Press.

22. Calne DB, Horowski R, McDonald RJ, Wuttke W. (Eds.). (1983). *Lisuride and Other Dopamine Agonists.* New York, Raven Press.

23. Fahn S, Calne DB, Shoulson I. (Eds.). (1983). *Experimental Therapeutics of Movement Disorders.* Adv. Neurol., Vol. 37, New York, Raven Press.

24. Calne DB, Lee RG. (Eds.). (1984). *Canad J Neurol Sci* (Suppl) 11: 89.

25. Hassler RG, Christ JF. (Eds.). (1984). *Parkinson-Specific Motor and Mental Disorders.* Adv. Neurol, Vol. 40. New York, Raven Press.

26. Fahn S, Marsden CD, Jenner P, Teychenne PF. (Eds.). (1986). *Recent Developments in Parkinson's Disease.* New York, Raven Press.

27. Vance ML, Evans WS, Thorner MO. (1984). *Ann Intern Med* 100: 78.

28. LeWitt PA, Calne DB. (1981). *J Neural Transm* 51: 175.

29. Quinn N, Illas A, L'Hermitte F, Agid Y. (1981). *Neurology* 31: 662.

30. Lander CM, Lees AJ, Stern GM. (1979). *Clin Exptl Neurol* 16: 197.

31. Maier Hoehn MM, Elton RL. (1985). *Neurology* 35: 199.

32. LeWitt PA, Burns RS, Newman RP. (1986). *Clin Neuropharmacol* 9: 293.

33. Jankovic J. (1981). *Ann Neurol* 10: 64.

34. Duvoisin RC, Mendoza MR, Yahr MD, Sweet RD. (1979). In: Fuxe K, Calne DB (Eds.), *Dopaminergic Ergot Derivatives in Motor Function.* New York, Pergamon Press.

35. Koller WC, Weiner WJ, Nausieda PA, Klawans HL. (1979). *Neurology* 29: 1439.

36. Jackson JA, Jankovic J, Ford J. (1983). *Ann Neurol* 13: 373.

37. LeWitt PA, Calne DB. (1983). In: Calne DB, Horowski R, McDonald RJ, Wuttke W (Eds.), *Lisuride and Other Dopamine Agonists.* New York, Raven Press.

38. Stern GM, Lees AJ. (1983). *Adv Neurol* 37: 17.

39. Rascol A, Montastruc JL, Rascol O. (1984). *Can J Neurol Sci* 11: 229.

40. Rinne UK. (1986). In: Fahn S, Marsden CD, Jenner P, Teychenne PF (Eds.), *Recent Developments in Parkinson's Disease.* New York, Raven Press.

41. Staal-Schreinemachers AL, Wesselring H, Kamphuis DJ, Burg WRD, Lakke JPWF. (1986). *Neurology* 36: 291.

42. Burns RS, Calne DB. (1981). In: Corsini GU, Gessa GL (Eds.), *Apomorphine and Dopaminimimetics: Clinical Pharmacology,* Volume II. New York, Raven Press.

43. Teychenne PF, Bergsrud D, Racy A. (1986). In: Fahn S, Marsden CD, Jenner P, Teychenne PF (Eds.), *Recent Developments in Parkinson's Disease.* New York, Raven Press.

44. Lees AJ, Haddad S, Shaw KM, Kohout LJ, Stern GM. (1978). *Arch Neurol* 35: 503.

45. Lieberman AN, Kupersmith M, Gopinathan G, Estey E, Goodgold A, Goldstein M. (1979). *Neurology* 29: 363.

46. Teychenne PF, Bergsrud D, Elton R, Vern B. (1982). *Neurology* 32: 577.
47. Stern G. (1986). In: Fahn S, Marsden CD, Jenner P, Teychenne PF (Eds.), *Recent Developments in Parkinson's Disease*. New York, Raven Press.
48. Grimes JD, Hassan MN. (1986). In: Fahn S, Marsden CD, Jenner P, Teychenne PF (Eds.), *Recent Developments in Parkinson's Disease*. New York, Raven Press.
49. Klawans HL, Goetz CG, Tanner CM, Glantz R. (1986). In: Fahn S, Marsden CD, Jenner P, Teychenne PF (Eds.), *Recent Developments in Parkinson's Disease*. New York, Raven Press.
50. Larsen TA, Newman RP, LeWitt PA, Calne DB. (1983). *Neurology* 31: 662.
51. LeWitt PA, Burns RS, Calne DB. (1983). *Adv Neurol* 37: 131.
52. LeWitt PA. (1986). In: Fahn S, Marsden CD, Jenner P, Teychenne PF (Eds.), *Recent Developments in Parkinson's Disease*. New York, Raven Press.
53. Parkes JD, Schachter M, Marsden CD, Smith B, Wilson A. (1981). *Ann Neurol* 9: 48.
54. Lieberman AN, Neophytides A, Leibowitz M, Gopinathan G, Pact V, Walker R, Goodgold A, Goldstein M. (1983). *Adv Neurol* 37: 95.
55. Obeso JA, Luquin MR, Martinez Lage JM. (1986). *Ann Neurol* 19: 31.
56. Mear J, Parroche G, de Smett Y, Weber M, L'Hermitte F, Agid Y. (1984). *Neurology* 34: 983.
57. Lieberman AN, Gopinathan G, Neophytides A, Nelson J, Hiesiger E, Walker R, Leibowitz M, Goldstein M. (1986). In: Fahn S, Marsden CD, Jenner P, Teychenne PF (Eds.), *Recent Developments in Parkinson's Disease*. New York, Raven Press.
58. Jankovic J. (1986). In: Fahn S, Marsden CD, Jenner P, Teychenne PF (Eds.), *Recent Developments in Parkinson's Disease*. New York, Raven Press.
59. Sage J, Duvoisin RC. (1986). *Clin Neuropharmacol* 9: 160.
60. Markstein R. (1983). *Eur J Pharmacol* 95: 101.
61. Pfeiffer RF. (1985). *Clin Neuropharmacol* 8: 64.
62. DeBono A, Marsden CD, Asselman P, Parkes JD. (1976). *Br J Clin Pharmacol* 3: 977.
63. Parkes JD, DeBono AG, Marsden CD. (1976). *J Neurol Neurosurg Psychiatr* 39: 1101.
64. Sibley WA, LaGuna F. (1981). Excerpta Medica. *Intern Congr Series* 548: 329–330.
65. Schran HF, Bhuta SI, Schwarz HJ, Thorner MO. (1980). In: Calne DB, Goldstein M, Lieberman A, Thorner MO (Eds.), *Ergot Compounds and Brain Function: Neuroendocrine and Neuropsychiatric Aspects*. New York, Raven Press.
66. Teychenne PF, Rosin AJ, Plotkin CN, Calne DB. (1980). *Br J Clin Pharmacol* 9: 47.
67. Blum I, Leiba S. (1980). *N Engl J Med* 303: 1418.
68. Jellinger K. (1982). *J Neurol* 227: 75.
69. Vardi J, Glaubman H, Rabey JM, Streifler M. (1978). *J Neurol* 218: 35.

70. Ayres J, Maisey MM. (1980). *N Engl J Med* 302: 806.
71. Gopinathan G, Calne DB. (1980). *Ann Neurol* 8: 204.
72. Wass JAH, Thorner MO, Besser GM. (1976). *Lancet* 1: 1135.
73. Delposa E, Maclay WP. (1976). *Lancet* 2: 906.
74. Van Loon GR. (1980). *Clin Invest Med* 2: 131.
75. Reid JL, Bateman N. (1979). In: Fuxe K, Calne DB (Eds.), *Dopaminergic Ergot Derivatives in Motor Function*. New York, Pergamon Press.
76. Brosens IA. (1977). *Lancet* 2: 224.
77. White AC, Murphy TJC. (1977). *Br J Psychiatr* 130: 104.
78. Pearson KC. (1981). *N Engl J Med* 305: 173.
79. Brook NM, Cookson IB. (1978). *Br Med J* 1: 790.
80. Stern Y, Mayeux R, Ilson J, Fahn S, Cote L. (1984). *Neurology* 34: 201.
81. Serby M, Angrist B, Lieberman A. (1978). *Am J Psychiatr* 135: 1227.
82. Goodwin FK. (1971). *JAMA* 218: 1915.
83. Nausieda PA, Tanner CM, Klawans HL. (1983). *Adv Neurol* 37: 23.
84. Leibowitz M, Lieberman A, Goldstein M. (1981). *Clin Pharmacol Ther* 30: 7180.
85. Tanner CM, Chhablani R, Goetz CG, Klawans HL. (1985). *Neurology* 35: 918.
86. Kurlan R, Miller C, Knapp R, Murphy G, Shoulson I. (1986). *Neurology* 36: 993.
87. Eisler T, Hall RP, Kalaver K, Calne DB. (1981). *Neurology* 31: 1368.
88. Olanow LW, Alberts MJ. (1986). In: Fahn S, Marsden CD, Jenner P, Teychenne PF (Eds.), *Recent Developments in Parkinson's Disease*. New York, Raven Press.
89. Demonet JF, Rostin M, Dueymes M, Ioualalen A, Monastruc JL, Rascol A. (1986). *Clin Neuropharmacol* 9: 200.
90. Sechi G-P, Tanda F, Mutandi R. (1984). *Neurology* 34: 249.
91. Esteguy M, Gershanik O, Leguardia R. *Adv Neurol* (in press, 1986).
92. Snider SR. (1985). *Neurology* (Suppl 1) 35: 203.
93. Lieberman AN, Goldstein M, Gopinathan G, Neophytides A, Nelson J. (1985). *Neurology* (Suppl 1) 35: 203.
94. Stoessl AJ, Maj E, Calne DB. (1985). *Lancet* 2: 1330.
95. Karobath M. (1986). In: Fahn S, Marsden CD, Jenner P, Teychenne PF (Eds.), *Recent Developments in Parkinson's Disease*. New York, Raven Press.
96. Nomoto M, Jenner P, Marsden CD. (1985). *Neurosci Lett* 57: 37.
97. Braun AR, Fabbrini G, Mouradian MM, Barone P, Chase TN. (1986). *Neurology* (Suppl 1) 36: 246.

22
Monoamine Oxidase Inhibitors

ANDREW JOHN LEES
National Hospitals for Nervous Diseases, London, England

The importance of deamination in the degradation of monoamines has been recognized for more than a century (Schmiedeberg, 1877), but it was not until 1928 that the enzyme tyramine oxidase was isolated from liver by Mary Hare. Blaschko's work in Cambridge (1937) on the fate of epinephrine led to the more generalized concept of an amine oxidase system and in 1938 the term monoamine oxidase (MAO) was proposed (Zeller, 1938) for a whole system of enzymes responsible for the oxidative deamination of catecholamines. By this time the oxidation of aliphatic monoamines by MAO in the brain had already been demonstrated (Pugh and Quastel, 1937).

The monoamine oxidases are spherical, stable, sulfydryl flavoproteins with molecular weights around 100,000 which are widely distributed in the animal kingdom. They are bound to the outer membranes of mitochondria and as well as being present in neurons and glial tissue they are found in liver, kidney, heart, intestine, lung, smooth muscle, salivary gland, and gonads. They are important in the regulation of intracellular monoamine concentration and in the biological inactivation of a number of chemical messengers. For example, dopamine is broken down by monoamine oxidase and catechol-O-methyl transferase to homovanillic acid (see Fig. 1). In contrast to the other enzymes involved in catecholamine metabolism, monoamine oxidase in human brain actually increases with age (Nies et al., 1973). In Parkinson's disease, brain MAO levels remain normal (Bernheimer et al., 1962; Lloyd et al., 1973) and it has been claimed that their activity is greatest in the afternoon (Birkmayer and Riederer, 1980). Abnormalities of both brain and platelet MAO activity have been reported in migraine, bipolar affective disorder, schizophrenia, levodopa-

Metabolic Pathways of Dopamine Biosynthesis and Catabolism.

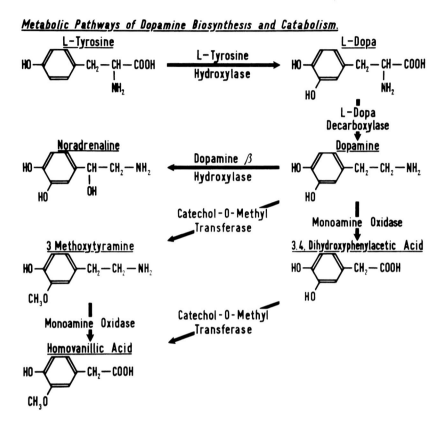

FIGURE 1 Metabolic pathways of dopamine biosynthesis and catabolism.

treated parkinsonian patients, and in alcoholics, although the significance of these findings is not understood. With the brain studies, interpretation is difficult in many instances because of possible associated neuronal loss.

In the 1950s iproniazid was used successfully in the treatment of tuberculosis, but it had one serious disadvantage: disinhibition and fatuous euphoria. One of the early papers describing its use reports patients "dancing in the halls" of the sanatorium. In 1955 Zeller and his colleagues showed the agent to be a monoamine oxidase inhibitor. Crane (1956) then suggested that this unwanted side effect might be put to good advantage in the treatment of depression. Despite considerable supportive evidence from clinical trials that monoamine oxidase inhibitors (MAOIs) could be useful in certain types of neurotic depression and phobic anxiety states, their use has remained controversial. This is partly due to their propensity to induce severe elevations in blood pressure when tyramine-containing foods such as cheese, pickled herrings, yeast extracts, and Chianti wine; phenylethylamine-containing foods such as chocolate; and broad beans, which are rich in dopa, are ingested. Adverse reactions also may occur when they are taken with over the counter remedies such as phenylpropanolamine.

In 1964 Knoll and colleagues synthesized a novel monoamine oxidase inhibitor, phenylisopropyl-N-methyl-propinylamine (deprenyl) with a substrate specificity for phenylethylamine and benzylamine (see Fig. 2). Promising uncontrolled studies in depression were reported from Hungary and the drug was claimed to have psychic energizing properties (Varga and Tringer, 1967). Subsequent controlled trials have produced conflicting results (Mendelewicz and Youdim, 1983; Mann and Gershon, 1980; Quitkin et al., 1984). In 1968 Johnston developed another MAOI, clorgyline (2:4 dichlorophenoxy propyl-N-methyl propinylamine), which, although structurally similar to deprenyl (see Fig. 2), had a completely different substrate specificity. The use of these two pharmacologic tools has led to the recognition of two types of MAO, type A and type B, which differ markedly in their relative concentrations from tissue to

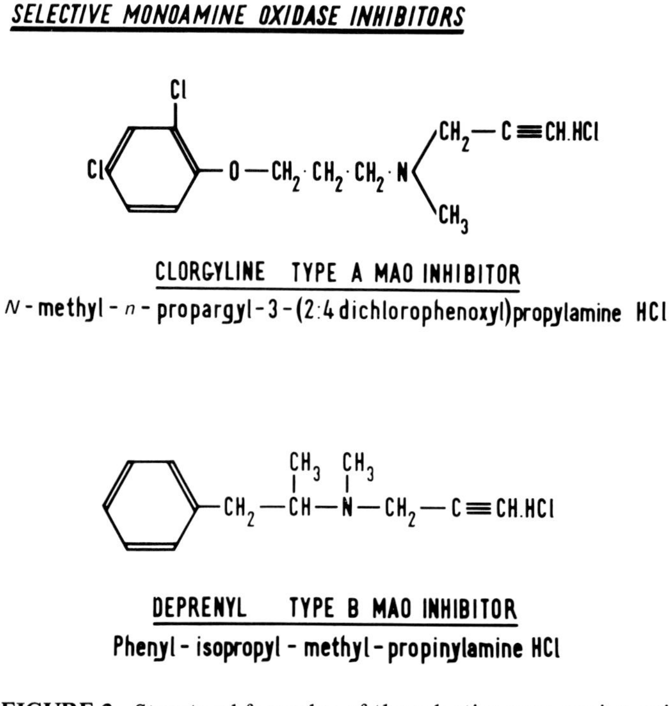

SELECTIVE MONOAMINE OXIDASE INHIBITORS

CLORGYLINE   TYPE A MAO INHIBITOR
N-methyl-*n*-propargyl-3-(2:4 dichlorophenoxyl)propylamine HCl

DEPRENYL   TYPE B MAO INHIBITOR
Phenyl-isopropyl-methyl-propinylamine HCl

FIGURE 2 Structural formulae of the selective monoamine oxidase inhibitors clorgyline and deprenyl.

tissue and species to species. It is now believed, for example, that most human brain MAO is type B and that much of it is localized within glial tissue. Brain MAO type A, on the other hand, is intraneuronal (Student and Edwards, 1977). The ratio of MAO-A/B varies considerably from one region of the human brain to another (e.g., pons B/A, 3.9:1; frontal cortex B/A, 0.9:1) (Oreland et al., 1983). Although dopamine was originally considered to be a substrate only for type B in human brain (Glover et al., 1977) it now seems likely that it may also be a substrate for type A (Tipton et al., 1983).

(-)DEPRENYL (SELEGILINE HYDROCHLORIDE)

Deprenyl has an extremely rapid therapeutic action, being metabolized by MAO-B to form a product that combines irreversibly with the center of the enzyme. It is catabolized almost quantitatively to (-)methylamphetamine and (-)amphetamine, which are excreted in the urine (Reynolds et al., 1978a). Amphetamine has also been demonstrated in postmortem brain tissue from deprenyl-treated parkinsonian patients (Reynolds et al., 1978b). In the 6-hydroxydopamine-lesioned turning rodent model deprenyl causes mild ipsilateral rotation when given alone, behaving like an amphetamine, but when administered with levodopa (L-dopa) it markedly enhances contraversive turning. It has also been shown to induce striking aphrodisiac effects in aging rodents (Knoll et al., 1983) and to increase the frequency of wakefulness and stage II sleep and decrease REM sleep and stages III and IV in healthy volunteers (Stern et al., 1978). Deprenyl has been shown to increase urinary (Rinne et al., 1978) and cerebrospinal fluid dopamine levels (Eisler et al., 1981). There are also changes in cerebrospinal fluid homovanillic acid levels (Rinne et al., 1978). Following the long-term administration of deprenyl, 70-90% inhibition of brain MAO is found when dopamine is used as the substrate whereas only 60-70% inhibition occurs with 5-hydroxytryptamine. This suggests that at dosages of 10 mg/day selectivity is preserved, whereas at much higher dosages (100 mg/day) selectivity appears to be lost (Riederer and Reynolds, 1980).

Deprenyl, at dosages of 10 mg/day is without "cheese effects." Oral loading tests have shown that it can be used safely in human volunteers and patients with Parkinson's disease without the need to restrict tyramine- or phenylethylamine-containing foods (Elsworth et al., 1978). Serial tyramine challenges given to four patients with Parkinson's disease who had taken deprenyl for 18 months also failed to produce any adverse pressor reactions with cumulative dosages of tyramine up to 250 mg. At higher dosages of deprenyl (40-60 mg/day) given for 3 weeks, although reduction in tolerance was seen in some individuals, all the patients could tolerate at least 150 mg tyramine (Stern et al., 1978). Sparing of intestinal MAO inhibition (Elsworth et al., 1978), inhibition of norepinephrine release, and inhibition of tyramine uptake may all be relevant factors in this absence of "cheese effect" (Knoll et al., 1978). Deprenyl also does not cause any significant rise in blood pressure when given with high dosages of levodopa either alone or in combination with a peripheral dopa decarboxylase inhibitor (Elsworth et al., 1978).

MONOAMINE OXIDASE INHIBITORS IN THE TREATMENT OF PARKINSON'S DISEASE

Carlsson et al. (1957) showed that pretreatment of reserpinized rodents with a monoamine oxidase inhibitor potentiated the anticataleptic action of dopa. Similar antiakinetic effects were then reported using iproniazid in the treatment of reserpine-induced parkinsonian (Degkwitz et al., 1960). This beneficial effect of monoamine oxidase inhibition was believed to be caused by prevention of the breakdown of dopamine within the central nervous system. The demonstration of dopamine deficiency in the corpus striatum of patients dying with Parkinson's disease then led to a series of trials in the early 1960s of monoamine oxidase inhibitors given either alone or with low dosages of L-dopa.

Birkmayer and Hornykiewicz (1962) gave isocarboxazid and a number of experimental monoamine oxidase inhibitors to patients with Parkinson's disease for 3–10 days before starting levodopa therapy. They reported a marked potentiation of the antibradykinetic effects of 50 mg intravenous L-dopa per week, but also commented on an increase in the frequency of side effects including nausea, vomiting, excessive sweating, and occasional collapse. These effects could be partly counteracted by caffeine or euphylline infused with the levodopa or by phentolamine 25 mg given intravenously 1 hr beforehand. Barbeau and colleagues (1962) gave tranylcypromine at a dosage of 30 mg/day to patients with Parkinson's disease and noted a modest beneficial effect on tremor after 2–3 days and a 40% reduction in the severity of rigidity after 1 month's treatment. Similar improvement was also noted in neuroleptic-induced parkinsonism.

In another study 27 patients were treated with 10–20 mg/day of isocarboxazid and another 18 were given experimental hydrazine MAOIs. About half the patients derived worthwhile benefit, which usually started to occur after about a week; those with mild disease improved the most. In this study tremor was the least responsive symptom and overall the authors considered that the benefits seen were less than those with low dosages of levodopa. Adverse side effects included toxic confusional states, irritability, postural tremor, insomnia, palpitations, and jaundice. Pretreatment of 20 patients with 2 weeks of isocarboxazid potentiated the antibradykinetic effects of 50 mg intravenous levodopa, but side effects including alarming rises in blood pressure were frequent (Gerstenbrand and Prosenz, 1985).

Although the early reports of MAOI/L-dopa therapy were promising it soon became clear that severe rises in blood pressure could occur even with the lowest dosages of L-dopa (Hunter et al., 1970) (see Fig. 3). Nonselective monoamine

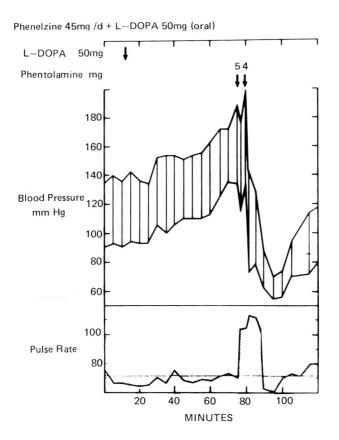

Phenelzine 45mg /d + L–DOPA 50mg (oral)

L–DOPA   50mg

Phentolamine mg

FIGURE 3   The pressor effect induced by 50 mg L-dopa given to a patient receiving phenelzine (a nonselective MAOI). (From Hunter et al., 1970.)

oxidase inhibitors had to be stopped for at least 14 days before levodopa treatment was introduced. Teychenne and colleagues (1975), however, were able to show that rises in blood pressure were appreciably less when levodopa was combined with a peripheral dopa decarboxylase inhibitor, suggesting that the pressor response was at least in part peripherally mediated. Levodopa/MAOI combinations have in fact been used with limited success in the treatment of parkinsonism with associated severe postural hypotension in an attempt to produce a controlled pressor response.

DEPRENYL (SELEGILINE) IN THE TREATMENT OF PARKINSON'S DISEASE SYMPTOMS

Deprenyl has a number of distinct pharmacologic actions that may facilitate dopamine modulation in the human brain and might therefore be beneficial in the control of Parkinson's disease symptoms (Knoll et al., 1978). It prevents the degradation of dopamine by selective monoamine oxidase B inhibition, it inhibits dopamine reuptake, and leads to the accumulation of amphetamine and the trace amine phenylethylamine, both of which may increase dopamine release from presynaptic terminals. There is also some evidence that monoamine oxidase inhibitors may increase the transport of dopa across the blood–brain barrier when central dopamine levels are depleted (Cotzias et al., 1974).

Birkmayer and colleagues (1975) first gave deprenyl to patients with Parkinson's disease and reported a potentiation of the antiparkinsonian effects of L-dopa when it was administered in combination with a peripheral dopa decarboxylase inhibitor. In further uncontrolled studies they also claimed that the drug might be useful in the treatment of end-of-dose deterioration (Birkmayer et al., 1977).

In a subsequent double-blind crossover trial, Lees and colleagues (1977) confirmed that the drug was useful in the management of mild L-dopa-induced motor oscillations and in the control of nocturnal and early morning disabilities. There was no improvement in patients with severe on–off disabilities (see Fig. 4) and no potentiation of antiparkinsonian effects in those individuals already receiving maximal tolerated dosages of L-dopa. No statistically significant improvement occurred in 15 patients who were rated as moderately or severely depressed on the Zung self-rating scale, although some patients described increased energy and well-being while receiving the drug. In dosages up to 15 mg daily deprenyl had no antiparkinson effects in five previously untreated patients. Adverse side effects included increased frequency of L-dopa-induced dyskinesias, nausea, dry mouth, dizziness, and psychotoxicity, but generally medication was easy to administer and relatively free from severe side effects at a dosage of 10 mg daily.

In further long-term studies these results were generally confirmed although only about half the patients derived initial benefit from wearing off and in even fewer was this sustained for longer than a year (Stern et al., 1978, 1983). These results were confirmed by a number of different groups (Yahr, 1978; Rinne et al., 1978; Csanda et al., 1978; Schachter et al., 1980).

Much more disappointing results, however, were reported by Eisler and colleagues (1981) on 11 carefully studied patients. The four patients who did derive benefit from 10 mg deprenyl appeared to do so as a result of coexisting euphoria. On this basis it was suggested that a nonselective antidepressant effect might be

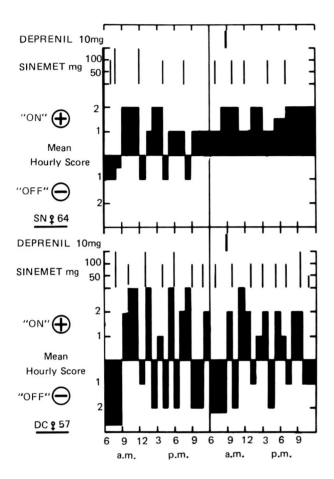

FIGURE 4 Beneficial effect of (−) deprenyl on mild oscillations in performance and its ineffectiveness in the on–off phenomenon. (From Lees et al., 1977.)

the explanation for the drug's antiparkinson effects. In support of this, the same group published biochemical results showing that deprenyl increased the excretion of phenylethylamine and tyramine, reduced the output of norepinephrine catabolites in the urine, but failed to alter the excretion of dopamine-deaminated metabolites. They attributed these alterations more to the conversion of deprenyl to amphetamine and methamphetamine than to inhibition of monoamine oxidase type B (Karoum et al., 1982).

To try to clarify the issue we conducted two separate double-blind studies. The urinary excretion of methamphetamine and amphetamine is pH dependent and the first approach was to modify the excretion rate following deprenyl administration. A more direct strategy was also used in which methamphetamine and amphetamine were substituted for deprenyl in the approximate dosage and proportion in which they appear in the urine after drug ingestion. The manipulation of urinary pH resulted in no detectable clinical change despite marked alterations in excretion rate of methamphetamine and amphetamine with a highly significant correlation with urinary pH. In the amphetamine substitution trial two patients suffered marked deterioration when placebo or methamphetamine/ amphetamine combinations were administered in place of deprenyl. No real change was seen in the other two patients completing the protocol (Reynolds et al., 1978a). It is reasonable to conclude that the beneficial effects of deprenyl in Parkinson's disease patients do not depend on the pharmacologic properties of its amphetamine metabolites. Some specific mood-elevating effects may still be important, however, in the therapeutic response. In current practice the most widely accepted indication for deprenyl would be in patients optimally controlled on L-dopa therapy who are developing wearing off effects when 5–10 mg a day may temporarily smooth over swings for periods up to 2 years.

MONOAMINE OXIDASE INHIBITION AND MPTP TOXICITY

1-Methyl-4-phenyl-1,2,3,6-tetrahydropyridine (MPTP), the "designer drug" used by California addicts can cause an irreversible parkinsonism and, when administered to monkeys, a behavioral syndrome closely resembling the human disease. Behavioral abnormalities may also be seen in the dog, rodents (particularly mice) and frog, but these animals seem to be less sensitive to the toxic effects than primates. The addicts who have developed MPTP-induced parkinsonism are exquisitely sensitive to dopaminergic agonists and, like postencephalitic parkinsonian patients, develop dyskinesias and motor oscillations early in the course of treatment. Pathologically the zona compacta of the substantia nigra takes the brunt of the damage with marked cell loss. In animals, at least, evidence for involvement of other catecholaminergic cell groups is accumulating, especially in old monkeys, and a few intraneuronal eosinophilic inclusion bodies have been seen. In contrast to Lewy body Parkinson's disease, however, the nucleus basalis of Meynert appears to be spared (Langston, 1985). The paucity of supportive evidence for major genetic factors in Parkinson's disease taken along with this alarming clinical observation has led Calne and Langston (1983) to propose that idiopathic Parkinson's disease might occur as a result of subliminal exposure to exogenous toxins in childhood or young adult life combined with the inexorable loss of the susceptible dopamine neuron that occurs with normal aging.

If this proposition proves true the mechanism underlying the toxicity of MPTP becomes of crucial importance. It has now been shown that MPTP is rapidly converted to its quaternary amine, a charged compound known as MPP+, and that this transformation occurs in all areas of the body except the eye. It is probable that when this conversion occurs in the central nervous system MPP+ is trapped intraneuronally. It has also been shown that when oxidation to MPP+ is prevented and the double bond is removed in the pyridine ring of MPTP the resultant compound is nontoxic, suggesting that conversion of MPP+ is vital for the observed toxic effects (Langston et al., 1984). Chiba and colleagues (1984) showed that monoamine oxidase in brain mitochondria converts MPTP to MPP+. It was then shown that [^{3}H] pargyline, an inhibitor of monoamine oxidase and [^{3}H] MPTP had a similar distribution of binding sites in the brain, suggesting that the "MPTP receptor" is actually the enzyme monoamine oxidase (Reznikoff et al., 1985). Pretreatment with type B MAO inhibitors abolished the behavioral effects of MPTP in both the mouse and monkey (Markey et al., 1984; Langston et al., 1984; Heikkila et al., 1984), and despite its improbable structural formula MPTP seems to act as a type B substrate for monoamine oxidase. Pargyline, a type B MAO inhibitor, has been shown to block the effect of MPTP on embryonic nigral neurons.

It is now known that MPTP is converted to MPP+ through an intermediate compound 1-methyl-4-phenyl-2,3-dihydropyridinium (MPDP+) (see Fig. 5) and it is also now known that MAO-B is involved in the first step of this two-step process. It remains possible therefore that MPDP+ rather than MPP is the toxin. It has now been demonstrated by [^{3}H] MPTP binding autoradiography (Javitch et al., 1984) and immunohistochemistry that MAO-B has discrete localization within the brain. In the rat at least it seems that the only neuronal cells that contain this enzyme are the serotonergic neurons in the raphé nucleus in the

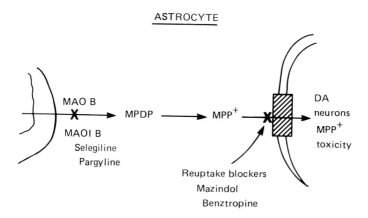

ASTROCYTE

FIGURE 5   Schematic diagram shows the mechanism underlying MPTP toxicity.

brain stem and that in other parts of the brain the enzyme is found in glial tissue and serotonergic terminals. On entering the brain MPTP binds selectively to MAO type B and is then transformed to MPDP, which can diffuse out and convert extracellularly to MPP+. Nigral cells, dopamine terminals, and norepinephrine terminals then accumulate MPP+ via an active catecholamine uptake system where it is then bound to neuromelanin within the neurons and gradually released, maintaining a toxic intracellular concentration. Therefore, dopamine uptake blockers such as benztropine and mazindol will also protect against MPTP toxicity (Ricaurte et al., 1985). It is probable that the handling of MPP+ in primates, where it disappears very slowly from the striatum, compared with the rapid disappearance in mouse, may explain the relative differences in cell damage between the two species, and this in turn may be related to MPP+ storage in neuromelanin.

The mechanism underlying MPP+ toxicity remains unknown but one possible explanation is the build up of toxic free radicals within the pigmented neurons. It is believed that other dopaminergic toxins such as 6-hydroxydopamine and manganese may lead to rapid oxidation in neurons, swamping the natural scavenging mechanisms, and MPP+ may be working along similar lines. If oxygen is built up within a cell it may induce direct toxic effects and also interreact with metal ions to increase hydroxyl (OH-) production. Acceptance of a single electron by the oxygen molecule forms the superoxide radical (O_2-) (see Fig. 6), which is a highly toxic species formed in vivo by the activity of mitochondrial and microsomal electron transport chains. The metal-ion-dependent oxidations of catecholamines also produce superoxide. When produced in small amounts this toxic radical is specifically scavenged by a superoxide dismutase enzyme system. Hydrogen peroxide (H_2O_2), although inert, crosses cell membranes and it decomposes to the highly noxious hydroxyl radical when it comes into contact with reduced forms of iron or copper (see Fig. 6). Two enzymes, catalase and glutathione peroxidase, are present in human tissue and destroy hydrogen peroxide thereby reducing the possibility of hydroxyl radical formation.

The brain, however, contains relatively little catalase but it is of interest that the small quantities present are concentrated in the substantia nigra and hypothalamus. Both superoxide and hydroxyl radicals attack the fatty acid side chains of membrane lipids causing lipid peroxidation in which polyunsaturated fatty acid side chains are converted into lipid peroxides. In the presence of metal complexes these compounds are broken down into reactive radicals that continue the chain reaction, leading to gradual loss of membrane fluidity and membrane potential with final loss of membrane integrity. This leads to inactivation of membrane-bound enzymes and receptors. Both lipofuscin and neuromelanin are end products of the oxidative degradation of lipids. Free radicals may also fragment DNA and react with proteins and carbohydrates. Increased

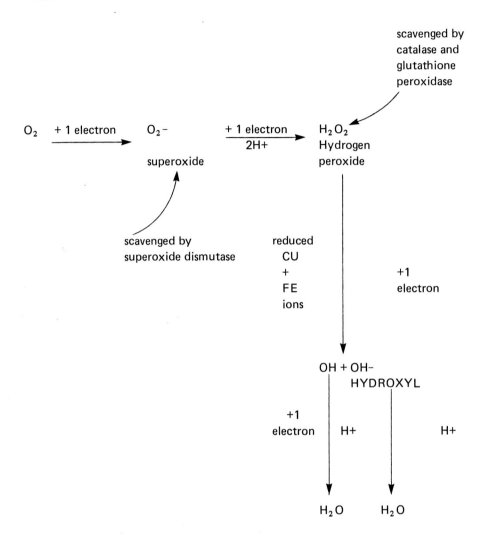

FIGURE 6 The four-step reduction of oxygen in dopaminergic neurons.

auto-oxidation or destruction of scavenging enzymes might therefore underlie the toxic effects of MPP+ once it has been concentrated in catecholamine neuronal uptake systems. The relationship of monoamine oxidase and MPTP has neurobiologic significance beyond MPTP toxicity: it suggests that oxidation of tetrahydropyridine rings may be an additional physiologic role for the enzyme. Pyridines are abundant in the environment and indeed MPP+ itself was field-tested as a herbicide. 4-Phenyl pyridine is a constituent of peppermint and spearmint tea and has been shown to deplete tyrosine hydroxylase in cell culture systems. The other possibility to explain MPP+ toxicity for which there is increasing biochemical and histological evidence is that the compound interferes directly with cytochrome systems disrupting intracellular energy mechanisms.

COULD TYPE B MONOAMINE OXIDASE INHIBITION IMPROVE THE NATURAL HISTORY OF PARKINSON'S DISEASE?

If one believes that an MPTP-like exogenous or endogenous toxin may be implicated in the genesis of Parkinson's disease, early treatment with a selective type B monoamine oxidase inhibitor would be logical. It is also probable that at least 5% of the normal population over the age of 60 have cryptic Parkinson's disease as judged by the presence of Lewy body disease at postmortem. If a way of picking out these individuals could be found in life, they too might be candidates for monoamine oxidase inhibitor treatment. Bradbury and colleagues (1985), however, have shown that the toxic effects of MPP+ injected intrastriatally into mice are actually enhanced by pretreatment with deprenyl whereas Mytilineou and Cohen (1985) demonstrated protection against the pyridinium ion by deprenyl in cell culture. These discrepancies need to be resolved but raise the possibility that pyridinium ion toxicity might actually be enhanced by deprenyl treatment. My own anecdotal experience using deprenyl in Parkinson's disease over the last 8 years would not indicate any dramatic effects on the natural history of the illness. Furthermore, benztropine and amantadine, two dopamine uptake inhibitors that prevent MPTP toxicity, also do not seem to have altered the course of Parkinson's disease in the past.

Birkmayer (1983) however, has suggested that deprenyl may prevent or retard the degeneration of striatal dopaminergic neurons and prolong the effect and duration of benefit from levodopa treatment. In an open, uncontrolled retrospective survey 377 patients treated with L-dopa in combination with benserazide alone were compared with 564 patients treated with L-dopa, benserazide, and deprenyl and followed up for periods up to 9 years (average length of deprenyl therapy 3.92 years). In 81 of these patients deprenyl was started at the same time as levodopa, but in the remainder it was added later with an increase in benefit occurring in the majority. The mean age at onset of therapy was 70 years in the levodopa-treated group and 67 years in the levodopa/deprenyl group. The pretreatment duration of disease was slightly longer in the levodopa/deprenyl group (3.9 years compared with 2.7 years) and the dosage of levodopa was also somewhat larger (627 mg compared with 524 mg). This latter observation may have been due to the Madopar/deprenyl group being more severely disabled and requiring higher dosages. The estimated survival times calculated from survival distribution curves gave a figure of 129.2 months for the levodopa and 144.5 months for the levodopa/deprenyl group. The authors concluded that there was a significant increase in survival regardless of whether demographic differences were taken into consideration, but the estimates were based on time from start of treatment to death, not from the time of diagnosis. To clarify this important issue further multicenter prospective studies are under way in both the United Kingdom, where L-dopa in combination with a peripheral dopa decarboxylase inhibitor is being compared with levodopa combined with deprenyl in patients of differing disease severity, and in the United States, where deprenyl will be compared against placebo and a nonspecific antioxidant, vitamin E, in mild untreated cases.

REFERENCES

Barbeau A, Sourkes TL, Murphy GF. (1962). Les catecholamines dans la maladie de Parkinson. In: Ajuriaguerra J (Ed.), *Monoamines et Système Nerveux Central*. Bal-Air Symposium, Genève. Paris, Masson.

Barbeau A, Dallaire L, Bull NT, Veilleux F, Poirier J. (1985). Comparative, behavioural, biochemical and pigmentary effects of MPTP, MPP+ and paraquat in rana pipiens. *Life Sci* 37: 1529–1538.

Bernheimer H, Birkmayer W, Hornykiewicz O. (1962). Verhalten der monoaminoxydase im gehirn des menschen nach therapie mit monoaminoxydase hemmern. *Wien Klin Wochenschr* 74: 558–559.

Birkmayer W. (1983). Deprenyl leads to prolongation of L-dopa efficacy in Parkinson's disease. *Mod Probl Pharmacopsychiatry* 19: 170–176.

Birkmayer W, Hornykiewicz O. (1962). Der L-3,4-dioxyphenylalanin (=DOPA) effekt beim Parkinson syndrom des menschen. *Arch Psychiatr Nervenkr* 203: 560–574.

Birkmayer W, Riederer P. (1980). In: *Parkinson's Disease Biochemistry, Clinical Pathology and Treatment*. Vienna, Springer.

Birkmayer W, Riederer P, Youdim MBH, Linauer W. (1975). The potentiation of the anti-akinetic effect after L-dopa treatment by an inhibitor of MAO-B, Deprenil. *J Neural Trans* 36: 303–326.

Birkmayer W, Riederer P, Ambrozi L, Youdim MBH. (1977). Implications of combined treatment with Madopar and L-deprenyl in Parkinson's disease. *Lancet* 1: 439–443.

Blaschko H, Richter D, Schlossmann H. (1937). The inactivation of adrenaline. *J Physiol* 90: 1–19.

Bradbury AJ, Costall B, Jenner PG, Kelly ME, Marsden CD, Naylor AJ. (1985). The neurotoxic actions of 1-methyl-4-phenylpyridine (MPP+) are not prevented by deprenyl treatment. *Neurosci Lett* 58: 177–182.

Burns RS, Chiueh CC, Markey SP, Ebert MH, Jacobowitz DM, Kopin JJ. (1983). A primate model of parkinsonism: selective destruction of dopaminergic neurons in the pars compacta of the substantia nigra by N-methyl-4-phenyl-1,2,3,6-tetrahydropyridine. *Proc Nat Acad Sci* 80: 4546–4550.

Calne DB, Langston JW. (1983). Aetiology of Parkinson's disease. *Lancet* 2: 1457–1459.

Carlsson A, Lindqvist M, Magnusson T. (1957). 3:4 Dihydroxyphenylalanine, 5-hydrotryptophan as reserpine agonists. *Nature* 180: 1200.

Chiba K, Trevor A, Castagnoli N. (1984). Metabolism of the neurotoxic tertiary amine MPTP by brain monoamine oxidases. *Biochem Biophys Res Commun* 120: 574-578.

Cotzias GC, Tang LC, Ginos JZ. (1974). Monoamine oxidase and cerebral uptake of dopaminergic drugs. *Proc Nat Acad Sci* 71: 2718-2719.

Crane GE. (1956). Psychiatric side-effects of iproniazid. *Am J Psychiatry* 112: 494.

Csanda E, Antal J, Antony M, Csanaky A. (1978). Experiences with L-deprenyl in parkinsonism. *J Neural Transm* 43: 263-269.

Degkwitz R, Frowein R, Kulenkampff C, Mohs U. (1960). Uber die wirkungen des L-dopa beim menschen und ihre. beeinflussung durch reserpin, chlorpormazin, iproniziad unde vitamin B6. *Klin Woschenschr* 38: 120-123.

Eisler T, Teravainen H, Nelson R, Krebs H, Weise V, Lake CR, Ebert MH, Whetzel N, Murphy DL, Kopin IJ, Calne DB. (1981). Deprenyl in Parkinson's disease. *Neurology* 31: 19-23.

Elsworth JD, Glover V, Reynolds GP, Sandler M, Lees AJ, Phuapradit P, Shaw KM, Stern GM, Kumar P. (1978). Deprenyl administration in man: a selective monoamine oxidase B inhibitor without the "cheese effect." *Psychopharmacology* 57: 33-38.

Gerstenbrand F, Prosenz P. (1965). Uber die behandlung des Parkinson syndroms mit monoamineoxidasehemmern allein und in kombination mit L-dopa. *Praxis* 54: 1373-1377.

Glover V, Sandler M, Owen F, Riley GJ. (1977). Dopamine is a monoamine oxidase B substrate in man. *Nature* 265: 80-81.

Hare MLC. (1928). Tyramine oxidase 1. A new enzyme system in liver. *Biochem* 22: 968-979.

Heikkila RE, Manzino L, Cabbat FS, Duvoisin RC. (1984). Protection against the dopaminergic neurotoxicity of 1-methyl-4-phenyl-1,2,3,6, tetrahydropyridine by monoamine oxidase inhibitors. *Nature* 311: 467-469.

Hunter KR, Boakes AJ, Laurence DR, Stern GM. (1970). Monoamine oxidase inhibitors and L-dopa. *Br Med J* 3: 388.

Javitch JA, Uhl GR, Snyder SH. (1984). Parkinsonism-induced neurotoxin, N-methyl-4-phenyl-1,2,3,6 tetrahydropyridine: characterisation and localisation of receptor binding sites in rat and human brain. *Proc Nat Acad Sci* 81: 4591-4595.

Markey SP, Johannsson JN, Chiuens CC, Burns RS, Herkenham MA. (1984). Intracranial generation of a pyridinium metabolite may cause drug-induced parkinsonism. *Nature* 31: 464-467.

Mendlewicz J, Youdim MBH. (1983). L-deprenyl monoamine oxidase type B inhibitor in the treatment of depression. A double blind evaluation. *Br J Psychiatry* 142: 508-511.

Mytilineou C, Cohen G. (1985). Deprenyl protects dopamine neurones from the neurotoxic effect of 1-methyl-4-phenylpyridinium ion. *J Neurochem* 45: 1951-1953.

Nies A, Robinson DS, Davis JM, Ravaris CL. (1973). Changes in monoamine oxidase with aging. In: Eisdorfer, Fann (Eds.), *Psychopharmacology and Aging*. New York, Plenum Press.

Oreland L, Arai Y, Stenstrom A, Fowler CJ. (1983). Monoamine oxidase activity and localisation in the brain and the activity in relation to psychiatric disorders. *Mod Probl Pharmacopsychiatry* 19: 246–254.

Pugh CEM, Quastel JH. (1937). Oxidation of aliphatic amines by brain and other tissues. *Biochem J* 31: 286–291.

Quitkin F, Liebowitz MR, Stewart JW, McGrath PJ, Harrison W, Rabkin JG, Markowitz J, Davies SO. (1984). L-deprenyl in atypical depressives. *Arch Gen Psychiatry* 777–781.

Reynolds GP, Elsworth JD, Blau K, Sandler M, Lees AJ, Stern GM. (1978a). Deprenyl is metabolised to methamphetamine and amphetamine in man. *Br J Clin Pharmacol* 6: 542–544.

Reynolds GP, Riederer P, Sandler M, Jellinger K, Seemann D. (1978b). Amphetamine and 2-phenylethylamine in postmortem Parkinsonian brain after (−)deprenyl administration. *J Neural Transm* 43: 271–277.

Reznikoff G, Manaker S, Parson B, Rhodes CH, Rainbow TC. (1985). Similar distribution of monoamine oxidase (MAO) and Parkinsonian toxin (MPTP) binding sites in human brain. *Neurology* 35: 1415–1419.

Ricaurte GA, Langston JW, Delanney LE, Irwin I, Brooks JD. (1985). Dopamine uptake blockers protect against the dopamine depleting effects of MPTP in the mouse striatum. *Neurosci Lett* 59: 259–264.

Riederer P, Reynolds GP. (1980). Deprenyl is a selective inhibitor of brain MAO-B in the long-term treatment of Parkinson's disease. *Br J Clin Pharmacol* 9: 98–99.

Rinne UK, Siirtola T, Sonninen V. (1978). L-deprenyl treatment of on–off phenomena in Parkinson's disease. *J Neural Transm* 43: 253–262.

Schachter M, Marsden CD, Parkes JD, Jenner P, Testa B. (1980). Deprenyl in the managment of response fluctuations in patients with Parkinson's disease on levodopa. *J Neurol Neurosurg Psychiatry* 43: 1016–1021.

Schmiedeberg O. (1877). Uber das verhaltnis des ammoniaks und der primaren monoaminbasen zur harnstoffbildung im theirkorper. *Naunyn-Schmiedebergs Arch Pharmacol* 8: 1–14.

Stern GM, Lees AJ, Sandler M. (1978). Recent observations on the clinical pharmacology of (−)deprenyl. *J Neural Transm* 43: 245–251.

Stern GM, Lees AJ, Hardie R, Sandler M. (1983). Clinical and pharmacological aspects of deprenyl treatment in Parkinson's disease. *Mod Probl Pharmacopsychiatry* 19: 215–219.

Student AK, Edwards DJ. (1977). Subcellular localisation of Types A and B monoamine oxidase in rat brain. *Biochem Pharmacol* 26: 2337–2342.

Teychenne PF, Calne DB, Lewis PJ, Findley LJ. (1975). Interactions of levodopa with inhibitors of monoamine oxidase and L-aromatic aminoacid decarboxylase. *Clin Pharmacol Ther* 18: 273–277.

Tipton KF, O'Carroll A-M, Mantle TJ, Fowler CJ. (1983). Factors involved in the selective inhibition of monoamine oxidase. *Mod Probl Pharmacopsychiatry* 19: 15-30.

Varga E, Tringer L. (1967). Clinical trial of a new type of promptly acting psychonergetic agent (phenyl-isopropyl-methyl-propinylamine Hci (E250)). *Acta Med Acad Sci Hung* 23: 289-295.

Yahr MD. (1978). Overview of present day treatment of Parkinson's disease. *J Neural Transm* 43: 273-278.

Zeller EA. (1938). Uber den enzymatischen abbau von histamin und diaminen. *Helv Chim Acta* 21: 881-890.

Zeller EA, Barsky J, Berman ER. (1955). Amine oxidase XI. Inhibition of monoamine oxidase by 1-isonicotinyl-2-isopropylhydrazine. *J Biol Chem* 214: 267-274.

23
Stereotactic Surgery

GEORGE SELBY
Royal North Shore Hospital, Sydney, New South Wales, Australia

HISTORY

Surgical attempts to relieve some of the symptoms of paralysis agitans began about 50 years ago. The first operations were based on the observation that tremor was arrested by a hemiparesis due to a cerebral vascular accident and on the erroneous assumption that the corticospinal tract conducted impulses essential for the production of tremor. Suppressor strips in the prefrontal cortex, since disproven, were also implicated in the pathophysiology of tremor.

The cortical motor area (Bucy and Case, 1939) and later the premotor cortex (Klemme, 1940) were excised, and the corticospinal tract was interrupted at the base of the cerebral peduncles (Walker, 1952) or in the cervical part of the spinal cord (Putnam, 1938; Oliver, 1953). These operations achieved control of tremor at the expense of a hemiparesis, but they had no effect on rigidity.

Surgical efforts were then directed at the basal ganglia and Russell Meyers extirpated the head of the caudate nucleus and the anterior third of the globus pallidus, and, a little later, sectioned pallidofugal fibers using a transventricular approach (Meyers, 1940, 1942). French neurosurgeons destroyed the medial pallidum and ansa lenticularis by electrocoagulation through a subfrontal and temporal craniotomy (Guiot and Brion, 1952). Stereotactic brain surgery, a technique that directs an instrument at a target within the cranial cavity with the aid of mathematical coordinates, was first used in the treatment of parkinsonian patients by Spiegel and Wycis in 1946 (Spiegel et al., 1946). They achieved relief from rigidity and tremor by electrolytic lesions confined to the globus pallidus and ansa lenticularis (Spiegel and Wycis, 1954). The successful results of stereotactic surgery aroused widespread interest throughout the world and many types of apparatus and operative methods were described between 1946 and 1965. Early pioneers in stereotactic brain surgery were Leksell (1949) in Sweden, Riechert and Wolff (1951) in Germany, Narabayashi and Okuma (1953) in Japan, Guiot (1958) in France, and Gillingham et al. (1960) in Scotland. Cooper (1954), who had previously discovered that ligation of the anterior choroidal artery, which supplies the medial globus pallidus and ansa lenticularis, achieves reduction of both tremor and rigidity, later created lesions in the basal ganglia by injecting alcohol or a mixture of alcohol and cellulose. The operation, called chemopallidectomy, did not rely strictly on stereotactic techniques, but the correct placement of the cannula was checked by injecting procaine or by inflating a small balloon at the tip of the cannula, thereby producing reversible effects.

In the first 5 years of basal ganglia surgery the medial globus pallidus and ansa lenticularis were the preferred targets, but then Hassler and Riechert (1954) selected the lateral ventral nucleus of the thalamus and this and its surrounding area are still the universally favored sites of the surgical lesion. While pallidotomy relieved rigidity, it had no lasting effect on tremor. The destruction of the posterior part of the ventrolateral nucleus of the thalamus (VIM or VOP of Hassler) has the best results on tremor, while destruction of the anterior segment of this nucleus (VOA of Hassler) has more effect on rigidity. Some surgeons prefer to place the lesion in the subthalamic area of the zona incerta and include the fields H1 and H2 of Forel (Mundinger, 1965).

Using chemopallidectomy, Cooper (1954) produced the lesion by injecting alcohol and cellulose. The direction and extent of flow of alcohol could not be accurately controlled and he improved his method by freezing the intended target area to −40 to −60°C using liquid nitrogen delivered through a vacuum-insulated cannula. This cryogenic surgery has now been largely replaced by controlled heat using high-frequency electrocoagulation. Sophisticated instruments to create a well-defined lesion of predetermined size are now available and provide for control of temperature, voltage, current intensity, and tissue resistance during coagulation. Other more complex methods of producing the lesion, such as implantation of radioisotopes, focused ultrasonic irradiation, and crossed proton beams directed at the target area have been abandoned for technical and economic reasons.

Autopsy correlation showed that the lesions produced by surgeons were not always at the intended target site and the correct placement of the tip of the electrode is now always confirmed either by observing the motor effects of electrical stimulation (Hassler et al., 1960; Mundinger and Riechert, 1963; Selby, 1967b), or by microelectrode recording from different thalamic subnuclei

(Albe-Fessard et al., 1961; Gillingham, 1966; Narabayashi, 1986). During the past 15 years instruments for stereotactic operations have been improved and computers are now used to assist in guiding the electrode toward the target. There are also significant advances in the apparatus used for neurophysiologic confirmation of the correct placement of the tip of the electrode at the target point and in applying the precise amount of heat for electrocoagulation, so that the lesion produced will be of the desired size.

METHOD

The target area—lateral ventral nucleus of thalamus or subthalamic zona incerta and fields H1 and H2 of Forel—is determined from a metrizamide ventriculogram with the aid of brain atlases for stereotaxis (Spiegel and Wycis, 1952; Schaltenbrand and Bailey, 1959). The place of the lateral ventral nucleus (Fig. 1), for example, can be calculated from reference points such as the anterior and posterior commissures and the septum pellucidum (interventricular septum) on the ventriculogram. The problem of directing the electrode at a small area within the irregular shape of the human skull is overcome by the base ring of the stereotactic instrument, which converts the skull into a regular sphere. The base ring is the equator of this sphere from which three coordinates—horizontal, sagittal, and coronal—can be established. The distance of the intended site of the surgical lesion from these coordinates is applied to the base ring of the instrument after corrections for distortion on the x-rays are made. An arc with an electrode holder that can be moved in various directions (Fig. 2) is next fixed onto the base ring. The exact direction, angle, and depth of the electrode used to be calculated with the aid of a "phantom" base ring that is not applied to the patient's skull, but can now be more speedily and accurately determined with a computer and "simulator."

After the electrode, which has a noninsulated tip, has been inserted through a burr hole in the skull, further x-rays are taken to show its position. The correct placement of the electrode is confirmed by electrical stimulation or by microelectrode recording from the cells of the lateral ventral nucleus or subthalamic area. After correct placement of the electrode has been established, the surgical lesion is made by radiofrequency thermocoagulation at a temperature of 70°C.

The operative procedure described above is that introduced by Riechert in Freiburg, West Germany, and later improved by Mundinger. Various stereotactic instruments and methods are employed in different parts of the world and most now achieve the aim of precise placement and size of the stereotactic lesion. It is thought that a correctly placed lesion 3-5 mm in diameter is sufficient to abolish tremor and rigidity.

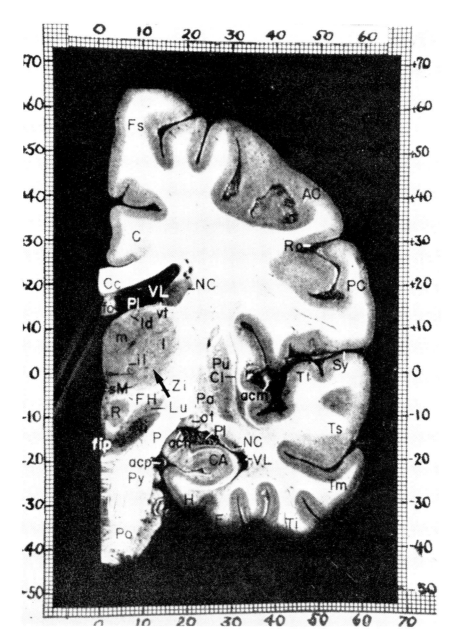

FIGURE 1 Coronal macroscopic section of the human brain at a level 15 mm anterior to the pineal gland. The arrow points to the basal part of the lateral ventral nucleus of the thalamus. (From Spiegel and Wycis, 1952.)

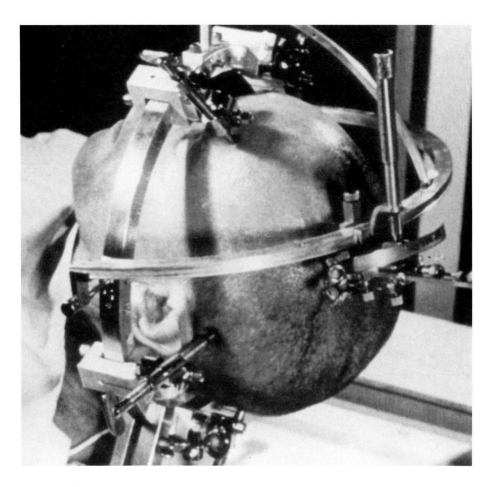

FIGURE 2 The stereotactic instrument of Riechert and Mundinger (1955). (From Selby, 1968.)

THERMOCOAGULATIVE LESION

Figures 3 and 4 illustrate the appearance of the thermocoagulative lesion at different intervals of time after the operation. Figure 3 is a coronal section of the brain of a woman, aged 69 years, who died 12 weeks after the operation from a coronary artery occlusion. The operation was uncomplicated and succeeded in relieving both rigidity and tremor of her left limbs. Figure 4 shows a coronal section of the brain of a man, aged 58 years, who died from malignant metastases 9 months after the operation, which had completely abolished both

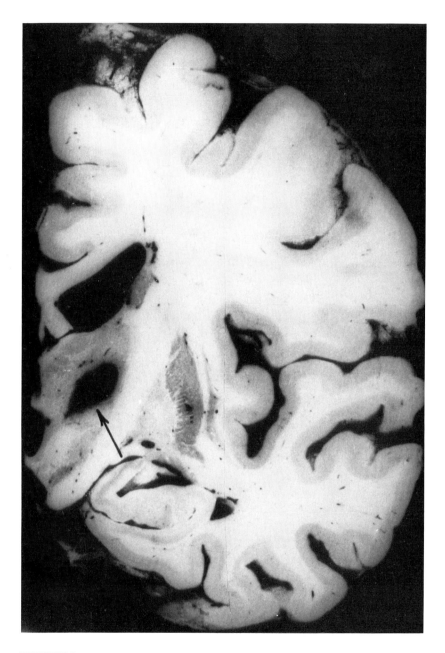

FIGURE 3   Coronal section showing electrocoagulative lesion in lateral ventral nucleus of thalamus 12 weeks after operation. (From Selby, 1967b.)

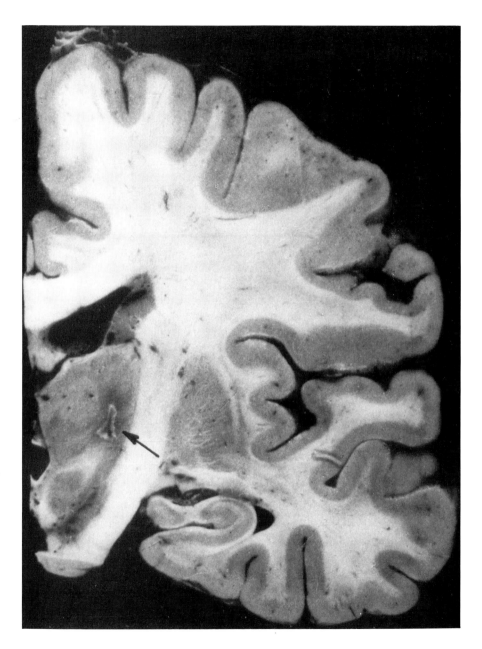

FIGURE 4 Coronal section showing electrocoagulative lesion in lateral ventral nucleus of thalamus 9 months after operation. (From Selby, 1967b.)

rigidity and tremor of his left limbs. The surgical lesion in the lateral ventral nucleus of the right thalamus was $2 \times 3 \times 3$ mm.

In the earlier days of stereotactic surgery, an autopsy study (Smith, 1967) revealed that the lesion was often not at the site the surgeon had intended. Smith (1967) showed that relief from tremor and rigidity had also been achieved by small lesions in the globus pallidus, in the anterior part of the posterior limb of the internal capsule, and in the field of Forel. This permits one to assume that destruction of fibers of the dentatorubrothalamic and pallidothalamic pathways, or of the nuclei associated with these fiber systems, which occupy a considerable part of the region of the basal ganglia, are essential for relief from tremor and rigidity. Mundinger and Meyer-Tuwe (1978) place their lesion in the subthalamic region including the field of Forel, while Narabayashi (1986) favors the ventralis intermedius part of the lateral ventral nucleus for the relief of tremor and the ventralis oralis anterior part of this nucleus for control of rigidity.

INDICATIONS

During the years 1952–1969 before treatment with levodopa (L-dopa) became available, various methods of stereotactic surgery had rapidly gained favor throughout the world. Before 1960 more than 5000 patients had been subjected to basal ganglia surgery and by 1969 this number had increased to at least 10,000 patients. It was then recognized that a correctly placed surgical lesion in the lateral ventral nucleus of the thalamus or in the subthalamic region could abolish tremor and rigidity of the limbs of the side opposite to it in over 80% of patients (Selby, 1967a) and that some improvement of manual dexterity and of gait disorders was observed in about 70% of patients. This beneficial effect on dexterity and gait was reasonably attributed to relief from rigidity and both akinesia and disorders of gait and equilibrium were found to progress in time even though tremor and rigidity did not recur. It is now recognized that over 50% of patients have no tremor and very little rigidity 20–25 years after successful surgery to the basal ganglia (Selby, 1984), while bradykinesia, disturbances of speech, dementia, and particularly problems in equilibrium and gait have shown the inevitable progression, despite continued treatment with L-dopa and a decarboxylase inhibitor or with bromocriptine or another dopa receptor site agonist (Kelly and Gillingham, 1980).

About 61% of parkinsonian patients treated with a dopa-containing preparation (Sinemet or Madopar) for 5 years or longer develop dopa-induced involuntary movements. These involve the head, lips, neck, and limbs and in a proportion of cases they are painful due to cramps or involuntary flexion and extension of the toes. The majority of patients prefer these dyskinetic movements to their parkinsonian disabilities and therefore refuse to reduce the dosage of L-dopa. A stereotactic thalamotomy can either abolish or greatly diminish the dyskinetic movements or abnormal dystonic postures of the limbs. It has, however, no influence on the occurrence of end-of-dose deterioration or on the "on-off" phenomenon.

In a study of 148 parkinsonian patients who had taken L-dopa for 2–5 years, prior stereotactic thalamotomies had been performed on 67 patients and 17 of those had bilateral operations. Although the deterioration in the degree of hypokinesia after 3–5 years of treatment with L-dopa involved a slightly lower proportion of patients who had a previous operation, the difference did not reach statistical significance. The study showed clearly that rigidity and tremor on the operated side did not recur and that dopa-induced dyskinetic movements were abolished or markedly reduced. On the other hand, dysarthria, akinesia, the various disorders of gait and equilibrium, the occurrence of temporary psychotic reactions, or the development of end-of-dose failure or the on–off phenomenon were not influenced by previous surgery (Selby, 1976).

Mundinger and Meyer-Tuwe (1978) succeeded in abolishing the rigidity of 93.2% of 260 extremities by a stereotactic lesion placed in the zona incerta and basis of the nucleus ventralis oralis and regard the surgical treatment of rigidity and of tremor as superior to the treatment with an L-dopa-containing preparation.

With the advent of pharmacologic treatment by a preparation containing L-dopa, or by dopa receptor site agonists such as bromocriptine, the use of surgery in the treatment of Parkinson's disease symptoms has declined to a dramatic extent. Whereas some 1,185 pallidotomies and thalamotomies were performed between 1952 to 1965 by Mundinger, Hassler, and Riechert in Freiburg, West Germany, they performed subthalamotomies on about 180 patients per year in 1977 (Mundinger and Meyer-Tuwe, 1978). Narabayashi in Tokyo did about 30–50 operations per year between 1977 and 1982 (Narabayashi, 1986) while Grant and Selby did no more than 10–15 stereotactic thalamotomies annually in the past 10 years. It should, however, be pointed out that the number of units performing surgery on Parkinson's disease patients has declined to less than 25% of such units in the world since about 1962.

The current indications for a stereotactic thalamotomy or subthalamotomy are:

1. Severe tremor or rigidity, not controlled by an L-dopa containing preparation or receptor site agonist or anticholinergic drug, or if pharmacologic treatment is not tolerated or produces unacceptable side effects. Surgical treatment is particularly indicated in the younger patient and in those with unilateral tremor and rigidity. A unilateral operation, however, does not protect the patient from the later development of tremor and rigidity on the unoperated side. It may be considered also in bilateral asymmetrical parkinsonism if tremor and rigidity on one side are the most disabling symptoms.

It is the most effective and permanent form of treatment for tremor and rigidity.
2. Severe dopa-induced dyskinetic movements or dystonic postures of the limbs, which limit the dosage of an L-dopa-containing preparation. (Narabayashi et al., 1984.)

BILATERAL OPERATIONS

The indications for bilateral surgical procedures are the same as for unilateral operations: severe tremor, dopa-induced dyskinetic movements and dystonic postures, and, to a lesser extent, severe rigidity on the unoperated side. Bilateral surgery is only rarely indicated and patients must be selected with great care. A time interval of several months between the first and second operation is generally allowed and some surgeons leave at least 12 months between the two operations (Narabayashi, 1986). Mundinger and Meyer-Tuwe (1978), however, are satisfied with a shorter time interval before performing a subthalamotomy on the second side. Postoperative changes in affect such as apathy and indifference and adverse changes in personality and intellect, as well as a high incidence of aggravation of dysarthria and dysphonia, rarely amounting to an almost complete anarthria after the operation on the second side, are the reasons for a widespread reluctance to perform bilateral surgical procedures. Twenty-five years ago it was recommended that the surgical lesion on the two sides be in a different position, such as a thalamotomy on one and a pallidotomy on the other side (Hassler et al., 1960), but other surgeons claimed that bilateral thalamotomies achieved better results without an increase in complications (Krayenbühl et al., 1963; Selby, 1967b). It is, however, widely agreed that the surgical lesion on the second side should be smaller than the first even if tremor, dyskinesias, and rigidity are only reduced and not completely abolished.

The age of the patient at bilateral surgery should be less than 60 years. Narabayashi (1986) performed most of his bilateral nucleus intermedius coagulations on patients in whom parkinsonian tremor began before the age of 40 years. None of his 25 patients who had operations on the second side performed between 1977 and 1982 had postoperative mental impairment or significant dysphonia or dysarthria. Before being accepted for a stereotactic operation on the second side a patient must have had a smooth postoperative course after the first operation, no past history of mental confusion or of transient psychoses, retain normal speech without loss of voice volume or dysarthria, have no evidence of significant cerebral atrophy on the computed tomographic (CT) brain scan, and a full neuropsychological evaluation and the electroencephalogram (EEG) must be normal. Only by strict adherence to these criteria can the common complications of bilateral operations, such as prolonged mental confusion and adverse effects on personality and intellect, as well as a permanent severe monotonous dysarthria be avoided.

Forty-four of 270 parkinsonian patients treated by the author for more than 5 years had bilateral stereotactic operations (Selby, 1984), the lesion being directed mainly at the lateral ventral nucleus of the thalamus. Progression of the negative symptoms of Parkinson's disease was recorded in 30% of 27 patients who had only bilateral stereotactic procedures without the addition of an L-dopa-containing preparation. Tremor and, to a lesser extent, rigidity remained abolished in almost all operated cases.

In an earlier series of 413 operations (Selby, 1967b) transient mental obscuration occurred in 64.3% of 84 operations on the second side and often lasted for a few days or weeks only. Permanent impairment of memory or mental concentration was reported by only 3 of the 59 patients who had bilateral procedures (5.1%). A permanent slurring dysarthria and reduction of volume of the voice was, however, observed in 27.6% of 29 patients with a preoperative normal speech and in 23.3% of 30 patients with preexisting dysarthria after bilateral surgical procedures. Two of these patients were rendered permanently anarthric as a direct result of the operation. It is, therefore, essential to warn patients and their relatives of the high risk of deterioration of their speech before one undertakes surgery on the second side.

RISKS AND ADVERSE EFFECTS

Mortality rates have been progressively reduced from about 2.7% in 1961 to less than 0.3% of operations at present. Death was usually the result of hemorrhage into the basal ganglia, but isolated patients died of more indirect postoperative complications such as pulmonary embolism or infection (Selby, 1968).

Impairment of consciousness, somnolence, mental confusion, and difficulties with concentration and memory occur frequently during the immediate postoperative period, but generally recover completely within 2 weeks. More rarely, intellectual defects may persist for up to 3 months.

A temporary minimal hemiparesis is not unusual after a stereotactic operation and is thought to be due to encroachment of the internal capsule by the zone of edema that surrounds the destructive lesion. A mild central facial weakness on the side of the operation is regarded by us as a good sign that the lesion was made in the correct place. The mild hemiparesis usually recovers within a few days, but the slight facial paresis may last for a few months and is hardly noticed by the patient. Lasting hemiparesis is a rare complication, usually attributed to hemorrhage or infarction in the vicinity of the surgical lesion. It can now be easily seen by a postoperative CT brain scan, which can give a useful guide to prognosis. Lasting hemiparesis occurred after 0.8-3.4% of the early operations before 1965 (Selby, 1967b), but is now only very rarely seen (less than 0.5% of cases).

A cerebellar ataxia of the operated limbs, or a temporary lateropulsion of the gait towards the operated side, occurs more frequently after surgical lesions in the posterior part of the lateral ventral nucleus of the thalamus (VOP of Hassler). Many of our patients lean or deviate a little toward the side of the operated limbs for the first few days after surgery. A lasting hemicerebellar ataxia is, however, very rare and is attributed to destruction of dentatothalamic fibers from the brachium conjunctivum.

Involuntary movements, ranging from irregular jerking to hemiballismus of the operated limbs, occurred in less than 1% of the early operations and always returned to normal completely within a few weeks. These findings were a little more frequent after bilateral thalamic procedures. Several patients have nocturnal myoclonic jerks for months after the surgical procedure, but this receives comment mainly from their spouses.

Partial or generalized convulsive seizures were observed during the immediate postoperative period in a few cases and may be due to slight cortical damage from insertion of the electrode. More recently some generalized convulsive seizures during the immediate postoperative period were attributed to the metrizamide used for the ventriculogram.

A transient deterioration of speech, mainly a slight slurring dysarthria and some loss of voice volume, may occur after some unilateral thalamotomies but always are corrected within the first few days or weeks. Permanent monotony and slurring of speech never occur after unilateral operations, but involve almost 25% of patients after bilateral surgery. It must be emphasized, however, that the patient's speech never improves after unilateral surgery, although some patients may speak a little more loudly. The speech of many patients is worse when they are examined 5 or more years after stereotactic surgery. This is entirely due to natural progression of the disease and cannot be blamed on the surgical intervention.

A significant proportion of patients, however, exhibit a temporary expressive dysphasia after operations on the dominant cerebral hemisphere. They have difficulties in finding the word they need to express their thoughts and their speech may be slow and hesitant for a few postoperative days. This expressive dysphasia always recovers completely and its cause is unknown; it was observed more often after pallidotomy than thalamotomy.

In the early days of surgery other transient complications such as sensory disturbances, defects of the visual fields, and disorders of eye movements were reported in isolated cases. They were due to misplacement of the lesion and have never occurred with the recent use of accurate thalamotomy or subthalamotomy. It can be concluded that the risks and potential side effects of surgical treatment are now less than the risks of pharmacologic therapy for Parkinson's disease.

CONCLUSIONS

The treatment of Parkinson's disease is still far from perfect and much research remains to be done to determine the causes and chemical and physiologic mechanisms of this common, progressive scourge. The medical world was excited 15 years ago at having found the first remedy for a "degenerative" neurologic disorder, but realized 5 years later that the beneficial therapeutic effect was not lasting and that various adverse reactions to treatment appeared and could not be remedied.

At the present time L-dopa-containing preparations and dopa-receptor site agonists relieve the "negative" symptoms of Parkinson's disease (hypokinesia, early disorders of gait) and, to a lesser extent and in relatively high dosages, they improve rigidity and tremor, the "positive" symptoms. As the disease gradually advances, both the negative and positive symptoms progress and various adverse effects of treatment, such as dyskinetic movements and fluctuations in patients' performance during the day, appear.

Stereotactic surgery has no effect on negative symptoms, but it can permanently abolish the positive symptoms of tremor and rigidity at least on one side and can control the drug-induced dyskinesias. It is a safe operation, with fewer long-term risks than pharmacologic treatment and should therefore be offered to all patients in whom tremor and rigidity are the predominant abnormalities. A frank discussion with the patient and his or her relatives about the operation must point out the high probability of permanently abolishing tremor and rigidity on one side and must explain that hypokinesia and disorders of speech, gait, and equilibrium are likely to appear and progress slowly in the future. Patients with unilateral tremor and rigidity should be informed that tremor and rigidity will also involve the other side after some years in about 60% of cases (Selby, 1984) and that a unilateral operation cannot prevent this.

When severe tremor appears on the second side but the patient is relatively healthy and less than 60 years old and has little or no negative symptoms, an operation on the second side can be considered after the patient is warned of the high risk of dysarthria. In some cases of parkinsonism with predominantly tremor beginning before the age of 50 years, early surgical treatment may delay the need for a dopa-containing preparation and thus reduce the development of long-term adverse effects of medical therapy. Some 10 years or more after the onset of Parkinson's disease about 40% of patients develop a progressive dementia. Surgical treatment has neither a beneficial nor adverse influence on this dementia.

In conclusion, it would therefore appear that thalamotomy or subthalamotomy at present is a relatively neglected avenue of treatment of Parkinson's disease symptoms.

REFERENCES

Albe-Fessard D, Arfel G, Guiot G, Hardy J, Vourc'h G, Hertzog E, Aleonard P. (1961). Identification et délimitation précise de certaines structures souscorticales de l'homme par l'électrophysiologie. Son intérêt dans la chirurgie stéréotaxique des dyskinésies. *C R Acad Sci* 253: 2412–2414.

Bucy PC, Case TJ. (1939). Tremor. Physiologic mechanism and abolition by surgical means. *Arch Neurol Psychiatry* 41: 721–746.

Cooper IS. (1954). Intracerebral injection of procaine into the globus pallidus in hyperkinetic disorders. *Science* 119: 417–418.

Gillingham FJ. (1966). Depth recording and stimulation. *J Neurosurg* 24: 382–387.

Gillingham FJ, Watson WS, Donaldson AA, Naughton JAL. (1960). The surgical treatment of parkinsonism. *Br Med J* 2: 1395–1402.

Guiot G. (1958). Le traitement des syndromes parkinsoniens par la destruction du pallidum interne. *Neurochirurgia* 1: 94–98.

Guiot G, Brion S. (1952). Traitement neuro-chirurgical des syndromes choréoathétosiques et parkinsoniens. *Sem Hôp Paris* 49: 2095–2099.

Hassler R, Riechert T. (1954). Indikationen und Lokalisationsmethode der gezielten Hirnoperationen. *Nervenarzt* 25: 441–447.

Hassler R, Riechert T, Mundinger F, Umbach W, Ganglberger JA. (1960). Physiological observations in stereotaxic operations in extrapyramidal motor disturbances. *Brain* 83: 337–350.

Kelly PJ, Gillingham FJ. (1980). The long-term results of stereotaxic surgery and L-dopa therapy in patients with Parkinson's disease. A 10-year follow-up study. *J Neurosurg* 53: 332–337.

Klemme RM. (1940). Surgical treatment of dystonia, paralysis agitans and athetosis. *Arch Neurol Psychiatry* 44: 926.

Krayenbühl H, Siegfried J, Yasargil MG. (1963). Résultats tardifs des opérations stéréotaxiques dans le traitement de la maladie de Parkinson. *Rev Neurol* 108: 485–494.

Leksell L. (1949). A stereotaxic apparatus for intracerebral surgery. *Acta Chir Scand* 99: 229–233.

Meyers R. (1940). Surgical procedure for postencephalitic tremor, with notes on the physiology of premotor fibres. *Arch Neurol Psychiatry* 44: 455–457.

Meyers R. (1942). Surgical interruption of the pallidofugal fibres. Its effect on the syndrome of paralysis agitans and technical considerations in its application. *NY State J Med* 42: 317–325.

Mundinger F. (1965). Die Subthalamotomie zur symptomatologischen Behandlung extrapyramidaler Bewegungsstörungen, insbesondere des Parkinson-syndroms. *Dtsch Med Wochenschr* 90: 2002–2007.

Mundinger F, Meyer-Tuwe W. (1978). Ergebnisse der stereotaktischen Behandlung des Parkinson-Rigors. In: Fischer PA (Ed.), *Langzeitbehandlung des Parkinson-Syndroms. Frankfurter Symposium über Ergebnisse und Probleme der Langzeitbehandlung des Parkinson-Syndroms am 10. und 11. Februar 1978*, Stuttgart, F.K. Schattauer Verlag.

Mundinger F, Riechert T. (1963). Die stereotaktischen Hirnoperationen zur Behandlung extrapyramidaler Bewegungsstörungen (Parkinsonismus und Hyperkinesen) und ihre Resultate. *Fortschr Neurol Psychiatr* 31: 1–120.

Narabayashi H. (1987). Surgical treatment in the era of levodopa and other pharmacological treatment. In: Stern G (Ed.), *Parkinson's Disease*. London, Chapman and Hall.

Narabayashi H, Okuma T. (1953). Procaine oil blocking of the globus pallidus for the treatment of rigidity and tremor of Parkinsonism. *Proc Jpn Acad* 29: 134–137.

Narabayashi H, Yokochi F, Nakajima Y. (1984). Levodopa-induced dyskinesia and thalamotomy. *J Neurol Neurosurg Psychiatry* 47: 831–839.

Oliver LC. (1953). *Parkinson's Disease and its Surgical Treatment*. London, Lewis.

Putnam TJ. (1938). Relief from unilateral paralysis agitans by section of the lateral pyramidal tract. *Arch Neurol Psychiatry* 40: 1049–1050.

Riechert T, Wolff M. (1951). Über ein neues Zielgerät zur intrakraniellen Ableitung und Ausschaltung. *Arch Psychiatr Nervenkr* 186: 225–230.

Schaltenbrand G, Bailey P. (1959). *Introduction to Stereotaxis with an Atlas of the Human Brain*. New York, Grune and Stratton.

Selby G. (1967a). Stereotactic surgery for the relief of Parkinson's disease. I. A critical review. *J Neurol Sci* 5: 315–342.

Selby G. (1967b). Stereotactic surgery for the relief of Parkinson's disease. II. An analysis of the results of a series of 303 patients (413 operations). *J Neurol Sci* 5: 343–375.

Selby G. (1968). Parkinson's disease. In: Vinken PJ, Bruyn GW (Eds.), *Handbook of Clinical Neurology*, Vol. 6. Amsterdam, North-Holland.

Selby G. (1976). The influence of previous stereotactic thalamotomy on l-dopa therapy in Parkinson's disease. *Proc Aust Assoc Neurol* 13: 55–60.

Selby G. (1984). The long-term prognosis of Parkinson's disease. *Clin Exp Neurol* 20: 1–25.

Smith MC. (1967). Stereotactic operations for Parkinson's disease—Anatomical observations. In: Williams D (Ed.), *Modern Trends in Neurology*. London, Butterworths.

Spiegel EA, Wycis HT. (1952). *Stereoencephalotomy (Thalamotomy and Related Procedures)*. Part I. *Methods and Stereotaxic Atlas of the Human Brain*. New York, Grune and Stratton.

Spiegel EA, Wycis HT. (1954). Ansotomy in paralysis agitans. *Arch Neurol Psychiatry* 71: 598–614.

Spiegel EA, Wycis HT, Marks M, Lee AJ. (1946). Stereotaxic apparatus for operations on the human brain. *Science* 106: 349–350.

Walker AE. (1952). Surgical treatment of involuntary movements. *Texas Rep Biol Med* 10: 105–129.

24
Brain Grafting

MARK J. PERLOW
University of Illinois Westside Veterans Administration Hospital,
Chicago, Illinois

Parkinson's disease is a clinical neurologic syndrome that has been known and identified for over 200 years. Although the illness has diverse causes and a variable clinical course, it is manifest by four major signs: tremor, cogwheel rigidity, akinesia, and loss of postural or balance reflexes. Other manifestations of the disorder include respiratory dysfunctions, eye movement abnormalities, autonomic dysfunctions, and dementia (1,2). During the natural course of this illness, an individual may have one or many of these clinical manifestations, and each to a variable extent. Although pathologic changes are observed throughout the nervous system, the most characteristic changes seem to be a neural cell loss in the zona compacta of the substantia nigra, the locus ceruleus, and the autonomic ganglia (3). Associated with these morphologic alterations are a number of biochemical abnormalities. Besides the reduction of acetylcholine and its synthetic enzymes in the nucleus basalis of Meynert, which correlates with the dementing aspects of this illness (4,5), and the reduction in dopamine and its metabolites in the caudate nucleus, which correlates with hypokinesia and rigidity (6,7), there does not seem to be a clear relationship between these compounds and most clinical symptoms. A reduction in the concentration of the peptides met- and leu-enkephalin, cholcystokinin, substance P, bombesin, and somatostatin has been measured in various portions of the brains of individuals dying with this illness (8). As is the case with norepinephrine (NE) and serotonin (5-HT), none of these biochemical changes seems to correlate with the clinical symptoms (6-8).

Based on these biochemical alterations, drugs have been administered to treat Parkinson's disease. It was hoped that the drugs would reverse the biochemical changes and at least some portion of the individual's symptoms. Included among the drugs are compounds that modify serotonin, norepinephrine, and acetyl-choline metabolism. Although success has been achieved with a number of pharmacologic compounds, replacement of dopamine and the administration of compounds that modify dopamine metabolism still remain the backbone of contemporary parkinsonian therapy.

The response to dopaminergic therapy has led scientists and clinicians to hypothesize that Parkinson's disease is primarily the result of a loss of dopamine in discrete or localized areas of the brain. Accordingly, pharmacologic investigations looking for new therapies have tended to emphasize dopamine metabolism abnormalities over abnormalities associated with other neurochemical systems. This approach has been successful in developing new medications. The ideal dopaminergic agent would accordingly be a direct-acting dopaminomimetic compound with full agonist activity on dopamine receptors; have good penetrability through the blood–brain barrier; be metabolically stable and produce prolonged effects on dopamine receptors; operate on discrete areas of the brain where dopamine activity is normally present; be released in response to normal physiologic needs rather than the timing, the amount, and route of drug administration; and not alter other brain and body systems in an unphysiologic manner. To fulfill the above pharmacologic criteria, the most logical treatment of the symptoms of Parkinson's disease would be a localized infusion of dopamine into portions of the brain that have a deficiency, similar to the manner normally achieved by the normal brain. Initial experiments on the transplantation of substantia nigra dopamine neurons by Perlow and colleagues (10) to treat a Parkinson-like syndrome induced in rats were based on a modification of this conceptualization: to infuse dopamine via dopamine-synthesizing neurons obtained primarily from the substantia nigra onto portions of the brain deficient in dopamine.

In order to determine if transplantation might be a useful therapy in humans, the effects of substantia nigra transplants were performed in experimental animals. At the time of the original experiments by Perlow (9,10) and Bjorklund (11,12) and their colleagues, the best animal model of Parkinson's disease was a unilaterally lesioned 6-hydroxydopamine (6-OHDA) rat. In this paradigm, the dopaminergic projecting systems from the substantia nigra to the corpus striatum are destroyed by intranigral injections of 6-OHDA. As a consequence of the loss of the dopaminergic neurons in the A9 and A10 regions in the ventral tegmentum of the brain stem, there is a reduction in the concentration of dopamine in the substantia nigra and its terminal projecting areas, the corpus striatum (primarily the caudate nucleus) and the mesolimbic cortex, including the nucleus accumbens and frontal cortex (13–15). Along with the loss of these neurons is a consequent degeneration of their axons and an increase in the number of dopamine receptors in the nucleus accumbens and the corpus striatum (14,16,17).

Clinical manifestations of this induced rodent illness are dependent on the extent of the lesions as well as on whether the 6-OHDA injection was performed unilaterally or bilaterally. When the injection is made on both sides of an animal's brain stem the animal becomes severely aphagic and adipsic. While it is possible to perform experiments on animals prepared in this manner, these disabilities are so severe that maintenance of large numbers of animals is very difficult (18,19). The rat model of unilateral injection of 6-OHDA in the rat striatum is an easier model to maintain and as a consequence is more commonly used in parkinsonian research today. Asymmetrical motor and sensory behaviors are the quantifiable clinical manifestations of the unilateral dopamine loss (9,10,12, 20–23). The motor behavior (i.e., walking in tight circles on a flat or curved surface) occurs spontaneously (toward or ipsilateral to the side of the lesion) as well as in response to dopamine-releasing drugs, such as amphetamine (ipsilateral walking or rotation), and dopamine-receptor activating drugs, such as apomorphine (contralateral walking or rotation). Asymmetrical posture and sensory inattention (sometimes called sensory neglect) toward stimuli applied to the side of the body contralateral to the lesion are the induced sensory deficits and they too can be quantified. Bilateral substantia nigra lesions reduce the animal's total response to environmental stimuli. The animals develop akinetic behavior, bilateral sensory inattention, cataplexy, a hunched posture, aphagia, and adipsia. We and other have used both models extensively (9,10,12,13,20–22).

In most studies the dopamine neurons used for transplantation were obtained from the ventral tegmenta of fetal animals (9,10,24–26). Cell blocks (0.5–1.0 mm^3) were dissected out of the mesencephalic flexure of 15–18-day rat fetuses, and transplanted to the brains of the adult animals with 6-OHDA-lesioned substantia nigra. Although not quite as functionally successful, tissue from fetal animals up to 19 days gestation can be used. If one subjects these cell blocks to an enzyme solution, commonly a trypsin solution, a suspension of neurons and glia is obtained and can be used for transplantation (27–36).

Investigators have found that the cells from 14–15-day fetal animals are easily suspended and provide an excellent source of tissues for behavioral restoration. Once these tissues are dissected free from the fetal animal and/or are dispersed, they are placed into the animal's brain via pipette or needle and stylet, commonly a modified lumbar puncture needle. These cell populations are transplanted either directly into the substance of the caudate nucleus, into the lateral ventricle adjacent to the denervated caudate nucleus, or on the surface of the caudate nucleus (9,12,18–22,28,31–42). This latter preparation, commonly called a "delayed cavity" preparation, is made by aspirating the cerebral cortex overlying the dorsal or lateral portion of the corpus striatum (22,31,43). This is followed 3–6 weeks later by intracavitary transplantation. The delayed cavity technique permits a larger number of cells to be transplanted but, because of the destructive nature of the making of the cavity, it is used primarily by basic scientists for experimental studies. While most experiments have used cells from the same species, successful transplants have also been obtained when a host and a donor are not of the same species (44–46). Immunosuppressants seem to enhance hetero- and xenotransplant survival (45,46).

Transplantation of these nigral cell populations has reversed most of the behavioral, biochemical, and anatomical abnormalities induced by dopamine-denervating lesions. The nature and degree of success of the transplants are in part dependent upon their position within the corpus striatum. Behaviorally, all of the abnormalities except adipsia and aphagia could be reversed by discrete transplants (9–12,18,19,21,22,27,31,38). Biochemically the transplants restored much, and in some cases up to 50%, of the lost caudate dopamine (35). Dopamine receptor concentration was reduced to normal levels in regions adjacent to the graft (16). Anatomically, the transplanted dopaminergic cells appeared normal and sprouted in a limited manner into the substance of the caudate. In most cases the axon terminals synapsed normally with the dendritic shafts and spine necks of the host's caudate medium spiny neurons (47). This efferent sprouting was occasionally abnormal, sometimes forming neuronal "baskets" around the host giant cholinergic striatal cells, making many synaptic contacts in the course. Dopamine in the striatum appears to function by reactivating intact neuronal machinery used for motion; whether this occurs on the basis of synaptic contact or on extracellular release of dopamine remains to be determined. Afferent projections to the transplant were less frequently observed; some of these projections synapsed with transplant neurons (9–12,41,47–50). It is presently unknown if any of the afferent projections are random occurrences or represent target-specific reinnervation.

Transplanted dopaminergic neurons in general sprouted only 0.5–1.5 m, up to a maximum of 3–4 mm, into the substance of the brain (9–12,27,29,41,51). This is much less than they do in an intact animal, and less than the total area of denervation (i.e., entire corpus striatum). The reasons for the limited reinnervation of the caudate are largely unknown. It does not, however, appear that it is because the grafted dopamine neurons are unable to extend their axons over long distances (48). Ingrowth of neurons and the pattern of ingrowth and reinnervation probably are the result of factors in both the fetal donor substantia nigra as well as in the adult host denervated striatum. As with other paradigms, this interaction may be relatively specifically dependent on the different types of cells in the graft as well as cells in the host. Caudate reinnervation is increased if early-gestation fetal substantia nigra are used as donor tissues, or if neonatal instead of adult rats are used as hosts (52,53).

Because of limited axonal growth into brain tissue and limited diffusion of dopamine into the surrounding brain, transplants seem to be most effective when they are adjacent to or within the experimental site itself, rather than at a distance from the site of action. Thus, transplants in diencephalic (lateral hypothalamus) or in mesencephalic brain stem (substantia nigra) sites, distant from the denervated caudate, do not cause an anatomical or biochemical reinnervation of the caudate nucleus, nor do they alter the animal's behavior (35,37). Practical techniques to increase the dopaminergic innervation of the denervated striatum at the present time are primarily limited to increasing the volume of the transplanted substantia nigra or distributing the transplants throughout the caudate nucleus in small patches (29). Small discrete injections of cell suspensions into multiple sites produce relatively little damage to either host or donor tissue. While additional growth was not obtained if the posttransplant recovery period was extended, transplants of dispersed fetal nigral cells intermixed with fetal caudate, increased the sprouting by 50% (54). Sprouting is also increased by prior frontal cortex decortication via as yet unspecified mechanisms (52).

Transplanted neurons from the substantia nigra contain two groups of dopaminergic neurons. One group, A9, located in the lateral portion of the nigra and projecting primarily to the corpus striatum, contains only dopamine. The other more medially placed group, A10, projects primarily to the nucleus accumbens, and in addition to having catecholamine enzymes, also contains the peptide cholecystokinin (CCK). Transplants containing a mixture of the monoamine and the monoamine-CCK neurons grow in the host brain. However, the axons that penetrate beyond 0.1 mm and sprout within the substance of the caudate nucleus are primarily those that contain only dopamine and not CCK (51). This observation suggests that regulatory mechanisms in the denervated neostriatum selectively favor the ingrowth of fibers from the appropriate A9 dopamine neuronal subset. A similar stimulation of growth and sprouting is seen in vitro when fetal substantia nigra is cultured with pieces of caudate tissue or with striatal or nigral glia (55-63). The absence of sprouting from A10 tegmental dopamine neurons to the dorsal striatum allows us to transplant mixed cell populations with less concern about the possibility of abnormal synapse formation. Although nature in this case seems to select the correct population of cells to support, an anatomically correct reinnervation pattern is not universally found. Abnormal growth and behavior are observed in some transplant paradigms (43, 64,65).

The substantia nigra and the corpus striatum are heterogeneous structures (66-72). As with a number of brain regions, afferent projections from the substantia nigra to the caudate are distributed topographically within the caudate nucleus. If we transplant substantia nigra cells to different areas of the caudate, selected aspects of the induced behavioral syndrome are reduced. Thus, when the transplants are placed in the dorsal portion of the unilaterally dopamine-denervative caudate-putamen, there is an amelioration of spontaneous and drug-induced rotation and the ipsilateral turning bias associated with exploration in an unbaited T-maze. Transplants have no effect on contralateral sensory inattention. Reinnervation of the ventral and lateral portion of the caudate-putamen by nigral transplants over that region of the caudate reduces sensory motor inatten-

tion and increases responsiveness of the contralateral side of the body to stimulation but does not alter spontaneous or drug-induced rotation (11,18–22,31,37,
38). Reinnervation of the nucleus accumbens and the prefrontal cortex
normalizes the locomotor response to the dopaminergic drugs amphetamine and
apomorphine (38,73,74). In total, most of the impairments noted with 6-OHDA
lesions are responsive to the substantia-nigra dopamine transplants. Nigral transplants can even reinnervate the dopamine-depleted neostriatum to sustain intracranial self-stimulation (48). Multiple grafts provide more extensive reinnervation of the dopamine denervated regions of the brain and result in a more complete recovery than is observed with any single graft. Only adipsia and aphagia in
bilaterally lesioned animals appear to be unresponsive to the present techniques
(18,19).

Before initiating transplantation as a method to treat humans with Parkinson's disease, we should be aware of a number of recently discovered features of
this illness and the role these may play in its pathophysiology. The normal degeneration of dopaminergic neurons that occurs with aging is accelerated in
parkinsonian patients (75). When the striatal content of dopamine declines to
approximately 30% of its normal value, parkinsonian symptoms may become apparent (6). Human and animal data suggest that other neurologic infirmities of
old age, especially those related to higher cortical functions, may in part be
secondary to a loss of dopamine. Pharmacologic reversal of some of these
deficits by dopaminergic compounds has been reported by both Cotzias and
Marshall (76–78). Likewise, Gage and Bjorklund (32,33,39,79) have reversed
age-dependent deficit in sensory motor coordination and swimming by the transplantation of fetal substantia nigra neurons. These presumably work by
dopaminergic mechanisms. Unfortunately, not all behavioral deficits associated
with aging were reversed by the drugs or the transplants.

Thus it appears that intercerebral grafts of substantia nigra cells reduce some
of the effects of central nervous system aging and some of the effects of ex-
perimentally induced substantia nigra lesions. The behavioral effect of the transplants appears to be specific and related to their location in the host brain. Their
effect seems to be mediated through direct action of the grafted neurons and/or
their secretions on the adjacent host brain parenchyma. However, since the
dopamine neurons contain other compounds besides dopamine and the transplants contain nondopaminergic cells and glia, it is conceivable that these and
other putative neurotransmitters and/or other cells contribute to the beneficial
behavioral response. The role of these nondopaminergic cells and their projections to the caudate nucleus in Parkinson's disease patients remain to be determined. Thus, efforts directed toward the development of methods of obtaining pure populations of dopaminergic cells as the ultimate nigral transplant
panacea may be both premature and ill founded.

While transplanted dopaminergic neurons project to the host brain, there is, using the present paradigms, at best only little evidence suggesting that host brain neurons project to the transplanted substantia nigra neurons (47,79). From a clinical perspective, it is hoped that these afferents make synaptic contact with the transplant neurons in a manner similar to that seen in the intact animal. Further studies are needed to determine the nature of these afferent axons in each of the experimental paradigms to determine which is best for experimental work and which one best applies to humans. If the relationship between brain transplants and the host is disorganized, it is possible that the transplant will add to the animal's disability. Since this can, in the final analysis, only be determined by investigation, careful experimentation should be performed in a number of paradigms prior to use of central nervous system transplantation in humans.

In the absence of afferents to the transplant, it is still possible to alter the firing rate and thus the secretory activity of the transplant itself (50,80-87). Dopamine neurons in the fetal substantia nigra, transplanted to the denervated caudate, respond to iontophoretically placed dopamine, dopaminergic agonists and antagonists, and amphetamine in a reliable manner similar to that observed in the intact animal (88). Behavioral motor response of the transplanted neurons to parenteral amphetamine substantiates their ability to function normally in a whole animal in the heterotopic environment of the denervated caudate nucleus.

When discussing the topic of transplantation of neural tissue in humans, one of the most commonly asked questions is "What will be the source of dopaminergic fetal tissue?" Although human tissue has been transplanted to rats and is probably the best source material for use in humans, human fetal neuronal tissues are not readily available for experimentation and/or for human transplantation. However, neonatal and adult human tissues are available and should be considered a source of nigral tissue. Unfortunately, transplanted adult neurons have not been very successful in reversing any of the biochemical, anatomical, or behavioral deficits described above. Another potential tissue source for transplantation into humans is fetal tissue from other animals.

Nonhuman primates seem to be the most appropriate nonhuman source of tissue. It is reasonable to assume that the substantia nigra from these two-legged, upright animals subserve motor functions similar to that seen in humans. Immunosuppression (45) coupled with the already privileged status of the brain compared with the remainder of the body (44,46,89,90) makes intra- and interspecies transplantation a realistic possibility. I believe that the clinical immunologic status of brain transplants is equal to or better than that presently existing for kidney transplants. For example, anatomically intact, functional substantia nigra grafts between mouse and rat have survived without immunologic rejection for over 3 months (44). Bovine chromaffin cells have also been transplanted to rat brain without being rejected (90). From a strictly biochemical point of view, other catecholamine tissues, especially dopaminergic tissues, such as autonomic ganglia (91), should be considered for transplantation. Although I think it is risky to use catecholamine-containing pheochromocytoma cell tumor cell lines or strains (such as PC 12 cells) for transplantation into humans, investigators are evaluating this possibility (92-94). Recently Freed and Olson et al. (95-102) have successfully transplanted adult adrenal chromaffin medullary tissue into unilaterally 6-OHDA-lesioned substantia nigra in rats. Although the data do not fully support this conclusion, the favorable long-term behavioral response as measured by rotation was hypothesized to be secondary to the release of dopamine from these transplants. The rotational response immediately following transplant surgery may be due to the acute release of norepinephrine and epinephrine.

The same experiment has been performed on individuals with Parkinson's disease. The adrenal medulla tissue in these clinical studies was obtained from each patient's own adrenal gland. The results of the first two human Parkinson's disease patients studied by Olson and colleagues (103-105) in whom the transplants were placed in the caudate nucleus were inconclusive. However, two additional patients in whom the adrenal chromaffin implants were made into the putamen instead of the caudate showed a clear improvement in the limbs contralateral to the transplant. Unfortunately, this good response lasted only 2-3 months. The failure to maintain behavior was not understood but, based on animal experiments, was thought to be secondary to the absence of nerve growth factor (NGF) in the substance of the caudate nucleus (102,106). Its presence may be needed to maintain and stimulate the chromaffin cell "axonal" sprouts or neurites. Extensive sprouting of the chromaffin cells is seen in vitro when cultured with NGF and when transplanted to the iris, where NGF is normally found in abundance (91,94,100,107-109). Since the human studies were uncontrolled experiments, the favorable behavioral response should be considered with caution. It is possible that the good response is not due to the secretion of dopamine but is the result of the reinitiation of dopaminergic drugs following a "drug holiday" or due to norepinephrine in the cells. A clearer picture will no doubt evolve as more studies are performed.

Prior to transplanting any neurons or cells to large numbers of Parkinsonian patients, it is necessary to visualize adequately and characterize biochemically the structures in the substance of the human brain. As suggested by Dunnett and Bjorklund's rat studies (11,18-22,31,37,38), in which specific behavioral responses to the transplants corresponded to specific areas of the caudate, it is important to correlate the human biochemical-anatomical changes with specific aspects of clinical symptoms in order to place grafts correctly. To achieve the greatest reduction in clinical symptoms from these grafts, it will probably be necessary to perform transplants with either small blocks of tissue or as suspension of cells in a sterotaxic fashion into "well-defined" anatomical locations or sites within the substance of the brain. Nonspecific or "shot-gun" transplantation in multiple, less defined, widely distributed sites may also be effective in reversing parkinsonian symptoms. As with different pharmacologic treatments of Parkinson's disease symptoms, I anticipate that some signs and symptoms will be more responsive to transplant treatment than others; for example, anticholinergics reduce tremor and rigidity with little effect on bradykinesis while L-dopa seems to be most effective in reducing bradykinesia and postural problems (65).

Although we have considered Parkinson's disease a "substantia nigra illness," it is clear that it is really a systemic disease that compromises many areas of the neuraxis and many biochemical systems. Each of these regions contributes in a unique way to an individual patient's medical problems. To increase the clinical effectiveness of brain grafts or transplants as a treatment for the symptoms of Parkinson's disease might also require the grafting of these other central nervous system tissues, such as, locus ceruleus or nucleus basalis of Meynert. If so, further investigations, especially using the positron emission tomographic scan (PET scan) or similar biochemical imaging techniques, will be needed to assist in the correlation of the neuroanatomical-biochemical basis with clinical phenomena (14,106,110,111).

The use of non-central-nervous-system (non-CNS) tissues, such as the adrenal chromaffin cell, as donor sources should be considered. These sources should be used with caution, and only after careful experimentation. The biochemical and morphologic expression of these non-CNS tissues, as well as CNS tissues transplanted into heterotopic locations (e.g., substantia nigra into caudate instead of brain stem), can lead to nontherapeutic and even deleterius results, as well as having unique benefits. For example, in Parkinson's disease there is a reduction in the concentration of met-enkephalin in the globus pallidus (8). An increase in the concentration of met-enkephalin might be achieved by transplantation of the adrenal medulla which normally has high levels of this compound. Unless there were a change in the biochemical expression of fetal substantia nigra to make met-enkephelin, as a result of transplantation, transplantation of these dopaminergic cells would be unlikely to increase the concentration of this peptide. Reversal of any enkephalin-related clinical signs and symptoms would probably not then be achieved by substantia nigra transplants, but rather by the medulla transplants that probably will continue to synthesize and secrete the peptide.

Progress toward the use of brain grafts to treat Parkinson's disease symptoms has been stimulated by the development of a new model system using primates (and other animals, including rodents) (112–114) that corresponds more closely to many aspects of the normal human condition and idiopathic Parkinson's disease. In this system a neurotoxic chemical, methyl-phenyl-tetrahydropyridine (MPTP), is injected parenterally. Over the course of a few days the monkeys develop some of the human features of Parkinson's disease, especially hypokinesia, rigidity, and postural instability (112). Associated with the clinical features is a dramatic reduction in the concentration of dopamine and dopamine metabolites in the basal ganglia, and a discrete loss of dopamine-containing neurons in the substantia nigra. Preliminary reports suggest that fetal nigral grafts into the striatum of these animals live for prolonged periods of time and reverse a significant portion of the neurobehavioral and neurochemical deficits (115). Further studies are being actively pursued by a number of investigators (113,115) with the hope of developing additional neurosurgical treatments of Parkinson's disease and its symptoms.

REFERENCES

1. Bannister R. (1981). *Brain's Clinical Neurology*, 2nd ed. Oxford, Oxford University Press.
2. Parkinson J. (1917). *An Essay on the Shaking Palsy*. London, Sherwood, Neely and Jones.
3. Forno LS. (1981). Pathology of Parkinson's disease. In: Marsden CD, Fahn S (Eds.), *Movement Disorders*. London, Butterworths.
4. Fuxe K, Agnati LF, Bentenati F, Celeni F, Zinc I, Zoli M, Mutt V. (1983). *J Neural Transm* (Suppl. 18) 165–179.
5. Whitehouse PJ, Hedreen JC, White CL III, Price OL. (1983). Basal forebrain neurons in the dementia of Parkinson's disease. *Ann Neurol* 13: 243–248.
6. Bernheimer H, Birkmayer W, Hornykiewicz O, Jellinger K, Seitelberger F. (1973). Brain dopamine and the syndromes of Parkinson's and Huntington. Clinical morphological and neurochemical correlations. *J Neurol Sci* 20: 415–455.
7. Schultz W. (1982). Depletion of dopamine in the striatum as an experimental model of Parkinsonism. Direct effects and adoptive mechanisms. *Prog Neurobiol* 18: 121–166.
8. Agid Y, Javoy-Agid F. (1985). Peptides and Parkinson's disease. *Trends Neurosci* 10: 378–383.
9. Freed WJ, Perlow MJ, Karoum F, Seiger A, Olson L, Hoffer BJ, Wyatt RJ. (1980). Restoration of dopaminergic function by grafting of fetal rat substantia nigra to the caudate nucleus: long-term behavioural, biochemical, and histochemical studies. *Ann Neurol* 8: 510–519.
10. Perlow MJ, Freed WJ, Hoffer BJ, Seiger A, Olson L, Wyatt RJ. (1979). Brain grafts reduce motor abnormalities produced by destruction of nigrostriatal dopamine system. *Science* 204: 643–647.
11. Bjorklund A, Dunnett SB, Stenevi U, Lewis ME, Iversen SD. (1980). Reinnervation of the denervated striatum by substantia nigra transplants: functional consequences as revealed by pharmacological and sensorimotor testing. *Brain Res* 199: 307–333.
12. Bjorklund A, Stenevi U. (1979). Reconstruction of the nigrostriatal dopamine pathway by intracerebral nigral transplants. *Brain Res* 177: 555–560.

13. Brundin P. (1986). Morphological and functional effects of single and multiple grafts of mesencephalic dopamine neurons in different striatal and limbic regions. In: Azmitia E, Bjorklund A (Eds.), *Cell and Tissue Transplantation into the Adult Brain.* New York, New York Academy of Sciences.

14. Creese I, Hamblin MW, Leff SE, Sibley DR. (1982). CNS dopamine receptors. In: Iversen LL, Iversen SD, Snyder SH (Eds.), *Handbook of Psychopharmacology. Vol. 17. Biochemical Studies of CNS Receptors.* New York, Plenum Press, pp. 81–138.

15. Ungerstedt U. (1976). 6-Hydroxydopamine-induced degeneration of the nigro-striatal dopamine pathway: the turning syndrome. *Pharmacol Ther* 2: 37–40.

16. Freed WJ, Ko GN, Neihoff DL, Kuhar M, Hoffer BJ, Olson L, Spoor E, Morihisa JM, Wyatt RJ. (1983). Normalization of spiroperidol binding in the denerevated rat striatum by homologous substantia nigra transplants. *Science* 222: 937–939.

17. Palacios JM, Niehoff DL, Kuhar MJ. (1981). (^{3}H) spiperone binding sites in brain: autoradiographic localization of multiple receptors. *Brain Res* 213: 277–289.

18. Dunnett SB, Bjorklund A, Schmidt RH, Stenevi U, Iversen SD. (1983). Intracerebral grafting of neuronal cell suspension. V. Behavioural recovery in rats with bilateral 6-OHDA lesions following implantation of nigral cell suspensions. *Acta Physiol Scand* (Suppl). 522: 39–48.

19. Dunnett SB, Bjorklund A, Stenevi U, Iversen SD. (1981). Behavioral recovery following transplantation of substantia nigra in rats subjected to 6-OHDA lesions of the nigro-striatal pathway. II. Bilateral lesions. *Brain Res* 229: 457–470.

20. Bjorklund A, Stenevi U, Dunnett SB, Iversen SD. (1981). Functional reactivation of the deafferented neostriatum by nigral transplants. *Nature* 289: 497–499.

21. Dunnett SB, Bjorklund A, Stenevi U, Iversen SD. (1981). Grafts of embryonic substantia nigra reinnervating the ventrolateral striatum ameliorate sensory motor impairments and akinesia in rats with 6-OHDA lesions of the nigro-striatal pathway. *Brain Res* 229: 209–217.

22. Dunnett SB, Bjorklund A, Stenevi U, Iversen SD. (1981). Behavioral recovery following transplantation of substantia nigra in rats subjected to 6-OHDA lesions of the nigro-striatal pathway. I. Unilateral lesions. *Brain Res* 215: 147–161.

23. Ungerstedt U, Arbuthnott G. (1970). Quantitative recording of rotational behaviour in rats after 6-hydroxydopamine lesions of the nigro-striatal dopamine system. *Brain Res* 24: 485–493.

24. Seiger A, Olson L. (1973). Late prenatal ontogeny of central monoamine neurons in the rat: Fluorescence histochemical observations. *Z Anat Entwicklungsgesch* 140: 281–318.

25. Specht LA, Pickel VM, Joh TH, Reis DJ. (1981). Light-microscopic immunocytochemical localization of tyrosine hydroxylese in prenatal rat brain. I. Early ontogeny. *J Comp Neurol* 199: 233–253.

26. Specht LA, Pickel VM, Joh TH, Reis DJ. (1981). Light-microscopic im-
    munocytochemical localization of tyrosine hydroxylese in prenatal rat
    brain. I. Late Ontogeny. *J Comp Neurol* 199: 255–276.
27. Bjorklund A, Schmidt RH, Stenevi U. (1980). Functional reinnervation of
    the neostriatum in the adult rat by use of intraparenchymal grafting of
    dissociated cell suspensions from the substantia nigra. *Cell Tissue Res* 212:
    39–45.
28. Bjorklund A, Stenevi U, Schmidt RH, Dunnett SB, Gage FH. (1983).
    Intracerebral grafting of neuronal cell suspensions. I. Introduction and
    general methods of preparation. *Acta Physiol Scand* (Suppl) 522: 1–8.
29. Bjorklund A, Stenevi U, Schmidt RH, Dunnett SB, Gage FH. (1983). Intra-
    cerebral grafting of neuronal cell suspensions. II. Survival and growth of
    nigral cell suspensions implanted in different brain sites. *Acta Physiol
    Scand* (Suppl). 522: 9–18.
30. Brundin, P, Isacson O, Bjorklund A. (1985). Monitoring of cell viability
    in suspensions of embryonic CNS tissue and its use as a criterion for intra-
    cerebral graft survival. *Brain Res* 331(2): 251–259.
31. Dunnett SB, Bjorklund A, Schmidt RH, Stenevi U, Iversen SD. (1983).
    Intracerebral grafting of neuronal cell suspension. IV. Behavioural recovery
    in rats with unilateral 6-OHDA lesions following implantation of nigral
    cell suspensions in different forebrain sites. *Acta Physiol Scand* (Suppl)
    522: 29–37.
32. Gage FH, Bjorklund A, Stenevi U, Dunnett SB. (1983). Intracerebral
    grafting of neuronal cell suspensions. VIII. Cell survival and growth of im-
    plants of nigral and septal cell suspensions in intact brains of aged rats.
    Acta Physiol Scand (Suppl) 522: 67–75.
33. Gage FH, Dunnett SB, Brundin P, Isacson O, Bjorklund A. (1983–84).
    Intracerebral grafting of embryonic neural cells into the adult host brain:
    an overview of the cell suspension method and its application. *Dev Neurosci*
    6: 137–151.
34. Schmidt RH, Bjorklund A, Stenevi U. (1981). Intracerebral grafting of
    dissociated CNS tissue suspensions: a new approach for neuronal transplan-
    tation to deep brain sites. *Brain Res* 218: 347–356.
35. Schmidt RH, Bjorklund A, Stenevi U, Dunnett SB, Gage FH. (1983). Intra-
    cerebral grafting of neuronal cell suspensions. III. Activity of intrastriatal
    nigral suspension implants as assessed by measurements of dopamine syn-
    thesis and metabolism. *Acta Physiol Scand* (Suppl) 522: 19–28.
36. Schmidt RH, Ingvar M, Lindvall O, Stenevi U, Bjorklund A. (1985). Func-
    tional activity of substantia nigra grafts reinnervating the striatum: neuro-
    transmitter metabolism and (14C)-2-deoxy-D-glucose autoradiography. *J
    Neurochem* 38: 737–748.
37. Bjorklund A, Stenevi U. (1984). Intracerebral neural implants: neuronal
    replacement and reconstruction of damaged circuitries. *Annu Rev Neurosci*
    7: 279–308.
38. Dunnett SB, Bunch ST, Gage FH, Bjorklund A. (1984). Dopamine-rich
    transplants in rats with 6-OHDA lesions of the ventral tegmental area. I.

Effects on spontaneous and drug-induced locomotor activity. *Behav Brain Res* 13: 71–82.

39. Gage FH, Bjorklund A, Stenevi U, Dunnett SB. (1983). Intracerebral grafting of neuronal cell suspensions. VIII. Cell survival and axonal outgrowth of dopaminergic and cholinergic cells in the aged brain. *Acta Physiol Scand* (Suppl) 522: 67–75.

40. Hoffer B, Freed W, Olson L, Wyatt RJ. (1983). Transplantation of dopamine-containing tissues to the central nervous system. *Clin Neurosurg* 31: 404–416.

41. Jaeger CB. (1985). Cytoarchitectonics of substantia nigra grafts: a light and electron microscopic study of immunocytochemically identified dopaminergic neurons and fibrous astrocytes. *J Comp Neurol* 231: 121–1935.

42. Stenevi U, Bjorklund A, Dunnett SB. (1980). Functional reinnervation of the denervated neostriatum by nigral transplants. *Peptides* (Suppl. 1): 111–116.

43. Bjorklund A, Stenevi U, Svendgaard NAa. (1976). Growth of transplanted monoaminergic neurones into the adult hippocampus along the perforant path. *Nature* 262: 787–790.

44. Bjorklund A, Stenevi U, Dunnett SB, Gage FH. (1982). Cross-species neural grafting in a rat model of Parkinson's disease. *Nature* 298: 652–654.

45. Brundin P, Nilsson OG, Gage FH, Bjorklund A. (1985). Cyclosporin A increases survival of cross-species intrastriatal grafts of embryonic dopamine-containing neurons. *Exp Brain Res* 60: 204–208.

46. Dymecki J, Jedizejewska A, Pucilowski O, Poltorak M. (1986). Effects of intracerebral transplantation of rabbit substantia nigra into the striatum of rats with experimental hemiparkinsonism. In: Azmitia E, Bjorklund A (Eds.), *Cell and Tissue Transplantation into the Adult Brain*. New York, New York Academy of Sciences.

47. Freund TF, Bolam JP, Bjorklund A, Stenevi U, Dunnett SB, Powell JF, Smith AD. (1985). Efferent synaptic connections of grafted dopaminergic neurons reinnervating the host neostriatum: a tyrosine hydroxylase immunocytochemical study. *J Neurosci* 5: 603–616.

48. Fray PJ, Dunnett SB, Iversen SD, Bjorklund A, Stenevi U. (1983). Nigral transplants reinnervating the dopamine-depleted neostriatum can sustain intracranial self-stimulation. *Science* 219: 416–419.

49. Mahalik TJ, Finger TE, Stromberg I, Olson L. Substantia nigra transplants into denervated striatum of the rat: ultrastructure of graft and host interconnections. *J Comp Neurol* 240: 60–70.

50. Stromberg I, Johnson S, Hoffer B, Olson L. (1985). Reinnervation of dopamine-denervated striatum by substantia nigra transplants: immunohistochemical and electrophysiological correlates. *Neuroscience* 14: 981–990.

51. Schultzberg M, Dunnett SB, Bjorklund A, Stenevi U, Hokfelt T, Dockray GJ, Goldstein M. (1984). Dopamine and cholecystokinin immunoreactive neurons in mesencephalic grafts reinnervating the neostriatum: evidence for selective growth regulation. *Neuroscience* 12: 17–32.

52. Freed WJ, Wyatt RJ. (1986). Effects of cortical injury on neurite growth from substantia nigra grafts. In: Azmitia E, Bjorklund A (Eds.), *Cell and Tissue Transplantation into the Adult Brain*. New York, New York Academy of Sciences.

53. Schwartz SS, Freed WJ. (1986). Neonatally transplanted brain tissue matures with the host brain to protect the adult rat from a lesion-induced syndrome of adipsia, aphagia and akinesia. In: Azmitia E, Bjorklund A (Eds.), *Cell and Tissue Transplantation into the Adult Brain*. New York, New York Academy of Sciences.

54. Brundin P, Nilsson OG, Gage FH, Bjorklund A. (1986). Intrastriatal grafting of dopamine-containing neuronal cell suspensions: Effects of mixing with target and non-target cells. Submitted.

55. Denis-Donini S, Glowinski J, Prochiantz A. (1983). Specific influence of striatal target neurons on the in vitro outgrowth of mesencephalic dopaminergic neurites: a morphological quantitative study. *J Neurosci* 3: 2292–2299.

56. Denis-Donini S, Glowinski J, Prochiantz A. (1983). Specific influence of striatal target neurons on the in vitro outgrowth of dopaminergic neurites: a morphological quantitative study. *J Neurosci* 3: 2292–2299.

57. Denis-Donini S, Glowinski J, Prochiantz A. (1984). Glial heterogeneity may define the three dimensional shape of mouse mesencephalic dopaminergic neurones. *Nature* 307: 641–643.

58. Di Porzio U, Daguet MC, Glowinski J, Prochiantz A. (1980). Effect of striatal cells on in vitro maturation of mesencephalic dopaminergic neurons grown in serum-free conditions. *Nature* 288: 370–373.

59. Hemmendinger LM, Garber BB, Hoffman PC, Heller A. (1981). Target neuron-specific process formation by embryonic mesencephalic dopamine neurones *in vitro*. *Proc Natl Acad Sci* (USA) 78: 1264–1268.

60. Hoffman PC, Hemmendinger LM, Kotake C, Heller A. (1983). Enhanced dopamine cell survival in reaggregates containing telencephalic target cells. *Brain Res* 274: 275–281.

61. Kotake C, Hoffman PC, Heller A. (1982). The biochemical and morphological development of differentiating dopamine neurons coaggregated with their target cells of the corpus striatum *in vitro*. *J Neurosci* 2: 1307–1315.

62. Prochiantz A, Barbin G, Mallat M, Isacson O, Brudin P, Bjorklund A. (1986). Transplantation of cultured CNS dopaminergic neurons into adult striatum. In: Azmitia E, Bjorklund A (Eds.), *Cell and Tissue Transplantation into the Adult Brain*. New York, New York Academy of Sciences.

63. Prochiantz A, Di Porzio U, Kato A, Berger B, Glowsinski J. (1979). *In vitro* maturation of mesencephalic dopaminergic neurons from mouse embryos is enhanced in presence of their striatal target cells. *Proc Natl Acad Sci* (USA) 76: 5387–5391.

64. Olson L, Seiger A, Taylor D, Freedman R, Hoffer B. (1980). Conditions for adrenergic hyperinnervation in hippocampus: I. Histochemical evidence from intraocular double grafts. *Exp Brain Res* 39: 277–288.

65. Perlow MJ. (1980). Functional brain transplants. *Peptides* 1 (Suppl. 1): 101–110.
66. Beckstead RM, Domesick VB, Nauta WJH. (1979). Efferent connections of the substantia nigra and ventral tegmental area in the rat. *Brain Res* 175: 191–217.
67. Faull RLM, Carman JB. (1968). Ascending projections of the substantia nigra in the rat. *J Comp Neurol* 132: 73–92.
68. Faull RLM, Mehler WR. (1978). The cells of origin of nigrotectal, nigro-thalamic and nigrostriatal projections in the rat. *Neurosci* 3: 989–1002.
69. Graybiel AM, Ragsdale CW Jr. (1981). Fibre connections of the basal ganglia. *Prog Brain Res* 51: 239–283.
70. Graybiel AM, Ragsdale CW. (1983). Biochemical anatomy of the striatum. In: Emson PC (Ed.), *Chemical Neuroanatomy*. New York Raven Press.
71. Grofava I. (1979). Extrinsic connections of the neostriatum. In: Divac I, Oberg RGE (Eds.), *The Neostriatum*. Oxford, Pergamon Press.
72. Nauta WJH, Domesick VB. (1984). Afferent and efferent relationships of the basal ganglia. *Ciba Found Symp* 107: 3–29.
73. LeMoal M, Herman JP, Choulli K, Taghzouti K, Simon H. (1986). Behavioral effects of mesencephalic dopamine neurons in rats with lesions of the meso-limbo-cortical dopamine system. In: Azmitia E, Bjorklund A (Eds.), *Cell and Tissue Transplantation into the Adult Brain*. New York, New York Academy of Sciences.
74. Nadaud D, Herman JP, Simon H, Le Moal M. (1984). Functional recovery following transplantation of ventral mesencephalic cells in rat subjected to 6-OHDA lesions of the mesolimbic dopaminergic neurons. *Brain Res* 304: 137–141.
75. McGeer EG. (1981). Neurotransmitter systems in aging and senile dementia. *Prog Neuropsychopharmacol* 5: 435–445.
76. Cotzias GC, Miller ST, Tang LC, Papavasiliou PS. (1977). Levodopa, fertility and longevity. *Science* 196: 549–551.
77. Marshall JF, Berrios N. (1979). Movement disorders of aged rats: reversal of dopamine receptor stimulation. *Science* 206: 447–479.
78. Papavasiliou PS, Miller ST, Thel LJ, et al. (1981). Age-related motor and catecholamine alterations in mice on levodopa supplemented diet. *Life Sci* 28: 2945–2952.
79. Gage NH, Dunnett SB, Stenevi U, Bjorklund A. (1983). Aged rats: recovery of motor impairments by intrastriatal nigral grafts. *Science* 219: 416–418.
80. Arbuthnott G, Dunnett S, Macleod N. (1985). Electrophysiological properties of single units in dopamine-rich mesencephalic transplants in rat brain. *Neurosci Lett*
81. Hoffer B, Rose G, Gerhardt G, Stromberg I, Olson O. (1985). Demonstration of monoamine release from transplanted-reinnervated caudate nucleus by in vivo electrochemical detection. In: Bjorklund A, Steveni U. (Eds.), *Neural Grafting in the Mammalian CNS*. Amsterdam, Elsevier, pp. 437–447.

82. Olson L, Vanderhaeghen JJ, Freedman R, Henschen A, Hoffer B, Seiger A. (1985). Combined grafts of the ventral tegmental area and nucleus accumbens in oculo. Histochemical and electrophysiological characterization. *Exp Brain Res* 59: 325-337.

83. Rose G, Gerhardt G, Stromberg I, Olson L, Hoffer B. (1985). Monoamine release from dopamine-depleted rat caudate nucleus reinnervated by substantia nigra transplants: An in vivo electrochemical study. 341: 92-100.

84. Taylor D, Freedman R, Seiger A, Olson L, Hoffer B. (1980). Conditions for adrenergic hyperinnervation in hippocampus: II. Electrophysiological evidence from intraocular double grafts. *Exp Brain Res* 39: 289-299.

85. Wuerthele SM, Freed WJ, Olson L, Morihisa J, Spoor L, Wyatt RJ, Hoffer B. (1981). Effect of dopamine agonists and antagonists on the electrical activity of substantia nigra neurons transplanted into the lateral ventricle of the rat. *Exp Brain Res* 44: 1-10.

86. Wuerthele SM, Olson L, Freed W, Wyatt R, Hoffer B. (1984). Electrophysiology of substantia nigra transplants. In: Usdin E, Carlsson A, Dahlstrom A, Engel J (Eds.), *Catecholamines. Part B. Neuropharmacology and Central Nervous System: Theoretical Aspects*. New York, Alan R. Liss, pp. 333-341.

87. Zetterstrom T, Brundin P, Gage FH, Sharp T, Isacson O, Dunnett SB, Ungerstedt U, Bjorklund A. (1986). In vivo measurement of spontaneously release and metabolism of dopamine from intrastriatal nigral grafts using intracerebral dialysis. *Brain Res*

88. Aghajanian GK, Bunney BS. (1973). Central dopaminergic neurons: neurophysiological identification and responses to drugs. In: Usdin E (Ed.), *Frontiers in Catecholamine Research*. New York, Pergamon Press.

89. Barker CF, Billingham RE. (1977). Immunologically privileged sites. *Adv Immunol* 25: 1-54.

90. Perlow MJ, Kumkura K, Guidotti A. (1980). Prolonged survival of bovine adrenal chromaffin cells in rat cerebral ventricles. *Proc Natl Acad Sci* (USA) 77: 5278-5281.

91. Olson L, Seiger A. (1983). Adrenergic nerve growth regulation: nerve fiber formation by the superior cervical ganglion, the adrenal medulla, and locus coeruleus: similarities and differences as revealed by grafting. In: Elfvin LG (Ed.), *Autonomic Ganglia*. Chichester, John Wiley, pp. 507-522.

92. Gash DM, Notter MFO, Bing G, Kordower JH. (1986). Neural implants into primates: Studies employing differentiated neuroblastoma cells. In: Azmitia E, Bjorklund A (Eds.), *Cell and Tissue Transplantation into the Adult Brain*. New York, New York Academy of Sciences.

93. Jaeger CB. (1986). Morphological and immunocytochemical characteristics of PC12 cell grafts in rat brain. In: Azmitia E, Bjorklund A (Eds.), *Cell and Tissue Transplantation into the Adult Brain*. New York, New York Academy of Sciences.

94. Notter MFD, Kordower JH, Gash DM. (1986). Differentiated neuronal cell lines as donor tissue for transplantation into the central nervous system. In: Azmitia E, Bjorklund A (Eds.), *Cell and Tissue Transplantation into the Adult Brain*. New York, New York Academy of Sciences.

95. Freed WJ, Hoffer B, Olson L, Wyatt RJ. (1984). Transplantation of catecholamine-containing tissues to restore the functional capacity of the damaged nigrostriatal system. In: Sladek J, Gash D (Eds.), *Neuronal Transplants, Development and Function*. New York, Plenum Press, pp. 373–406.

96. Freed WJ, Morihisa JM, Spoor E, Hoffer B, Olson L, Seiger A, Wyatt RJ. (1981). Transplanted adrenal chromaffin cells in rat brain reduce lesion-induced rotational behaviour. *Nature* 292: 351–352.

97. Herrera-Marschitz M, Stromberg I, Olsson D, Olson L, Ungerstedt U. (1984). Adrenal medullary implants in the dopamine-denervated rat striatum. II. Acute behavior as a function of graft amount and location and its modulation by neuroleptics. *Brain Res* 297: 53–61.

98. Olson L, Bjorklund H, Hoffer B. (1984). Camera bulbi anterior: new vistas on a classical locus for neural tissue transplantation. In: Sladek J, Gash D (Eds.), *Neuronal Transplants, Development and Function*. New York, Plenum Press, pp. 125–165.

99. Olson L, Seiger A, Freedman R, Hoffer B. (1980). Chromaffin cells can innervate brain tissue: evidence from intraocular double grafts. *Exp Neurol* 70: 414–426.

100. Olson L, Stromberg I, Herrera-Marschitz M, Ungerstedt U, Ebendel T. (1985). Adrenal medullary tissue grafted to the dopamine-denervated rat striatum: Histochemical and functional effects of additions of nerve growth factor. In: Bjorklund A, Stenevi U (Eds.), *Neural Grafting in the Mammalian CNS*. Amsterdam, Elsevier, pp. 505–525.

101. Stromberg I, Herrera-Marschitz M, Hultgren L, Ungerstedt U, Olson L. (1984). Adrenal medullary implants to the dopamine-denervated rat striatum. I. Acute catecholamine levels in grafts and host caudate as determined by HPLC-electrochemistry and fluorescence histochemical image analysis. *Brain Res* 297: 47–51.

102. Stromberg I, Herrera-Marschitz M, Ungerstedt U, Ebendal T, Olson L. (1985). Chronic implants of chromaffin tissue into the dopamine-denervated striatum. Effects of NGF on graft survival, fiber growth and rotational behavior. *Exp Brain Res* 60: 335–349.

103. Backlund EO, Olson L, Seiger A, Lindvall O. (1986). Towards a transplantation therapy in Parkinson's disease: A progress report from ongoing clinical experiments. I. Surgical procedures. In: Azmitia E, Bjorklund A (Eds.), *Cell and Tissue Transplantation into the Adult Brain*. New York, New York Academy of Sciences.

104. Backlund EO, Grandberg PO, Hamberger B, Knutsson E, Martensson A, Sedvall G, Seiger A, Olson L. (1985). Transplantation of adrenal medullary tissue to striatum in parkinsonism: First clinical trials. *J Neurosurg* 62: 169–173.

105. Lindvall O, Olson L, Seiger A, Backlund E-O. (1986). Towards a transplantation therapy in Parkinson's Disease: A progress report from ongoing clinical experiments. II. Neurological Assessment. In: Azmitia E, Bjorklund A (Eds.), *Cell and Tissue Transplantation into the Adult Brain*. New York, New York Academy of Sciences.

106. Garrett ES, Nahmias C, Firnau G. (1984). Central dopaminergic pathways in hemiparkinsonism examined by positron emission emission tomography. *Can J Neurol Sci* 11: 174–198.
107. Ebendal T, Olson L, Seiger A. (1980). Nerve growth factors in the rat iris. *Nature* 286: 25–28.
108. Olson L. (1970). Fluorescence histochemical evidence for axonal growth and secretion from transplanted adrenal medullary tissue. *Histochemie* 22: 1–7.
109. Olson L, Seiger A. (1972). Brain tissue transplanted to the anterior chamber of the eye. I. Fluorescence histochemistry of immature catecholamine and 5-hydroxytryptamine neurons reinnervating the rat iris. *Z Zellforsch Mikrosk Anat* 135: 175–194.
110. Wagner HN Jr, Burns HD, Dannals RF, et al. (1983). Imaging dopamine receptors in the human brain by positron tomography. *Science* 221: 1264–1266.
111. Wong DF, Wagner HN Jr., et al. (1984). Effects of age on dopamine and serotonin receptors measured by positron tomography in the living human brain. *Science* 226: 1393–1396.
112. Burns RS, Chiueh CC, Markey SP, Ebert MH, Jacobowitz DM, Kopin IJ. (1983). A primate model of parkinsonism: Selective destruction of dopaminergic neurons in the pars compacta of the substantia nigra by N-methyl-4-phenyl-1,2,3,6-tetrahydro-pyridine. *Proc Natl Acad Sci* (USA) 8: 4546–4550.
113. Hallman H, Olson L, Jonsson G. (1984). Neurotoxicity of the meperidine analogue 1-methyl-4-phenyl-1,2,5,6-tetrahydropyridine on brain catecholamine neurons in the mouse. *Eur J Pharmacol* 97: 133–136.
114. Heikkila RE, Hess A, Duvoisin R. (1984). Dopaminergic neurotoxicity of 1-methyl-4-phenyl-1,2,5,6, tetrahydropyridine in mice. *Science* 224: 1451–1453.
115. Redmond DE, Sladek JR Jr, Roth RH, Collier TJ, Elsworth JD, Deutch AY, Haber S. (1986). Fetal neuronal grafts in monkeys given methyl-phenyltetrahydropyridine. *Lancet* 1: 1125–1127.
116. Barrow DL, Bakay R, Fiandoca MS. (1986). Biochemical and behavioral correction of MPTP Parkinson's like syndrome by fetal cell transplantation. In: Azmitia E, Bjorklund A (Eds.), *Cell and Tissue Transplantation into the Adult Brain*. New York, New York Academy of Sciences.

25
Rehabilitation Approach

SUSAN E. KASE
Parkside Home Health Services, Park Ridge, Illinois

CHERYL A. O'RIORDAN
Edward Hines, Jr. Veterans Administration Hospital, Hines, Illinois

Parkinson's disease is common, ranking closely behind cerebral vascular disease and arthritis in frequency as chronic diseases of late adulthood (1,2). It has been estimated that 22–25% of these patients become severely disabled or die within 5 years. Sixty percent become disabled or die within 10 years and the number advances to 80% for those living approximately 15 years or more (3,4). People are living longer, and during the past decade a great deal of attention has been directed toward the aged population in terms of their economic, physiological, social, psychological, and philosophic, as well as, medical needs.

Despite the multiple medical problems associated with Parkinson's disease, the authors believe that the basic human needs of the patient must be met if the process of rehabilitation is to be effective. These needs include acceptance, independence, and maintenance of control. Parkinson's disease, like many other chronic diseases, presents a challenge for rehabilitation therapists. This challenge is answered by sustaining the quality of life through the amelioration of physical limitations, by understanding preexisting family relationships, and by providing support.

The intent of rehabilitation is to restore the patient to the highest level of independent function. Goal planning should be designed jointly with the patient and family to include the patient's mental attitude, family involvement, multidisciplinary factors, treatment, and self-care.

MENTAL ATTITUDE

It has been reported that a significant progressive decline in intellectual functioning occurs in 41% of the patients afflicted for more than 10–15 years with

455

Parkinson's disease. This progressive dementia is associated with mental confusion, apathy, loss of recent memory, and lack of interest in the environment
(4). Rehabilitation therapists cannot ignore the fact that dementia will influence
the type of treatment approach designed for a specific patient based on his or
her ability to participate.

Asnis reports that a high incidence of depression is seen in the early stages of
this disease. This symptom occurs even when the disability is mild. Depression is
sometimes present in many other medical, gynecologic, and surgical disabilities
as well as in spinal cord injuries. But Asnis states that the incidence of depression
is higher in Parkinson's disease (5). Depression may develop from increased
dependency and frustration, or in response to a chronic disease or a biochemical
reaction (2,6).

Since Parkinson's disease leads to progressive impairment, depression has to
be addressed. If not, it will intensify the progressive decline of any gains already
achieved. Feelings of inadequacy, loss of self-esteem, hopelessness, withdrawal,
dependency, and lack of interest are all common to the parkinsonian patient.
The patient may often be seen blending into the backround without participation. He or she appears to be an "inanimate object" (3).

Minnigh refers to parkinsonian patients as introverted by nature. They are
usually older people who probably have become more inactive and less vigorous
(7). It is no wonder that a lack of motivation and overall lack of interest may
occur. For a patient beset by frustration and embarrassment, it often becomes
easier to withdraw than be a responsive, functioning person.

Ideally, a rehabilitation regimen is planned with a full circle effect in mind.
That is, it addresses physical components that have a direct effect on personal
body image, such as facial exercises, gait training, improved posture, mobility,
and self-care. If these physical components are restored, an increase in self-
esteem may occur. Subsequently there may be greater socialization and participation in life, thereby reducing depression and rounding out the circle through
continued physical conditioning.

Motivation then becomes the key to productive rehabilitation (8). Unless the
patient assumes responsibility for his or her treatment regimen and desires to
remain active and involved in life, rehabilitation efforts will be frustrating and
ineffective.

FAMILY INVOLVEMENT

In keeping with the recent emphasis on family/patient relationships, it is appropriate that rehabilitation be addressed with the family in mind. Indeed, the
family's importance and how it relates to therapy goals cannot be overstated.
Families play a major role in establishing the proper environment for the patient

with a debilitating disease. Often, far more critical than the disability itself are the reactions, attitudes, and quality of the relationships within this ecosystem in determining the success of rehabilitation and the acceptance by the patient and caregiver of life-style changes. Families are dynamic entities with established relationships, ways of dealing with everyday problems, and various attitudes toward illness (9).

Supporting members must willingly uphold the patient's role in the family structure. This is most important in stimulating the patient's motivation. The foundation of motivation rests on the premise of family cooperation through maintenance and restoration of the patient in his or her role as an active participant. It is equally important that the patient meet his or her responsibility in making a voluntary effort to achieve maximal gains (3,9).

Since Parkinson's disease affects the aging population, the patient often becomes dependent on an ailing spouse or middle-aged children occupied with rearing their own families (8). The patient experiences dependency on others in addition to suffering physical losses (3).

It is not abnormal for additional family stresses and depression to result from these interactions (8). A critical issue is the ability of the family unit to organize itself during this crisis. Versluys states that "organized families usually have: had previous experience and success in mediating family members; good marital adjustment; a family history of meeting problems through interfamily discussions and problem solving." They will be supportive by challenging and encouraging the patient to continue his or her role in the family and involving the patient in the decision-making process. Spouses or caregivers who communicate attitudes of essential worth to the patient help to stabilize self-concept, foster a positive attitude toward the future, and facilitate the maintenance of rehabilitation gains (9).

According to Versluys, an inadequately organized family does not demonstrate the ability to manage stress. The rigid behavior of its members may create more problems. Lack of organization is present as well as lack of concern for others. These caregivers' responses will be negative "leading to overprotectiveness, encouragement of dependency, neglect, avoidance of future planning, excessive and/or inappropriate demands and punitive action towards the patient" (9).

The patient is often abused knowingly or unknowingly by both family members and health professionals. The type of failure most often manifested is known as passive neglect. Examples of this include the omission of assistive follow-through with a home exercise program, or treatment of the patient as a nonentity in family discussions. Verbal whipping is the next most common form of abuse followed by active neglect. Examples would be withholding bathroom assistance, or noncompliance in utilizing an assistive device to aid in independence. Actual physical abuse may also be seen (10).

Understanding and cooperation on the part of patient and family are important in maintaining a quality of life that is meaningful for all. Support groups assisting in this effort are available throughout the country. Literature can be obtained through national Parkinson's disease associations. Local groups provide opportunities for socialization and education as well as disseminating additional supportive information.

TEAM APPROACH

"Rehabilitation staff are nurturing people" (9). They are healing, caring people dedicated to the relief of pain and discomfort. They can provide the means to a safe and productive life within the limits of the patient's disability.

Through the practice of administering and serving, the staff is dedicated to the commitment involved in long-term treatment. Innocently enough, they may automatically expect caregivers to accommodate and cooperate readily to their every suggestion. Values, attitudes, and family dynamics may not have been considered. So often neglected in this plan is the realization that not all families have the coping mechanisms required to comprehend the initial diagnosis of a chronic disabling disease. Subsequently, they may appear as uncooperative or unmotivated in their attempts to deal with it (9).

Inquiring families often are made to feel guilty about their inadequacies, intrusions, reluctance, and anxieties by the busy ward staff and crowded therapy departments. "Staff make value judgements concerning family relationships, note neurotic tendencies, call attention to the refusal to make necessary home adjustments or to order equipment on time" (9). Subsequently staff, while intending to be attentive to the patient and realizing the adjustment needs of that individual, may also expect the family to cope instantly and respond positively. Many are unable to do so (9). Though different from the patient's, a family's adjustment may be as painful and long.

There must be a cooperative effort among the entire rehabilitation team to improve the patient's capacity to interact physically and emotionally with his or her environment and to include the family as active, informed team members (1).

Therapists should be available and empathetic with caregivers and be able to identify and appreciate their feelings. Families need to realize the value of short-term goals, such as providing a built-up spoon handle to facilitate independent eating. If the physical and emotional environment does not support bringing the patient home, the caregivers should not be made to feel guilty about placement decisions, but be encouraged to maintain as much of a relationship as possible. Team members should be available to offer genuine support and understanding. They should also keep families informed of treatments, tests, procedures, and facts about the disease and fill in the information gaps left by others.

TREATMENT

Rehabilitation as an adjunct to medication focuses on maintaining or improving the quality of life in persons with acute or chronic disease. It also strives to keep that person safely functional within the limits of his or her disability.

In the treatment of Parkinson's disease, occupational and physical therapists are concerned with the primary issues of rigidity, bradykinesia, and the loss of postural reflexes. Tremor that presents more as a social embarrassment to the patient does not in itself limit the patient physically except in rare instances.

Rigidity is the most common impairment produced by the disease (15). It is estimated that between 78 and 85% of patients will develop rigidity (2). Lead-pipe or cogwheel rigidity involves the extrapyramidal system and produces increased muscle tone in both agonist and antagonist muscle groups, leading the patient to complain of stiffness and heaviness in the arms and legs. This alteration of tone exists not only peripherally but also involves the face and trunk and results in a simian posture, facial masking, slurred and monotonous speech, along with suppressed shallow breathing. Contractures may be present in neck, hands, and feet.

Bradykinesia, slowness of movement, and loss of agility often result in the inability to initiate motor activities or adjust movements already in progress. As control of precise motor skills diminishes so does the ability to perform daily routines independently. Even the simplest of activities require concentrated effort to complete: grooming, rolling over in bed, handling money, rising from a chair, dressing, manipulating fasteners, walking through a doorway, chewing, and swallowing. Fine hand coordination is noticeably affected, resulting in micrographia. Precise repetitive activities such as tying shoes and buttoning clothes are extremely taxing.

This general immobility and paucity of movement can result in great frustration for the patient's family since virtually every task attempted becomes time-consuming and burdensome. It is important that the caregiver become aware, when planning activities, of the abrupt losses of response relative to doses of levodopa (L-dopa) preparations. The patient's performance can fluctuate from complete control to no control. These fluctuations are of two basic types (a) wearing off type in which the effectiveness of the medication wears off, for example after 3 rather than 4 hours; and (b) on–off phenomena or yo-yoing type in which there is acute worsening then improvement followed by worsening. On the other hand, the positive effects of L-dopa are noticeable: diminished rigidity, reduced contractures, and improved balance and coordination (6).

Along with rigidity and bradykinesia, postural instability is the third criterion therapists consider in establishing a plan of care (1). Postural instability results in the patient's inability to compensate quickly enough for changes in direction secondary to impairment of postural reflexes. Gautherier's study "showed postural instability to be the most significant cause of activities of daily living impairment" (11). The center of gravity tends to be displaced forward secondary to the rigidly flexed head and trunk posture. This makes the patient feel insecure. Most patients are unable to correct a loss of balance forward or backward by the quickly needed arm or leg adjustments. Subsequently and unpredictably frequent falls occur. Protective or righting reactions are not exhibited.

Gait, one of the most noticeable of the deteriorations, is described as robot-like and automatic. There is little or no arm swing or head, trunk, and pelvic rotation. Steps are slow, shuffling, and festinating. Patients complain of start hesitation, stalling, or the feeling of being frozen to one spot with heaviness in the legs. Canes and walkers may be unsafe and become a handicap to the patient, while wheelchairs may be therapeutically indicated but emotionally undesirable.

Considering the above-mentioned problems, the authors' primary rehabilitation goals are as follows.

1. To maintain or increase active and passive range of motion, especially extension, and to prevent contractures by stretching tight muscles
2. To improve speed, flexibility, dexterity, and coordination of motor movements and repetitive tasks
3. To enhance awareness of posture and balance losses and correct where possible
4. To restore chest expansion/contraction not only as an end in itself, but to encourage relaxation and increase voice volume
5. To review gait with particular emphasis on increasing step length, widening the base of support, increasing the range of hip flexion, enhancing reciprocal arm movements, and improving stops, starts, and turns
6. To upgrade activities of daily living, teach simplification of tasks and conservation of energy techniques for the patient and caregiver
7. To function as a support, teacher, and information source for the patient, family, and medical team

The following secondary gains of rehabilitation are obtained through increased activity: decreasing the incidence of constipation, pneumonia, and osteoporosis; increasing peripheral circulation, which decreases thrombi and prevents decubiti and urinary calculi.

Despite current pharmacologic regimens, patients with Parkinson's disease do experience impairments in activities of daily living that increase as the disease advances (11). Rehabilitation approaches to this disease are extensive. One approach involves one-to-one techniques, such as proprioceptive neuromuscular facilitation (PNF), Rood, or Bobath theoretical applications (11). This type of treatment program is best suited to meet the patient's particular needs when stress may affect performance and inhibit group interaction (12–14). Another treatment direction is group therapy sessions. These provide a social milieu where patients relearn how to interact and practice skills in a safe, supportive environment with peer group reinforcement (8). Lastly, there is the instruction and support afforded by home care organizations which address particular problems in the home situation. No matter which approach is assumed, motivation of the patient becomes the key to his or her rehabilitation.

Some of the specialized treatment procedures to achieve rehabilitation goals focus on electrical muscle stimulation, proprioceptive stimulation, sensory integration, and PNF techniques.

Some examples of PNF include use of rhythmic initiation to improve the patient's ability to initiate movement (14). Slow reversal techniques are used to enhance the patient's awareness of movement and to minimize cocontraction of muscle groups. Patterning techniques are used to incorporate diagonal and rotational components into coordinated movement.

Wroe and Greer present an excellent example of incorporating neck and trunk rotation exercises into treatment (14). They promote using wide arcs of motion with the patient seated in an armless swivel rocker. This positioning increases mobility and extension of the neck and trunk, improves sitting balance, reduces tone in the limbs, and stimulates the semicircular canals.

Repetitive exercises with the trunk can be used to facilitate a total associated extensor response, thereby decreasing a flexed posture. To encourage motivation and participation, activities such as ball throwing, balance exercises, trunk rotation and gait training, possibly to music or a metronome, can be performed with several patients together (12,14). Activities that initiate and halt movement—getting in and out of a chair, sitting up from a supine position, and rolling over into a prone position—should be incorporated, not only as a flexibility routine, but also as a facilitator to activities of daily living (1,14).

Davis uses timed evaluations of the patient's activities such as writing, dressing, moving, and repeated rapid movements (1). Pulleys are used for upper extremity reciprocal movements and active and passive range of motion in a posture that facilitates trunk extension rather than flexion. In addition to repeated movements, pulleys can also be used for limb and trunk rotation and balance by placing the patient in diagonal patterns.

Static and dynamic balance activities are facilitated in group performance. Some examples are standing in a circle holding hands, standing on one leg, or rocking back and forth on heels and then toes while the group holds hands. Games that require coordination and interaction between groups of patients are excellent (1).

It is recommended that patients who are mildly impaired participate in senior exercise groups at local community facilities. Moderately or severely involved patients should participate in a hospital or rehabilitation program with follow-through utilizing a home program. Home health therapists can design individual programs while working directly with the patient in a home setting. Gordon and Oster state that fatigue occurs as a result of frustration and expenditure of maximum effort against tremors, rigidity, and bradykinesia (15). Therefore, frequent rest periods should be included in the treatment program both in the hospital setting and at home.

The patient must be encouraged at all times to maintain independence. There is a natural tendency for friends and family to be overprotective and to foster reduction in general mobility. This overprotectiveness often decreases achievable levels of independence (9,12,13).

SELF-CARE

A structured exercise session each day administered by the patient, family member, or therapist is necessary and an ideal expectation. One can also think in terms of improving joint range of motion, flexibility, and balance through activities of daily living. These in themselves are miniexercise routines. Every posture or task performed during the day can have its own exercise component. Often these are more pleasurable, meaningful, and instantly rewarding to perform than structured isolated routines designed by therapists. Thus, it becomes essential to orient the patient to these activities of daily living exercise concepts in the hope that a twofold purpose will be realized: rehabilitation goals will be accomplished and the patient will achieve a sense of productive functioning and independence. Activities of daily living might be as "simple" as getting dressed, eating, walking from the bedroom to the kitchen table, shaving, combing hair, folding laundry, doing dishes, playing cards, writing letters, reading the paper. Other skills can be more "complex" such as gardening, making beds, and cleaning house. The efforts of the therapists should center on making these tasks as attainable as possible with the least amount of energy expenditure and the greatest amount of safety.

Often, solutions involve adaptations or additions to a patient's environmental setting, such as removal of clutter, scatter rugs, door sills, fragile objects, sharp-cornered furniture, or the addition of built-up handles on pens and utensils, wheelchairs, bath benches, raised toilet seats, grab bars, reachers, button hooks, plate guards, rocker knives, high chairs, and well-lit hallways and rooms.

Writing letters and doing word games and puzzles can be excellent and functional exercises for fine hand coordination and mental stimulation. It would be simpler and more efficient to place loose change in a coin purse before placing in the pocket, or just filling a glass half full to avoid spills. What better way to do range-of-motion exercises than to dress daily. Playing catch with a dog or children can improve coordination and flexibility.

It will be helpful for the family to work out a satisfactory time schedule for the patient to allow for independent completion of tasks. Individuals with

Parkinson's disease cannot be hurried since this hinders performance. Assisting the patient with dressing, feeding, and washing may occasionally be imposed simply to save time but does tend to promote dependency. This requires great patience and cooperation on the part of the caregivers. Pacing activities throughout the day to allow for a combination of rest and activity becomes important in the face of fluctuating energy levels. Often it helps to have a plan for the day written out in detail that includes all activities from rising in the morning to retiring at night.

Duvoisin reported that "one patient complained to me that getting out of a deep upholstered chair required 'a campaign of instruction to every muscle involved'" (17). The plight of the parkinsonian patient is a desperate one, fraught with frustration, embarrassment, and loneliness. Physical and occupational therapists can serve as a new beginning for these people by breaking down the barriers that create this desperation. Therapists recognize the reality of Parkinson's disease as a progressive entity. However, there is optimism within the limitations of this disease. Even the smallest gains made through the combined rehabilitation efforts of the family, patient, and medical team can be integrated into a more meaningful life.

REFERENCES

1. Davis JC. (1977). Team management of Parkinson's disease. *Am J Occup Ther* 31: 300–308.
2. Perlik SJ, Koller WC, Weiner WJ, Nausieda PA, Klawans HL. (1980). Parkinsonism: Is your treatment appropriate? *Geriatrics* 35: 65–70, 74.
3. Greer M. (1976). How to achieve maximum benefit for the patient with Parkinson's disease. *Geriatrics* 31: 89–96.
4. Selby G. (1977). The natural history of Parkinson's disease. *Aust Fam Physician* 13: 1–3.
5. Asnis G. (1977). Parkinson's disease, depression and ECT: a review and case study. *Am J Psychiatry* 134: 191–195.
6. Stewart RM. (1981). Parkinson's disease: new treatments. *Compr Ther* 7: 38–44.
7. Minnigh EC. Part II. (1971). The Northwestern University concept of rehabilitation through group physical therapy. *Rehab Lit* 32: 38–39, 50.
8. Szekely BC, Neiberg Kosanovich N, Sheppard W. (1982). Adjunctive treatment in Parkinson's disease: physical therapy and comprehensive group therapy. *Rehab Lit* 43: 72–76.
9. Versluys H. (1980). Physical rehabilitation and family dynamics. *Rehab Lit* 41: 56–58.
10. Hickey T, Douglass RL. (1981). Mistreatment of the elderly in the domestic setting: an exploratory study. *Am J Publ Health* 71: 500–507.
11. Gauthier L, Gauthier S. (1983). Functional rehabilitation of patients with Parkinson's disease. *Physiother Can* 25: 220–222.

12. Godwin-Austen R. (1975). The treatment of parkinsonism. *Practitioner* 215: 445–451.
13. McFarland RH. (1975). Treating parkinsonism in the era of levodopa. *Am Fam Pract* 12: 99–104.
14. Wroe MA, Greer M. (1973). Parkinson's disease and physical therapy. *Physical Ther* 53: 849–855.
15. Gordon VC, Oster C. (1974). Rehabilitation of the patient with Parkinson's disease. *J Am Osteopath Assoc* 74: 307.
16. Marx JL. (1979). Parkinson's disease: search for better therapies. *Science* 203: 737–738.
17. Duvoisin RC. (1978). *Parkinson's Disease: A Guide for Patient and Family*. New York, Raven Press.

26
Psychosocial Aspects

BONNIE E. LEVIN and WILLIAM J. WEINER
University of Miami School of Medicine, Miami, Florida

When an individual develops a chronic, degenerative disease, he or she not only must face a myriad of physical changes, but must also confront significant psychologic and social changes (Davis, 1963). These changes are often subtle and difficult for the patient to express to his or her physician. Yet research investigating the impact of chronic illness has shown that psychologic and social factors may significantly increase disability and interfere with acceptance and adjustment to the disease (Cobb, 1976). These observations have led many to conclude that more attention must be directed toward certain psychosocial factors because their neglect will interfere with even the best medical therapeutic programs (Hyman, 1972).

Although there is a large current literature describing the motor symptoms of Parkinson's disease, relatively few investigations have dealt with the psychosocial aspects of the disorder. Even less attention has been paid to the patient's family and the psychosocial changes they inevitably face as a result of their spouse's or loved one's physical condition (Miles, 1979). The paucity of literature in these areas may be due to the widespread belief that if motor symptoms are pharmacologically remediated, social and psychological functions will improve as well. However, research has not shown this to be the case. Although treatment with dopaminergic agents significantly decreases mortality and remediates motor symptoms, levodopa (L-dopa) alone does not reverse the decline in social functioning (Singer, 1974). Furthermore, the effect of levodopa on the level of functioning may even be reduced by a number of social and psychologic aspects of chronic illness.

465

This chapter reviews the psychosocial aspects of Parkinson's disease. Practical intervention strategies directed toward maximizing physicial, psychologic and social wellbeing of patients and their families are proposed for three different stages of Parkinson's disease.

NEWLY DIAGNOSED AND MILDLY AFFECTED PATIENTS

In unilateral stage 1 Parkinson's disease, facial expression is usually normal and the posture is erect. The most common initial manifestation is an involuntary resting tremor of one extremity. The tremor is often quite disturbing to patients and usually brings them to the attention of their physician. Even though the early tremor rarely interferes with the activities of daily living, the involuntary nature of the movement is quite distressing and often embarrasses the patient. Patients often report that they are unable to button their shirts, write accurately, or cut their food. However if one closely observes these patients, it is usually apparent that when the patient attempts to use the involved extremity other parkinsonian signs besides tremor, such as bradykinesia and rigidity, underlie the disability.

Another common complaint of early Parkinson's disease patients is difficulty using an extremity, particularly the upper limbs. When patients walk, they may note that the arm of the affected side does not swing as readily. They may also report that the lower extremity drags. Limb complaints may include stiffness or tightness of the fingers, difficulty manipulating the fingers for activities that require fine finger dexterity, alterations in handwriting or a sense of slowness when attempting to use the extremity. These symptoms have often been present for several years but will be better tolerated than involuntary movements such as tremor.

In stage 2 Parkinson's disease (bilateral involvement) there may be a masked face, and decreased eye blinking. A slight simian posture may be present when the patient stands and there is usually decreased arm swing. Patients usually report some slowness associated with their daily activities such as increased time for dressing, hygienic activities, rising from chairs, and feeding themselves.

Drug therapy should be administered according to the severity of symptoms. Anticholinergics are administered for control of tremor but they often produce side effects such as dry mouth, blurred vision, urinary hesitancy, and occasional forgetfulness. Amantadine hydrochloride is the treatment of choice for bradykinesia. Amantadine has little effect on normal renal function and its most common side effect is the appearance of livido reticularis. When the patient's symptoms are more severe, levodopa/carbidopa (Sinemet) and bromocriptine (Parlodel) are started. Short-term administration of levodopa/carbidopa may initially produce some nausea and anorexia, but the long-term administration may produce more severe complications such as dyskinesias, "on-off," and a behavioral syndrome including vivid nightmares and paranoid confusional states. Bromocriptine is often useful if side effects with levodopa/carbidopa are noted. Both drugs can be titrated together for maximum motor improvement and minimal side effects.

Depressive symptoms are also common among these patients. Estimates of parkinsonian-related depression range from 30% (Liberman, 1979) to 90% (Mindham, 1970). It has been noted that depression is often an initial misdiagnosis in the early stages of the disease (Rabins, 1982; Paulson, 1981). This may be due to a number of overlapping symptoms shared by both parkinsonism and depression. Both disorders may present with motor retardation, apathy, weight loss, intellectual decline, diminished energy, memory difficulties, and a depressed or saddened appearance.

It has often been stated that the depression experienced by a Parkinson's disease patient is reactive: a realistic response to knowing that one has a chronic, progressive disease. This may be true for many patients but more recent evidence suggests that for at least some patients, depression may be due to an underlying organic process (Levin, Rodriguez and Weiner, 1986). In depth, prospective neuropsychological testing is needed to determine whether depressive symptoms and other cognitive impairments are reactive or specific to the disease process.

Psychosocial Adjustments

The way patients react to the diagnosis of Parkinson's disease depends in part on factors such as their ability to handle stress and previous response to life crises. A common reaction may be denial, which may lead the individual to get a second opinion or, seek out multiple experts in an effort to obtain less threatening medical advice (Blumenfield, 1977). Others may superficially accept the diagnosis but remain unwilling to learn about the problems associated with the disease or think about the need for future adjustment.

In early Parkinson's disease, the psychologic changes a patient experiences may be more devastating and disabling than the actual motor disability. At a time when other people are getting ready to retire and enjoy their independence and freedom, parkinsonian patients must face the prospect of being physically and economically dependent (Nanton, 1985). For many, the illness represents a significant life change and it is a time when feelings of loss of control and competence may predominate. Feelings of anger and guilt associated with becoming a burden may also be expressed.

For the spouse, the effect of a husband or wife's chronic illness superimposed on the often difficult aging process can be a confusing and overwhelming experience. Feelings of loss of control and helplessness may arise because the cause of Parkinson's disease is unknown and the illness is a progressive, degenerative condition with an unpredictable course. The spouse or caregiver may express sadness, disappointment, or fear over the prospect of psychosocial adjustments.

In the early stages, a family's needs and feelings of distress are often only superficially acknowledged because it is easy for others to rationalize that their distress is a "natural" response to hearing that their loved one is afflicted with a serious illness. However, recognition of a family's needs and early intervention are necessary if the family is to become the primary and emotionally healthy support system for the patient. Furthermore, patients who are most successful in handling their parkinsonism have been shown to have a good working relationships with health care professionals (Duvoisin, 1984).

A thorough and frank discussion of the diagnosis, the progressive nature of the illness and realistic prognosis is essential for both the patient and his or her family. A willingness to discuss issues related to the disease by exhibiting a frank and open attitude will minimize feelings of alienation and helplessness. Furthermore, building an open and trusting relationship in the early stage of the illness will become an important source of support during more critical phases of the disease.

Intervention Strategies

In a recent article, Geronemus (1980) outlined several goals for early intervention strategies for a group of chronic multiple sclerosis patients. Multiple sclerosis patients are younger than Parkinson's disease patients, but the intervention strategies used are relevant because both groups share a number of common features: both have a chronic, progressive degenerative disease with an uncertain future characterized by increasing immobility and dependency on others. For patients with these illnesses, it is important for health care professionals to bring out and support the healthy and productive aspects of patient–family interactions while minimizing helpless and dependent "patient" behaviors. A second goal is to help the individual and family confront the diagnosis and explore its meaning for the individual and the family unit. Third, by being directed away from feelings of continual crisis and more toward openly expressing feelings and apprehensions associated with the disease, the family will be in a better position to learn about parkinsonism and establish a reality from which the patient and family may begin to adjust.

Most investigators agree that these issues can best be addressed by group therapy (support groups). The group may consist of either patients alone or patients with their spouses or other family members. Group treatment permits the individual to become involved in a social support system in which patients may learn to adjust to the diagnosis of Parkinson's disease and share their experience with others in similar situations. Nanton (1985) reported that support groups also increase motivation and willingness to pursue self-care. A second function of a treatment group is to disseminate information. The group can serve as a vital educational resource, addressing issues such as availability of services in the community, how to deal effectively with health care professionals in the medical system, medication side effects, and how to overcome many of the physical inconveniences associated with Parkinson's disease.

MODERATELY DISABLED PATIENTS

Parkinsonian patients with moderate disability (stages 3 and 4) are beginning to experience difficulties with gait and balance. They report difficulty walking and note that their stride has become shorter. They occasionally may shuffle and experience difficulty with turning and balance. Postural balance difficulties may also present as frequent falls with no warning. These patients also note the progressive development of an inability to stop their forward or backward progress (propulsion and retropulsion). Patients in this group walk forward but are unable to stop without the support of an object, such as a wall or a chair. Patients also report difficulty maneuvering out of corners of rooms, and entering and exiting through doors. They note that slight postural perturbations such as back slaps or jostling lead to a fall.

Many patients with stage 4 disease experience the side effects of chronic dopaminergic medication. The most troublesome long-term side effect for patients is the "on–off effect" characterized by sudden motor fluctuations. This phenomenon is often disabling and fear provoking. During the "on" phase patients are quite mobile and able to carry out activities outside the home such as shopping. However, during the "off" phase, the same patient becomes fully disabled and cannot walk, rise from a chair, or use his or her hands meaningfully. Since the "on–off" effect is unpredictable, the patient must plan ahead without knowing when he or she will be able to perform certain activities. Patients may find themselves in dangerous situations such as crossing the street when the off phenomenon occurs.

Dyskinesias are another important drug-induced problem in stage 3-4 Parkinson's disease. These are usually choreiform in nature: patients report "dance-like" movements of the limbs, chewing movements of the lower jaw, a darting tongue, swaying when walking, and to and from movements of the head and neck. These dyskineasias are a symptom of dopaminergic overactivity. Usually the family is more concerned about these movements and the patient often associates them with "good" nonparkinsonian times.

Drug-induced behavioral problems include insomnia, vivid nightmares, nocturnal vocalizations, nonthreatening visual hallucinations, delusions, and paranoid confusional states. The insomnia can involve both difficulty falling asleep and frequent night-time awakenings. Patients will often report that although they did not normally remember their dreams, they are now extraordinarily vivid. Nocturnal vocalizations are reported by the bed partner and consist of loud shouting during sleep often associated with flailing of the arms and/or legs. These events can interrupt sleep. Nonthreatening visual hallucinations are the most common type of hallucination seen in Parkinson's disease patients. These are often described as involving family members, strangers, animals, and shadows that become animate objects.

Psychosocial Adjustments

Once Parkinson's disease symptoms are clearly present to the point of reducing the patient's capacity to maintain an independent lifestyle, it becomes necessary to restructure the goals and expectations placed on patients by themselves and their families. It becomes necessary to restructure roles and role relationships, a task that produces considerable conflict for everyone involved (Geroremus, 1980). It is a time when the distinction between a normally functioning adult and a disabled patient with a chronic disease may become blurred.

The variability of parkinsonian symptoms will also create stress and tension in the patient's caregiver: one minute the patient may be able to do something for himself, the next moment he cannot (Szkeley et al., 1962). These situations are often frustrating and cause a partner to lose his or her temper, resulting in increased guilt for not being patient with someone who is afflicted with a chronic disease. In addition, secondary effects of Parkinson's disease such as speech impairment, fatigue, and loss of facial expression often make communication with family members and friends difficult. Mild cognitive difficulties such as slowed reaction time, attentional difficulties, difficulty switching set and short-term memory problems will also interfere with communication skills.

This situation is further compounded by depressive symptoms experienced by as many as 40% of Parkinson's disease patients. Feelings of depression expressed by parkinsonian patients may present as increased distractibility, irritability, apathy, lethargy, pessimism, or feelings of dissatisfaction. These emotional changes will negatively affect interpersonal relationships and ultimately interfere with the feelings of intimacy shared by a couple. This places considerable strain on both the patient and his or her partner, whose resources for coping are already stressed. Although increased emotional support is needed, Nanton (1985) points out that a more likely trend is a general tendency toward loss of friends and social and recreational activities.

Families of Parkinson's disease patients often feel just as isolated and in need of support as patients. Feelings of anger and resentment at their new roles and responsibilities are frequently expressed. During this time there may be economic concerns along with anxiety and fear of anticipated changes.

Intervention Strategies

The type of therapeutic intervention at this stage depends upon the patient's and family's needs. At a time when social withdrawal and isolation frequently occur, group therapy permits the individual to interact and express frustrations with others in a safe, nurturant environment with peer group support (Szekely et al., 1982). Long-term goals should include helping patients to (a) accept their disability and physical limitations while promoting a healthy self image; (b) accept changing role relationships while maintaining feelings of independence and self-esteem; (c) develop effective strategies for coping with emotionally stressful situation (Geronemus, 1980); (d) express fears and concerns about parkinsonism while correcting myths and misconceptions about the disease.

Treatment programs for family groups offer them a unique opportunity to interact with other physically healthy individuals who must confront similar issues with their loved ones. Long-term therapeutic goals for members of Parkinson's disease family groups are (a) understanding the patients' disability and the accompanying behavioral changes while assisting nondisabled family members in developing effective methods for coping with these changes and with feelings such as anger and distress; (b) recognizing and alleviating guilt felt by nonaffected individuals who are healthy and who feel helpless as they watch a loved one suffer from a chronic disease; (c) understanding that other non-affected family members have equally important and valid needs that require attention; (d) learning how to set limits on the patient while still promoting feelings of independence and self-esteem.

To those who would not benefit from group treatment, individual therapy using the same goals outlined above can also be used as an effective means of intervention. This would be the treatment of choice for those who have a pre-existing psychiatric problem that would either disrupt or resist group dynamics or when the family is dysfunctional and cannot tolerate the effect of a group. Other individuals may be so socially isolated that a group may be perceived as threatening and cause the family to withdraw even more.

SEVERELY DISABLED PATIENTS

Patients with Parkinson's disease who have reached stage 5 are severely disabled. These patients are wheelchair or bed-bound and require great assistance in standing. Even then, they may be unable to take any steps by themselves. They may not be able to stand independently. Stage 5 patients may be totally dependent for their activities of daily living on support personnel, either family or medical staff. Speech difficulties with these patients are often pronounced, and it is often difficult to understand their speech because of the low tonal volume and the monotonous quality. These patients may eventually develop mild contractures, and are subject to decubitus ulcers and recurrent urinary tract infections.

Other symptoms of Parkinson's disease prevalent in patients with all levels of disability include a sense of fatigue. Patients often note that they feel more tired than usual, and it seems to take more effort to perform certain tasks. Patients often describe a sense of discomfort in the posterior cervical region, low back, and shoulders, which consists of a dull-tight aching pain. As Parkinson's disease progresses, patients often report symptoms of autonomic instability, including extreme sensations of heat and cold; diaphoresis, unrelated to physical activity, often of a drenching nature; a flushing of the skin, which at times can be alarming to the patients and their family.

Since the advent of effective drug therapy, all Parkinson's disease patients do not become totally dependent or bed-bound. However, as the disease progresses, patients experience less and less "on" time and more totally dependent time. "End stage" Parkinson's disease does not itself lead to death. However Parkinson's disease patients often experience increasing dysphagia that can lead to recurrent aspiration pneumonia, a possible cause of death. In addition poor respiratory excursion can also contribute to fatal pneumonia. Other contributing terminal events can include systemic infections secondary to decubitus ulcers and urinary tract infections. Although in earlier stages of Parkinson's disease physical therapy and speech therapy can be useful, in end-stage Parkinson's disease these treatment modalities are less effective.

Psychosocial Adjustments

The end stage of Parkinson's disease often requires that major decisions and adjustments be made at a time when the stress and strain associated with chronic disease appear insurmountable. It is a time when the long-term effects of the illness are felt most strongly and may result in real social, economic, and psychological changes. Previously held roles may have to be substantially modified or given up altogether. For younger Parkinson's disease patients, this may mean unanticipated financial difficulties (Nanton, 1985).

It may also be necessary to turn to community-based services for additional assistance. Sitter services, day and/or night attendants, private nurses, home help services may be necessary if the patient is to remain at home. In other cases, the patient with advanced Parkinson's disease may become too much of a burden for an elderly spouse and placement in a custodial or chronic care facility may have to be considered.

As symptoms progress, self-imposed social isolation and withdrawal may increase. The disease, once only a minor disruption to the patient's and caregivers' lives, becomes a prime focus of their day-to-day existence (Nanton, 1985). As practical solutions to daily problems become difficult to find, feelings of helplessness, depression, and despair abound.

The health care professional should frequently reassess the patient's and family's resources and capacity for coping with the physical and emotional concomitants of far advanced Parkinson's disease. Intervention at this stage involves several levels: (a) to identify real or potential crises and propose solutions to resolve or alleviate them; (b) to assist the family in reaching the healthiest solution while simultaneously dealing with real and imagined fears and feelings of guilt involved in planning for change; and (c) to help the family carry through difficult decisions (Geronemus, 1980).

Patients with stage 5 Parkinson's disease and their families will continue to benefit greatly from education regarding patient care and treatment. For patients who are mobile, group therapy is still the best opportunity to learn more about advanced Parkinson's disease and to socialize with other severely disabled patients and their families. Unlike the other earlier stages of the disease, the group may focus on issues related to survival and creative solutions to accomplish daily activities. Chafetz (1955) reported that group members who were incapacitated but able to carry out productive activities stimulated other patients to strive for better adjustment.

For immobile patients, home visits may be the only resource for health care information and individual psychotherapy. When staff time and expenses are limited and do not permit individual visits, every effort should be made by the family member either to join a group or seek out individual therapy. The need for ongoing emotional support is critical. Feeling of ambivalence, conflict, anger, and guilt are normal and need to be ventilated. The group experience will provide an opportunity to air feelings and fears, while learning how others are handling the same experiences.

REFERENCES

Blumenfield MD. (1977). The psychological reactions to physical illness. In: Simmons R, Pardes H (Eds.), *Understanding Human Behavior in Health and Illness*. Baltimore, Williams and Wilkins Co.

Chafetz ME, Bernstein N, Sharpe W, Schwab R. (1955). Short-term group therapy of patients with Parkinson's disease. *N Engl J Med* 253(22): 961–964.

Cobb S. (1976). Social support as a moderator of life stress. *Psychoso Med* 38(5): 300–314.

Davis F. (1963). *Passage Through Crisis*. New York, Bobbs-Merrill.

Duvoisin RC. (1984). *Parkinson's Disease. A Guide for Patient and Family*. New York, Raven Press.

Geronemus F. (1980). The role of the social worker in the comprehensive long-term care of multiple sclerosis patients. *Neurology* 30(2): 48–54.

Hyman MD. (1972). Sociopsychological obstacles to L-dopa therapy that may limit effectiveness in parkinsonism. *J Am Geriatr Soc* 20: 200–208.

Levin BE, Rodriguez ML, Weiner WJ. (1986). Depression in Parkinson's disease. *Neurology* 36; 134 (abst).

Liberman A, Dziatolowski M, Kupersmith M, Serby M, Goodgold A, Korein J, Goldstein M. (1979). Dementia in Parkinson's disease. *Ann Neurol* 6: 355–359.

Miles A. (1972). Some psycho-social consequences of multiple sclerosis: problems of social interaction and group identity. *Br J Med Psychol* 552: 321–331.

Mindham RHS. (1970). Psychiatric syndromes in parkinsonism. *J Neurol Neurosurg Psychiatry* 30: 88–91.

Nanton V. (1985). The consequences of Parkinson's disease–needs, provisions and initiatives. *J R Soc Health* 105(2): 52–54.

Paulson GW. (1981). The psychological aspects of parkinsonism. *Ohio State Med J* 77: 711–717.

Rabins P. (1982). Psychopathology of Parkinson's disease. *Compr Psychiatr* 23: 421–429.

Singer E. (1973). Social costs of Parkinson's disease. *J Chron Dis* 26: 243–254.

Singer E. (1974). The effect of treatment with levodopa on Parkinson patients' social functioning and outlook on life. *J Chron Dis* 27(11): 581–584.

Szkely BC, Kosanovich NN, Sheppard W. (1982). Adjunctive treatment in Parkinson's disease: physical therapy and comprehensive group therapy. *Rehab Lit* 43: 72–76.

Appendix

HOEHN AND YAHR SCALE OF CLINICAL STAGES

Stage	Signs
0	No clinical signs evident
1	Unilateral involvement only
2	Bilateral involvement only
3	First evidence of impaired postural and righting reflexes by examination or a history of poor balance, falls, etc. Disability is mild to moderate.
4	Fully developed severe disease; disability marked
5	Confinement to bed or wheelchair

Source: Hoehn MM, Yahr MD. (1967). *Neurology* 17(5): 427–442.

EVALUATION OF DISABILITY IN PARKINSON'S DISEASE

All points are graded on a scale of 0-4 of increasing severity (0.5 values can be used if patient's condition falls between the following categories).

1. Facial expression:
    A. Facial Masking:
        0 – none
        1 – decreased or absent eye blinking
        2 – mild facial masking

          3 – moderate facial masking

          4 – no movements of face

   B. Convergence and Upward Gaze:

          0 – normal

          1 – mild

          2 – moderate

          3 – severe

          4 – no movement

2.   Seborrhea:

          0 – normal

          1 – slightly increased oiliness of skin

          2 – oiliness of skin with dry, scaly patches

          3 – moderate seborrheic dermatitis

          4 – severe seborrheic dermatitis

3.   Salivation:

          0 – normal

          1 – slightly increased saliva in mouth

          2 – occasional drooling, especially at night

          3 – severe intermittent drooling

          4 – drooling all the time

4.   Speech:

          0 – normal

          1 – slightly monotonous and/or soft, with tendency to fade

          2 – marked monotony and/or softness with occasional dysarthria, but still easily understood

          3 – severe monotony, softness, and dysarthria; difficult to understand

          4 – no comprehensible speech

5.9.   Tremor:

          0 – absent

          1 – slight and intermittent

          2 – mild

          3 – moderate

          4 – very severe

          S – tremor on sustension

          R – tremor at rest

          I – tremor greatly increased at the end of an intentional movement

10-14.   Rigidity:

          0 – absent

          0.5 – present only with synkinetic movements of the opposite extremity

          1 – mild

          2 – moderate

          3 – severe but range of movement full or only slightly impaired

          4 – severe rigidity with marked limitation of full range of passive movement

15-16. Finger Tapping:
Thumb and middle finger with range of at least 2-3$''$ and speed equal to examiner's.
0 — normal
1 — slow, especially when tapping repeated ten or more times
2 — slow with decreased range of movement
3 — very slow, range of movement decreased to less than one inch, very irregular
4 — unable to do the task at all

17-18. Secession and Alternating Movements:
Alternating pronation and supination movements of the hand on patient's knee.
0 — slowing after repetitive movements (approximately 10) and/or unable consistently to hit the same spot on the knee with the palmar and sorsal aspects of the hand
2 — slow from onset of test plus inaccuracy in hitting the same spot
3 — very slow, inaccuracy in hitting the same spot, irregular, inability to pronate the hand fully
4 — unable to perform the task

19-20. Foot Tapping:
With knee flexed at right angles, heel on floor, tapping toe.
0 — normal
1 — slow, especially when tapping repeated 10 or more times
2 — slow with decreased range of movement
3 — very slow, range of movement decreased to less than one inch, very irregular
4 — unable to do the task at all

21. Arising from Hard Side Chair with Outstretched Arms:
0 — normal
1 — slow
2 — several attempts but able to perform task
3 — unable to arise from the chair without pushing himself up with his hands from the seat or other object
4 — unable to arise from a chair without assistance

22. Standing Posture:
0 — normal erect
1 — slight forward protrusion of the head, and/or one shoulder dropped slightly, very slight flexion of the elbows and pronation of the forearms
2 — mildly stooped posture, moderate flexion of elbows with hands held across the upper thighs or lower abdomen
3 — moderately stooped posture with forward flexion of 45° or more, moderate flexion of the elbows with the hands held in front of the body, some ulnar deviation of the hands with adduction of the thumbs, flexion of the M. P. joints, and hyperextension of the I. P. joints, possible scoliosis, and/or some flexion of the hips and knees

4 – abnormalities of posture such as $90°$ forward flexion on the hips, sub-
luxation of the I. P. joints in hyperextension, etc.

23. Stability:
    0 – normal
    1 – clear instability when turning or on other abrupt changes of posture.
        Patient takes one or two steps backward when given a sharp push on
        the sternum when standing with feet $6''$ apart and eyes closed; he or
        she is unable to correct this tendency to take steps backwards
    2 – patient takes three or more steps backwards when given a sternal push
        but still able to save self from falling
    3 – patient takes many steps backwards and is unable to stop from falling
        after a sternal push; or patient takes no steps backward after a sternal
        push and must be caught to prevent falling
    4 – patient unable to stand unassisted with eyes closed and feet $6''$ apart

24. Gait:
    Patient must walk at least 20 feet away from observer and back as quickly
    as possible.
    0 – freely ambulatory, good stepping, turns readily
    1 – slow but regular with or without slightly decreased stride length
    2 – slow, decreased stride length, unable to perform pivotal turns, shuffles
        or drags one leg, especially after some distance; rare flexion, festina-
        tion, and/or pulsion, does not require help
    3 – very slow, with very short stride length, with or without any of the fol-
        lowing: marked shuffling, festination, flexing, pulsion; requires con-
        siderable help
    4 – unable to walk at all

25. General Bradykinesia:
    Special reference to quantity and quality of associated and spontaneous
    movements, as well as slowness and ability to sustain movements or to do
    more than one motor task at a time.
    0 – none
    1 – slow in all movements
    2 – slow in all movements, with decreased quantity of spontaneous and
        associated movements
    3 – extremely slow; almost no spontaneous or associated movements; un-
        able to perform two or more motor tasks at the same time
    4 – unable to move

26. Dysphagia:
    0 – normal
    1 – some subjective difficulty swallowing
    2 – occasionally chokes, no limitation of diet
    3 – frequent choking, diet limited
    4 – unable to swallow

27. Handwriting:
    Signature, and outward spiraling circles, made with both right and left
    hands.

0 – normal

1 – almost normal speed and legibility of signature; some slowing and difficulty making circles

2 – writes slowly, with or without some tremor; letters and circles tend to be small

3 – writes very slowly, moderate to severe tremor, signature may be barely legible

4 – handwriting is illegible, or patient cannot write at all

NEW YORK UNIVERSITY FUNCTIONAL STAGING SCALE FOR PARKINSON'S DISEASE (PD)

Stage	Status	Description
0	No symptoms	
1	Fully employed	Transportation: goes alone
	Symptoms	Work schedule: full
		Work assistance: none
2	Partially employed	Transportation: may go alone
	Reduced schedule	Walking: goes out alone
	Assistance at work	Activities of daily living: independent
3	Independent	Transportation: may/may not go alone
	Retired, non-PD re-lated	Walking: goes out alone
		Activities of daily living: independent (but slow)
	Retired, PD-related	
4	Semidependent	Walking: may/may not go out alone
		Activities of daily living: mostly independent
		No aide or parttime aide
5	Dependent	Walking: does not go out alone
	Living at home	Activities of daily living: mostly dependent
	Institutionalized	Full-time aide

NORTHWESTERN UNIVERSITY DISABILITY SCALES

Scale A: Walking
Never walks alone

0 Cannot walk at all, even with maximum assistance

1 Needs considerable help even for short distances; cannot walk outdoors with help

2 Requires moderate help indoors; walks outdoors with considerable help

3 Requires potential help indoors and active help outdoors

Sometimes walks alone

4 Walks from room to room without assistance, but moves slowly and uses external support; never walks alone outdoors

5 Walks from room to room with only moderate difficulty; may occasionally walk outdoors without assistance

6 Walks short distances with ease; walking outdoors is difficult but often accomplished without help; rarely walks longer distances alone

Always walks alone

7 Gait is extremely abnormal; very slow and shuffling; posture grossly affected; there may be propulsion

8 Quality of gait is poor and rate is slow; posture moderately affected; there may be a tendency toward mild propulsion; turning is difficult

9 Gait only slightly deviant from normal in quality and speed; turning is the most difficult task; posture essentially normal

10 Normal

Scale B: Dressing

Requires complete assistance

0 Patient is a hindrance rather than a help to assistant

1 Movements of patient neither help nor hinder assistant

2 Can give some help through bodily movements

3 Gives considerable help through bodily movements

Requires partial assistance

4 Performs only gross dressing activities alone (hat, coat)

5 Performs about half of dressing activities independently

6 Performs more than half of dressing activities alone, with considerable effort and slowness

7 Handles all dressing alone with the exception of fine activities (tie, buttons)

Complete self-help

8 Dresses self completely with slowness and great effort

9 Dresses self completely with only slightly more time and effort than normal

10 Normal

Scale C: Hygiene

Requires complete assistance

0 Unable to maintain proper hygiene even with maximum help

1 Reasonably good hygiene with assistance, but does not provide assistant with significant help

2 Hygiene maintained well; gives aid to assistant

Requires partial assistance

3 Performs a few tasks alone with assistant nearby

4 Requires assistance for half of toilet needs

5 Requires assistance for some tasks not difficult in terms of coordination

6 Manages most of personal needs alone; has substituted methods for accomplishing difficult tasks (electric razor)

Complete self-help

7 Hygiene maintained independently, but with effort and slowness, accidents are not infrequent; may employ substitute methods

8 Hygiene activities are moderately time consuming; no substitute methods; few accidents

9 Hygiene maintained normally, with exception of slight slowness
10 Normal

Scale D: Eating and Feeding[a]

Eating

0 Eating is so impaired that a hospital setting is required for adequate nutrition
1 Eats only liquids and soft food; these are consumed very slowly
2 Liquids and soft foods handled with ease; hard foods occasionally eaten, but require great effort and much time
3 Eats some hard food routinely, but these require time and effort
4 Follows a normal diet, but chewing and swallowing are labored
5 Normal

Feeding

0 Requires complete assistance
1 Performs only a few feeding tasks independently
2 Performs most feeding activities alone, slowly and with effort; requires help with specific tasks (cutting meat, filling cup)
3 Handles all feeding alone with a moderate slowness; still may get assistance in specific situation (cutting meat in restaurant); accidents not infrequent
4 Fully feeds self with rare accidents; slower than normal
5 Normal

Scale E: Speech

0 Does not vocalize at all
1 Vocalizes but rarely for communicative purposes
2 Vocalizes to call attention to self
3 Attempts to use speech for communication, but has difficulty in initiating vocalization; may stop speaking in middle of phrase and be unable to continue
4 Uses speech for most communication, but articulation is highly unintelligible; may have occasional difficulty in initiating speech; usually speaks in single words or short phrases
5 Speech always employed for communication, but articulation is still very poor; usually uses complete sentences
6 Speech can always be understood if listener pays close attention; both articulation and voice may be defective
7 Communication accomplished with ease, although speech impairment detracts from content
8 Speech easily understood, but voice or speech rhythm may be disturbed
9 Speech entirely adequate; minor voice disturbances present
10 Normal

---

[a]Eating and feeding are figured separately and the two scores added.

Source: Canter GJ, DeLa Torre R, Mier M. (1961). *J Nerv Ment Dis* 122: 143-147.

UNIFIED RATING SCALE FOR PARKINSONISM
VERSION 2.0 – DECEMBER 1985

Definitions of 0–4 Scale

I. Mentation, Behavior, and Mood
    1. Intellectual Impairment:
        0 = None.
        1 = Mild. Consistent forgetfulness with partial recollection of events and no other difficulties.
        2 = Moderate memory loss, with disorientation and moderate difficulty handling complex problems. Mild but definite impairment of function at home with need of occasional prompting.
        3 = Severe memory loss with disorientation for time and often to place. Severe impairment in handling problems.
        4 = Severe memory loss with orientation preserved to person only. Unable to make judgements or solve problems. Requires much help with personal care. Cannot be left alone at all.
    2. Thought Disorders (due to dementia or drug intoxication)
        0 = None.
        1 = Vivid dreaming.
        2 = "Benign" hallucinations with insight retained.
        3 = Occasional to frequent hallucinations or delusions; without insight; could interfere with daily activities.
        4 = Persistent hallucinations, delusions, or florid psychosis. Not able to care for self.
    3. Depression:
        0 = Not present.
        1 = Periods of sadness or guilt greater than normal, never sustained for days or weeks.
        2 = Sustained depression (1 week or more).
        3 = Sustained depression with vegetative symptoms (insomnia, anorexia, weight loss, loss of interest).
        4 = Sustained depression with vegetative symptoms and suicidal thoughts or intent.
    4. Motivation/Initiative:
        0 = Normal.
        1 = Less assertive than usual; more passive.
        2 = Loss of initiative or disinterest in elective (nonroutine) activities.
        3 = Loss of initiative or disinterest in day to day (routine) activities.
        4 = Withdrawn, complete loss of motivation.
II. Activities of Daily Living (determine for "On/Off")
    5. Speech:
        0 = Normal.
        1 = Mildly affected. No difficulty being understood.
        2 = Moderately affected. Sometimes asked to repeat statements.
        3 = Severely affected. Frequently asked to repeat statements.
        4 = Unintelligible most of the time.

6. Salivation:
   0 = Normal.
   1 = Slight but definite excess of saliva in mouth; may have nighttime drooling.
   2 = Moderately excessive saliva; may have minimal drooling.
   3 = Marked excess of saliva with some drooling.
   4 = Marked drooling, requires constant tissue or handkerchief.
7. Swallowing:
   0 = Normal.
   1 = Rare choking.
   2 = Occasional choking.
   3 = Requires soft food.
   4 = Requires NG tube or gastrotomy feeding.
8. Handwriting:
   0 = Normal.
   1 = Slightly slow or small.
   2 = Moderately slow or small; all words are legible.
   3 = Severely affected; not all words are legible.
   4 = The majority of words are not legible.
9. Cutting Food and Handling Utensils:
   0 = Normal.
   1 = Somewhat slow and clumsy, but no help needed.
   2 = Can cut most foods, although clumsy and slow; some help needed.
   3 = Food must be cut by someone, but can still feed slowly.
   4 = Needs to be fed.
10. Dressing:
    0 = Normal.
    1 = Somewhat slow, but no help needed.
    2 = Occasional assistance with buttoning, getting arms in sleeves.
    3 = Considerable help required, but can do some things alone.
    4 = Helpless.
11. Hygiene:
    0 = Normal.
    1 = Somewhat slow, but no help needed.
    2 = Needs help to shower or bathe; or very slow in hygienic care.
    3 = Requires assistance for washing, brushing teeth, combing hair, going to bathroom.
    4 = Foley catheter or other mechanical aids.
12. Turning in Bed and Adjusting Bed Clothes:
    0 = Normal.
    1 = Somewhat slow and clumsy, but no help needed.
    2 = Can turn alone or adjust sheets, but with great difficulty.
    3 = Can initiate, but not turn or adjust sheets alone.
    4 = Helpless.
13. Falling (Unrelated to Freezing):
    0 = None.
    1 = Rare falling.

       2 = Occasionally falls, less than once per day.

       3 = Falls an average of once daily.

       4 = Falls more than once daily.

14. Freezing When Walking:

       0 = None.

       1 = Rare freezing when walking; may have start-hesitation.

       2 = Occasional freezing when walking.

       3 = Frequent freezing. Occasionally falls from freezing.

       4 = Frequent falls from freezing.

15. Walking:

       0 = Normal.

       1 = Mild difficulty. May not swing arms or may tend to drag leg.

       2 = Moderate difficulty, but requires little or no assistance.

       3 = Severe disturbance of walking, requiring assistance.

       4 = Cannot walk at all, even with assistance.

16. Tremor:

       0 = Absent.

       1 = Slight and infrequently present.

       2 = Moderate; bothersome to patient.

       3 = Severe; interferes with many activities.

       4 = Marked; interferes with most activities.

17. Sensory Complaints Related to Parkinsonism

       0 = None.

       1 = Occasionally has numbness, tingling, or mild aching.

       2 = Frequently has numbness, tingling, or aching; not distressing.

       3 = Frequent painful sensations.

       4 = Excruciating pain.

III. Motor Examination:

18. Speech:

       0 = Normal.

       1 = Slight loss of expression, diction and/or volume.

       2 = Monotone, slurred but understandable; moderately impaired.

       3 = Marked impairment, difficult to understand.

       4 = Unintelligible.

19. Facial Expression:

       0 = Normal.

       1 = Minimal hypomimia, could be normal "Poker Face."

       2 = Slight but definitely abnormal diminution of facial expression.

       3 = Moderate hypomimia; lips parted some of the time.

       4 = Masked or fixed facies with severe or complete loss of facial expression; lips parted 1/4 inch or more.

20. Tremor at Rest:

       0 = Absent.

       1 = Slight and infrequently present.

       2 = Mild in amplitude and persistent. Or moderate in amplitude, but only intermittently present.

      3 = Moderate in amplitude and present most of the time.

      4 = Marked in amplitude and present most of the time.

21. Action or Postural Tremor of Hands:

      0 = Absent.

      1 = Slight; present with action.

      2 = Moderate in amplitude, present with action.

      3 = Moderate in amplitude with posture holding as well as action.

      4 = Marked in amplitude; interferes with feeding.

22. Rigidity: (Judged on passive movement of major joints with patient relaxed in sitting position. Cogwheeling to be ignored.)

      0 = Absent.

      1 = Slight or detectable only when activated by mirror or other movements.

      2 = Mild to moderate.

      3 = Marked, but full range of motion easily achieved.

      4 = Severe, range of motion achieved with difficulty.

23. Finger Taps: (Patient taps thumb with index finger in rapid succession with widest amplitude possible, each hand separately.)

      0 = Normal.

      1 = Mild slowing and/or reduction in amplitude.

      2 = Moderately impaired. Definite and early fatiguing. May have occasional arrests in movement.

      3 = Severely impaired. Frequent hesitation in initiating movements or arrests in ongoing movement.

      4 = Can barely perform the task.

24. Hand Movements: (Patient opens and closes hands in rapid succession with widest amplitude possible, each hand separately.)

      0 = Normal.

      1 = Mild slowing and/or reduction in amplitude.

      2 = Moderately impaired. Definite and early fatiguing. May have occasional arrests in movement.

      3 = Severely impaired. Frequent hesitation in initiating movements or arrests in ongoing movement.

      4 = Can barely perform the task.

25. Rapid Alternating Movements of Hands: (Pronation-supination movements of hands, vertically or horizontally, with as large an amplitude as possible, both hands simultaneously.)

      0 = Normal.

      1 = Mild slowing and/or reduction in amplitude.

      2 = Moderately impaired. Definite and early fatiguing. May have occasional arrests in movement.

      3 = Severely impaired. Frequent hesitation in initiating movements or arrests in ongoing movement.

      4 = Can barely perform the task.

26. Foot Agility: (Patient taps heel on ground in rapid succession, picking up entire foot. Amplitude should be about 3 inches.)

      0 = Normal.

1 = Mild slowing and/or reduction in amplitude.

2 = Moderately impaired. Definite and early fatiguing. May have occasional arrests in movement.

3 = Severely impaired. Frequent hesitation in initiating movements of arrests in ongoing movement.

4 = Can barely perform the task.

27. Arising from Chair: (Patient attempts to arise from a straightback wood or metal chair with arms folded across chest.)

0 = Normal.

1 = Slow; or may need more than one attempt.

2 = Pushes self up from arms of seat.

3 = Tends to fall back and may have to try more than one time, but can get up without help.

4 = Unable to arise without help.

28. Posture:

0 = Normal erect.

1 = Not quite erect, slightly stooped posture; could be normal for older person.

2 = Moderately stooped posture, definitely abnormal; can be slightly leaning to one side.

3 = Severely stooped posture with kyphosis; can be moderate leaning to one side.

4 = Marked flexion with extreme abnormality of posture.

29. Gait:

0 = Normal.

1 = Walks slowly, may shuffle with short steps, but no festination or propulsion.

2 = Walks with difficulty, but requires little or no assistance; may have some festination, short steps, or propulsion.

3 = Severe disturbance of gait, requiring assistance.

4 = Cannot walk at all, even with assistance.

30. Postural Stability: (Response to sudden posterior displacement produced by pull on shoulders while patient erect with eyes open and feet slightly apart. Patient is prepared.)

0 = Normal.

1 = Retropulsion, but recovers unaided.

2 = Absence of postural response; would fall if not caught by examiner.

3 = Very unstable, tends to lose balance spontaneously.

4 = Unable to stand without assistance.

31. Body Bradykinesia and Hypokinesia: (Combining slowness, hesitancy, decreased armswing, small amplitude, and poverty of movement in general.)

0 = None.

1 = Minimal slowness, giving movement a deliberate character; could be normal for some persons. Possibly reduced amplitude.

2 = Mild degree of slowness and poverty of movement which is definitely abnormal. Alternatively, some reduced amplitude.

        3 = Moderate slowness, poverty or small amplitude of movement.

        4 = Marked slowness, poverty or small amplitude of movement.

IV. Complications of Therapy (In the past week)

    A. Dyskinesias

        32. Duration: What proportion of the waking day are dyskinesias present? (Historical information)

            0 = None

            1 = 1–25% of day.

            2 = 26–50% of day.

            3 = 51–75% of day.

            4 = 76–100% of day.

        33. Disability: How Disabling Are the Dyskinesias? (Historical information, may be modified by office examination.)

            0 = Not disabling.

            1 = Mildly disabling.

            2 = Moderately disabling.

            3 = Severely disabling.

            4 = Completely disabled.

        34. Painful Dyskinesias: How Painful Are the Dyskinesias?

            0 = No painful dyskinesias.

            1 = Slight.

            2 = Moderate.

            3 = Severe.

            4 = Marked.

        35. Presence of Early Morning Dystonia: (Historical information)

            0 = No

            1 = Yes

    B. Clinical Fluctuations

        36. Are any "off" periods predictable as to timing after a dose of medication?

            0 = No

            1 = Yes

        37. Are any "off" periods unpredictable as to timing after a dose of medication?

            0 = No

            1 = Yes

        38. Do any of the "off" periods come on suddenly (e.g., over a few seconds?)

            0 = No

            1 = Yes

        39. What proportion of the waking day is the patient "off" on average:

            0 = None

            1 = 1–25% of day.

            2 = 26–50% of day.

            3 = 51–75% of day.

            4 = 76–100% of day.

    C. Other Complications

        40. Does the patient have anorexia, nausea, or vomiting?
            0 = No
            1 = Yes

        41. Does the patient have any sleep disturbances (e.g., insomnia or hypersomnolence?
            0 = No
            1 = Yes

        42. Does the patient have symptomatic orthostasis?
            0 = No
            1 = Yes

RECORD THE PATIENT'S BLOOD PRESSURE, PULSE, AND WEIGHT ON THE SCORING FORM.

  V. Hoehn and Yahr Staging

    Stage 0 = No signs of disease.
    Stage 1 = Unilateral disease.
    Stage 2 = Bilateral disease, without impairment of balance.
    Stage 3 = Mild to moderate bilateral disease; some postural instability; physically independent.
    Stage 4 = Severe disability; still able to walk or stand unassisted
    Stage 5 = Wheelchair bound or bedridden unless aided.

  VI. Schwab and England Activities of Daily Living Scale

    100% Completely independent. Able to do all chores without slowness, difficulty, or impairment. Essentially normal. Unaware of any difficulty.

    90% Completely independent. Able to do all chores with some degree of slowness, difficulty and impairment. Might take twice as long. Beginning to be aware of difficulty.

    80% Completely independent in most chores. Takes twice as long. Conscious of difficulty and slowness.

    70% Not completely independent. More difficulty with some chores. Three to four times as long in some. Must spend a large part of the day with chores.

    60% Some dependency. Can do most chores, but exceedingly slowly and with much effort. Errors; some impossible.

    50% More dependent. Help with half, slower, etc. Difficulty with everything.

    40% Very dependent. Can assist with all chores, but few alone.

    30% With effort, now and then does a few chores alone or begins alone. Much help needed.

    20% Nothing alone. Can be a slight help with some chores. Severe invalid.

    10% Totally dependent, helpless. Complete invalid.

    0% Vegetative functions such as swallowing, bladder and bowel functions are not functioning. Bedridden.

Anticholinergic Compounds Used in the Symptomatic Treatment of Parkinson's Disease

Brand (trade) name	Generic name	Formulations
Artane	Trihexyphenidyl	2- and 5-mg white tablets and 5-mg long-acting capsules
Tremin	Trihexyphenidyl	2-mg white tablet
Kemadrin	Procyclidine	2 and 5 mg white tablets
Pagitane	Cycrimine	1.25 mg orange and 2.5 mg brown sugar-coated capsules
Akineton	Biperiden	2 mg white tablet
Cogentin	Benztropine	0.5 and 2 mg round white tablets and 1 mg long, elliptical white tablets
Parsidol	Ethopropazine	10 and 50 mg white tablets

Levodopa Compounds Used in the Symptomatic Treatment of Parkinson's Disease

Name	Description
Larodopa	Pink tablets
	100 mg (elliptical, scored)
	200 mg (round)
	500 mg (oblong, scored)
	Capsules
	100 mg (pink and scarlet)
	250 mg (pink and beige)
	500 mg (pink)
Dopar	Capsules only
	100 mg (small, opaque green)
	250 mg (medium, opaque green and white)
	500 mg (large, opaque green)

Levodopa-decarboxylase inhibitor combinations

Sinemet	Elliptical tablets (scored)
(carbidopa/levodopa)	10/100 mg (dark dappled blue)
	25/100 mg (yellow)
	25/250 mg (light dappled blue)
Madopar[a]	Capsules
(benserizide/levodopa)	25/100 mg (pink and blue)
	50/200 mg (caramel and blue)

---

[a]Madopar is not available in the United States.

Other Drugs Used in the Symptomatic Treatment of Parkinson's Disease

Trade name	Generic name	Description
Parlodel	Bromocriptine	2.5 mg tablets and 5 mg capsules (caramel and white)
Symmetrel	Amantadine HCl	100 mg (bright red capsules)

Cost of Antiparkinsonian Drugs

Sinemet
   10/100 mg, 200 @ $49.95; 500 @ $121.88
   25/100 mg, 200 @ $74.88; 500 @ $181.44
   25/250 mg, 200 @ $78.75; 500 @ $193.68
Symmetrel
   100 mg, 100 @ $38.60; 200 @ $75.97; 500 @ $186.45
Cogentin
   0.5 mg, 200 @ $21.98
   1 mg, 200 @ $24.78
   2 mg, 200 @ $28.99
Benztropine mesylate (generic Cogentin)
   0.5 mg, 200 @ $12.65
   1 mg, 200 @ $12.78
   2 mg, 200 @ $14.40
Artane
   2 mg, 200 @ $15.69
   5 mg, 200 @ $30.78
Trihexyphenidyl (generic Artane)
   2 mg, 200 @ $3.64
   5 mg, 200 @ $6.13
Benadryl
   25 mg, 200 @ $18.49
   50 mg, 200 @ $25.48
Diphenhydramine (generic Benadryl)
   25 mg, 200 @ $6.98
   50 mg, 200 @ $7.98
Parlodel
   2.5 mg:
   60 @ $40.74; 90 @ $57.94; 150 @ $93.44; 300 @ $182.46; 600 @ $360.88
   5 mg:
   100 @ $103.64; 200 @ $204.98; 500 @ $508.75

Source: Mr. Jim Roth, Rx Allstates Pharmacy, 360 West Superior Street, Chicago, Illinois, 60610. These estimates may be lower than in other pharmacies. These prices were quoted as of August 1986.

National Organizations Concerned with Parkinson's Disease

United Parkinson Foundation (International)
360 West Superior Street
Chicago, Illinois 60610

The American Parkinson Disease Association, Inc.
116 John Street
New York, New York 10034

The Parkinson Disease Foundation
William Black Medical Research Building
640 West 168th Street
New York, New York 10032

National Parkinson Foundation, Inc.
1501 Ninth Avenue NW
Miami, Florida 33136

The Parkinson Foundation of Canada
Suite 232 ManuLife Centre
55 Bloor Street West
Toronto, Ontario Canada M4W 1A6

Since clinicians reading this text may feel, as I do, that the Parkinson's disease patient and his family are usually more cooperative and more receptive to suggestions of various forms of therapy once they understand the disorder and its ramifications, they may wish to refer patients to lay organizations for printed information. Having worked with the staff of the United Parkinson Foundation in Chicago and being familiar with their materials, I can recommend the organization for this purpose. Their materials are prepared under the supervision of and include essays by members of their Medical Advisory Board, many of whom are authors of this book's chapters.

Contact the UPF at 360 West Superior Street, Chicago, Illinois 60610 (USA), and for similar materials in Canada, the Parkinson Foundation at 55 West Bloor Street, Suite 232, Toronto, Ontario M4W 1A6. Both organizations also support research in Parkinson's disease and related disorders and should be contacted directly for guidelines.

Support groups exist in many cities in North America. Either of the national organizations can direct patients to local groups for such programs as they may individually provide.

Books about Parkinson's Disease for Lay Persons

Parkinson's Disease: A Guide for Patient and Family
Second Edition (1984)
Roger C. Duvoisin
Raven Press
1140 Avenue of the Americas
New York, NY 10036
Hardcover and paperback — 197 pages

Backus Strikes Back (1984)
Jim and Henry Backus
Stein and Day/Publishers
Scarborough House
Briarcliff Manor, NY 10520
Hardcover — 124 pages

Living with Chronic Neurologic Disease: A Handbook for Patients and Family
(1976)
I.S. Cooper
W.W. Norton & Company
New York, NY
Hardcover and paperback — 318 pages

Awakenings (1974)
Oliver Sacks
Doubleday & Company
Garden City, NY
Hardcover — 249 pages

Parkinson's Disease: The Facts
Gerald Stein and Andrew Lees
Oxford University Press
New York, NY
Hardcover — 74 pages

Index

About the Editor

WILLIAM C. KOLLER is Professor of Neurology and Pharmacology, Department of Neurology and Pharmacology, Loyola University Stritch School of Medicine, Maywood, Illinois, and Director of the Parkinson Disease Center at Loyola Medical Center. A member of the American Academy of Neurology, Movement Disorder Society, and Society for Neurosciences, Dr. Koller is the author or coauthor of more than 100 articles in medical and scientific journals. He received the M.S. (1971), Ph.D. (1974) in pharmacology, and M.D. (1976) degrees from Northwestern University Medical School, Chicago, Illinois. A Pillsbury Fellow from 1979-80, Dr. Koller completed his residency in neurology (1977-80) at Rush-Presbyterian St. Luke's Medical Center in Chicago.